Surgical Management of Venous Disease

SESHADRI RAJU, M.D.
Professor Emeritus of Surgery
University of Mississippi
Jackson, Mississippi

J. LEONEL VILLAVICENCIO, M.D.
Professor of Surgery
Uniformed Services University of Health Sciences
Bethesda, Maryland

Surgical Management of Venous Disease

Williams & Wilkins
A WAVERLY COMPANY

BALTIMORE • PHILADELPHIA • LONDON • PARIS • BANGKOK
BUENOS AIRES • HONG KONG • MUNICH • SYDNEY • TOKYO • WROCLAW

Editor: Carroll C. Cann
Managing Editor: Susan L. Hunsberger
Marketing Manager: Diane M. Harnish
Production Coordinator: Cindy Park
Book Project Editor: Kathy Gilbert
Designer: Maria Karkucinski
Illustration Planner: Cindy Park
Cover Designer: Maria Karkucinski
Typesetter: University Graphics, Inc.
Printer: Edwards Brothers, Inc.
Digitized Illustrations: University Graphics, Inc.
Binder: Edwards Brothers, Inc.

351 West Camden Street
Baltimore, Maryland 21201-2436 USA

Rose Tree Corporate Center
1400 North Providence Road
Building II, Suite 5025
Media, Pennsylvania 19063-2043 USA

Accurate indications, adverse reactions and dosage schedules for drugs are provided in this book, but it is possible that they may change. The reader is urged to review the package information data of the manufacturers of the medications mentioned.

Printed in the United States of America

First edition, 1997

Library of Congress Cataloging-in-Publication Data

Surgical management of venous disease / [edited by] Seshadri Raju, J. Leonel Villavicencio
p. cm.
Includes index.
ISBN 0-683-07111-4
1. Veins—Surgery. 2. Veins—Diseases. I. Raju, Seshadri. II. Villavicencio, J. Leonel.
[DNLM: 1. Veins—physiopathology. 2. Veins—surgery. 3. Vascular Surgery—methods. WG 600 S9615 1997]
RD598.7.S87 1997
617.4′14—dc20
DNLM/DLC
for Library of Congress 96-31993
CIP

The publishers have made every effort to trace the copyright holders for borrowed material. If they have inadvertently overlooked any, they will be pleased to make the necessary arrangements at the first opportunity.

97 98 99 00
1 2 3 4 5 6 7 8 9 10

To three great surgical teachers:

Dr. H.S. Bhat, whose brilliant and artful mastery of surgery awed and inspired his students;

Dr. James D. Hardy, whose energy and pioneering skill motivated a generation of surgeons in the South; and

Dr. Robert Kistner, who inaugurated a new branch of vascular surgery by questioning conventional wisdom.

S.R.

To my wife Suzie, and my children John, Andrew and Suzanne in recognition for their many hours of solitude. They have shared my burdens and joys and represent what is really valuable in life.

J.L.V.

Preface

Concepts and beliefs have a tendency to gain credibility simply because they have the weight of tradition behind them. It is remarkable that the ideas of Trendelenburg and Virchow, propounded more than 100 years ago, still have currency today. To a great extent this is due to the power behind the men and their concepts, but to some degree, it is indicative of failure to critically analyze principles that have been accepted simply because they are considered well established dogma. Venous disease has been recognized since ancient times. Patients suffering from some form of venous disease, constitute the large majority of the patient population attending the vascular clinics of Europe, Latin America, Canada, and Australia. In a recent communication, N. Bosanquet has called venous disease "the new international challenge" (Phlebology 1996; 11:6–9). He estimates that the cost of treatment of venous diseases of the lower extremities as a percentage of costs for all conditions ranges from 5% in France to 1.5% in Germany. This represents the total spending on physician services and prescription medicines. In addition, there are long-term direct and indirect costs related to disability and lost work. The available figures for Europe revealed that the disability costs were 1.2% of the total expenditure on health services in Germany, and 0.4% in the UK (953 million DM, and 73 million pounds, respectively for 1987). In his Presidential Address: A Venous Renaissance?, the late Michael Hume, MD, a founding member and President of the American Venous Forum wrote . . . . "two examples (of venous disease) both quite widespread, offer distinctly different challenges: varicose veins and leg ulcers. The cost of health care in this country is ballooning; the "system" of care for venous leg ulcers is an extravagant example. Yes, ... a venous renaissance is needed. The scope of the problem in this country is vast, and academically, it is not an overcrowded field—at least not yet. It will fall to vascular surgeons, however, to lead the post-graduate education of the health care team . . . . if any impact is to be made on the problem at national level." (J Vasc Surg 1992; 15:947–951). It is estimated that there are eight patients with venous disease for every patient with an arterial disorder. Nonetheless, interest in venous problems dwindled during the last three decades. The advent of direct arterial surgery, with its brilliant techniques and dramatic results, boosted vascular surgery into a highly respected status, but relegated the care of venous diseases to a neglected corner in the basement of the vascular building.

A survey conducted by one of us among 60 vascular fellowship programs approved by the American Board of Surgery revealed that, even though all of them had a strong arterial surgical schedule, only six programs had a dedicated clinic devoted to the care of venous diseases . . . . and two of them were Canadian! It is clear that the vascular surgeons graduating from such programs have a large gap in their vascular training. Fortunately, several events have come to the rescue of the "Cinderella" of vascular diseases. A true technological revolution has provided us with new tools to investigate the venous system. Now, it is possible to obtain precise information about the hemodynamics of most venous problems. Duplex scanning, new plethysmographic techniques, endovascular visualization of venous structures and dramatic advances in imaging techniques have rekindled interest in longstanding venous problems and contributed to create a multidisciplinary approach to the field. A cornerstone in the management of chronic venous insufficiency was the development of venous valve reconstruction and transplantation. The pioneering work of Kistner reconstructing "floppy" femoral venous valves, and the subsequent development of axillary vein valve transplantation by Taheri and Raju, stirred renewed interest in the study and understanding of the challenging pathophysiology behind chronic venous insufficiency and leg ulceration. Parallel to the technologic and surgical advances has been the progress of interventional radiology. The introduction of precise catherization and balloon dilatation techniques, endovascular embolization, stent utilization, and other radiological procedures has revolutionized the diagnosis and management of complex venous problems such as congenital vascular malformations, stenosis of large veins, acute venous thrombosis, portal hypertension, and many others. The pioneer investigators of this field faced a difficult challenge because new information and knowledge that is contrary to tradition and old dogma are not accepted easily. The foundation of the American Venous Forum, an academic society devoted to the study of venous disorders, has contributed to stimulate the interest in this field and . . . . to nurture the venous renaissance of Michael Hume. The Forum forms an important part of the rescue team of our Cinderella. Its members are represented by a cadre of dedicated physicians whose contributions and experience in the field of venous disorders form the core of this book. A great deal of concepts expressed in its chapters are here to stay. Others will continue evolving as the progress of our knowledge continues. The editors have witnessed the dramatic changes that occurred in vascular surgery during the last three decades. The amount of new information covering a wide spectrum of the venous pathology that has come forward in a relatively short time is astonishing. New information has brought changes. . . . but conventional ideas have a tendency to resist changes and oppose progress. There is wisdom in the words of Maeterling, "At every crossroad of the path leading to progress there are a thousand men assigned to defend the past." In the chapters of this book, the reader will find the rationale for the changes that led to progress. The inevitable overlapping observed in most multiauthored books has been kept to a minimum by the editors who wrote nearly one third of the book chapters themselves. It is their hope that in the pages of this book, the readers find the excitement of a rapidly evolving field of knowledge and the factual basis for a better understanding and treatment of their patients with venous disorders.

Seshadri Raju, MD
Jackson, Mississippi

J. Leonel Villavicencio, MD
Bethesda, Maryland

Contributors

FREDERICK A. ANDERSON, JR., PH.D.
Research Associate Professor
Department of Surgery
University of Massachusetts Medical School
Worcester, MA

GIOVANNI BELCARO, M.D.
Microcirculation Laboratory, Cardiovascular Institute,
G. D'Annunzio University
Chieti, Italy and
Irvine Laboratory for Cardiovascular Investigation and Research
St. Mary's Hospital
London, U.K.

ERIC BERENS, M.D.
Fellow
Division of Vascular Surgery; Department of Surgery
Mayo Clinic and Foundation
Rochester, MN

JOHN J. BERGAN, M.D.
Clinical Professor of Surgery
Scripps Memorial Hospital
La Jolla, CA

D. CHRISTOPOULOS, M.D.
Academic Vascular Surgery
Irvine Laboratory for Cardiovascular Investigation and Research
St. Mary's Hospital
London, U.K.

ANTHONY J. COMEROTA, M.D., FACS
Department of Surgery; Section of Vascular Surgery
Temple University Hospital
Philadelphia, PA

CASS W. CONAWAY, M.D.
Peripheral Vascular Surgery Service
Walter Reed Army Medical Center
Washington, D.C.

ROBERT CRANLEY, M.D., FACS
Faculty and Attending Staff; Good Samaritan Hospital
Associate, The Cranley Surgical Associates, Inc.
Cincinnati, Ohio
Co-Director; Kachelmacher Memorial Clinic
Logan, Ohio

SILKE DURHOIT, M.D.
International Guest Scholar
Department of Surgery
Uniformed Services University of the Heath Sciences
National Naval Medical Center
Bethesda, MD

BO EKLOF, M.D.
Director
Straub Foundation and Clinics
Clinical Professor of Surgery
University of Hawaii Medical School
Honolulu, HI

SABRINA EWALD, M.D.
Mercy Hospital Anderson
Cincinnati, OH

MARK X. GANNON, M.D.
International Guest Scholar
Department of Surgery
Uniformed Services University of the Health Sciences
Bethesda, MD

DAVID L. GILLESPIE, M.D., MAJ., MC, USA
Division of Vascular Surgery; Department of Surgery
F. Edward Heben School of Medicine
Uniformed Services University of the Health Sciences
Bethesda, MD

PETER GLOVICZKI, M.D.
Consultant and Associate Professor of Surgery
Department of Surgery
Mayo Medical School
Mayo Clinic and Foundation
Rochester, MN

JAMES M. GOFF, M.D., MAJ., MC, USA
Division of Vascular Surgery; Department of Surgery
F. Edward Hebert School of Medicine
Uniformed Services University of the Health Sciences
Bethesda, MD

MITCHEL P. GOLDMAN, M.D.
Assistant Professor of Dermatology/Medicine
University of California
San Diego, CA

LAZAR J. GREENFIELD, M.D.
Frederick A. Coller Professor and Chairman
Department of Surgery
University of Michigan Medical School
Ann Arbor, MI

JOERG D. GRUSS
F.A. Coller Professor of Surgery
Chairman of the Department of Surgery
University of Michigan Medical School
Ann Arbor, MI

CLARENCE M. JABS, PH.D.
Faculty of Medicine and Health Sciences
Department of Surgery
United Arab Emirates University
Al Ain, Abu Dhabi, United Arab Emirates

MARK R. JACKSON, M.D., FACS, MAJ., MC, USA
Division of Vascular Surgery; Department of Surgery
F. Edward Hebert School of Medicine
Uniformed Services University of the Health Sciences
Bethesda, MD

GEORGE JOHNSON, JR., M.D.
Roscoe B.C. Cowper Distinguished Professor of Surgery
Department of Surgery
University of North Carolina at Chapel Hill School of Medicine
Chapel Hill, NC

W. HEIMER
Department of Vascular Surgery
University of Kassel
Federal Republic of Germany

RICHARD F. KEMPCZINSKI, M.D.
Division of Vascular Surgery; Department of Surgery
University of Cincinnati Medical Center
Cincinnati, OH

ROBERT L. KISTNER, M.D.
Clinical Professor of Surgery
Department of Vascular Surgery, University of Hawaii
Department of Vascular Surgery, Straub Clinic and Hospital
Honolulu, HI

JOANN M. LOHR, M.D., FACS
Medical Director, John J. Cranley Vascular Lab
Faculty and Associate Attending Staff, Good Samaritan Hospital
Associate, The Cranley Surgical Associates, Inc.
Cincinnati, Ohio
Co-Director, Kachelmacher Memorial Clinic
Logan, Ohio

JOHN C. MAYBERRY, M.D.
Division of Vascular Surgery; Department of Surgery
Oregon Health Sciences University
Portland, OR

GREGORY L. MONETA, M.D.
Division of Vascular Surgery; Department of Surgery
Oregon Health Sciences University
Portland, OR

JAMES U. MORANO, M.D.
Professor of Radiology
Director of Vascular and Interventional Radiology
University of Mississippi
Jackson, MS

PETER NEGLÉN, M.D., PH.D.
Professor of Surgery
Faculty of Medicine and Health Sciences
United Arab Emirates University
Al Ain, Abu Dhabi, United Arab Emirates

A.N. NICOLAIDES, M.D.
Academic Vascular Surgery
Irvine Laboratory for Cardiovascular Investigation and Research
St. Mary's Hospital Medical School
London, U.K.

SEAN D. O'DONNELL, M.D., FACS, MAJ., MC, USA
Division of Vascular Surgery; Department of Surgery
F. Edward Hebert School of Medicine
Uniformed Services University of the Health Sciences
Bethesda, MD

THOMAS F. O'DONNELL, M.D., FACS
Professor of Surgery
Chair, Vascular Surgery Section
Department of Surgery
Tufts-New England Medical Center
Boston, MA

HUGO PARTSCH, M.D.
Professor and Chairman
Dermatological Department
Wilhelminen Hospital
Vienna, Austria

JOHN R. PFEIFER, M.D.
Director of Surgical Research, Providence Hospital, Southfield, MI
Associate Clinical Professor, Wayne State University, Detroit, Michigan
Adjunct Professor of Health Sciences, Oakland University, Rochester, MI

EMMANOUIL PIKOULIS, M.D.
Assistant Professor of Surgery
Department of Surgery
Uniformed Services University of the Health Sciences
Bethesda, MD

JOHN M. PORTER, M.D.
Division of Vascular Surgery; Department of Surgery
Oregon Health Sciences University
Portland, OR

SESHADRI RAJU, M.D., FACS
Professor Emeritus of Surgery
Department of Surgery
The University of Mississippi Medical Center
Jackson, MS

NORMAN M. RICH, M.D., FACS
Vascular Surgery Service; Department of Surgery
Walter Reed Army Medical Center
Washington, DC

AGUSTIN A. RODRIGUEZ, M.D.
Vascular Surgery Research Fellow
Department of Surgery; Section of Vascular Surgery
Tufts-New England Medical Center
Boston, MA

DAVID L. ROLLINS, M.D.
Private Practice
Willoughby, OH

RONALD A. SAVRIN, M.D.
Chief of Division Vascular Surgery
Associate Program Director General Surgical Residency
Medical Director Vascular Laboratory
St. Luke's Medical Center
Cleveland, OH

CAROLYN M. SEMROW, BSEE
Vascular Assistant
St. Vincent's Hospital
Cleveland, OH

RICHARD K. SPENCE, M.D.
Director of Surgery
Staten Island University Hospital
Staten Island, NY

DAVID S. SUMNER, M.D.
Distinguished Professor of Surgery and Chief, Section of Peripheral Vascular Surgery
Department of Surgery
Southern Illinois University School of Medicine
Springfield, IL

OLAV THULESIUS, M.D.
Department of Clinical Physiology
University Hospital
Linkoping, Sweden

ANDERS THURIN, M.D.
Department of Clinical Physiology
University Hospital
Linkoping, Sweden

PAUL S. VAN BEMMELEN, M.D., PH.D.
Fellow in Peripheral Vascular Surgery
Department of Surgery
Southern Illinois University School of Medicine
Springfield, IL

J. LEONEL VILLAVICENCIO, M.D., FACS
Director, Venous and Lymphatic Surgical Clinics;
Walter Reed Army and National Naval Medical Centers
Washington, DC
Uniformed Services University of the Health Sciences
Bethesda, MD

H. BROWNELL WHEELER, M.D.
Harry M. Haidak Distinguished Professor and Chairman
Department of Surgery
University of Massachusetts Medical School
Worcester, MA

THOMAS A. WHITEHILL, M.D.
Lecturer in Surgery
Department of Surgery
University of Michigan Medical School
Ann Arbor, MI

Contents

section I

History and Physiology of Venous Surgery

chapter 1

History of Venous Surgery in the United States

J. Leonel Villavicencio and Emmanouil Pikoulis

HISTORY OF VENOUS SURGERY IN THE UNITED STATES*

There is a long and honorable tradition of history and interest in the study of the venous system in the United States. Every field of medicine progresses continuously due to the contributions of distinguished individuals who devote their time and effort to the noble discipline of medicine.

Progress in the management of venous diseases has been uneven over the years. In reviewing the most important events that contributed to the evolution of surgery for varicose veins in America, we place special emphasis on those developments that can be considered as cornerstones in the progress of venous surgery.

It is generally recognized that the operation that Friedrich Von Trendelenburg (Fig. 1.1) introduced in 1860 and published in 1890 (1) was the beginning of modern surgery for varicose veins. The operation consisted of a transverse incision at the junction of the upper and middle third of the thigh with double ligation and section of the saphenous vein. Trendelenburg made it clear that the procedure applied only to cases in which the saphenofemoral valve was incompetent as determined by his compression test. In his publication, Trendelenburg recognized Sir Benjamin Brodie for stressing the importance of mid-thigh ligation of the saphenous vein. Brodie (1783–1862), from London, was the first to demonstrate reflux in the saphenous vein (2). He described the tourniquet test by which reflux is prevented by placing a tourniquet below the saphenofemoral junction.

*The opinions or assertions contained herein are those of the authors and are not to be construed as official or as reflecting the view of the Department of Defense, Department of the Army, or the Uniformed Services University of the Health Sciences.

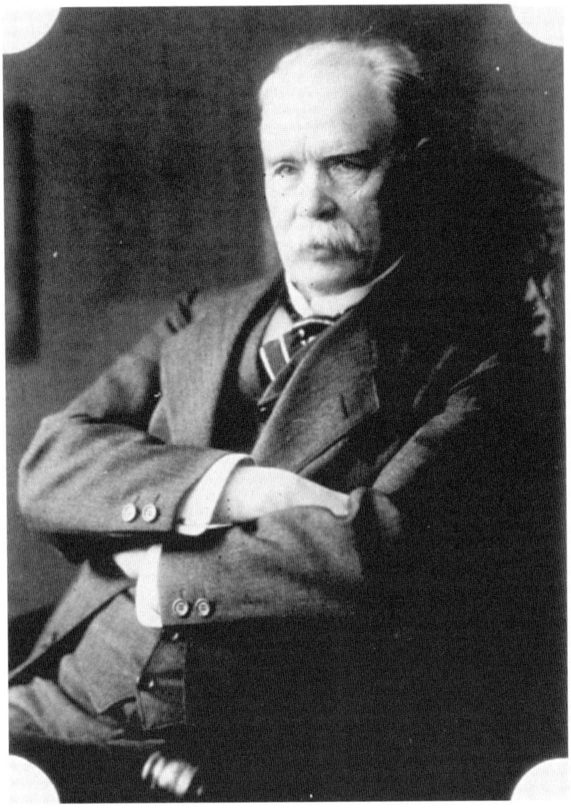

FIG. 1–1. In 1890, Friedrich Von Trendelenburg published a technique for division of the greater saphenous vein in the upper third of the thigh. It was the beginning of modern surgery for varicose veins. (Courtesy of Dr. H. Loeprecht.)

Trendelenburg did not advocate ligation of the saphena magna at the saphenofemoral junction.

An Australian surgeon, William Moore, recommended ligation at the saphenofemoral junction at the groin. He was the first to perform ambulatory venous surgery under cocaine anesthesia (32). Flush ligation of the saphenofemoral junction, as it is practiced at the present time, is credited to John Homans who described the procedure in his classic paper in 1916 (3).

In the United States, Charles H. Mayo (Fig. 1.2), in 1888, performed the first operation on a patient with varicose veins at St. Mary's Hospital in Rochester, Minnesota, shortly after graduating from medical school (4). Mayo excised the saphenous vein through a single incision extending from the groin to just below the knee. During the last decade of the 1800s, Mayo had operated on 53 more patients using the technique described. In 1904, he reported 125 patients operated on for varicose veins through a long incision (5). Before Mayo's approach, the operations described by Trendelenburg and Schede were the most popular surgical procedures for the management of varicose veins. Schede performed a circular incision around the leg down to the fascia with the concept of interrupting the proximal reflux (6).

The long incision used by the Mayo technique required considerable time for closure. He described a special extraluminal stripper with which the saphenous trunk could be removed through shorter incisions placed along the saphenous trunk. When Charles Mayo published his paper in 1906, he wrote: "We have operated on 185 cases of varicose veins. The complete Schede operation we have not made for several years. We have always liked to excise the long saphenous vein. Earlier operations were by long incisions over the vein. It required considerable time to close the wound. This was partially overcome some years ago by using a ring-vein enucleator" (7). In this paper, Mayo described the stripper in more detail and included a sketch (Fig. 1.3).

Interest in the surgical management of varicose veins grew considerably after the publications of Mayo. Keller, in 1905, described a surgical procedure that may be considered as the first intraluminal stripping for removal of varicose veins (8). Keller wrote: "The saphenous vein was removed in segments by passing a twisted wire through its lumen. This wire was tied to one end of the vein and then pulled out while the vein inverted itself and came out." Surgeons have always felt the need to redesign, modify, or improve instruments or procedures that other colleagues have earlier conceived. Babcock was no exception. In 1907, he published a report on the stripping of the saphenous vein and other varicosities utilizing a vein stripper of his own design. This was the prototype of the intraluminal strip-

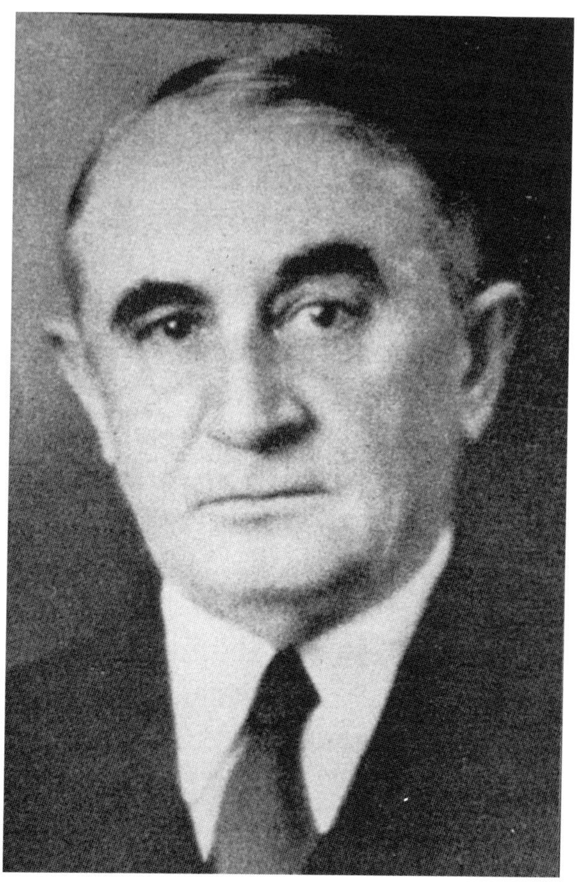

FIG. 1–2. Shortly after graduating medical school in 1888, Charles Mayo performed the first operation for varicose veins in a patient at St. Mary's Hospital in Rochester, Minnesota. In 1906, he described the ring-vein enucleator for external stripping of the saphenous vein. (Courtesy of the Mayo Clinic.)

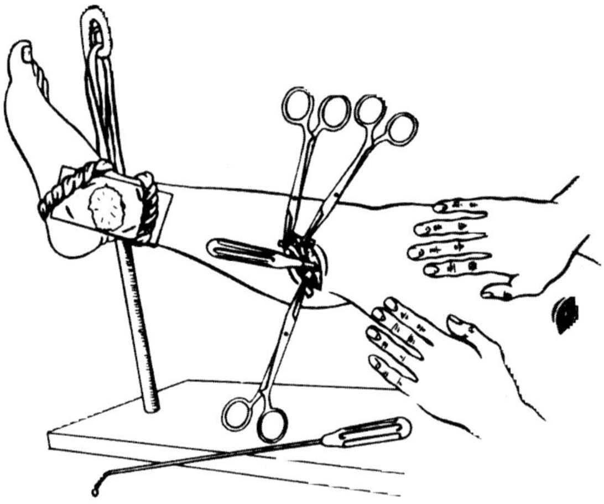

FIG. 1–3. Extraluminal vein stripper designed by Charles Mayo. This instrument is still in use. (Reproduced by permission from Lofgren K. Management of varicose veins, Mayo Clinic experience. In: Bergan JJ, Yao JST, eds. Venous problems. Chicago: Yearbook Medical Publishers, 1978:72.)

pers. Babcock described his procedure as follows: "The most promising of the operations advocated, are those aiming to extirpate the venous trunks involved. Charles H. Mayo finally devised an ingenious method in which the internal saphenous vein is exposed through a small incision, double ligated, divided and an instrument shaped like a dull ring is slipped over the vein. Unfortunately, in our experience, the method is valuable but fragile, and very tortuous or adherent vessels, often embarrass the operator. We, therefore, devised a procedure by means of which almost the entire saphenous vein may be removed through two small incisions. This method is one of the simplest and most expeditious of any thus far devised" (9). Babcock used an intraluminal stripper with an acorn-shaped head that pleated the vein as it removed it. However, the instrument was rigid and too short. After Babcock's publication, many others followed, both in Europe and America. Babcock's method was again modified by others, including Sir Henry Gray, who, in 1909, modified Babcock's instrument by varying the size of the acorn bulbs and adding a joint in the middle of the shaft, lengthening the size of the stripper (33).

During the period between 1907–1927, the saphenofemoral junction was not flush ligated and recurrence from residual varicosities was not uncommon. In the preantibiotic era, surgery had been accompanied by considerable morbidity, sepsis and pulmonary embolism. It was a common routine to have patients on bedrest for 8–10 days after surgery for varicose veins.

INTRODUCTION OF SCLEROTHERAPY

The Mayo operation for varicose veins and the Babcock stripping were employed by general surgeons in the United States and the Mayo Clinic staff for more than two decades. The suboptimal results obtained by surgery were responsible for the enthusiastic adoption of sclerotherapy as a promising new therapeutic modality for varicose veins. After the introduction of sclerotherapy by Linser of the Tübingen Clinic in 1911, sclerotherapy became very popular in Europe and was considered the ideal method for the treatment of varicose veins. In the United States, McPheeters (10) and Dixon (11) utilized extensively a solution of quinine and urethane. In 1931, sodium morrhuate was introduced in the United States, and sclerotherapy was extensively used either as a single form of treatment or in combination with ligation of the saphenous vein. Geza De Takats (Fig. 1.4), a pioneer vascular surgeon of Chicago, practiced high ligation of the saphenous vein at the groin, followed by distal injection of a sclerotherapy agent (12). He placed special emphasis on the ligation of the tributaries of the saphenous vein and a flush saphenofemoral junction ligation. By 1939, it had become evident from the reports of McPheeters, De Takats, and Smith (13), as well as from the report of another pioneer of vascular surgery, Dr. Alton Ochsner of New Orleans (14), that the recurrence rate following the use of sclerotherapy alone or in combination with high ligation was unacceptably high. These poor results were later confirmed by Waugh (15) who reviewed 101 patients several years after the original ligation and injection. Sixty percent of the patients had poor or fair results, and 36% of the entire group needed additional surgery.

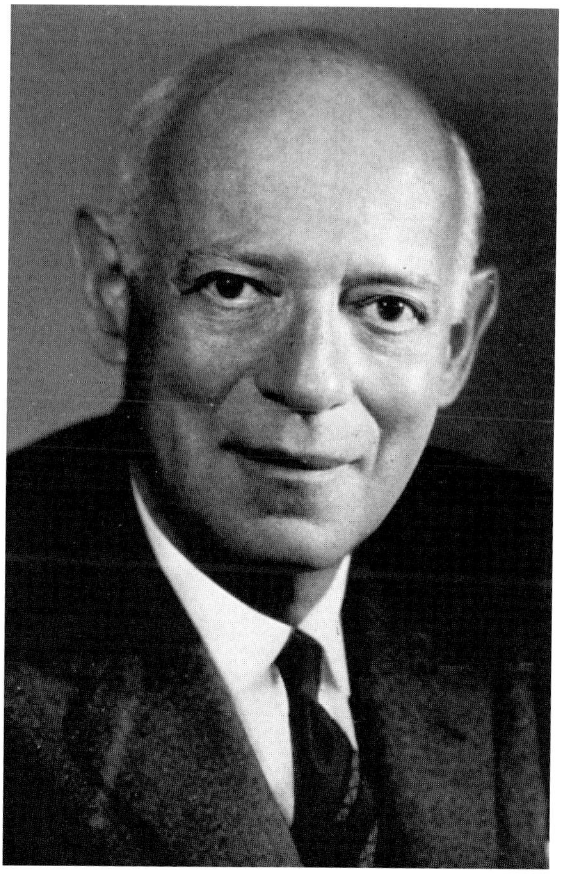

FIG. 1–4. Geza De Takats was a pioneer vascular surgeon who made numerous and important contributions to vascular surgery. He emphasized the flush saphenofemoral junction ligation and division of the tributaries of the saphenous vein at the junction. (Courtesy of Dr. Geza De Takats.)

THE PERIPHERAL VEIN SURGERY SECTION OF THE MAYO CLINIC

The reports of failure in the treatment of varicose veins by the surgical procedures of Mayo and Babcock and by sclerotherapy, either alone or in combination with high ligation, paved the way for the next stage in the search for improvement in the long-term results of surgery. A great impetus in renewing the interest in the surgical treatment for varicose veins came from Thomas T. Myers (Fig. 1.5), who, in 1947, not only developed an excellent intraluminal flexible stripper, but also designed a radical method of surgical treatment for varicose veins. The new intraluminal strippers were available in different sizes and had exchangeable tips so that veins of various lengths and sizes could be removed. The varicose clusters were directly excised. The thorough, extensive long- and short-stripping operation produced better long-term results when performed completely from foot to groin than when done from knee to groin. The extensive operation has been the treatment of choice for varicose veins since 1950. It has been performed in nearly 30,000 operations in more than 18,000 patients at the Mayo Clinic alone, and has provided good-to-excellent long-term control of the disease

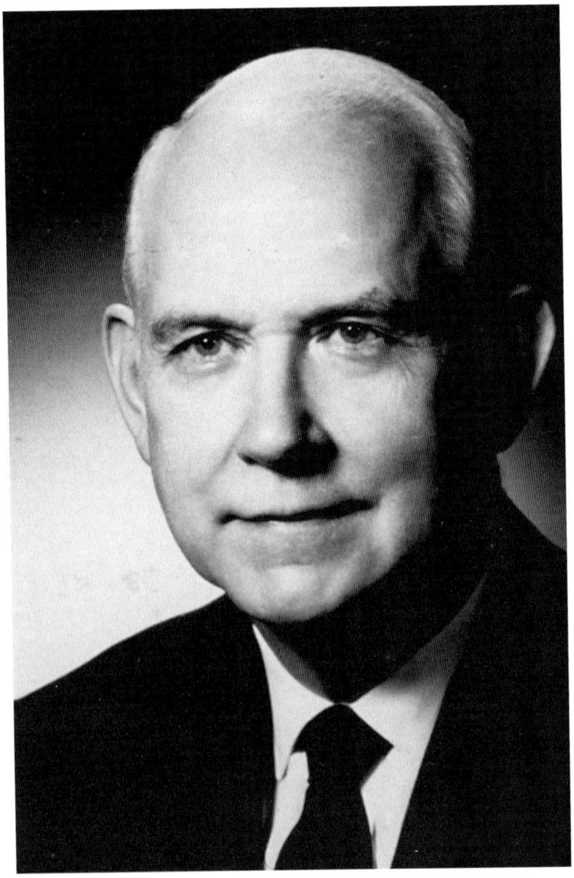

FIG. 1–5. Thomas T. Myers, under whose leadership the peripheral vein surgery of the Mayo Clinic became known worldwide. Myers designed a radical method of surgical treatment for varicose veins and new instruments that are still in use around the world. (Courtesy of Dr. Karl Lofgren.)

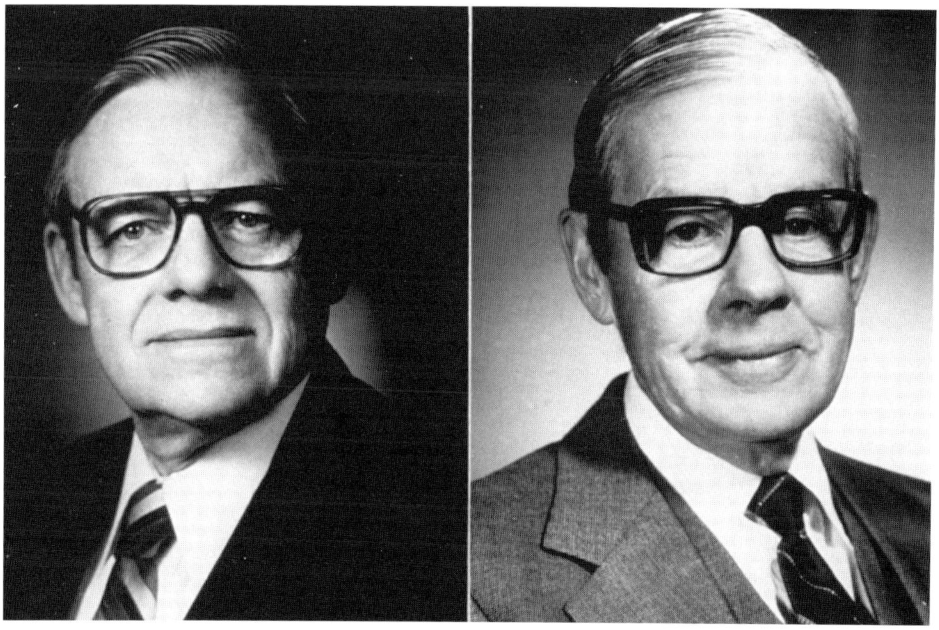

FIG. 1–6. The brothers Eric (*left*) and Karl Lofgren (*right*). Drs. Eric and Karl Lofgren operated on more than 18,000 patients with varicose veins at the Mayo Clinic alone. Their careful technique and excellent results contributed to the prestige of the Peripheral Vein Surgery Section of the Mayo Clinic. (Courtesy of Dr. Karl Lofgren.)

for 10 or more years after surgery in 85% of the patients (16). To a great extent, the good results and large clinical experience of the Mayo Clinic in venous surgery have been the result of the leadership of T.T. Myers and the continued and dedicated work of Eric and Karl Lofgren (Fig. 1.6) (17).

A cornerstone in the understanding and management of the postthrombotic sequelae was the publication of Robert Linton (Fig. 1.7), a surgeon at Massachusetts General Hospital in Boston. Linton described the operation of subfascial ligation of the medial lower leg communicating veins (18). The role of the incompetent large perforating veins found under the ulcer bed in many patients with severe reflux and venous ulceration was stressed by Linton. His operation consisted in the division of all the perforating veins encountered in the medial aspect of the leg. His approach was a long incision extending from behind the medial malleolus to just below the knee. In his original paper, Linton recommended the ligation of the superficial femoral vein to prevent reflux to the lower extremity. Many surgeons considered the Linton operation "too radical," but few denied that Linton's observations were pivotal in the understanding of the disease. Fifteen years after the Linton publication, Cockett and Dodd modified the radical operation and in 1953 described the "ankle blow-out syndrome." Their paper revived interest in the surgical management of the postthrombotic syndrome and venous ulceration. These two operations were, for many years, the mainstay in surgical management of the challenging problem of the postthrombotic leg and venous ulceration.

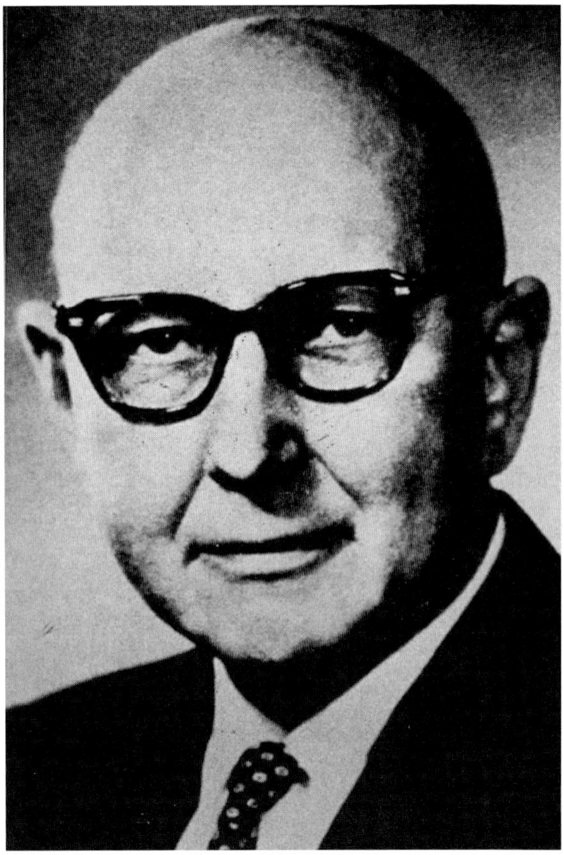

FIG. 1–7. Robert Linton, a distinguished surgeon at the Massachusetts General Hospital of Boston. Among the many contributions of Dr. Linton to the field of vascular surgery is his description of subfascial ligation of the leg communicating veins for the postthrombotic sequelae. (Reproduced by permission from Schumacker HB. The Society for Vascular Surgery. A history: 1945–1983. Manchester, MA: The Society for Vascular Surgery, 1984.)

The attack on the postthrombotic sequelae and venous obstruction continued with the classic paper of Richard Warren in 1954 (Fig. 1.8) (19). Warren published the first description of the use of the saphenous vein for bypassing a postthrombotic occlusion of the superficial femoral vein. It was the beginning of reconstructive venous surgery. He reported 14 patients with a follow-up of up to 3 years. Six had evidence of patency by venography and nine had improvement in their ambulatory venous pressures. Dr. Warren's important contribution was a stimulus in the development of reconstructive venous surgery. In 1960, the Uruguayan surgeon, Eduardo Palma, published his work on vein transplants and grafts in the surgical treatment of the postphlebitic syndrome (20). Palma described for the first time the use of the femoro-femoral crossover venous bypass to alleviate symptoms of venous obstruction in the proximal segments. The Palma approach to venous reconstruction was popularized in the United States by Andrew Dale (Fig. 1.9) (21). Dale's interest in reconstructive venous surgery began in the early 1960s with a series of canine experiments that convinced him that venous anastomosis and grafts could remain patent for long periods of time and that a refined, delicate surgical technique was needed. Dale's series reported a long-term patency rate of 75% (22). Dale was a strong advocate of the use of synthetic material for large venous reconstruction and, in 1984, reported several cases of long-term suc-

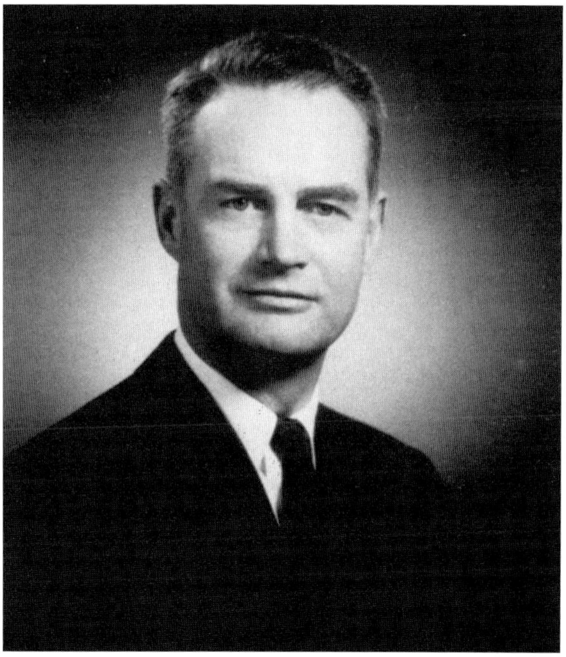

FIG. 1–8. An illustrious surgeon from Boston, Richard Warren described, for the first time, the use of the saphenous vein as a bypass of a postthrombotic occlusion of the superficial femoral vein. His contribution was a stimulus to the development of reconstructive venous surgery. (Reproduced by permission from Schumacker HB. The Society for Vascular Surgery. A history: 1945–1983. Manchester, MA: The Society for Vascular Surgery, 1984.)

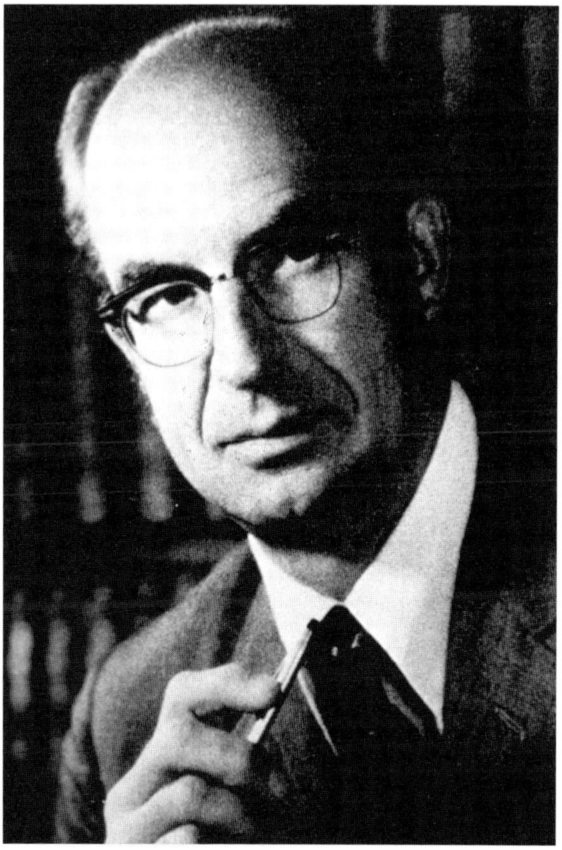

FIG. 1–9. Andrew Dale's interest in reconstructive venous surgery began in the early 1960s and continued throughout his entire life. He popularized the femorofemoral bypass (Palma operation) and reported on the long-term success of replacement of the inferior vena cava using prosthetic material. (Reproduced by permission from Schumacker HB. The Society for Vascular Surgery. A history: 1945–1983. Manchester, MA: The Society for Vascular Surgery, 1984.)

cess of replacement of the inferior vena cava using externally supported PTFE grafts (23).

Throughout history, it has been recognized that important surgical progress occurs during periods of armed conflict when surgeons are confronted with large numbers of injured patients within a relatively short period of time. Venous injuries had been treated by ligation during World War II, and this practice extended to the Korean War. The high morbidity that followed routine ligation of venous injuries during the Korean War stimulated Spencer and Hughes to repair injured veins. Norman Rich, during the Viet Nam War, established the importance of primary venous injury repair, emphasizing the benefits of the repair and the decreased morbidity observed in patients in whom the popliteal vein had been repaired versus those in whom the vein had been ligated (24, 25). The experimental and clinical work of Rich and collaborators has provided stimulus to several generations of vascular surgeons for a continued application of the principle of venous reconstruction in major vein trauma.

A monumental step forward in reconstruction of the venous system began in 1975 with Kistner's report on the surgical repair of the incompetent femoral vein valve (26). Kistner's pioneer work was performed in patients with primary valve incompetence. A second report, in 1979, described the transposition of a vein segment for patients with incompetent valves due to postthrombotic valve injury (27).

Kistner's reports stimulated other investigators such as Raju, Taheri, O'Donnell, Schanzer, Sottiurai, Glovizski, and Perrin in France to begin in their own centers the surgical reconstruction of the venous valve, often modifying and improving the surgical technique. The axillary vein transplantation technique was simultaneously developed by Raju and Taheri independent of each other (28).

Great progress has been made in the field of venous surgery. The long-term results of venous valve surgery for primary valvular disease approach a competency of nearly 80% (34). Most of these patients have had perforator interruption in addition to valve surgery. Initial results in patients with postthrombotic damage who have received valve segment transplantation or transposition are not as good as in the primary valvular insufficiency. However, there is no doubt that future improvements in the present techniques will lead to better results in this challenging group. A recent report from Raju (29) indicates that excellent long-term results in postthrombotic patients can be achieved by utilizing multiple valve reconstructions.

MODERN VEIN SURGERY: NEW TRENDS

The introduction of sophisticated noninvasive technology has provided us with fascinating tools that allow for an accurate and objective examination of the anatomy, physiology, and pathophysiology of the venous system. These methods have made exploration and investigation of the venous system more objective and scientific. Even though the classic methods of palpation and percussion of the veins and the tourniquet test are still used in certain special cases, there is no doubt that the introduction of the bidirectional Doppler duplex scanner, air plethysmography, and magnetic resonance imaging have provided objective information on the venous hemodynamics and pathophysiology of most venous disorders. In experienced hands, the bidirectional Doppler ultrasound has been effective in the diagnosis of venous obstruction and in the localization of points of reflux. It is the least expensive and most popular diagnostic method in the study of varicose veins. Duplex scanning with the addition of color can quantify reflux in a given venous territory and is the most valuable test in the evaluation of venous and arterial disease. Air plethysmography provides information on the performance of the calf pump mechanism and the hemodynamics of the superficial and deep venous systems.

For several decades, the extensive operation of the Mayo Clinic became the indiscriminate method of treatment for most forms of varicose veins. Many thousands of patients have had their saphenous veins removed. The extensive scarring of the operation, the loss of the most important autogenous conduit, together with the introduction of sophisticated technological advances of noninvasive diagnostic methods, have revived interest in the preservation of the saphenous vein. The greater saphenous vein is the most frequently used autogenous vascular conduit for peripheral arterial and coronary bypass surgery. Its importance is magnified as the limitations of the prosthetic vascular grafts have become evident. Large wrote: "Whether it is worth preserving the saphenous trunk as potential arterial bypass graft is arguable. It would seem irrational, however, to remove anything which is performing normally its assigned task without a good reason" (30).

SELECTIVE VENOUS SURGERY

In brief, this technique implies careful detection of the reflux site, based on bidirectional Doppler and duplex scanner examinations. The principles utilized in the Venous Clinics at Walter Reed Army Medical Center and the National Naval Medical Center to study patients with primary varicose veins are illustrated in Figure 1.10.

The clinical and Doppler examinations with the patient standing may reveal a competent or incompetent saphenofemoral junction. The objective of the noninvasive examination is to identify those patients with incompetent saphenofemoral junction who have a normal saphenous trunk by duplex scanning. Mapping of the entire saphenous trunk may reveal a dilated, aneurysmal varicose trunk that must be removed. However, if the examination reveals a healthy venous trunk, the saphenous vein is preserved. In this case, the saphenofemoral junction and its tributaries are ligated and divided, and the incompetent perforators localized and divided. Additionally, the clusters of varicose veins are removed by direct dissection using the "crochet hook" technique (31). One of the most frequent criticisms of the surgical management of varicose veins has been the postoperative scarring. With the traditional extensive stripping procedure developed at the Mayo Clinic, numerous surgical incisions were necessary. The cosmetic aspect of the wounds has been greatly improved with the introduction of the "crochet hook" technique. The special set of vein hooks of different sizes has been very useful to excise the tortuous varicose veins through 2–3-mm incisions. The tiny wounds become practically invisible a few months after surgery.

Following the principle of selective venous surgery, the greater and lesser saphenous veins have been stripped in 57% and 10%, respectively, of all cases op-

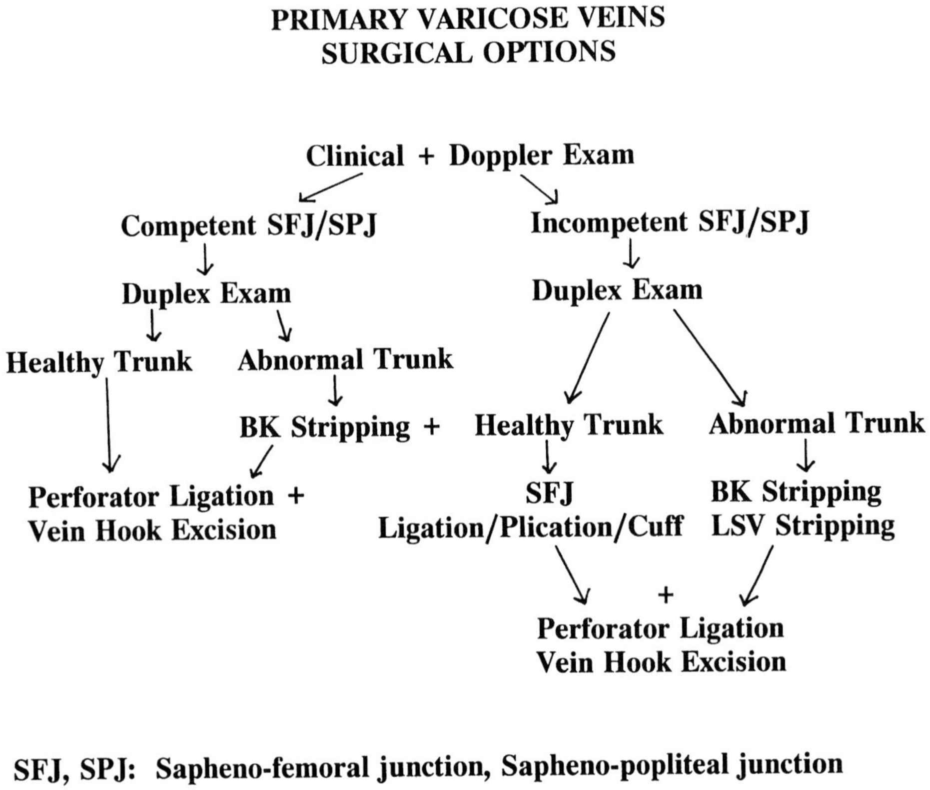

FIG. 1–10. Algorithm describing the use of Doppler ultrasound and duplex scanning in the selection of patients for surgery for primary varicose veins. Patients with incompetent saphenous veins by Doppler have their entire saphenous trunks examined by duplex scanning. If the saphenous trunk is found dilated and irregular, it is removed. However, if the examination reveals a healthy venous trunk, the saphenous vein is preserved. Incompetent perforating veins are identified and divided.

erated on during the last 5 years. The current trend to preserve the long saphenous vein for possible later use as an autogenous arterial substitute is not justified if the venous trunk is demonstrated to be diseased.

REFERENCES

1. Trendelenburg F. Über die Unterbindung der Vena Saphena Magna bei Unterschenkelvaricen. Berl Klin Chir 1890;7:195.
2. Brodie BC. Lectures illustrative of various subjects in pathology and surgery. London: Longmans, Green, 1846.
3. Homans J. The operative treatment of varicose veins and ulcers based upon a classification of these lesions. Surg Gynec Obstet 1916;22:143.
4. Mayo CH. Varicose veins of the lower extremity. St Paul Med J 1900;2:595.
5. Mayo CH. The surgical treatment of varicose veins. St Paul Med J 1904;6:695.

6. Schede M. Über die operative Behandlung der Unterschenkelvaricen. Beitr Klin Wochenschr 1877;14:85–89.
7. Mayo CH. Treatment of varicose veins. Surg Gynec Obstet 1906;2:385.
8. Keller WL. A new method of extirpating the internal saphenous and similar veins in varicose conditions. A preliminary report. NY Med J 1905;82:385.
9. Babcock WW. A new operation for the extirpation of varicose veins of the legs. NY Med J 1907;86:153.
10. McPheeters HO. Injection treatment of varicose veins by the use of sclerosing solutions. Surg Gynec Obstet 1927;45:541.
11. Dixon CF. The result of injection treatment of varicose veins. Proc Staff Meet Mayo Clin 1930;5:42.
12. De Takats G. Ambulatory ligation of the saphenous vein. JAMA 1930;94:1194.
13. Smith FL. Varicose veins: complications and results of treatment of 5,000 patients. Milit Surg 1939;85:514.
14. Ochsner A, Mahorner RH. The modern treatment of varicose veins. Surgery 1937;2:889.
15. Waugh JM. Ligation and injection of great saphenous veins. Proc Staff Meet Mayo Clin 1941;16:832.
16. Myers TT. Results and technique of stripping operation for varicose veins. JAMA 1957;163:87.
17. Lofgren KA. Management of varicose veins: Mayo Clinic experience. In: Bergan JJ, Yao JST, eds. Venous problems. Chicago: Yearbook Medical Publishers, 1978:71–84.
18. Linton RR. The communicating veins of the lower leg and the operative technique for their ligation. Ann Surg 1938;107:582.
19. Warren R. Transplantation of the saphenous vein for post-phlebitic stasis. Surgery 1954;35:867.
20. Palma EC, Esperon R. Vein transplants and grafts in the surgical treatment of the post-phlebitic syndrome. J Cardiovasc Surg 1960;1:94.
21. Dale WA. Reconstructive venous surgery. In: Veith FJ, ed. Critical problems in vascular surgery. New York: Appleton Century-Crofts, 1982:199–213.
22. Dale WA. Venous bypass surgery. Surg Clin N Am 1982;62:391.
23. Dale WA, Harris J, Terry RD. Polytetrafluoroethylene reconstruction of the inferior vena cava. Surgery 1984;95:625.
24. Rich NM, Hughes CW. Viet Nam Vascular Registry. A preliminary report. Surgery 1969;65:218.
25. Rich NM, Hughes CW, Baugh JG. Acute arterial injuries in Viet Nam: 1,000 cases. J Trauma 1970;10:359.
26. Kistner RL. Surgical repair of the incompetent femoral vein valve. Arch Surg 1975;110:1336.
27. Kistner RL. Surgery in acute and chronic venous disease. Surgery 1979,85.31.
28. Raju S. Discussion after Johnson ND, Queral LA, Flinn WR, Yao JST, Bergan JJ. Late objective assessment of venous valve surgery. Arch Surg 1981;116:1461.
29. Raju S, Fredericks RK, Neglen PN, Bass JD. Durability of venous valve reconstruction techniques for "primary" and postthrombotic reflux. J Vasc Surg 1996;23:357–366.
30. Large J. Doppler testing as an important consideration measure in the treatment of varicose veins. Aust NZ J Surg 1984;54:357.
31. Villavicencio JL, Collins GJ, Youkey JR, et al. Non-surgical management of lower extremity venous problems. In: Bergan JJ, Yao JST, eds. Surgery of the veins. New York: Grune & Stratton, 1985:323–345.
32. Moore W. The operative treatment of varicose veins with special reference to a modification of Trendelenburg operation. Intercolonial Med J Aus 1896;1:393.
33. Gray H. The medical magazine. 1919; Gray H, Jour RAMC, eds. 1909;xviii:272.
34. Masuda EM, Kistner RL. Long-term results of venous valve reconstruction: a 4 to 21 year follow-up. J Vasc Surg 1994;19:391–403.

chapter 2

Hemodynamics of the Venous System: Calf Pump and Valve Function

David S. Sumner and Paul S. van Bemmelen

The primary and most obvious function of the venous system is to return blood to the heart after it has passed through the arteries and capillaries, thus completing the circuit that begins in the left ventricle. But veins are not merely passive conduits. They serve a vital function as capacitance vessels, buffering changes in blood volume to maintain blood pressure at physiologic levels. They also assist in the propulsion of blood during exercise, acting much like a "peripheral heart." Because of their proximity to the skin, superficial veins play an important role in thermoregulation.

In many respects, the physiology of veins is more complex than that of the arterial system. Unlike arteries, veins are thin-walled, collapsible tubes. There are two large systems, superficial and deep, that are connected at various points by "perforating" or "communicating" veins. Although deep veins parallel arteries with the same name, superficial veins have no arterial counterpart. Similarly, there is no arterial counterpart to the large, saccular veins (sinusoids) that are deeply imbedded in the muscles of the calf. Veins have a larger diameter than their accompanying arteries and in peripheral locations are duplicated. Veins are seldom completely distended; even so, large and small veins contain approximately two-thirds of the blood in the body. Only about 15% of the blood is in the arterial system, the remainder being distributed between the capillaries, lungs, and heart. At comparable sites in the circulation, blood pressure in the veins is always lower than that in arteries; and, unlike the situation in arteries, the hydrostatic component of the total pressure in veins is often proportionally larger than the dynamic component. In contrast to arteries, in which blood flow is pulsatile but relatively constant from one cardiac cycle to the next, blood flow in veins is intermittent, varying with respiration and muscular activity. Perhaps the anatomic feature most responsible for differences in the physiology of the two systems is the presence of venous valves, which, when functioning properly, ensure unidirectional flow.

Although venous diseases are less dramatic than peripheral arterial diseases and attract less attention, deep venous thrombosis and chronic venous insufficiency are responsible for more disability than arterial obstruction, and pulmonary emboli are a major cause of death. Obstruction of venous flow, valvular incompetence, and abnormalities of the calf muscle pump mechanism are among the factors that contribute to the pathophysiology of the venous system. How hemodynamic aberrations instigate the microvascular changes that are ultimately responsible for the manifestations of venous disease remains incompletely understood, but, thanks to advances in cellular and molecular biology, inroads are being made.

This chapter reviews some of the key aspects of normal venous hemodynamics and their relationship to the pathophysiology of venous disease.

NORMAL HEMODYNAMICS

Four areas are of concern: (a) venous pressure and the role of gravity; (b) venous volume and its relationship to compliance; (c) pressure-flow phenomena in collapsible tubes; and (d) venous valves and their contribution to the venous pump mechanism.

Venous Pressure

There are two major components to the systemic venous pressure (P_v): dynamic pressure (P_d) and hydrostatic pressure (P_h). Under certain circumstances, static filling pressure (P_s) must be considered as well.

$$P_v = P_d + P_h \qquad (1)$$

Dynamic Pressure. Dynamic pressure is produced by contraction of the left ventricle, which forces blood to enter the vascular bed against resistances that are distributed throughout the entire vascular circuit. Thus, most of the work done in moving blood from the left side to the right side of the heart is performed by the left ventricle. Because a large portion of the dynamic pressure is dissipated in terminal arterioles and capillaries, the dynamic component of pressure in the venous system is markedly lower than that in the arterial tree. In the normal circulation, under resting conditions, the dynamic pressure in the venules hovers around 15–20 mmHg, falling to 5–10 mmHg in the major veins, and to 0–6 mmHg in the right atrium. Calf muscle contraction and respiration also contribute to the dynamic pressure.

Hydrostatic Pressure. Hydrostatic pressure represents the weight of the uninterrupted column of blood that extends from the point of measurement to a "zero" reference point, which is approximately at the level of the right atrium. It is equivalent to the product of the density of blood (ρ 1.056 gm/cm^3), the acceleration due to gravity (g, 980 cm/sec^2), and the vertical distance between the site of measurement and the reference point (h, cm).

$$P_h = -\rho g h \quad (2)$$

For example, the hydrostatic pressure 131 cm below the right atrium (at the ankle in a 6-foot tall person) would be about 135,569 dynes/cm^2 or 102 mmHg (since 1333 dynes/cm^2 is equivalent to 1 mmHg). *(A negative sign precedes the vertical distance because the measurement site is below the reference point. If it were above the reference point, a positive sign would be required.)*

$$P_h = 1.056\ gm/cm^3 \times 980\ cm/\sec \times -131\ cm = 135{,}569\ dynes/cm^2 = 102\ mmHg \quad (3)$$

Below the heart, hydrostatic pressure is the same in arteries, capillaries, and veins at the same level, provided there is no interruption of the column of blood in these vessels (Fig. 2.1). As a result, the hydrostatic pressure at ankle level in a quietly standing subject greatly exceeds the dynamic pressure in veins and capillaries and often approximates the dynamic pressure in arteries.

Above the heart, in which hydrostatic pressure in a standing subject has a negative value, the situation is more complicated. Because the dynamic pressure on the arterial side of the circulation is relatively high, total arterial pressure remains positive despite a negative hydrostatic pressure (Fig. 2.1). On the venous side of the circulation, in which the dynamic pressure is low compared to the negative hydrostatic pressure, total pressure in unsupported veins, such as those in subcutaneous tissues or muscles, falls below the surrounding tissue pressure, and the veins collapse. This increases venous resistance, thereby raising the dynamic pressure just enough to permit blood flow to continue, and the total pressure in these veins becomes slightly positive (Fig. 2.2). In supported veins, such as the dural

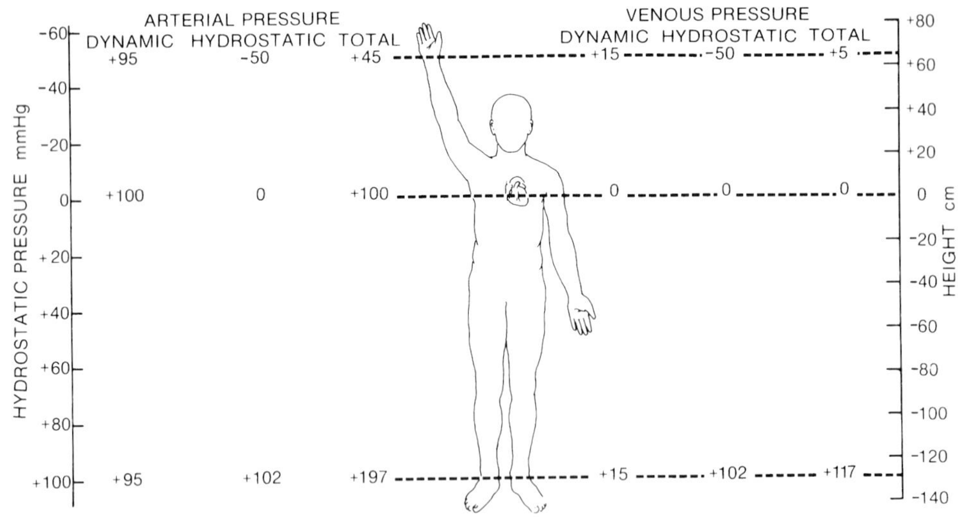

FIG. 2–1. Hydrostatic and dynamic venous and arterial blood pressures in a standing subject. The zero reference point is at the level of the right atrium. (Reproduced by permission from Sumner DS. Hemodynamics and pathophysiology of venous disease. In: Rutherford RB, ed. Vascular surgery. 4th ed. Philadelphia: WB Saunders Co., 1995:1673–1695.)

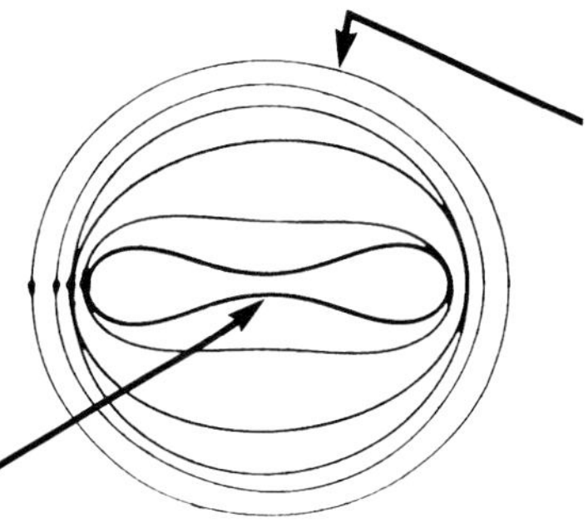

FIG. 2–2. Cross-section of venous lumen at various transmural pressures. At pressures below 0 mmHg, the lumen assumes a dumbbell configuration; at low pressures, the lumen is elliptical; and at high pressures, it becomes circular. Stretching of the circumference of the wall occurs with increasing transmural pressure. (Reproduced by permission from Sumner DS. Hemodynamics and pathophysiology of venous disease. In: Rutherford RB, ed. Vascular surgery. 4th ed. Philadelphia: WB Saunders Co., 1995:1673–1695.)

sinuses, in which the surrounding tissues prevent venous collapse, the total venous pressure becomes negative. Opening these veins when the apex of the skull is above the heart (as in a neurosurgical procedure) subjects the patient to the danger of an air embolism, because atmospheric pressure exceeds intravenous pressure. Even large neck veins, such as the jugular, may "suck air" when they are opened.

Static Filling Pressure. Static filling pressure (P_s) is the result of the atmospheric pressure, the pressure exerted by the surrounding tissues, and the elastic recoil of the venous wall acting on the enclosed volume of blood. It is analogous to air pressure in an inflated rubber balloon. As a separate entity, static filling pressure assumes importance when there is no blood flow in a venous segment isolated by valve closure at both ends.

Venous Volume and Control of Venous Capacity

The volume of blood contained within a segment of vein is a function of the transmural pressure (P_{TM}), the mechanical properties (elasticity) of the venous wall, and the contractile state of the smooth muscles within the media. Transmural pressure is the difference between the intravascular pressure acting to expand the vein and the pressure in the surrounding tissues that compresses the vein from the outside. (Interstitial fluid pressures in normal limbs are usually subatmospheric, averaging -2.5 mmHg with a range of -5 to 1 mmHg (1).)

Venous volume compliance (C_V) may be defined as the ratio of the change in venous volume (ΔV) to the change in transmural pressure (ΔP_{TM}):

$$C_v = \frac{\Delta V}{\Delta P_{TM}} \tag{4}$$

The venous pressure/volume curve is S-shaped (Fig. 2.3). At subatmospheric transmural pressures (when the outside pressure exceeds that of the blood on the inside) and at high transmural pressures, venous compliance is low and little change in volume occurs in response to a relatively large change in transmural pressure. Between these extremes, veins are very compliant (2). Large changes in venous volume occur in response to relatively little change in venous pressure.

When transmural pressure is very low (−10 to −15 mmHg), veins collapse almost completely, and venous volume approaches zero. The opposing venous walls are approximated except at the points of greatest curvature, where small channels remain (Fig. 2.3). With increasing transmural pressure, the cross-sectional configuration at first becomes dumbbell-shaped, then elliptical, and finally circular (2). Although the perimeter of the venous wall increases somewhat as the transmural pressure rises, the great increase in venous volume observed during this phase of expansion is largely attributable to changes in the venous cross-section. Because much less force is required to bend the venous wall than to stretch it, volume compliance is high (3, 4).

At zero transmural pressures, veins are only slightly elliptical (provided external forces are distributed equally around the circumference of the wall). This is immediately evident when one observes the roughly circular configuration of a venous segment immersed in a glass of water. With increasing transmural pressure, the cross-section becomes completely circular and any further changes in

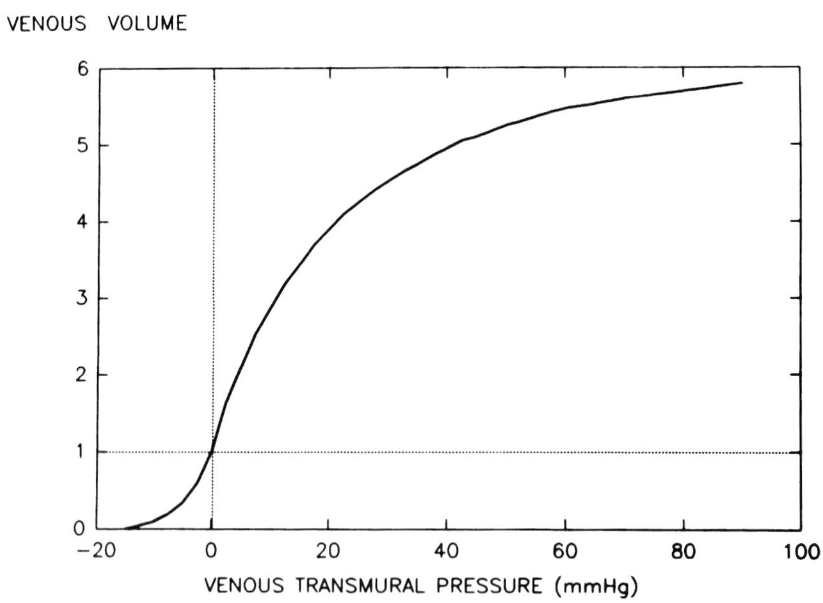

FIG. 2–3. Typical venous pressure—venous volume compliance curve. Venous volume at zero transmural pressure is considered to be unity. Veins are stiff at pressures below 0 mmHg and at pressures greater than 40 mmHg, but are very compliant at 0 to 20 mmHg.

venous volume are the result of stretching the wall itself. At first, most of the load is sustained by the structural protein, elastin, which is relatively easily stretched; but as the transmural pressure rises, the much stiffer collagen fibers are called into play. As a result, veins become quite stiff at high transmural pressures. In fact, at arterial pressures, veins are no more compliant than arteries and perhaps somewhat less so (2, 5, 6).

The shape of the venous pressure/volume curve has important physiologic implications. A change in position from supine to standing greatly increases the hydrostatic pressure in dependent portions of the leg. Because the extravascular (tissue) pressure does not change, the resulting increase in transmural pressure allows blood to accumulate to the limit of the venous compliance. In a typical individual, the volume of blood in each leg increases by approximately 250 ml (7). It is well-known that uncompensated translocation of 500 ml of blood from the central circulation to the legs may occasionally result in syncope. The muscle pump mechanism, which is ordinarily activated in the standing position, helps return blood to the more proximal veins and diminishes the quantity stored in the legs. Owing to the shape of the venous pressure/volume curve, the volume of blood in the legs increases more when a supine subject assumes a sitting position than when the subject shifts from a sitting to a standing position.

Abdominal and Thoracic Compartments. Throughout the abdomen, transmural venous pressure remains virtually constant regardless of position (7). Because the abdominal contents have a specific gravity similar to that of blood, the increased hydrostatic pressure within veins at all levels of the abdomen in a standing individual is balanced by a similar increase in intra-abdominal pressure at the same level. In all positions, supine or upright, blood pressure in the vena cava must exceed the intra-abdominal pressure to prevent venous collapse and to allow blood to flow. This results in a venous transmural pressure that is usually only slightly positive, placing the venous pressure/volume curve in the most compliant region.

Because intrathoracic pressure is subatmospheric, ranging from about -4 to -8 mmHg during quiet respiration to -30 mmHg during deep inspiration, central venous transmural pressures remain slightly positive despite intravascular pressures that are just above or just below atmospheric. Therefore, intrathoracic veins, as well as those in the abdomen, function in the most compliant region of the pressure/volume curve. This permits large shifts in venous blood volume to occur with little change in central venous pressure. Were it not for this feature, the body would be ill-equipped to handle blood loss, transfusions, intravenous fluid administration, and the large translocation of blood to the legs that accompanies assumption of a standing position. (Approximately three-quarters of the blood that accumulates in the legs comes from the intrathoracic vasculature [8].) Thus, within physiologic ranges, the system buffers changes in intravascular fluid volume. When, however, central venous pressures are elevated due to heart failure or pulmonary disease, excess fluid will be poorly tolerated. Similarly, a nearly empty circulatory system may be critically sensitive to sudden blood loss.

Active Constriction. When veins are filled sufficiently to have a roughly circular cross-section, contraction of smooth muscle within the vessel wall has an important effect on venous volume (9). Venous tone is minimal under normal resting conditions and is largely controlled by sympathetic alpha adrenergic activity (10, 11). (The local metabolic environment has little influence on venous contractility.) Peripheral veins constrict more intensely to sympathetic stimuli than do the more centrally located veins and have thicker walls and a higher smooth muscle content.

In general, veins contract in response to stimuli that increase cardiac output (12). During exercise, venoconstriction accelerates venous return and transfers blood from the legs and splanchnic capacitance vessels to the central circulation, where it is required to maintain an increased cardiac output. The elevated venous resistance is more than offset by metabolically induced dilatation of the arterioles in the exercising muscle so that total resistance is decreased. Unlike other peripheral veins, the intramuscular sinusoids, which lack sympathetic innervation, do not constrict (13). Constriction of these vessels would be counterproductive, since they constitute the major "bellows" of the muscle pump mechanism.

Cutaneous veins serve a thermoregulatory function. Heat is conserved when veins constrict and is dissipated when they dilate. Both direct cold exposure and the increased sympathetic activity mediated by a reduction in core temperature cause venous constriction (14). Warmth increases venous diameter both directly by relaxing the vascular smooth muscle and indirectly by decreasing sympathetic activity. During strenuous exercise, the excess heat generated overcomes the reflex vasoconstriction normally present and results in cutaneous venous dilatation. This, in turn, causes increased demands on the heart.

Although constriction of leg veins in response to standing would counteract the tendency for blood to pool in the lower extremities, this does not occur (15). Some protection, however, is afforded by reflex arteriolar constriction, which decreases limb blood flow and reduces the rate of venous filling. As mentioned previously, the muscle pump provides the major mechanism for diminishing gravitationally induced fluid shifts.

Pressure-Flow Phenomena

In an ideal (frictionless) system, fluid, once it is in motion, would continue to move without the dissipation of energy. Because this never occurs, blood—like all fluids—moves from one point to another in the venous system in response to an energy gradient. There are two components of the total fluid energy that need to be considered in order to understand the dynamics of venous blood flow: potential energy and kinetic energy. Potential energy is represented by the dynamic (P_d) and hydrostatic pressures ($P_h = -\rho gh$) (which were discussed previously) and by gravitational potential energy (E_g). The latter is the energy that a body possesses by virtue of its height above the surface of the earth. Thus, gravitational potential energy is equivalent to hydrostatic pressure but has an opposite sign:

$$E_g = +\rho gh \tag{5}$$

As the hydrostatic pressure increases, gravitational potential energy decreases, and vice versa. In many (but not all) physiologic situations, these two forms of energy cancel each other and can be neglected. This explains why there is no overall energy gradient between the water at the top of a glass and that at the bottom of the glass (Fig. 2.4).

Kinetic energy (E_k) represents the energy associated with a body (or particle of fluid) in motion:

$$E_k = \frac{1}{2}\rho v^2 \tag{6}$$

where v represents velocity in cm/sec. Because the kinetic energy of blood traveling at a velocity of 50 cm/sec is roughly equivalent to a pressure of only 1.0 mmHg, kinetic energy in the arterial system ordinarily contributes little to the overall fluid energy; but in the venous system where pressures may be low, the kinetic fraction may be appreciable.

The one-dimensional Bernoulli equation provides a simplified but convenient way of understanding the relationships between these various components of fluid energy:

$$P_{d1} + P_{h1} + \rho g h_1 + \frac{1}{2}\rho v_1^2 = P_{d2} + P_{h2} + \rho g h_2 + \frac{1}{2}\rho v_2^2 + heat \tag{7}$$

In this equation, the subscripts indicate two points along the vascular conduit, and "heat" represents the energy dissipated by friction as blood moves from point 1 to point 2.

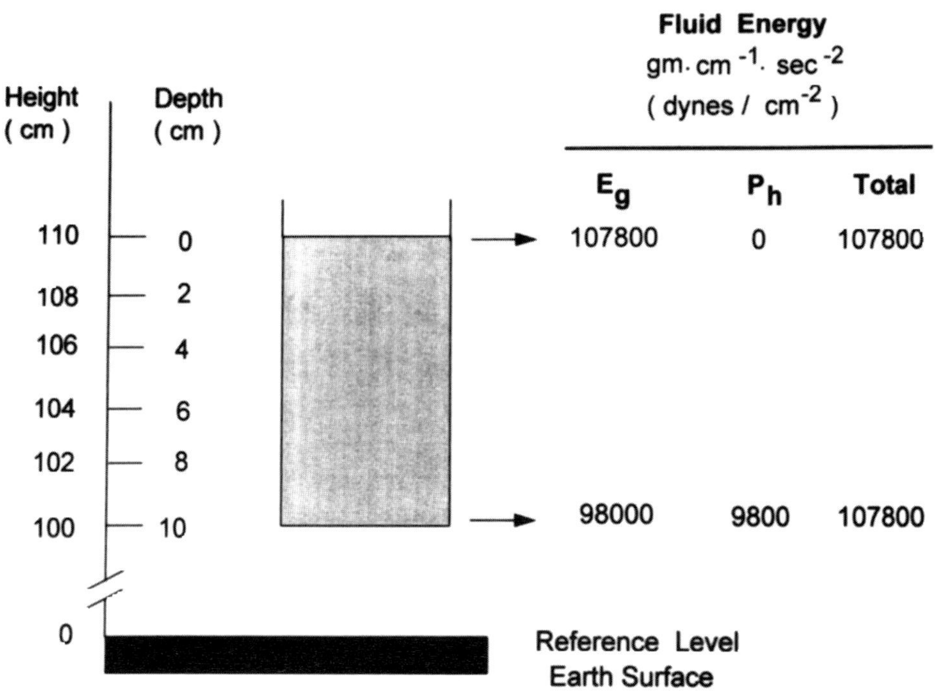

FIG. 2–4. Energy relationships in a glass of water. Because the difference between the gravitational potential energy (E_g) at the top and bottom of the glass is exactly counterbalanced by the difference in hydrostatic pressure (P_h), the total fluid energy at all levels is constant.

When a person is lying supine in a horizontal position, hydrostatic pressures are identical at all points equidistant from the horizontal plane and vary by only a few millimeters of mercury from the anterior to the posterior aspects of the body. The same is true of gravitational potential energy. In this situation, dynamic pressure and, to a much lesser extent, kinetic energy are the only parameters that need to be considered. That hydrostatic pressure and gravitational potential energy cancel when blood vessels are filled explains some of the apparent paradoxes of energy relationships in the standing position. For example, blood moves from the heart, in which the mean blood pressure may be 100 mmHg, against a pressure gradient to the ankles, in which the mean arterial pressure may be 197 mmHg; but, since the hydrostatic pressure and the gravitational potential energy cancel at all levels, the actual driving force is provided by the dynamic pressure at the heart, which is 5 mmHg greater than that at the ankle (Fig. 2.1). Similarly, the energy gradient returning blood from the ankle to the heart in the venous system is only 15 mmHg (the dynamic pressure gradient) and not the total pressure gradient of 117 mmHg. Thus, during quiet standing, only the dynamic pressure component needs to be considered.

Venous Resistance. The "resistance" (R_v) that a segment of vein has to blood flow is given by the ratio of the total energy gradient ($E_1 - E_2$) across the segment to the quantity of blood flowing through the segment (Q_v):

$$R_v = \frac{E_1 - E_2}{Q_v} \approx \frac{P_{d1} - P_{d2}}{Q_v} \tag{8}$$

For most purposes, however, the dynamic pressure gradient ($P_{d1} - P_{d2}$) can be substituted for the total energy gradient. This formula is analogous to Ohm's law in electrical circuits; but, unlike electrical resistance (which is relatively constant throughout a wide range of current and voltage), venous resistance varies with the velocity of blood flow, the cross-sectional configuration and diameter of the vein, and blood viscosity. Nonetheless, the concept of venous resistance is helpful in discussing the dynamics of venous blood flow.

Although veins are usually considered to be low-resistance vessels, the energy gradient from the venules to the heart is similar to that from the left ventricle to the arterioles. Because veins carry the same amount of blood as arteries and have a potential cross-sectional area that is three or four times as large, this observation seems somewhat incongruous. Veins, however, are often partially collapsed and are seldom completely distended. The resulting slit-like or elliptical cross-section offers more resistance to blood flow than does a circular cross-section (3). As veins distend, their resistance is markedly decreased, permitting relatively large increases in blood flow to be accommodated with little increase in the energy gradient.

Influence of Central Pressure Fluctuation. Whereas, in the arterial system, blood pressure, vascular volume, and blood flow usually change in the same direction, in veins the opposite often occurs (Fig. 2.5). Venous pressure and volume may decrease as flow increases or may increase as flow decreases or reverses. In the resting state, the rate and direction of blood flow in the venous system are determined by the pressure (energy) gradient between the peripheral (P_{pv}) and cen-

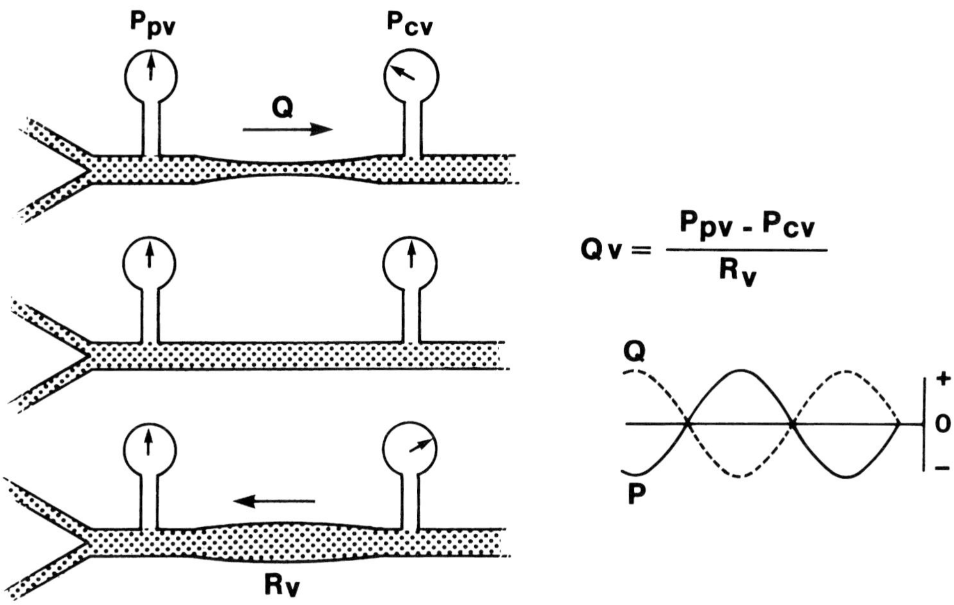

FIG. 2–5. Relationship between blood flow (Q) in a venous segment, the resistance (R) of the segment, and the peripheral (P_{pv}) and central (P_{cv}) venous pressures. Increasing pressure is indicated by a clockwise movement of the arrows on the meters. When P_{pv} and P_{cv} are equal, there is no flow. As centrally directed flow increases, pressure (P) at the midpoint of the vein decreases and the segment collapses. When flow reverses, the opposite occurs: pressure increases and the vein expands. (Reproduced by permission from Sumner DS. Applied physiology in venous problems. In: Bergan JJ, Yao JST, eds. Surgery of the veins. Orlando, FL: Grune & Stratton, 1985:3–23.)

tral (P_{cv}) veins. Because the peripheral venous pressure remains relatively constant while the central venous pressure fluctuates, changes in venous flow and pressure are largely the result of variations in central venous pressure. When the central venous pressure falls, the pressure gradient rises, and blood flow increases (provided the venous resistance does not change appreciably). Blood pressure in the venous segment, which must lie somewhere between the peripheral and central pressures, also decreases. This, in turn, leads to a reduction in venous volume. On the other hand, an increase in central venous pressure reduces the pressure gradient, flow decreases, pressure in the venous segment rises, and the vein expands. Fluctuations in the volume of neck veins are easily observed and reflect changes in central venous pressure related to the phase of the cardiac cycle. Similar pulsatile variations in venous blood flow velocity may be detected on Doppler examination of upper extremity veins in normal subjects who are resting quietly in a warm room (Fig. 2.6) (16). Cardiac-induced variations in lower extremity venous blood flow are usually masked by the much larger velocity fluctuations that accompany respiration, but may be evident in patients with elevated central venous pressure.

Flow Through Collapsible Tubes. The mechanics of fluid flow through a horizontally oriented collapsible tube (such as a Penrose drain) passing through

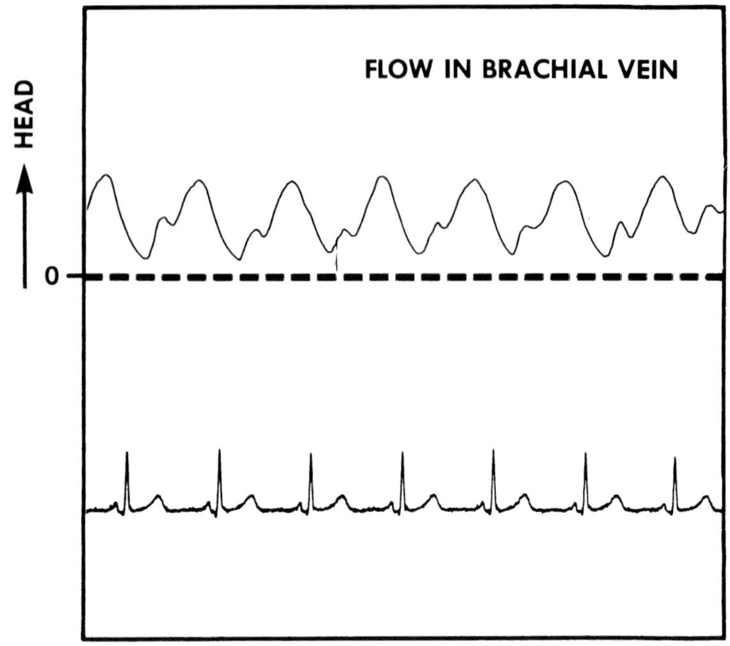

FIG. 2–6. Doppler recording of flow in a brachial vein (*upper panel*) and the corresponding EKG (*lower panel*). During each cardiac cycle, venous flow velocities vary with pressure changes that occur in the right atrium. (Reproduced by permission from Sumner DS. Noninvasive vascular laboratory assessment. In: Machleder HJ, ed. Vascular disorders of the upper extremity. 2nd ed. Mount Kisco, NY: Futura Publishing, 1989:9–57.)

a pressurized closed container are best understood in a model system (Fig. 2.7**A**) (4, 17–20). In this illustration, the driving pressure is 15 cm H_2O, the container pressure is 5 cm H_2O, and the outflow pressure at the end of the tube, which is open to the atmosphere, is 0 cm H_2O. Within the container, the tube remains collapsed until the pressure of the fluid in the tube exceeds that in the container by a slight amount (>5 cm H_2O). Thus, the pressure gradient driving fluid through the model is 10 cm H_2O (15 cm H_2O − 5 cm H_2O), not 15 cm H_2O − 0 cm H_2O. Obviously, increasing or decreasing the inflow pressure will increase or decrease the pressure gradient in a linear fashion and will have a similar effect on flow through the system (Fig. 2.7**B**). When the inflow-container pressure gradient is low, most of the tube remains partially collapsed. As the pressure gradient increases, more of the tube opens and eventually only that portion at the distal end of the closed container remains collapsed. As fluid flows though the system, the collapsed portion of the tube will flutter, opening and closing in response to pressure fluctuations, much like the rubber device that one blows into to make noise at parties or like the reed of a clarinet (20). When the tube is collapsed, there is no flow, and the fluid pressure rises until the tube opens. As the velocity of flow increases, the pressure in the tube falls in accordance with Bernoulli's principle (eq. 6); and the tube collapses, reopening again when the pressure rises.

Raising the end of the tube to increase outflow pressure will have no effect on flow until the outflow pressure exceeds that in the closed container (>5 cm H_2O), at which point the collapsible tube will remain distended throughout its length. Further increases in outflow pressure will decrease the pressure gradient, which now depends on the difference between the inflow and outflow pressures and is independent of the pressure in the closed container. Flow, of course, responds in a similar fashion (Fig. 2.7**C**). Raising the container pressure while the inflow pressure remains constant will decrease the pressure gradient and decrease flow, provided the outflow pressure is less than the container pressure (Fig. 2.7**D**). This model explains many of the peculiarities of venous blood flow.

Effect of Respiration. Because of their collapsible nature, pressure in the iliac veins and inferior vena cava must exceed that in the abdominal cavity (a closed container) to maintain a lumen and to allow blood to flow from the legs into the thorax. Therefore, the pressure gradient propelling blood from the legs

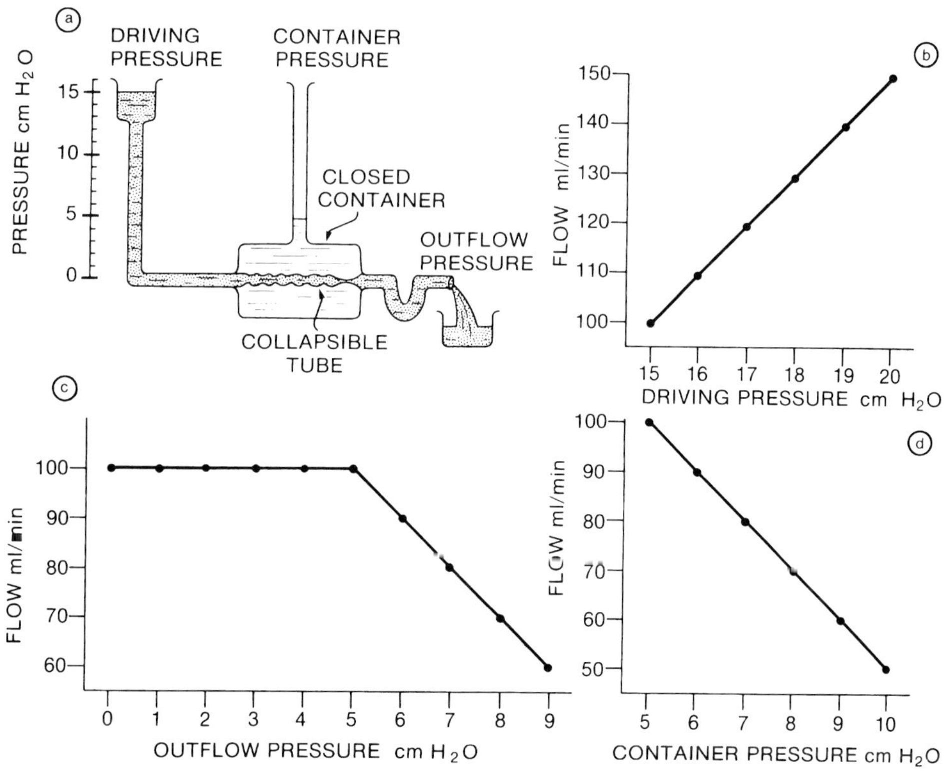

FIG. 2–7. A. Model illustrating flow through a collapsible tube passing through a closed container. **B.** Effect of elevating the "driving pressure," while "container pressure" and "outflow pressure" are held constant. **C.** Effect of elevating "outflow pressure," other pressures constant. **D.** Effect of elevating "container pressure," other pressures constant. (Reproduced by permission from Sumner DS. Hemodynamics and pathophysiology of venous disease. In: Rutherford RB, ed. Vascular surgery. 4th ed. Philadelphia: WB Saunders Co., 1995:1673–1695.)

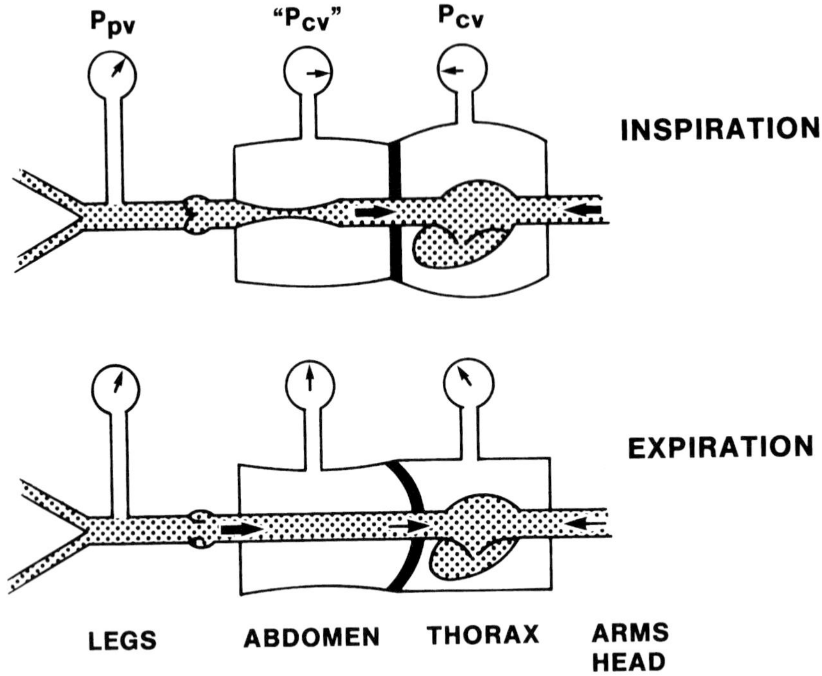

FIG. 2–8. Effect of respiration on venous blood flow from the lower extremities, abdomen, and brachiocephalic area. Abdomen and thorax are considered to be "closed compartments," through which the collapsible veins pass. With inspiration, abdominal pressure increases while thoracic pressure decreases. With expiration, the opposite occurs. (Reproduced by permission from Sumner DS. Applied physiology in venous problems. In: Bergan JJ, Yao JST, eds. Surgery of the veins. Orlando, FL: Grune & Stratton, 1985:3–23.)

to the thorax is not the difference between the peripheral venous pressure and that in the thorax (as might be expected) but rather it is the difference between the peripheral and intraabdominal pressures. When a person lying supine breathes in, the diaphragm descends, compressing the abdominal viscera. This in turn raises intra-abdominal pressure (Fig. 2.8). The intra-abdominal veins collapse, and blood flow from the legs ceases temporarily (Fig. 2.9) (21). During this period, venous pressure in the legs rises. Then when the person exhales, the diaphragm rises, the intraabdominal pressure falls, and blood is propelled out of the legs into the abdomen by the increased pressure gradient between the legs and abdominal veins (Figs. 2.8 and 2.9). If, on the other hand, the inspiration is maintained for more than a few seconds, venous pressure in the legs will increase until it exceeds that in the abdomen, allowing blood to flow out of the legs into the abdomen. Exhaling against a closed glottis (Valsalva maneuver) causes the abdominal pressure to exceed that in the leg veins, thereby reversing the venous pressure gradient. Blood flow from the legs comes to a standstill or may reverse, maintaining a retrograde direction down the leg until a competent valve is encountered (Fig. 2.9) (21).

During inspiration, intrathoracic pressure falls while that in the abdomen rises, causing blood to flow from the upper abdomen into the chest. Like the tube in the closed container model, the inferior vena cava tends to collapse just below the diaphragm. In the upper extremity and neck, the extrathoracic tissues correspond to the closed container (Fig. 2.8). Because the intrathoracic pressure is lower than the extrathoracic tissue pressure, respiration has less effect on venous outflow from the arms and cephalic circulation. In general, blood flow increases with inspiration as the intrathoracic pressure falls and decreases with expiration as the pressure rises (Fig. 2.10) (16). As predicted by the collapsible tube model, a rapid, deep inspiration will "suck" the subclavian vein closed just as it crosses the first rib to enter the thorax. The narrowing of the subclavian vein at this point seen on upper extremity phlebograms is sometimes misinterpreted as a stenosis.

Vertical Tubes. Fluid flowing downward in a vertically oriented collapsible tube open at the lower end to the atmosphere acts as if it were in a "free fall." Pressure within the tube at all levels is equal to the atmospheric pressure (transmural pressure equals zero). Thus, there is no pressure gradient from the top to the bottom of the tube. The force propelling fluid downward is equivalent to the gravitational potential energy gradient (ΔE_g), which is determined by the vertical distance ($h_1 - h_2$) between the upper and lower ends of the tube (17):

$$\Delta E_g = \rho g(h_1 - h_2) \tag{9}$$

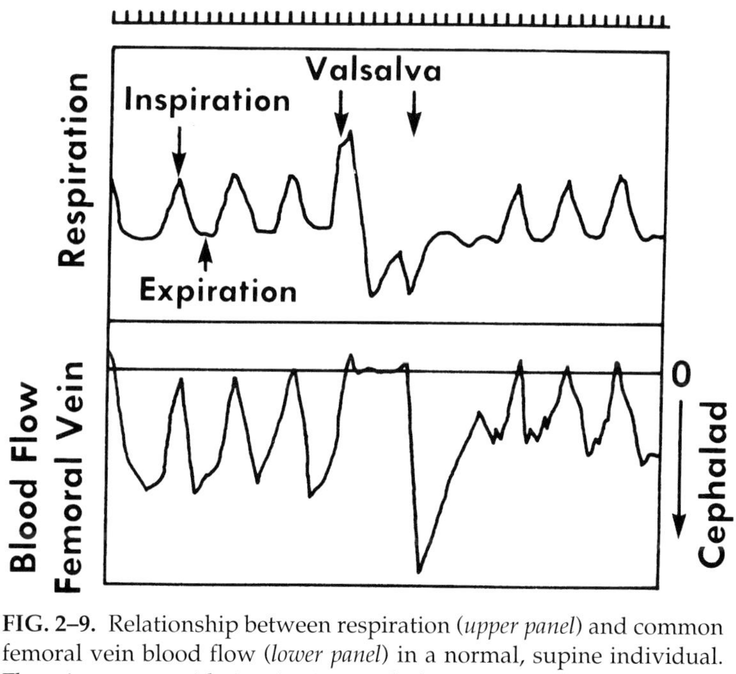

FIG. 2–9. Relationship between respiration (*upper panel*) and common femoral vein blood flow (*lower panel*) in a normal, supine individual. Flow increases with inspiration and decreases with expiration. A Valsalva maneuver causes flow to cease without reversing direction. (Reproduced by permission from Sumner DS. Diagnosis of venous thrombosis by Doppler ultrasound. In: Bergan JJ, Yao JST, eds. Venous problems. Chicago: Year Book Medical Publishers, 1978:159–185.)

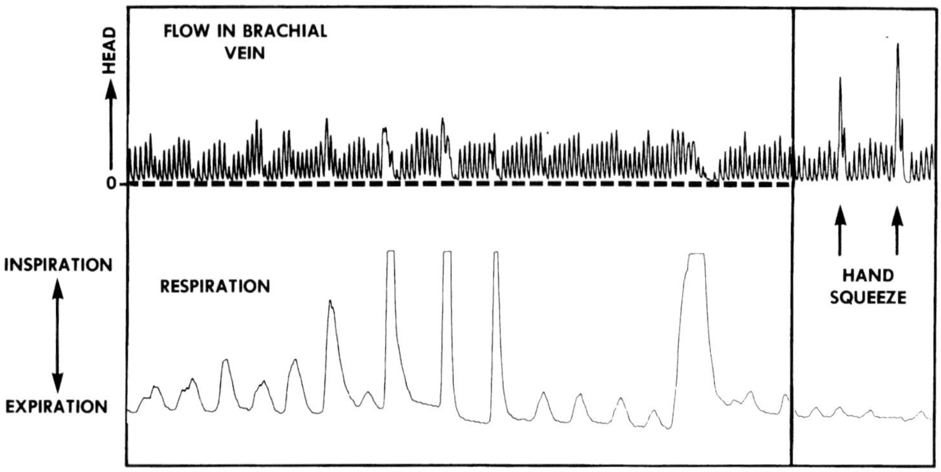

FIG. 2–10. Relationship between respiration and blood flow in a normal brachial vein. Flow increases with quiet inspiration and with slow deep inspiration but ceases temporarily with forcible rapid inspiration, which "sucks" the subclavian vein closed. Superimposed cardiac pulsations are prominent. Hand squeeze increases flow. (Reproduced by permission from Sumner DS. Noninvasive vascular laboratory assessment. In: Machleder HJ, ed. Vascular disorders of the upper extremity. 2nd ed. Mount Kisco, NY: Futura Publishing, 1989:9–57.)

Clearly, the "loss" of energy is independent of the volume of flow as long as the tube remains partially collapsed. As flow increases, the cross-section becomes circular, viscous losses appear, and a pressure gradient develops. These principles apply to retrograde flow in the legs of patients with venous valvular incompetence and to the return of blood from the hand to the heart when the arm is elevated.

Uphill flow in a collapsible tube causes the tube to assume a circular cross-section. In this situation, viscous effects are operative and a pressure gradient is present. Therefore, flow up the leg in a person who is standing is determined by the dynamic pressure gradient.

Venous Valves and the Muscle Pump Mechanism

Return of blood to the heart is facilitated by venous valves and the muscle pump mechanism, which acts like a peripheral "heart." In fact, during strenuous exercise as much as 30% of the energy required to circulate blood may be furnished by the muscle pump (22). Of more importance to the circulation is the ability of the muscle pump to reduce peripheral venous volume and pressure in dependent portions of the legs. This in turn decreases the rate of edema formation. Failure of the muscle pump is ultimately responsible for the constellation of symptoms and signs that constitute the syndrome of chronic venous insufficiency.

The veins themselves constitute the "bellows" of the pump, and muscle contraction provides the force required to compress the bellows. By restricting retrograde flow, valves increase the efficiency of the pump. Although the basic structure of the pump is conceptually simple, the hemodynamic relationships between venous pressure, flow, volume, resistance, and compliance before, during, and after muscle contraction are complicated and are poorly understood—even in normal extremities. Concomitant fluctuations in arterial inflow and precapillary blood pressure add to the complexity. Furthermore, anatomic relationships between venous conduits, muscles, and the investing fascia vary at different levels of the leg, as does the influence of gravity. The measurements necessary to comprehend the dynamic interaction among these factors are difficult (or impossible) to obtain. Descriptions of the mechanism, therefore, must rely on observations made by many investigators using different methods, supplemented by experiments on models and assumptions based on physical principles.

Functional Anatomy. Both the superficial and deep veins are components of the muscle pump and are squeezed during muscle contraction. The superficial veins, however, are less directly affected since they lie outside the investing fascia and must be compressed against the skin. Lacking the extrinsic support that the deep veins have, they tend to have relatively thick muscular walls. Deep veins, which parallel arteries of the same name, are thin-walled and less muscular. As a rule, their cross-sectional area is roughly three times that of the adjacent artery (23). Large, thin-walled, spindle-shaped veins (sinusoids) lie within the calf muscles, where they constitute a major component of the bellows. These vessels are typically 5–10 cm long and have a diameter of 1.0 cm (24). The soleal sinusoids drain into the posterior tibial veins, and the gastrocnemius sinusoids usually empty into the popliteal veins. At various levels of the leg, veins "perforate" the fascia to connect the deep and superficial systems. These so-called perforating or communicating veins are more frequent in the calf than in the thigh. Of particular interest to the surgeon are the perforators located just above the ankle that connect the posterior tibial vein and a network of tributaries of the greater saphenous vein known as the posterior arch vein (25). The terminal segments of the greater and lesser saphenous veins, which drain into the common femoral and popliteal veins, respectively, represent the two largest perforators. In the region of the adductor canal, a large perforating vein (the Hunterian vein) connects the superficial femoral and greater saphenous veins.

Distributed at intervals in the veins of both systems are a series of delicate, but extremely strong, bicuspid valves. Each valve lies at the base of a localized dilatation referred to as a sinus (Fig. 2.11). This arrangement permits the valves to open widely without coming in contact with the venous wall and allows closure to occur rapidly (usually within 0.5 seconds) when flow begins to reverse (26, 27). (Reversed flow velocities in excess of 30 cm/sec may be necessary for complete closure of the valves to occur [28].) Valves are numerous and closely spaced in the distal portions of the leg, where the hydrostatic pressure is greatest when the subject stands, and are few and widely spaced in the more proximal parts of the leg, where the hydrostatic pressure is less. The posterior tibial vein contains roughly 9 to 19 valves; the anterior tibial, 9 to 11; and the peroneal, about 7. There is usually one valve in the popliteal and three in the superficial femoral vein. In

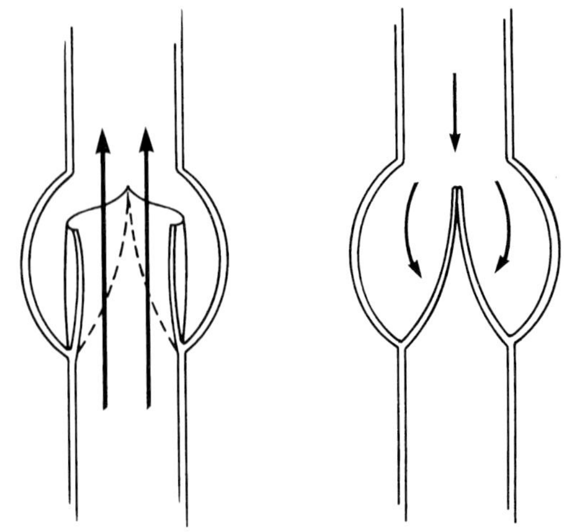

FIG. 2–11. Longitudinal section through a venous valve illustrating the role of the valve sinus in facilitating rapid closure of the valve cusps. (Reproduced by permission from Sumner DS. Applied physiology in venous problems. In: Bergan JJ, Yao JST, eds. Surgery of the veins. Orlando, FL: Grune & Stratton, 1985:3–23.)

two-thirds of the common femoral veins, a valve is present at the upper end. Only one-fourth of the external iliac veins and one-tenth of the hypogastric veins have a valve. Valves are rare in the common iliac veins. As a rule, valves are less frequent in the superficial veins than at comparable levels in the deep veins. The greater and lesser saphenous veins contain about 7 to 9 valves. In tributary veins, a valve is usually located just proximal to the junction with a larger venous conduit. Valves are found in veins of all sizes, including venules with diameters as small as 0.15 mm (23).

Valves in the deep and superficial veins are oriented to direct flow centrally toward the heart. Although it is generally taught that valves in normal perforating veins permit blood to flow only from the superficial to the deep system, recent studies suggest that flow in the opposite direction can occur in about one-fifth of normal limbs under certain conditions (29). There is also some controversy regarding the orientation of valves in perforating veins of the foot. The conclusion reached by earlier investigators that these veins carry blood from the deep to the superficial system has been challenged by more recent studies (30).

Physiology of the Muscle Pump. In a quietly standing motionless subject, veins are passive conduits, simply collecting blood from the capillaries and transporting it to the heart. Under these conditions, the energy required to overcome the resistance to fluid flow is supplied totally by the left ventricle. Because valves at all levels are open, there is an uninterrupted column of blood extending from the leg to the right atrium. At any given level, the venous pressure equals the sum of the hydrostatic and dynamic pressure (Fig. 2.1). Thus, the total venous pressure at the ankle exceeds that at the groin by the difference in hydrostatic and dynamic pressure. Because the dynamic pressure gradient is ordinarily low (a few millimeters of mercury), the pressure differences are largely a function of the hydrostatic component.

Effect of Muscle Contraction. With calf muscle contraction, pressure in the muscular compartments rises sharply, reaching 40–200 mmHg (31–33). Venous transmural pressure is reduced in proportion to the rise in extravascular pressure (Fig. 2.12). As dictated by the venous volume/transmural pressure compliance curve (Fig. 2.2), blood is displaced from the venous segment and the calf venous volume decreases. (Thus, it is not necessary for muscle pressures to exceed intravenous pressures in order to pump blood.) Retrograde flow is prevented by closure of valves located below the site of venous compression; but even in the absence of functioning valves, there would be little retrograde flow owing to the high resistance imposed by the microvascular bed. Antegrade flow, on the other hand, is impeded only by the resistance of the proximal venous segment, the inertia of the blood, and the downward force exerted by pressure in the central veins—all of which are relatively low in normal subjects. These impediments to venous outflow are, however, sufficient to raise intravenous pressure transiently (34). The total quantity of blood ejected during muscle contraction depends on the rate at which muscle tension develops, the ultimate strength of the contrac-

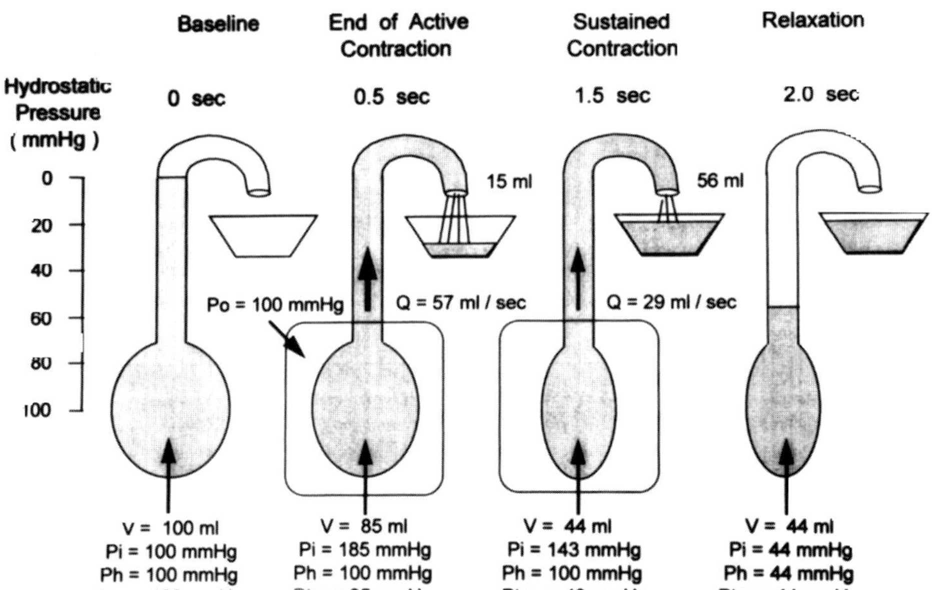

FIG. 2–12. Computer model of the calf venous pump mechanism. Calf veins are represented by an ellipsoidal collapsible container with a compliance of 1.0 ml/mmHg. The outflow tube has a resistance of 1.5 mmHg/ml/sec. Pressure developed by calf muscles during contraction (100 mmHg) is represented by the closed container. Transmural pressure (Ptm) is the difference between the pressure in the calf veins (Pi) and that of the surrounding muscles (Po), which is zero at baseline and during relaxation. Gravitational potential energy (Eg) (not shown), which is 100 mmHg greater at the top of the tube than it is at the bottom, cancels the hydrostatic pressure (Ph) at baseline and during muscle contraction. During calf muscle contraction, blood is propelled upward by the interaction between the decreasing transmural pressure and the venous compliance. Pi is elevated above Ph by the product of flow (Q) and the venous outflow resistance (R). Upon relaxation, calf vein pressure is reduced consistent with the residual volume of blood. Arterial inflow is assumed to be zero.

tion (i.e., the maximum increase in intramuscular pressure), the duration of contraction, and the outflow impedance. In normal limbs, ejection volumes average 90 ml and the ejection fraction (EF) usually exceeds 60% of the volume of blood that accumulated in the calf during quiet standing (35–37).

During sustained muscle contraction, antegrade flow decreases rapidly as intravenous pressure returns to precontraction levels, transmural pressure remains low, and the veins remain in a state of partial or complete collapse (Fig. 2.12).

When the muscles relax, pressure in the volume-depleted veins falls precipitously, again in accordance with the venous volume/transmural pressure compliance curve (Fig. 2.12). Although this produces an energy differential conducive to retrograde flow, little blood traverses the venous valves before they close. Because valves are arranged in tandem, the column of blood is no longer continuous from the periphery to the heart but is, in effect, segregated into shorter columns delimited by valve closure at the upper and lower ends. Unless the veins have been completely evacuated by muscle contraction, these segments are not defined by an area of collapse and, except for some reduction in diameter, the phlebographic appearance is not perceptually different from that seen when the veins are completely filled. The pressure, however, in these volume-depleted segments is reduced (38). Hydrostatic pressure at the bottom of each segment is equivalent to the length of the hydrostatic column; but at the top, just below the site of valve closure, it is effectively zero. Thus, static filling pressure, which depends on venous volume and compliance of the venous wall, is slightly greater at the bottom of the segment than at the top. As long as the top of the venous segment is not completely collapsed, the pressure at the bottom is greater than the hydrostatic pressure defined by the length of the subtended venous segment and exceeds that at the top of the segment immediately below (38). In other words, immediately after cessation of muscle contraction, the pressure above each valve is somewhat higher than that below (Fig. 2.13).

Within each segment, venous pressure gradually rises as the veins are refilled by arterial inflow and by flow up the leg from veins located distal to the area of compression (39). Once the pressure below a valve rises to exceed that immediately above the valve, the valve opens and blood again flows cephalad (Fig. 2.13). Although this immediately extends the length of the hydrostatic column to the next site of valve closure (or perhaps even to the heart if all proximal valves have reopened), there are no sudden jumps in total pressure during venous refilling (38). In normal limbs, refilling requires about 18–40 seconds (35, 40, 41).

Because pressure in the superficial veins ordinarily exceeds that in the deep veins at the same level, there is usually some flow from the superficial to the deep system through perforating veins during the refilling process (22, 39). The difference in pressure may be in part related to the relatively longer length of the venous segments in the superficial compared to the deep system, where valves are more closely spaced. In normal limbs, the quantity of inward flow is relatively small, since the caliber of the perforating veins is far less (1.0 mm) than that of the superficial veins (5.0 mm). These events are summarized in Figure 2.14.

Repeated Contractions. If, as in normal walking, muscle contraction is repeated before refilling is completed, the veins remain in a state of partial collapse. With each subsequent contraction, an additional bolus of blood is propelled centrally and the venous volume decreases until the volume of blood replenished by

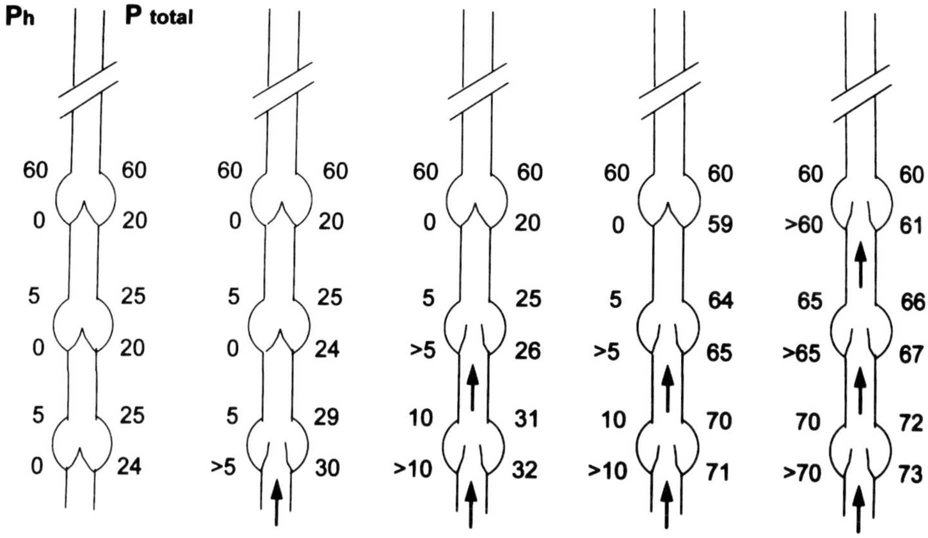

FIG. 2–13. Sequential refilling of calf veins during the relaxation phase following muscle contraction. Model assumes refilling from arterial inflow coming from below only. Hydrostatic pressures (Ph, mmHg), which are shown to the *left* of each figure, are determined by the lengths of the segregated blood columns between closed valves. Total venous pressures (P total, mmHg), which are shown on the *right*, depend on the hydrostatic pressure and also on the pressure developed due to the interaction between venous compliance and the amount of blood in each segment. Pressures are shown just above and below each valve. Valves remain closed until the pressure below exceeds that above. Thus, pressures measured at any point rise gradually throughout the refilling process.

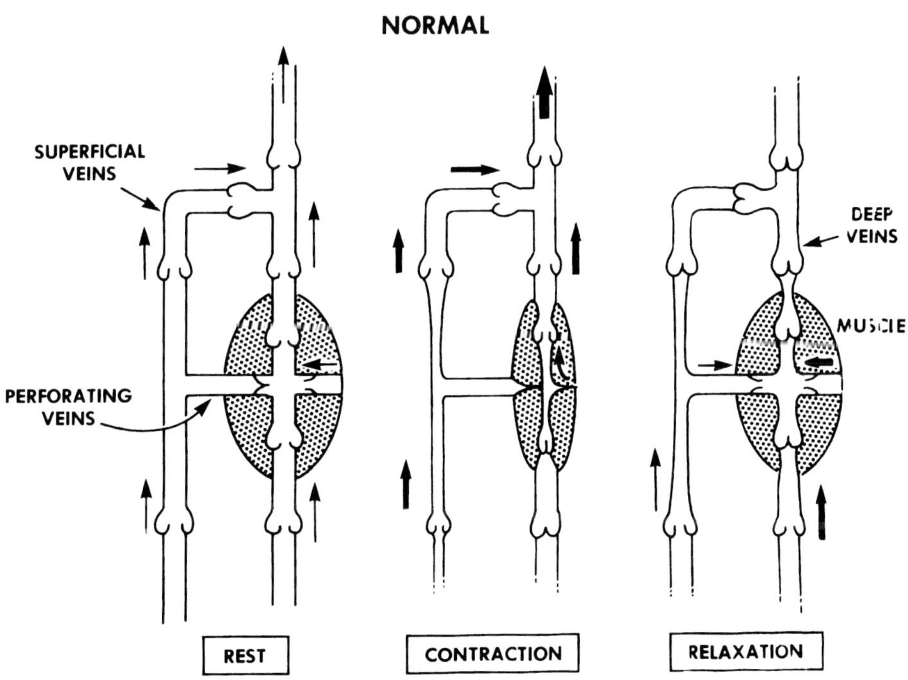

FIG. 2–14. Venous blood flow patterns in a normal limb before, during, and after calf muscle contraction. (Reproduced by permission from Sumner DS. Venous dynamics—varicosities. Clin Obstet Gynecol 1981;24:743.)

the increased arterial inflow equals that ejected with each contraction. The volume of blood remaining in the limb once a steady state is reached (the residual volume, RF) is usually less than 30% of that present prior to exercise (37). (This ratio is known as the residual volume fraction or RVF.) Because transmural venous pressure is a function of venous volume and compliance, RVF and venous pressure are correlated (37). Ambulatory venous pressure (the lowest steady-state pressure measured during or just after exercise) is ordinarily 15–30 mmHg in normal limbs and may reach values as low as 5 mmHg (Fig. 2.15) (22, 42, 43).

Compression of the plantar veins discharges blood into the deep veins of the calf and may initiate the pumping process (30). During normal walking, the events are synchronized in the following order: first, dorsiflexion of the foot empties the distal calf veins; then weight-bearing empties the foot; and finally, plantar flexion empties the proximal calf veins (44). Blood transmitted to the thigh is accelerated further during thigh muscle contraction (32).

Arterial inflow is increased by two mechanisms. First, arterioles in the exercising muscle dilate in response to the accumulation of metabolites, thereby reducing the resistance of the microvascular bed. Second, the reduction in venous pressure increases the arterial-venous pressure gradient across the interposed arterioles and capillaries. Gravity assists in this process, since the arterial pressure at any level is the sum of the dynamic pressure produced by contraction of the left ventricle and the hydrostatic pressure, which is determined by the vertical distance between the arteries and the heart (Fig. 2.1). Unlike the venous pressure, arterial pressure remains fairly constant and is not reduced by calf muscle contraction. In fact, there is usually some increase in systemic arterial pressure, which acts in turn to further increase the pressure gradient across the capillary bed.

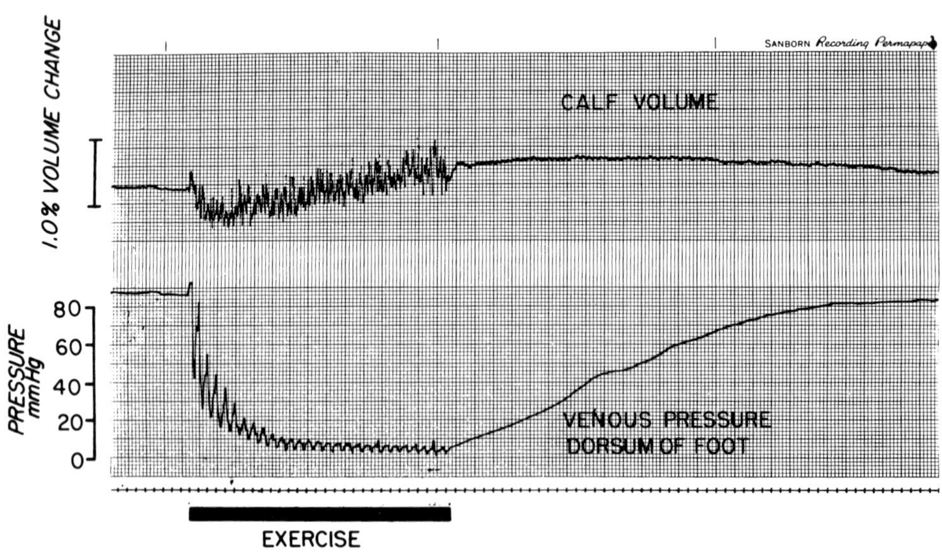

FIG. 2–15. Venous pressure response to treadmill exercise at foot level in a normal subject 5 feet 8 inches tall. (Reproduced by permission from Strandness DE Jr, Sumner DS. Hemodynamics for surgeons. New York: Grune & Stratton, 1975:138–139.)

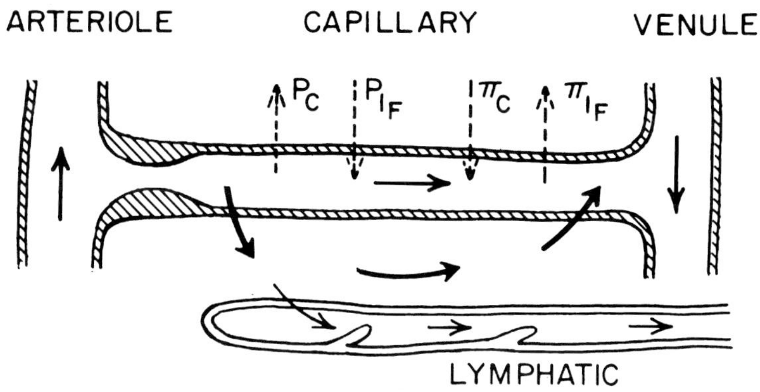

Pressures (mm. Hg)

	Arteriolar	Mean capillary	Venular
P_C	35	25	15
P_{IF}	5	5	5
π_C	25	25	25
π_{IF}	5	5	5
P	+10	0	−10

FIG. 2–16. Starling hypothesis: dynamics of fluid exchange in the capillary bed. *Solid arrows* indicate direction of fluid and blood flow; *dashed arrows* show direction of pressure gradients. (Reproduced by permission from Strandness DE Jr, Sumner DS. Hemodynamics for surgeons. New York: Grune & Stratton, 1975:112.)

Importance of Orthostatic Venous Pressure Reduction. Aside from augmenting the pressure gradient across the capillary bed, ambulatory venous pressure reduction markedly decreases venous congestion in the dependent limb. By translocating blood from peripheral to central veins, the muscle pump serves to enhance cardiac output. Moreover, because blood pressure in the capillaries must exceed that in the venules, decreasing venous pressure slows the rate of edema formation.

According to the Starling concept, most of the fluid leaving the arteriolar end of a capillary (where the intravascular pressure is relatively high) returns to the circulation at the venular end (where the pressure is relatively low) (45, 46). Excess fluid is removed by lymphatics (Fig. 2.16). Fluid is driven from the capillary by intracapillary pressure (P_c) and by the osmotic pressure of the interstitial fluid (π_{IF}) and is returned by forces exerted by the interstitial fluid pressure (P_{IF}) and the osmotic pressure of the blood (π_c). The net pressure (P) forcing fluid out of the capillary is:

$$P = P_c + \pi_{IF} - P_{IF} - \pi_c \qquad (10)$$

In the supine position, mean intracapillary blood pressure (P_c) is exactly balanced by the sum of the other pressures (Fig. 2.16), and little fluid is lost to the surrounding tissues. The equilibrium, however, is disturbed in dependent parts of the leg in the standing position. Capillary pressure at all levels is increased in proportion to the corresponding hydrostatic pressure. For example, at ankle level, the mean capillary pressure increase might approach or exceed 100 mmHg in a 6-foot tall subject (Fig. 2.1). Under the influence of the elevated pressure gradient, fluid escapes from the capillaries until tissue pressure (P_{IF}) rises sufficiently to restore the equilibrium (46). The rate of fluid transfer depends on capillary surface area and permeability and on the compliance of the surrounding tissues.

In limbs with normal venous valvular function, the marked reduction in venous pressure that accompanies ordinary calf muscle activity is sufficient to minimize interstitial fluid accumulation.

HEMODYNAMICS OF VENOUS DISEASE

The pathophysiologic effects of venous disease are not only attributable to vascular obstruction but are also the result of valvular incompetence. Thus, there are no arterial counterparts to many of the functional aberrations associated with venous disorders.

Venous Valvular Incompetence and Failure of the Muscle Pump Mechanism

Failure of the venous valve cusps to coapt properly allows blood to reflux down the veins in a retrograde fashion when the peripheral to central fluid energy gradient is reversed. This can occur in response to a Valsalva maneuver or in response to any abrupt increase in intra-abdominal pressure. Reversed flow detected during a Valsalva maneuver by Doppler interrogation of the common femoral vein in a supine patient identifies incompetence of the iliac and proximal femoral veins. Reflux continues down the leg until the first competent valve is encountered. Below this level, venous valvular incompetence cannot be assessed by the Valsalva maneuver. In patients in whom all proximal and distal valves are incompetent, however, the Valsalva maneuver may produce reversed flow to the posterior tibial vein at the ankle.

When a person shifts from a supine to a standing position, the gravitational potential energy in the abdominal and pelvic veins increases relative to that in the distal part of the legs. In the absence of functioning valves, blood essentially falls downward until the pressure in the dependent veins rises sufficiently to neutralize the energy gradient (Fig. 2.17). At any level, venous compliance dictates the volume of blood that must accumulate before the sum of the venous pressure and gravitational energy is equivalent to that in the veins immediately above. The rapidity with which the calf veins fill (venous filling time) is a measure of the severity of valvular incompetence and is a key element in the assessment of chronic venous insufficiency by the air plethysmographic technique (37, 47, 48). In severely incompetent limbs, filling may occur in only a few seconds. On the other hand, the actual volume increase after a period of quiet standing is determined by venous compliance and typically is larger in limbs with varicose veins than in normal limbs (37).

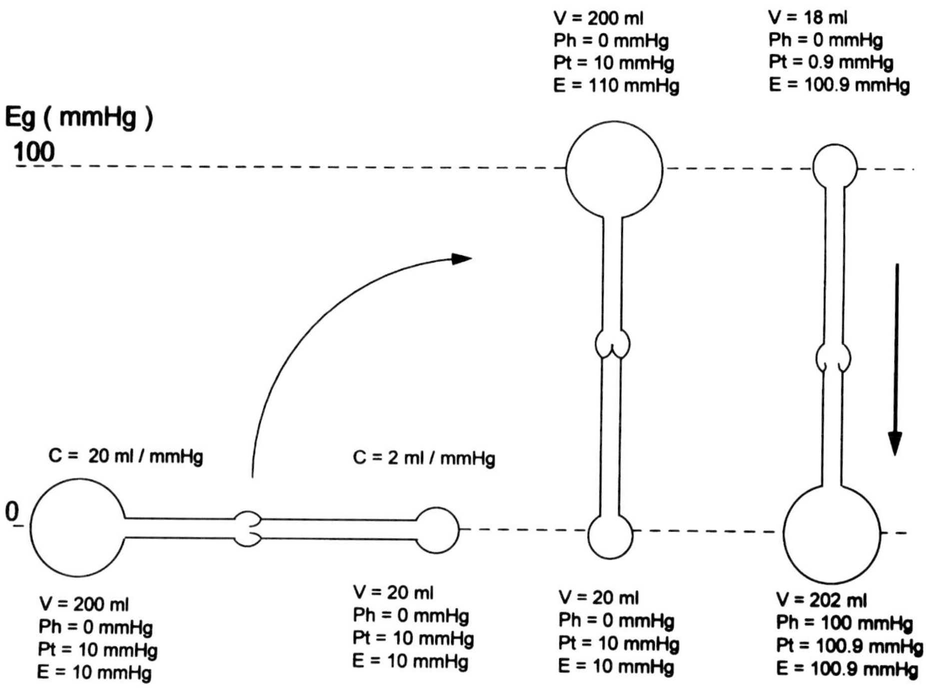

FIG. 2–17. Model illustrating mechanism of reflux flow that occurs when a person shifts from a horizontal to a vertical position. Two spherical balloons are connected by a rigid tube containing a valve. In the middle panel, reflux flow is prohibited by valve closure despite a total energy gradient of 100 mmHg. The incompetent valve in the right hand panel permits reflux flow to occur until the energy gradient is erased. *V* = volume of fluid in balloons; *C* = compliance of the balloons; *Ph* = hydrostatic pressure at center of the balloons; *Pt* = total pressure in the balloons; and *E* = the total fluid energy (Pt + Eg).

Of more importance, however, is the reversal of the energy gradient that develops during the relaxation phase following muscle contraction. In limbs with valvular incompetence, calf muscle contraction forces blood up the leg, just as it does in normal limbs (Fig. 2.12). For reasons that are not entirely understood, the volume of blood displaced with a single contraction (the ejection fraction) in limbs with chronic venous insufficiency is less than that displaced in normal limbs (37). (Possible explanations include stiffer, less compliant venous bellows; a shift of the venous volume to the more superficial veins in which compression is less efficient; edema; residual venous obstruction; and impaired muscle function [49].) At any rate, the dependent veins are at least partially depleted of blood after muscle contraction and the venous pressure is reduced, albeit to a lesser extent than that observed in normal limbs at the same anatomic level. Because gravitational potential energy remains relatively constant during exercise as long as the upright position is maintained, the total fluid energy in the distal veins is reduced while that in the proximal veins is unaffected, allowing blood in the proximal venous reservoirs to fall down the leg unimpeded by functioning valves. As a result, once the muscles relax, venous pressure and venous volume rapidly rise toward precontraction levels (35, 40).

If muscle contraction is repeated before the distal veins are completely refilled by reflux flow or by inflow from the arterial system, an additional (but smaller) increment of blood is forced cephalad. After several successive contractions, an asymptote is reached and the distal venous volume and pressure remain essentially constant as long as exercise is continued. The quantity of blood remaining in the distal veins (residual volume) and the blood pressure in these veins (ambulatory venous pressure) after cessation of walking or tip-toe exercise is typically greater in limbs with chronic venous insufficiency than in normal limbs (Fig. 2.18) (35, 37, 40, 48). When valvular incompetence is extensive, there may be little reduction in venous volume or venous pressure. As in the case of a single muscle contraction, the dependent veins refill rapidly once the exercise is terminated (41).

Thus, unlike normal limbs in which the calf muscle pump protects the distal tissues from the adverse effects of hydrostatic pressure, limbs with chronic venous insufficiency are constantly subjected to venous congestion and an elevated venous pressure (as long as the upright position is maintained). This leads to elongation and dilatation of the cutaneous and subcutaneous capillaries and venules (50–52). Because capillary pressure must exceed venous pressure, the Starling

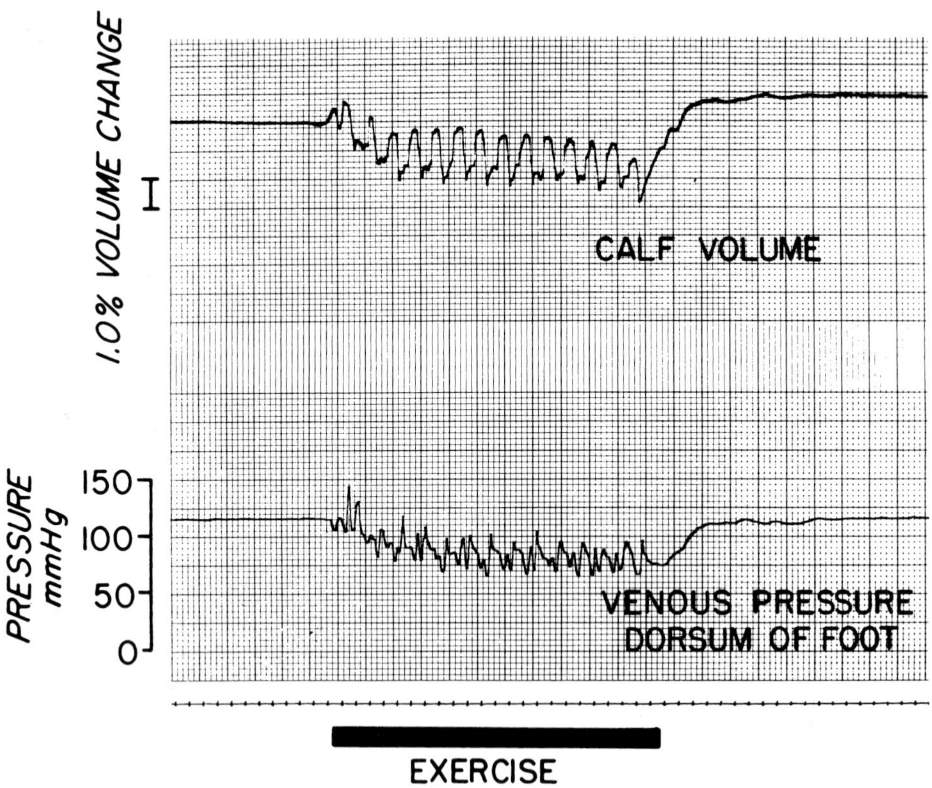

FIG. 2–18. Effect of exercise on calf volume and foot venous pressure in a patient with chronic venous insufficiency. (Reproduced by permission from Strandness DE Jr, Sumner DS. Hemodynamics for surgeons. New York: Grune & Stratton, 1975:397.)

TABLE 2-1

INCIDENCE OF ULCERATION IN LIMBS WITH CHRONIC VENOUS INSUFFICIENCY; RELATIONSHIP TO AMBULATORY VENOUS PRESSURE*

Pressure (mmHg)	Limbs with ulcer (%)
<30	0
31–40	11
41–50	22
51–60	38
61–70	59
71–80	68
>80	73

*Adapted from Nicolaides AN, Hussein MK, Szendro G, et al. The relation of venous ulceration with ambulatory venous pressure measurements. J Vasc Surg 1973;17:414–419.

equilibrium is upset, allowing a net transfer of fluid from the intravascular to the extravascular compartments (raising the interstitial fluid pressure) (1). Edema, therefore, is the initial clinical manifestation of chronic venous insufficiency. With time, leakage of protein and red-blood cells instigates changes in the surrounding tissues that eventually result in hyperpigmentation, lipodermatosclerosis, and ulceration (52–54). Although these changes occur on the microvascular and molecular levels and involve white blood cells, cytokines, fibrin deposition, and other incompletely understood mechanisms that are the subject of intense investigation, all changes are ultimately attributable to venous hypertension (55–58). Although ulcers may occur in limbs with little or no elevation of the ambulatory venous pressure (48, 59, 60), in general there is a fairly close correlation between the incidence of ulcers and postexercise venous hypertension (Table 2.1) (61).

Varicose Veins. In patients with simple, primary varicose veins, valvular incompetence is predominantly confined to the superficial system. The entire greater saphenous vein may be involved or only the above- or below-knee segments. Incompetence of the lesser saphenous vein may be isolated or coexist with incompetence of the greater saphenous vein.

As described earlier, varicose veins, when compressed during calf muscle contraction, propel blood cephalad, albeit not as efficiently as do normal superficial veins. During the relaxation phase between muscle contractions, blood refluxes down the leg, rapidly restoring the length of the hydrostatic column (which in the case of patients in whom the entire greater saphenous vein is involved extends from the ankle to the heart) (62, 63). Because the postcontraction pressure in normally valved deep veins is markedly reduced, a pressure gradient develops causing blood to flow from the superficial to the deep system through perforating veins located in the distal part of the leg. As a result, a "private circulation" or circular movement of blood is established in the exercising leg (Fig. 2.19) (62, 64–66). Part of the blood pumped from the deep veins of the calf reverses direction upon reaching the common femoral vein and flows down the function-

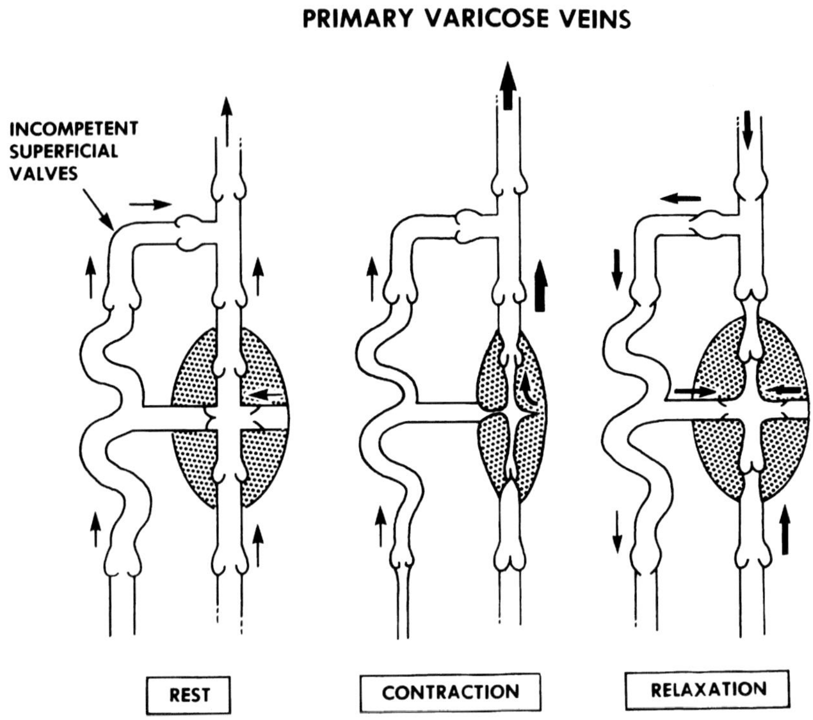

FIG. 2–19. Venous blood flow patterns in a limb with primary varicose veins, before, during, and after calf muscle contraction. (Reproduced by permission from Sumner DS. Venous dynamics—varicosities. Clin Obstet Gynecol 1981;24:743.)

ally valveless saphenous vein to the lower part of the leg, where it reenters the deep system, thus completing the parasitic circuit.

Although exercise tolerance does not appear to be adversely affected by the circular blood flow pattern (52), reflux flow (together with the elevated ambulatory pressure) contributes to the progressive distension and elongation of tributary veins, producing unsightly varicosities (67). Edema, heaviness, and tightness of the leg, symptoms often experienced by patients with varicose veins, are attributable to the elevated venous pressure. Interestingly, many patients with longstanding massive varicosities have no symptoms; in others, small, scattered varicosities are symptomatic.

Compressing varicose veins manually or with a tourniquet prevents reflux flow during exercise and allows the muscle pump to return ambulatory venous pressure to near normal levels, provided the deep system is competent (64, 68). Normalization of the plethysmographically measured venous filling time by the application of a tourniquet distinguishes superficial from deep venous incompetence and identifies those limbs that are likely to benefit most from high ligation and stripping of varicose veins.

Deep Venous Incompetence. Following an episode of acute deep venous thrombosis (DVT), venous valves may become incompetent as a result of valve destruction or fibrotic distortion that occurs during the process of clot shrinkage, organization, and lysis (69–72). Incompetence may be detected as early as 7 days, but is more likely to occur in veins in which the process of resolution is prolonged (73, 74). Through mechanisms that are not entirely clear, major deep venous segments not directly involved with clot may also become incompetent (75). Additionally, preexisting collateral veins distend to accommodate flow diverted from partially or completely obstructed axial veins; as a result, valves in these veins fail to coapt properly and become incompetent. When incompetent collaterals are located in the superficial tissues, they are often referred to as "secondary varicose veins."

About two-thirds of patients with deep venous incompetence don't recall having had DVT (76–78). Moreover, there may be no phlebographic or duplex scan evidence of a previous thrombosis. In such cases, venous valvular incompetence or the predisposition to develop incompetence may have been present since birth. In other cases, a subclinical episode of DVT may be responsible.

As a rule, the calf muscle pump mechanism is less efficient in limbs with deep venous reflux than in limbs with varicose veins (79). The ejection fraction is lower and the residual venous volume and ambulatory venous pressure are even higher than in patients with primary varicose veins. During exercise, venous pressure may actually rise due to the higher outflow resistance imposed by partially or completely obstructed proximal veins (80–83). When valves located below the major calf muscle mass are incompetent, blood may be propelled retrograde into the distal leg during the contraction phase (Fig. 2.20). Additionally, blood from the deep system may be forced into the superficial system through incompetent perforating veins, temporarily raising pressure in the cutaneous capillaries (80). This, in part, may be responsible for the predilection of ulcers to develop in the region just above the medial malleolus, where several prominent perforators are located (84). When superficial venous incompetence is also present, the circular blood flow pattern described under "Varicose Veins" may be present and may contribute to the inefficiency of the muscle pump.

Location of Incompetent Valves. Clinical and physiologic observations suggest that below-knee valves are functionally more important than those in the thigh, groin, or pelvis (43, 64, 65, 85). As discussed earlier, venous valves are much more numerous and closely spaced in the infrapopliteal veins than in the veins above the knee. From a teleologic point of view, valves are strategically placed to ameliorate the effects of hydrostatic pressure and to facilitate the action of the calf muscle pump mechanism.

Reflux detected in the common femoral vein by Doppler examination is found in about 15% of otherwise normal limbs (63, 86), and descending phlebography has repeatedly confirmed the benign nature of reflux to the level of the knee (87). On the other hand, many investigators using plethysmographic tests and ambulatory venous pressure measurements have shown that peripheral venous refilling times and postexercise pressures are more likely to be abnormal when popliteal or calf veins are incompetent than when incompetence is confined to the above-knee veins (88–94). Studies that have used directional Doppler flow detection or duplex scanning to identify the location of venous valvular incompetence in limbs with ulcers and lipodermatosclerosis have demonstrated that combined

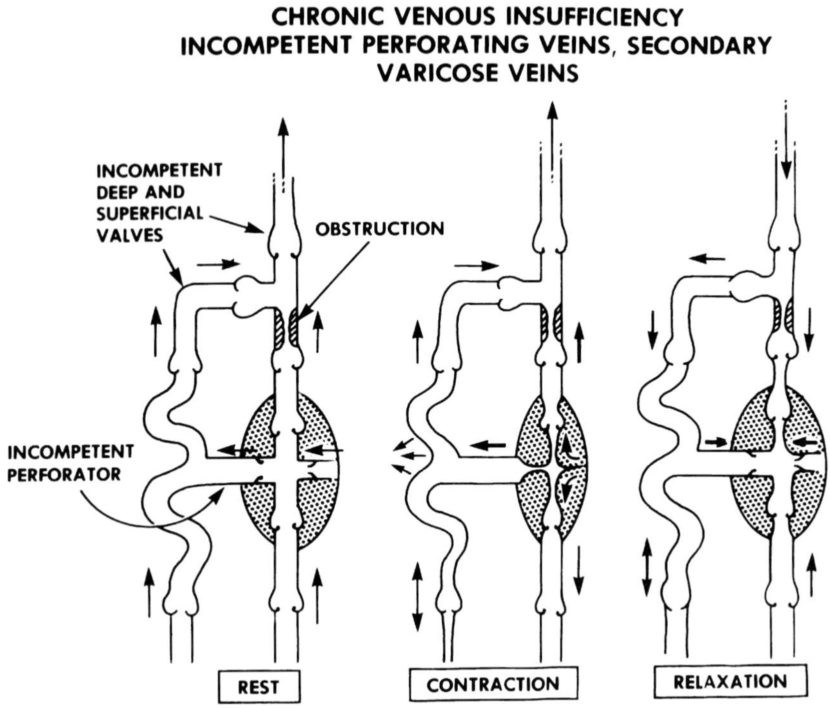

FIG. 2–20. Venous blood flow patterns in a limb with chronic deep venous insufficiency, secondary varicose veins, and incompetent perforating veins, before, during, and after calf muscle contraction. (Reproduced by permission from Sumner DS. Venous dynamics—varicosities. Clin Obstet Gynecol 1981;24:743.)

above-knee and below-knee incompetence is the most common pattern (Fig. 2.21) (76–78, 95). Isolated below-knee incompetence is less frequently observed, but most reports indicate that it is somewhat more frequent than isolated above-knee incompetence. The opposite is true in patients with less severe manifestations of chronic venous insufficiency (edema, venous flares) in whom incompetence isolated to the above-knee veins is more common than incompetence isolated to the calf veins. The reported incidence of popliteal and deep calf vein incompetence in limbs with stasis ulcers or lipodermatosclerosis (42–68%) is appreciably higher than that in less severely affected limbs (3–35%) (48, 77, 95, 96). Moreover, incompetence of the distal superficial veins (below-knee greater saphenous vein and lesser saphenous vein), either alone or in conjunction with above-knee greater saphenous venous incompetence, appears to be more strongly associated with ulcer development than incompetence limited to the proximal superficial veins (76, 78, 94, 96). In one study, only 4% of limbs with reflux confined to the above-knee saphenous veins exhibited skin changes and none had ulcers (93).

Although the importance of distal venous incompetence is generally accepted, the relative importance of superficial and deep venous incompetence remains controversial. Combined superficial and deep venous incompetence, the most common pattern, has been reported in 20–88% of legs with ulcers or lipodermatosclerosis (Table 2.2) (97, 98). In some studies, isolated superficial venous

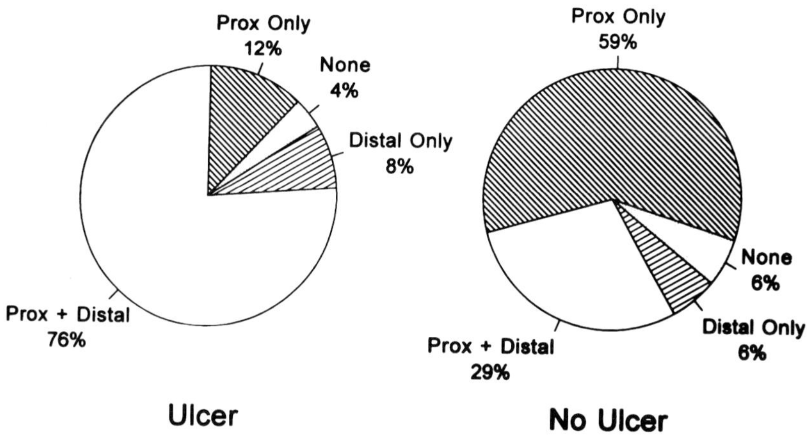

FIG. 2–21. Distribution of valvular incompetence in patients with venous ulcers and in patients with chronic venous disease but no ulcers. (Adapted from data reported by van Bemmelen PS, Bedford G, Beach K, Strandness DE Jr. Status of the valves in the superficial and deep venous system in chronic venous disease. Surgery 1991;109:730.)

TABLE 2-2

DISTRIBUTION OF VENOUS VALVE INCOMPETENCE IN LIMBS WITH ULCERS OR LIPODERMATOSCLEROSIS

Authors	Number of Limbs	SVI Only	SVI + DVI	DVI Only	Perf Only	None
Araki, et al. (1994) (98)	25*	0%	71%	20%	—	4%‡
Moore, et al. (1986) (77)	35	3%	69%	23%	—	6%
van Bemmelen, et al. (1991) (95)	25	4%	84%	8%	4%	0%
Neglén, Raju (1993) (48)	31	6%	65%	29%	0%	0%
Araki, et al. (1994) (98)	18†	6%	88%	6%	—	0%
Weingarten, et al. (1993) (99)	192	10%	42%	19%	—	20%
Hanrahan, et al. (1991) (78)	95	36%	43%§	6%§	8%	6%
Myers, et al. (1995) (96)	96	38%	48%	8%	2%	4%
Labropoulos, et al. (1995) (76)	112	44%	39%	11%	3%	4%
Lees, Lambert (1993) (100)	25	52%	44%	4%	0%	0%
Shami, et al. (1993) (101)	79	53%	32%	15%	0%	0%
van Rij, et al. (1994) (97)	120	70%	20%	8%	2%	<1%

*Active ulcers
†Healed ulcers
‡Authors' figures do not equal 100%
§Deep calf veins not studied
SVI = superficial venous insufficiency; DVI = deep venous insufficiency
Perf = incompetent perforating veins

incompetence was rarely observed (48, 77, 95, 98), but in others the majority of limbs demonstrated this pattern (Table 2.2) (97, 100, 101). Isolated deep venous incompetence is somewhat less frequently reported. On the other hand, reflux confined to the superficial veins is common in legs with minimal signs of chronic venous insufficiency (edema, venous flares), whereas isolated deep venous incompetence is relatively rare (48, 96, 100). Patients with massive varicose veins that have been present for many years often have normal skin and soft, pliable, subcutaneous tissues in the gaiter area. This alone is a strong argument against the theory that superficial venous incompetence alone is sufficient to cause stasis changes.

The location of stasis ulcers in the gaiter area of the leg suggests that incompetent perforating veins are implicated in the genesis of stasis ulcers, especially since skin breakdown is most common just above the medial malleolus where several large perforating veins communicate with the posterior arch veins. Although incompetent perforating veins are present in approximately two-thirds of limbs with stasis ulcers or lipodermatosclerosis, they are usually associated with incompetent superficial or deep veins (48, 76, 96, 100). Isolated perforator incompetence is rare in limbs with stasis changes (Table 2.2). Because it is difficult to disassociate the adverse effects of perforator incompetence from those of superficial and deep venous disease, the importance of perforator incompetence is debated. (In one study, no incompetent perforating veins were found in 46% of the ulcer beds that were examined [78].) Nonetheless, clinical observations generally support the therapeutic benefit of perforator ligation.

These observations, however, are difficult to interpret. Lacking are basic data concerning the incidence of various patterns of venous incompetence in the general population. For example, superficial venous incompetence is almost certainly far more common than deep venous incompetence; yet, the proportion of ulcerated limbs with superficial incompetence does not differ appreciably from the proportion with deep venous incompetence, suggesting that the odds for developing an ulcer are higher with deep venous disease than when incompetence is localized to the superficial system (Fig. 2.22). Although the hemodynamic aberrations associated with venous incompetence occur immediately, their clinical effect is gradual, and overt signs and symptoms may not become evident for several years. Thus, studies that attempt to correlate valve function with a given stage of chronic venous insufficiency are obtaining a "snapshot" of a dynamic process. They can only be interpreted as showing that virtually any pattern of venous incompetence can be present in any of the stages of chronic venous insufficiency (76). Longitudinal studies are needed to put the picture in the proper perspective.

Hypothetical Effects of Different Patterns of Venous Incompetence. Models that incorporate considerations discussed in this chapter can be used to predict the effect of various patterns of venous incompetence on ambulatory venous pressure (Fig. 2.23). These models assume that the postexercise pressure at the distal end of a partially evacuated venous segment is at least equal to the length of the hydrostatic column of blood subtended by functional valves at either end (90). In normal limbs, and in limbs with competent distal but incompetent proximal valves, postexercise venous pressures at the ankle are low because the segmented column of blood extends only to the first competent valve, which

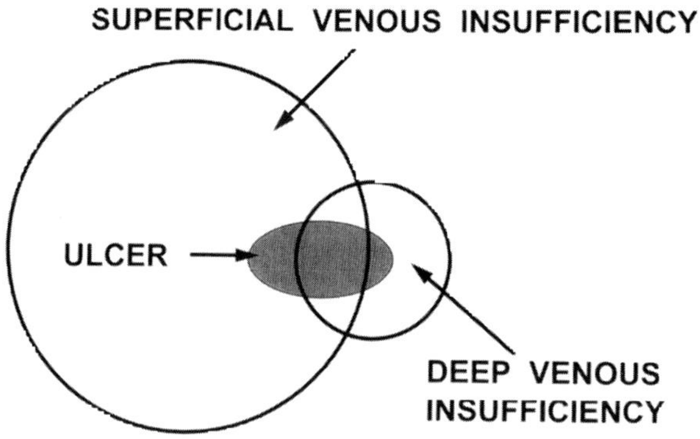

FIG. 2–22. Venn diagram correlating ulcer development with the relative prevalence of superficial and deep venous insufficiency.

is located well below the knee. When, however, the proximal valves are competent but the distal valves are incompetent, the postexercise column is relatively long, extending from the ankle to the mid or upper thigh. In this situation, ambulatory venous pressures are high. If perforating veins are also incompetent, the superficial system will refill rapidly, even when valves in this system are com-

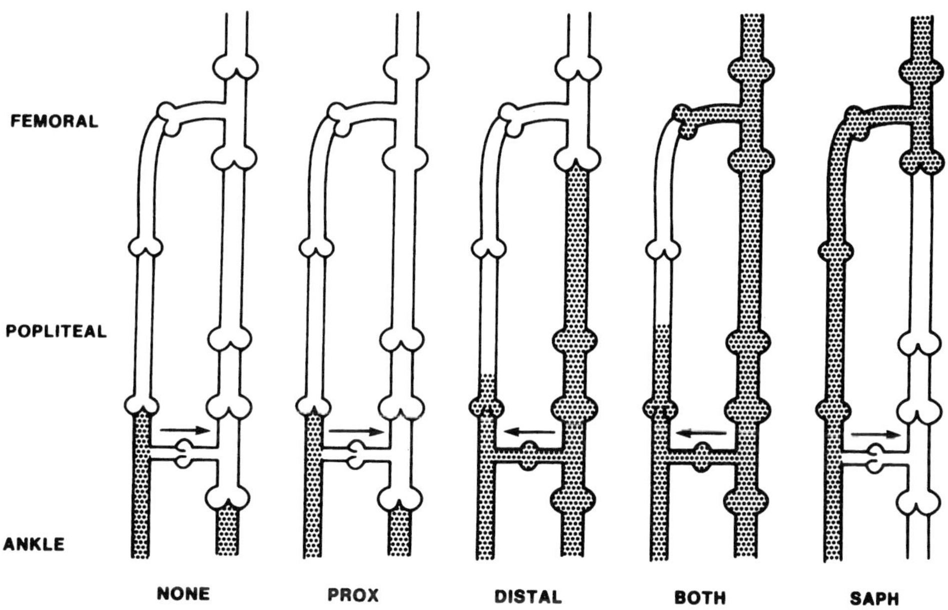

FIG. 2–23. Comparison of the length of the hydrostatic column of blood measured from the ankle (*stippled areas*) after exercise in limbs with no incompetent valves (*none*), incompetence limited to the proximal deep veins (*prox*), incompetence limited to the distal deep veins (*distal*), incompetence of both proximal and distal deep veins (*both*), and incompetence of the greater saphenous vein only (*saph*). Saphenous veins are on the left and deep veins on the right. *Arrows* indicate direction of flow in perforating veins. (Reproduced by permission from Gooley NA, Sumner DS. Relationship of venous reflux to the site of venous incompetence: implications for venous reconstructive surgery. J Vasc Surg 1988;7:50.)

petent. Incompetence of all valves in both above-knee and below-knee veins subjects the ankle veins to the entire weight of an uninterrupted column of blood extending to the heart. There is little reduction in ambulatory venous pressure, deep veins are rapidly refilled by reflux flow, and refilling of the superficial system via incompetent perforating veins is accelerated. In limbs with isolated superficial venous valvular incompetence extending the entire length of the saphenous system, ambulatory venous pressures are again high, but flow from the superficial veins through perforators into the competent deep system tends to ameliorate the pressure rise by hastening the evacuation of distended superficial veins. In the superficial system, ambulatory venous pressure is higher when distal valves are incompetent than when incompetence is isolated to the proximal saphenous vein (for the same reasons that are operative in the deep system).

Thus, these models predict that isolated deep venous incompetence should have a more adverse effect on postexercise hemodynamics than isolated superficial venous incompetence and that the combination of superficial and deep incompetence should be the most detrimental to venous function. They also predict that incompetence of both below-knee and above-knee valves is somewhat worse than below-knee incompetence alone and that isolated proximal venous incompetence may be compatible with near normal venous function.

Therapeutic Implications. When stasis ulcers, lipodermatosclerosis, and other manifestations of chronic venous insufficiency remain recalcitrant to conventional treatment (elevation, elastic stockings, Unna boots, etc.), operative therapy may be an attractive option. In those patients in whom valvular incompetence is isolated to the superficial system, ligation and stripping of the saphenous veins may be sufficient to reduce venous congestion and ambulatory venous pressure (36, 76, 78, 102, 103). Although stripping of incompetent superficial veins is occasionally beneficial in selected patients with combined deep and superficial incompetence, the hemodynamic defect is only partially corrected. Ligation of incompetent perforating veins has little effect on ambulatory venous hypertension but does prevent, at least theoretically, the transmission of high-pressure impulses to the subcutaneous capillaries.

When deep venous incompetence is the primary anatomic defect, restoration of valvular competence is appealing as a logical approach to correct the pathophysiologic abnormalities. Superficial femoral valvuloplasty and autotransplantation of a competent valve to the popliteal vein are among the operations that have been devised for this purpose. The rationale for these procedures is based on the premise that a single competent valve placed at or above the popliteal level in an otherwise incompetent system will reduce ambulatory venous hypertension. Despite generally favorable clinical results, hemodynamic abnormalities are seldom completely corrected (60, 104–108). The models discussed above provide a plausible explanation for this apparent contradiction (Fig. 2.23) (90, 95). Although a valve placed in the proximal superficial femoral vein interrupts the continuous column of blood to the heart, a long uninterrupted segment of blood remains above the ankle at the cessation of calf muscle contraction. A valve at the popliteal level further reduces the length of the hydrostatic column but not as efficiently as the multiple competent valves present in normal calf veins, which have the potential of segregating the column of blood into segments only a few centimeters long. Nonetheless, these operations may provide a margin of protection sufficient to permit ulcers to heal.

Venous Obstruction

Venous obstruction may be acute or chronic, partial or complete, localized or extensive, thrombotic or due to extrinsic compression. In patients with DVT, outflow resistance is increased in proportion to the extent of the thrombotic process (109, 110). Small, nonocclusive clots and clots confined to one of a pair of duplicated veins have little effect. Because the tibial veins are invariably paired and duplication of the superficial femoral and popliteal veins is not uncommon, these sites can be involved without raising venous resistance appreciably. Thrombi that occlude the orifices of major collateral veins elevate venous resistance more than those that are restricted to segments without large tributaries. (For example, a clot confined to the superficial femoral vein would have less effect on venous resistance than a clot in the common femoral vein that obstructs the junctions of the profunda femoris and greater saphenous veins.) Near-total occlusion of all the major deep veins in the leg and pelvis plus the superficial and deep venous collaterals produces a critical elevation of venous resistance and is responsible for the dread condition known as *phlegmasia cerulea dolens.*

With time, clots become firmly attached to the venous wall, some organize and remain totally occlusive, and others undergo partial or complete lysis (70, 73). Preexisting collateral channels dilate to accommodate flow diverted from completely or partially occluded major veins. Thus, after an episode of acute DVT, outflow resistance is at first rapidly and then more slowly reduced as the process enters the chronic phase. In many cases, venous resistance approaches that of a normal leg (81, 83, 111–115). Persistent obstruction, however mild, may have adverse pathophysiologic consequences, compounding the effects of venous valvular incompetence and restricting venous outflow during exercise.

Tumors, cysts, enlarged lymph nodes, hematomas, and other causes of extrinsic compression ordinarily affect only a small segment of the venous outflow; but when strategically located, they may result in an appreciable increase in venous resistance. In some patients, compression of the left iliac vein by the right iliac artery (May-Thurner syndrome) appears to be at least partially responsible for the development of DVT, which is proportionally more frequent in the left leg than the right.

Hemodynamics of Venous Obstruction. The hemodynamic effects of venous obstruction are all ultimately attributable to the increase in venous outflow resistance (R_v). Because venous outflow (Q_v) must equal arterial inflow (which is seldom affected by venous obstruction), and because the mean central venous pressure (P_{CV}) remains constant, venous pressure in the limb peripheral to the site of obstruction (P_{PV}) is increased in proportion to the outflow resistance (*cf.* eq. 7):

$$P_{PV} = R_V Q_V + P_{CV} \tag{11}$$

As a result of the increased venous pressure, distal limb veins become distended (eq. 3), dilated superficial veins may be clinically evident, and the limb takes on a bluish hue. Because blood pressure in the capillaries must exceed that in the venules and veins, the Starling equilibrium is upset, resulting in a net transfer of fluid from the capillary lumen to the surrounding tissues (Fig. 2.24). Thus, edema of some degree is a constant feature of acute and chronic venous obstruction (109). Edema fluid will continue to accumulate until tissue pressure rises sufficiently to restore the Starling equilibrium. It follows that the amount of edema reflects the elevation of capillary pressure, which, in turn, is proportional to the outflow resistance.

In limbs with phlegmasia cerulea dolens, the extremely high venous resistance leads to massive loss of fluid into the extravascular space and a correspondingly high tissue pressure (Fig. 2.25). Venous pressures may increase 16-fold within 6 hours (116); fluid loss may reach 6–10 liters within 5–10 days (117); and tissue pressures may rise to 48 mmHg within 1 or 2 days (116, 118). As the sum of the arterial, arteriolar, capillary, and venous resistance rises, arterial inflow is compromised. Ischemia of the distal limb occurs as a consequence of the elevated vascular resistance and the accompanying compression of resistance vessels (42, 118). Unless the major venous channels can be reopened promptly by surgical thrombectomy or by thrombolysis, the limb will succumb to venous gangrene.

Although residual venous obstruction is usually responsible for only a modest increase in the outflow resistance of postthrombotic limbs, the increase may ad-

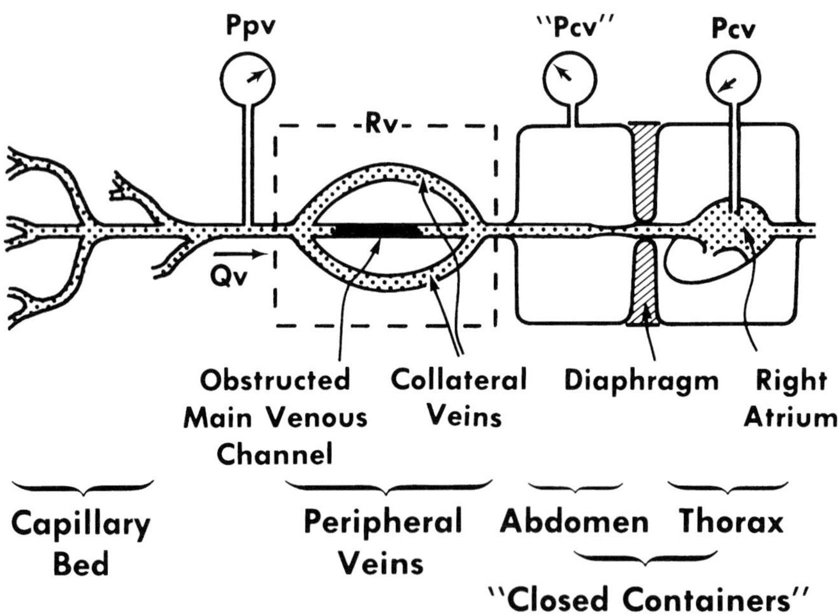

FIG. 2–24. Effect of venous obstruction on blood flow from the legs (*Qv*) and on peripheral venous pressure (*Ppv*). *Rv* represents the parallel resistances of the occluded venous segment and the collateral veins. *Pcv* is the central venous pressure and "*Pcv*" is the intra-abdominal pressure. (Reproduced by permission from Sumner DS. Hemodynamics and pathophysiology of venous disease. In: Rutherford RB, ed. Vascular surgery. 4th ed. Philadelphia: WB Saunders Co., 1995:1673–1695.)

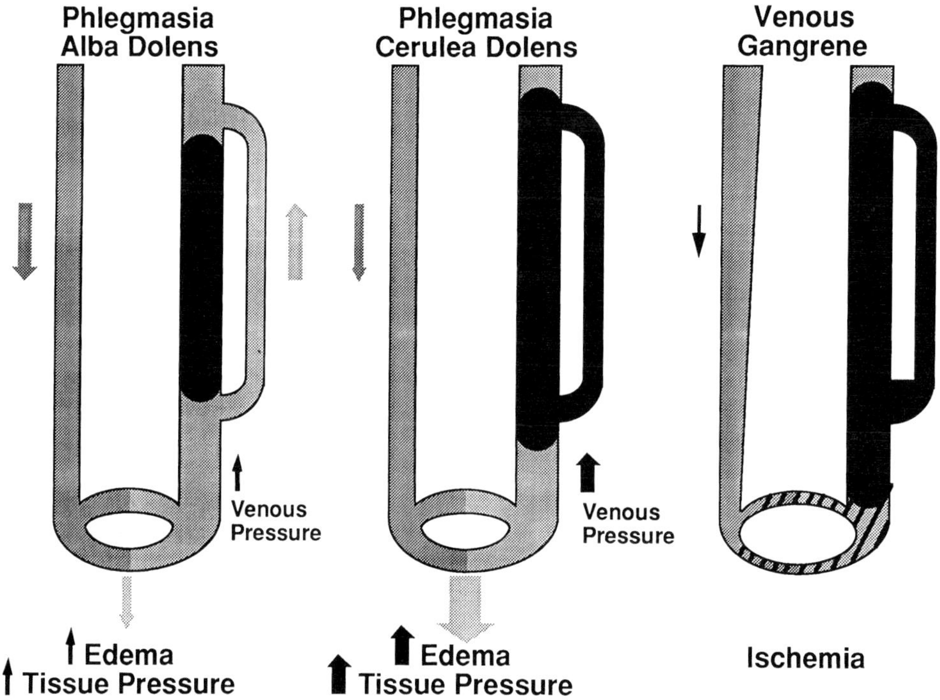

FIG. 2–25. Pathophysiology of increasingly severe venous obstruction. In each diagram, arterial inflow is shown on the *left* and venous outflow on the *right*. Location and extent of venous thrombosis is depicted in *black*. In phlegmasia alba dolens, clots are confined to the major deep veins; in phlegmasia cerulea dolens, collateral veins are also involved; and in venous gangrene, thrombosis extends to the small veins and capillaries. *Arrow size* indicates the relative magnitude of arterial and venous flow, venous and tissue pressure, and edema. (Reproduced by permission from Sumner DS. Hemodynamics and pathophysiology of venous disease. In: Rutherford RB, ed. Vascular surgery. 4th ed. Philadelphia: WB Saunders Co., 1995:1673–1695.)

versely affect calf muscle pump function. The quantity of blood forced out of the leg with each muscle contraction (Q_V) is inversely proportional to the venous resistance (eq. 12):

$$Q_V = \frac{P_{PV} - P_{CV}}{R_V} \qquad (12)$$

Thus, the ejection fraction will be reduced unless the pressure generated in the venous bellows (P_{PV}) by calf muscle contraction is increased sufficiently to compensate for the elevated outflow resistance. In most cases, there is a concomitant decrease in ejection fraction and an increase in ambulatory venous pressure (80–83). Pressure swings with calf muscle contraction and relaxation also tend to be exaggerated (82). These events further aggravate the effects of venous valvular incompetence, which is usually present as well. The combination of residual obstruction and valvular incompetence is especially frequent in limbs with stasis ulcers (48, 49, 72, 119).

Patients with chronic proximal venous obstruction may experience a deep "bursting-type" pain in the leg during exercise. This pain, which is often called "venous claudication," is caused by the increased venous pressure and congestion that occur in response to the combination of exercise-induced hyperemia and increased outflow resistance (120). Infrainguinal veins are often radiologically normal and valvular insufficiency is not a prominent feature. In these cases, claudication my be alleviated by a femoral-femoral venous bypass.

Implications for Noninvasive Testing. Because venous pressure peripheral to a clotted vein (P_{PV}) is elevated, the effect of central venous pressure fluctuations (P_{CV}) on the pressure gradient driving blood out of the leg ($P_{PV} - P_{CV}$) is reduced (Fig. 2.24). Consequently, respiratory variations characteristic of normal venous blood flow are minimized (in proportion to severity of the obstruction), and blood flow becomes less phasic and more continuous (eq. 12). Finding a "continuous" Doppler signal in a patent vein is, therefore, highly suggestive of a more centrally located venous obstruction and is an important feature to be noted in the course of noninvasive examinations (21, 121).

Plethysmographic tests for proximal (above-knee) venous obstruction depend on measurements of the rate at which blood flows out of the calf under the influence of a predetermined pressure gradient. In practice, a pneumatic cuff placed around the thigh of a supine patient is inflated to a standard pressure (40–60 mmHg), which exceeds that in the underlying veins but is less than that in the arteries. (This collapses the veins but has little effect on arterial inflow.) Venous outflow ceases and calf volume, which is recorded continuously with a plethysmograph (air, impedance, or mercury strain gauge), increases until the peripheral venous pressure rises to equal or exceed that in the cuff (Fig. 2.26). After a

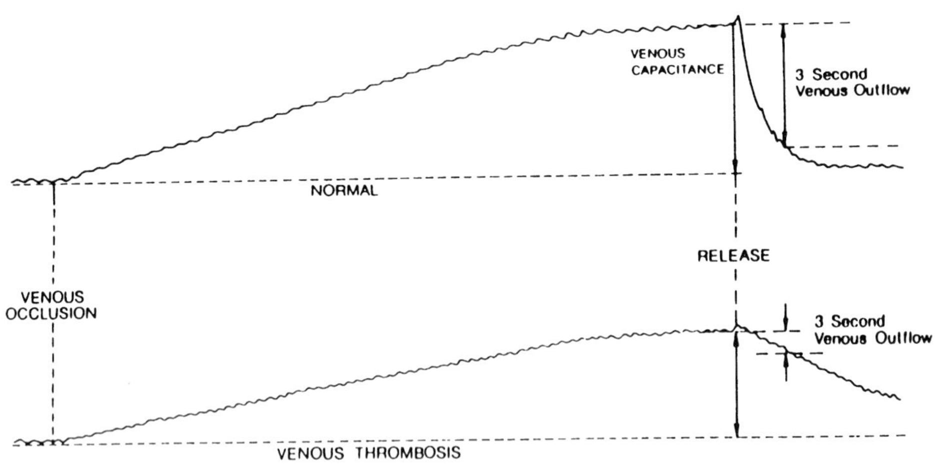

FIG. 2–26. Impedance plethysmographic tracings from a normal limb and a limb with proximal deep venous thrombosis. Three-second venous outflow is markedly reduced in the abnormal limb. (Reproduced by permission from Wheeler HB, Anderson FA Jr. Diagnosis of deep vein thrombosis by impedance plethysmography. In: Bernstein EF, ed. Vascular diagnosis. 4th ed. St. Louis: CV Mosby, 1993:820–829.)

stable calf volume is reached, the cuff is suddenly deflated, allowing blood trapped in the calf veins to flow out, propelled by a pressure gradient equivalent to the difference between the cuff pressure (P_{PV}) and the central venous pressure (P_{CV}). The initial rate at which blood flows out of the calf (the "maximum venous outflow" or MVO) is, therefore, inversely proportional to the venous resistance (eq. 12). In limbs with acute proximal DVT, MVO may be only one-third to one-fifth as great as in normal limbs (111–115).

Because the peripheral venous pressure (P_{PV}) in limbs with acute proximal DVT is usually elevated compared to that in normal limbs, the actual increase in calf venous pressure with cuff inflation is reduced. This, together with the reduced compliance of veins that are already partially distended, diminishes calf volume expansion. In normal legs, maximum calf volume expansion (also called "venous capacitance") averages about 2–4% of the baseline calf volume; but in legs with acute DVT, expansion may be restricted to only <0.5–2% of the baseline volume (112, 114).

MVO is often difficult to determine precisely because it requires accurate measurement of the initial slope of the calf volume curve at the point of cuff deflation. This has led to the use of timed venous outflow, defined as the volume decrease that occurs 2 or 3 seconds after cuff deflation (Fig. 2.26) (122, 123). Timed venous outflow, however, is not only a function of venous resistance but also depends on venous compliance, which—as pointed out earlier—is usually reduced in limbs with acute DVT. The venous outflow curve is steepest immediately after cuff release and becomes progressively more gradual as the calf venous pressure declines. As blood exits the calf, the rate at which venous pressure declines is determined by the venous compliance (C).

Analogous to the discharge of an electrical capacitor, timed venous outflow (ΔV_t) is directly proportional to the venous capacitance (V_o), provided that the venous resistance and compliance remain constant (42, 121, 124, 125):

$$\Delta V_t = V_o\left(1 - e^{\frac{t}{CR}}\right) \tag{13}$$

In this equation e represents the base of the natural logarithm and t is the time in seconds after cuff release. Thus, for a given V_o, ΔV_t decreases as the resistance and compliance increase. Because venous compliance increases as the venous pressure falls, equation 13 is only an approximation. Nonetheless, it emphasizes the need to consider venous capacitance when timed venous outflow is used to diagnose DVT and justifies the use of a discriminant line based on both parameters for separating normal limbs from those with DVT (Fig. 2.27) (122).

SUMMARY

Accurate diagnosis and effective treatment of venous disease depend on a basic understanding of normal venous physiology and the hemodynamic aberrations associated with venous obstruction and venous valvular incompetence. Although much has been learned, in many areas our knowledge remains inadequate. Few topics in medicine are more interesting or present a greater challenge for future research.

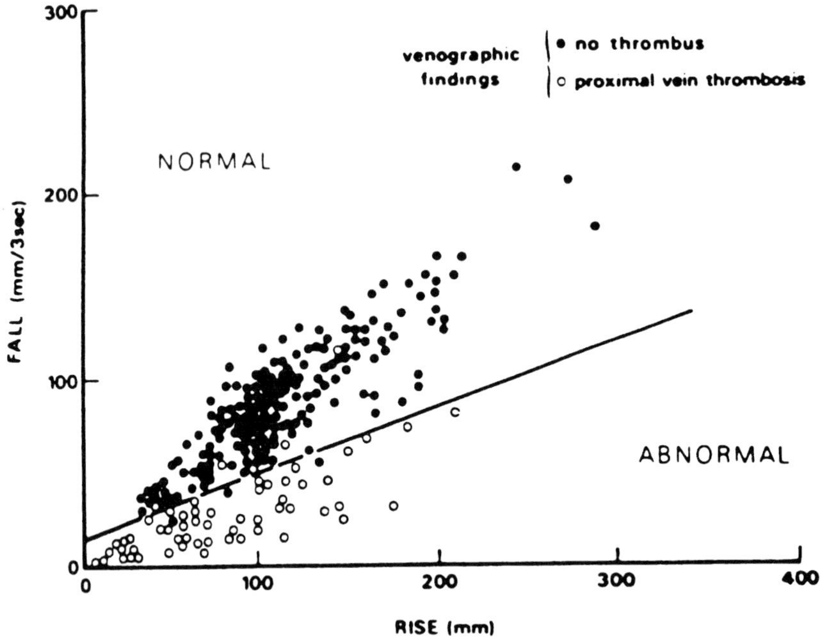

FIG. 2–27. Results of impedance plethysmography in patients with normal limbs and in patients with recent proximal deep venous thrombosis (*abnormal*). Three-second venous outflows (*fall*) are plotted as a function of the venous capacitance (*rise*). A discriminant line accurately divides normal from abnormal limbs. (Reproduced by permission from Hull R, van Aken WG, Hirsh J, et al. Impedance plethysmography using the occlusive cuff technique in the diagnosis of venous thrombosis. Circulation 1976;53:696.)

REFERENCES

1. Pflug JJ, Zubac DP, Kersten DR, Alexander NDE. The resting interstitial tissue pressure in primary varicose veins. J Vasc Surg 1990;11:411.
2. Moreno AH, Katz AI, Gold LD, Reddy RV. Mechanics of distension of dog veins and other thin walled tubular structures. Circ Res 1970;27:1069.
3. Caro CG, Pedley TJ, Schroter RC, Seed WA. The systemic veins. The mechanics of the circulation. Oxford: Oxford University Press, 1978:434–475.
4. Fung YC. The veins. In: Biodynamics, circulation. New York: Springer-Verlag, 1984:166–223.
5. Attinger EO. Wall properties of veins. IEEE Trans Biomed Eng 1969;16:253.
6. Lye CR, Sumner DS, Hokanson DE, Strandness DE Jr. The transcutaneous measurement of the elastic properties of the human saphenous vein femoropopliteal bypass graft. Surg Gynecol Obstet 1975;141:891.
7. Rushmer RF. Effects of posture. In: Cardiovascular dynamics. 3rd ed. Philadelphia: WB Saunders Co., 1970:192–219.
8. Sjöstrand T. Volume and distribution of blood and their significance in regulating the circulation. Physiol Rev 1953;33:202.
9. Öberg B. The relationship between active constriction and passive recoil of the veins at various distending pressures. Acta Physiol Scand 1967;71:233.
10. Ludbrook J, Loughlin J. Regulation of volume in postarteriolar vessels of the lower limb. Am Heart J 1964;67:493.

11. Webb-Peploe MM, Shepherd JT. Response of large hindlimb veins of the dog to sympathetic nerve stimulation. Am J Physiol 1968;215:299.
12. Shepherd JT. Role of the veins in the circulation. Circulation 1966;33:484.
13. Shepherd JT. Reflex control of the venous system. In: Bergan JJ, Yao JST, eds. Venous problems. Chicago: Year Book Medical Publishers, 1978:5–23.
14. Vanhoutte PM, Shepherd JT. Thermosensitivity and veins. J Physiol (Paris) 1970;63:449.
15. Samueloff SL, Browse NL, Shepherd JT. Response of capacity vessels in human limbs to head up tilt and suction on lower body. J Appl Physiol 1966;21:47.
16. Sumner DS. Noninvasive vascular laboratory assessment. In: Machleder HJ, ed. Vascular disorders of the upper extremity. 2nd ed. Mount Kisco, NY: Futura Publishing, 1989:9–57.
17. Holt JP. Flow through collapsible tubes and through in situ veins. IEEE Trans Biomed Eng 1969;16:274.
18. Lyon CK, Scott JB, Wang CY. Flow through collapsible tubes at low Reynolds numbers. Circ Res 1980;47:68.
19. Shapiro AH. Steady flow in collapsible tubes. J Biomechanical Eng Trans ASME August 1977:126.
20. Cancelli C, Pedley TJ. A separated-flow model for collapsible tube oscillations. J Fluid Mech 1985;157:375.
21. Sumner DS. Diagnosis of venous thrombosis by Doppler ultrasound. In: Bergan JJ, Yao JST, eds. Venous problems. Chicago: Year Book Medical Publishers, 1978:159–185.
22. Stegall HF. Muscle pumping in the dependent leg. Circ Res 1966;19:180.
23. Conrad MC. Functional anatomy of the circulation to the extremities. Chicago: Year Book Medical Publishers, 1971.
24. Kiely PE. A phlebographic study of the soleal sinuses. Angiology 1973;24:230.
25. Sherman RS Sr. Varicose veins: anatomy, reevaluation of Trendelenburg tests, and an operative procedure. Surg Clin N Am 1964;44:1369.
26. van Bemmelen PS, Bedford G, Beach K, Strandness DE. Quantitative segmental evaluation of venous reflux with duplex ultrasound scanning. J Vasc Surg 1989;10:425.
27. Masuda EM, Kistner RL. Prospective comparison of duplex scanning and descending venography in the assessment of venous insufficiency. Am J Surg 1992;164:254.
28. van Bemmelen PS, Beach K, Bedford G, Strandness DE. The mechanism of venous valve closure. Its relationship to the velocity of reverse flow. Arch Surg 1990;125:617.
29. Sarin S, Scurr JH, Coleridge Smith PD. Medial calf perforators in venous disease: the significance of outward flow. J Vasc Surg 1992;16:40.
30. Koslow AR, DeWeese JA. Anatomical and mechanical aspects of a plantar venous plexus. Presented at the Jobst symposium on current issues in venous disease. Chicago, 1988.
31. Ludbrook J. The musculovenous pumps of the human lower limb. Am Heart J 1966;71:635.
32. Ludbrook J. Aspects of venous function in the lower limbs. Springfield IL: Charles C Thomas, 1966:51–78.
33. Alimi YS, Barthelemy P, Juhan C. Venous pump of the calf: a study of venous and muscular pressures. J Vasc Surg 1994;20:728.
34. Arnoldi CC. Venous pressure in the leg of healthy human subjects at rest and during muscular exercise in the nearly erect position. Acta Chir Scand 1965;130:570.
35. Nicolaides AN, Sumner DS. Investigation of patients with deep venous thrombosis and chronic venous insufficiency. London: Med-Orion, 1991.
36. Christopoulos D, Nicolaides AN, Galloway JMD, Wilkinson A. Objective noninvasive evaluation of venous surgical results. J Vasc Surg 1988;8:683.
37. Christopoulos DG, Nicolaides AN, Szendro G, et al. Air-plethysmography and the effect of elastic compression on venous hemodynamics of the leg. J Vasc Surg 1987;5:148.

38. Raju S, Fredericks R, Lishman P, et al. Observations on the calf pump mechanism: determinants of postexercise pressure. J Vasc Surg 1993;17:459.
39. Almén T, Nylander G. Serial phlebography of the normal lower leg during muscular contraction and relaxation. Acta Radiol 1962;57:364.
40. Nicolaides AN, Zukowski AJ. The value of dynamic venous pressure measurements. World J Surg 1986;10:919.
41. Fernandes é Fernandes J, Horner J, Needham T, Nicolaides A. Ambulatory calf volume plethysmography in the assessment of venous insufficiency. Br J Surg 1979;66:327.
42. Strandness DE Jr, Sumner DS. Hemodynamics for surgeons. New York: Grune & Stratton, 1975:138–139.
43. Höjensgård IC, Stürup H. Static and dynamic pressures in superficial and deep veins of the lower extremities in man. Acta Physiol Scand 1952;27:49.
44. Gardner AMN, Fox RH. The return of blood to the heart: venous pumps in health and disease. London: John Libbey Eurotext Ltd., 1989.
45. Starling EH. On the absorption of fluids from the connective tissue spaces. J Physiol 1896;19:312.
46. Taylor AE. Capillary fluid filtration, Starling forces and lymph flow. Circ Res 1981;49:557.
47. Christopoulos D, Nicolaides AN, Szendro G. Venous reflux: quantification and correlation with the clinical severity of chronic venous disease. Br J Surg 1988;75:352.
48. Neglén P, Raju S. A rational approach to detection of significant reflux with duplex Doppler scanning and air plethysmography. J Vasc Surg 1993;17:590.
49. van Bemmelen PS, Mattos MA, Hodgson KJ, et al. Does air plethysmography correlate with duplex scanning in patients with chronic venous insufficiency. J Vasc Surg 1993;18:796.
50. Browse NL. The pathogenesis of venous ulceration. A hypothesis. J Vasc Surg 1988;7:468.
51. Fragrell B. Local microcirculation in chronic venous incompetence and leg ulcers. Vasc Surg 1979;13:217.
52. Arenander E. Hemodynamic effects of varicose veins and results of radical surgery. Acta Chir Scand 1960;260(Suppl):1.
53. Burnand KG, Whimster I, Naidoo A, et al. Pericapillary fibrin in the ulcer-bearing skin of the leg. The cause of lipodermatosclerosis and venous ulcerations. Br Med J 1982;285:1071.
54. Falanga V, Moosa HH, Nemeth AJ, et al. Dermal pericapillary fibrin in venous disease and venous ulceration. Arch Dermatol 1987;123:620.
55. Thomas PRS, Nash GB, Dormandy JA. White cell accumulation in dependent legs of patients with venous hypertension: a possible mechanism for trophic changes in the skin. Br Med J 1988;296:1693.
56. Wilkinson LS, Bunker C, Edwards JCW, et al. Leukocytes: their role in the etiopathogenesis of skin damage in venous disease. J Vasc Surg 1993;17:669.
57. Leu AJ, Leu H-J, Franzeck UK, Bollinger A. Microvascular changes in chronic venous insufficiency—a review. Cardiovasc Surg 1995;3:237.
58. Pappas PJ, Fallek SR, Garcia A, et al. Role of leukocyte activation in patients with venous stasis ulcers. J Surg Res 1995;59:553.
59. Raju S, Fredericks R. Hemodynamic basis of stasis ulceration—a hypothesis. J Vasc Surg 1991;13:491.
60. Raju S, Fredericks R. Valve reconstruction procedures for nonobstructive venous insufficiency: rationale, techniques, and results in 107 procedures with two- to eight-year follow-up. J Vasc Surg 1988;7:301.
61. Nicolaides AN, Hussein MK, Szendro G, et al. The relation of venous ulceration with ambulatory venous pressure measurements. J Vasc Surg 1993;17:414.

62. Bjordal RI. Simultaneous pressure and flow recordings in varicose veins of the lower extremity. A hemodynamic study of venous dysfunction. Acta Chir Scand 1970;136:309.
63. Folse R. The influence of femoral vein dynamics on the development of varicose veins. Surgery 1970;68:974.
64. Ludbrook J. Valvular defect in primary varicose veins, cause or effect? Lancet 1963;2:1289.
65. Arnoldi CC. Venous pressure in patients with valvular incompetence of the veins of the lower limb. Acta Chir Scand 1966;132:628.
66. McPheeters HO, Merkert CE, Lundblad RA. The mechanics of the reverse flow in varicose veins as proved by blood pressure readings. Surg Gynecol Obstet 1932;55:298.
67. Somerville JJF, Byrne PJ, Fegan WG. Analysis of flow patterns in venous insufficiency. Br J Surg 1974;61:40.
68. Warren R, White EA, Belcher CD. Venous pressures in the saphenous system in normal, varicose, and postphlebitic extremities. Surgery 1949;26:435.
69. Edwards EA, Edwards JE. The effect of thrombophlebitis on the venous valve. Surg Gynecol Obstet 1937;65:310.
70. Killewich LA, Bedford GR, Beach KW, Strandness DE Jr. Spontaneous lysis of deep venous thrombi: rate and outcome. J Vasc Surg 1989;9:89.
71. Markel A, Manzo RA, Bergelin RO, Strandness DE Jr. Valvular reflux after deep vein thrombosis: incidence and time of occurrence. J Vasc Surg 1992;15:377.
72. Welkie JF, Comerota AJ, Katz ML, et al. Hemodynamic deterioration in chronic venous disease. J Vasc Surg 1992;16:733.
73. Meissner MH, Manzo RA, Bergelin RO, et al. Deep venous insufficiency: the relationship between lysis and subsequent reflux. J Vasc Surg 1993;18:596.
74. Markel A, Meissner MH, Manzo RA, et al. A comparison of the cuff deflation method with Valsalva's maneuver and limb compression in detecting venous valvular reflux. Arch Surg 1994;129:701.
75. Caps MT, Manzo RA, Bergelin RO, et al. Venous valvular reflux in veins not involved at the time of acute deep vein thrombosis. J Vasc Surg 1995;22:524.
76. Labropoulos N, Leon M, Geroulakos G, et al. Venous hemodynamic abnormalities in patients with leg ulceration. Am J Surg 1995;169:572.
77. Moore DJ, Himmel PD, Sumner DS. Distribution of venous valvular incompetence in patients with the postphlebitic syndrome. J Vasc Surg 1986;3:49.
78. Hanrahan LM, Araki CT, Rodriguez AA, et al. Distribution of valvular incompetence in patients with venous stasis ulceration. J Vasc Surg 1991;13:805.
79. Husni EA, Ximenes JO, Goyette EM. Elastic support of the lower limbs in hospital patients—a critical study. JAMA 1970;214:1456.
80. Arnoldi CC, Linderholm H. On the pathogenesis of the venous leg ulcer. Acta Chir Scand 1968;134:427.
81. DeCamp PT, Schramel RJ, Roy CJ, et al. Ambulatory venous pressure determinations in postphlebitic and related syndromes. Surgery 1951;29:44.
82. Hjelmstedt A. Pressure decrease in the dorsal pedal veins on walking in persons with and without thrombosis. Acta Surg Scand 1968;134:531.
83. Negus D, Cockett FB. Femoral vein pressures in postphlebitic iliac vein obstruction. Br J Surg 1967;54:522.
84. Cockett FB, Jones DEE. The ankle blowout syndrome, a new approach to the varicose ulcer problem. Lancet 1953;1:17.
85. Vasdekis SN, Clarke GH, Nicolaides AN. Quantification of venous reflux by means of duplex scanning. J Vasc Surg 1989;10:670.
86. Reagan B, Folse R. Lower limb venous dynamics in normal persons and children of patients with varicose veins. Surg Gynecol Obstet 1971;132:15.

87. Thomas ML, Keeling FP, Ackroyd JS. Descending phlebography: a comparison of three methods and an assessment of the normal range of deep vein reflux. J Cardiovasc Surg 1986;27:27.
88. Shull KC, Nicolaides AN, Fernandes é Fernandes J, et al. Significance of popliteal reflux in relation to ambulatory venous pressure and ulceration. Arch Surg 1979;114:1304.
89. Lindner DJ, Edwards JM, Phinney ES, et al. Long-term hemodynamic and clinical sequelae of lower extremity deep vein thrombosis. J Vasc Surg 1986;4:436.
90. Gooley NA, Sumner DS. Relationship of venous reflux to the site of venous incompetence: implications for venous reconstructive surgery. J Vasc Surg 1988;7:50.
91. Pearce WH, Ricco J-B, Queral LA, et al. Hemodynamic assessment of venous problems. Surgery 1983;93:715.
92. Rosfors S, Lamke L-O, Nordström E, Bygdeman S. Severity and location of venous valvular insufficiency: the importance of distal valve function. Acta Chir Scand 1990;156:689.
93. Labropoulos N, Leon M, Nicolaides AN, et al. Superficial venous insufficiency: correlation of anatomic extent of reflux with clinical symptoms and signs. J Vasc Surg 1994;20:953.
94. Labropoulos N, Leon M, Nicolaides AN, et al. Venous reflux in patients with previous deep venous thrombosis: correlation with ulceration and other symptoms. J Vasc Surg 1994;20:20.
95. van Bemmelen PS, Bedford G, Beach K, Strandness DE Jr. Status of the valves in the superficial and deep venous system in chronic venous disease. Surgery 1991;109:730.
96. Myers KA, Ziegenbein RW, Zeng GH, Mathews PG. Duplex ultrasonography scanning for chronic venous disease: patterns of venous reflux. J Vasc Surg 1995;21:605.
97. van Rij AM, Solomon C, Christie R. Anatomic and physiologic characteristics of venous ulceration. J Vasc Surg 1994;20:759.
98. Araki CT, Back TL, Padberg FT, et al. The significance of calf muscle pump function in venous ulceration. J Vasc Surg 1994;20:872.
99. Weingarten MS, Branas CC, Czeredarczuk M, et al. Distribution and quantification of venous reflux in lower extremity chronic venous stasis disease with duplex scanning. J Vasc Surg 1993;18:753.
100. Lees TA, Lambert D. Patterns of venous reflux in limbs with skin changes associated with chronic venous insufficiency. Br J Surg 1993;80:725.
101. Shami SK, Sarin S, Cheatle TR, et al. Venous ulcers and the superficial venous system. J Vasc Surg 1993;17:487.
102. Darke SG, Penfold C. Venous ulceration and saphenous ligation. Eur J Vasc Surg 1992;6:4.
103. McEnroe CS, O'Donnell TF Jr, Mackey WC. Correlation of clinical findings with venous hemodynamics in 386 patients with chronic venous insufficiency. Am J Surg 1988;156:148.
104. Dalsing MC, Lalka SG, Unthank JL, et al. Venous valvular insufficiency: influence of a single venous valve (native and experimental). J Vasc Surg 1991;14:576.
105. Johnson ND, Queral LA, Flinn WR, et al. Late objective assessment of venous valve surgery. Arch Surg 1981;116:1421.
106. O'Donnell TF, Mackey WC, Shephard AD, et al. Clinical, hemodynamic, and anatomic follow-up of direct venous reconstruction. Arch Surg 1987;122:474.
107. Taheri SA, Heffner R, Meenaghan MA, et al. Technique and results of venous valve transplantation. In: Bergan JJ, Yao JST, eds. Surgery of the veins. Orlando, FL: Grune & Stratton, 1985:219–231.
108. Welch HJ, McLauglin RL, O'Donnell TF Jr. Femoral vein valvuloplasty: intraoperative angioscopic evaluation and hemodynamic improvement. J Vasc Surg 1992;16:694.

109. DeWeese JA, Rogoff SM. Phlebographic patterns of acute deep venous thrombosis of the leg. Surgery 1963;53:99.
110. Ellwood RA, Lee WB. Pedal venous pressure: correlation with presence and site of deep venous abnormalities. Radiology 1979;131:73.
111. Barnes RW, Collicott PE, Mozersky DJ, et al. Noninvasive quantitation of maximum venous outflow in acute thrombophlebitis. Surgery 1972;72:971.
112. Barnes RW, Collicott PE, Sumner DS, Strandness DE Jr. Noninvasive quantitation of venous hemodynamics in postphlebitic syndrome. Arch Surg 1973;107:807.
113. Dahn I, Eiriksson E. Plethysmographic diagnosis of deep venous thrombosis of the leg. Acta Chir Scand 1968;398(Suppl):33.
114. Hallböök T, Göthin J. Strain gauge plethysmography and phlebography in diagnosis of deep venous thrombosis. Acta Chir Scand 1971;137:37.
115. Sakaguchi S, Ishitobi K, Kameda T. Functional segmental plethysmography with mercury strain gauge. Angiology 1972;23:127.
116. Snyder MA, Adams JT, Schwartz SI. Hemodynamics of phlegmasia cerulea dolens. Surg Gynecol Obstet 1967;125:342.
117. Haller JA Jr. Effects of deep femoral thrombophlebitis on the circulation of the lower extremities. Circulation 1963;27:693.
118. Brockman SK, Vasko JS. The pathologic physiology of phlegmasia cerulea dolens. Surgery 1966;59:997.
119. Johnson BF, Manzo RA, Bergelin RO, Strandness DE Jr. Relationship between changes in the deep venous system and the development of the postthrombotic syndrome after an acute episode of lower limb deep vein thrombosis: a one- to six-year follow-up. J Vasc Surg 1995;21:307.
120. Tripolitis AJ, Milligan EB, Bodily KC, Strandness DE Jr. The physiology of venous claudication. Am J Surg 1980;139:447.
121. Sumner DS. Diagnosis of deep venous thrombosis. In: Rutherford RB, ed. Vascular surgery. 4th ed. Philadelphia: WB Saunders Co., 1995:1698–1743.
122. Hull R, van Aken WG, Hirsh J, et al. Impedance plethysmography using the occlusive cuff technique in the diagnosis of venous thrombosis. Circulation 1976;53:696.
123. Wheeler HB, Anderson FA Jr. Diagnosis of deep venous thrombosis by impedance plethysmography. In: Bernstein EF, ed. Vascular diagnosis. 4th ed. St. Louis: CV Mosby, 1993:820–829.
124. Sumner DS. Diagnosis of deep vein thrombosis by strain-gauge plethysmography. In: Bernstein EF, ed. Vascular diagnosis. 4th ed. St. Louis: CV Mosby, 1993:811–819.
125. Lundgren PO, Thulesius O. Maximal venous outflow in the diagnosis of deep venous thrombosis, new principles for its determination. Vasa 1985;14:346.

section II

Diagnostic Techniques

chapter 3

Diagnosis of Venous Disease: Duplex Imaging

David L. Rollins, Carolyn M. Semrow, Ronald A. Saurin, and Sabrina Ewald

The clinical manifestations of venous disease have been recorded for over 2000 years. Clinical characteristics of varicose veins, leg ulcerations, and acute venous thrombosis have been well described since early times and many theories as to their causes have been proposed (1). Yet many aspects of venous pathophysiology remain unknown or poorly understood. Important recent technical advances in the noninvasive diagnosis of acute deep venous thrombosis (DVT) and chronic venous disease (CVD) have both improved diagnostic accuracy and increased our knowledge of venous pathophysiology. The newer diagnostic tests have limited the need for contrast venography (2–6). Over the last decade, evolution of sophisticated real-time ultrasound technology and computer software have produced imaging systems with color Doppler capabilities. In the hands of experienced sonographers, much of the venous system can be visualized and acute and chronic disease diagnosed with a high degree of accuracy, challenging contrast venography as the prevailing "gold standard" (7–13). Ultrasonic venography (UV) provides precise anatomic location of venous abnormalities and reliably identifies acute and chronic venous pathology (14–17). Quantification of venous reflux using pulsed Doppler provides physiologic measurements that can distinguish venous outflow obstruction and reflux (18–20).

EQUIPMENT AND TECHNIQUES

Evaluation of the venous system by ultrasonic venography has been characterized by many names. Each name generally refers to the equipment and techniques employed. For example, "compression ultrasound" generally refers to diagnosis of acute thrombosis utilizing B-mode ultrasonic imaging and external compression of the veins. "Duplex ultrasound" indicates that B-mode imaging is performed in conjunction with Doppler ultrasound, fast Fourier transformations (FFT), and/or color.

EQUIPMENT

The extent of the procedure performed and diagnostic criteria employed dictate which equipment is required. Today, most laboratories utilize Duplex imagers with color Doppler capabilities. This technology allows greater flexibility and utilization of many diagnostic criteria. The color Doppler is particularly useful for rapid identification of vessels, determination of the origin of venous reflux, and assessment of acute calf vein thrombosis and chronic venous disorders.

Most systems utilize linear array transducers that provide a wide ultrasonic footprint and simultaneity of image and Doppler data. The choice of transducer frequency is dependent on the site to be examined. In general, 5 MHz transducers are adequate for lower extremity assessments. However, 7.5 MHz transducers provide better resolution, which is essential in assessment of calf veins, upper extremity, the saphenous system, and valve function. Transducers of 3.5 MHz are used to evaluate pelvic and abdominal veins. If precise measurements of vein size are needed, then a system that employs M-mode capabilities can be used.

Optimum patient positioning is important to assure accuracy of ultrasound examination. Examinations should be performed with the patient either sitting in an examination chair or in a bed placed in 15–20° degree reverse Trendelenburg position. Acutely ill, bedridden patients can be examined easily on a transport cart, but ambulatory patients are best examined in an adjustable chair (Fig. 3.1). Identification of reflux in chronic venous insufficiency is optimally performed with the patient standing.

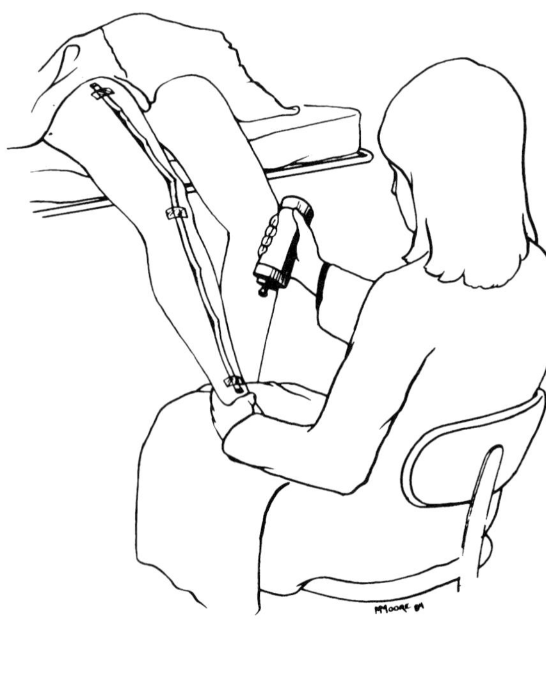

FIG. 3–1. Venous imaging in the ambulatory patient is performed with the patient seated and foot resting on examiner's knee. A tape measure may be applied to the anterior aspect of the limb for anatomic location of pathology. (Reproduced by permission from Semrow CM, Friedell ML, Buchbinder D, Rollins DL. Characterization of lower extremity venous disease using real-time B-mode ultrasonic imaging. J Vasc Tech 1987;9:187–191.)

TECHNIQUE

Many centers evaluate only the proximal venous system (common femoral to popliteal) for acute deep venous thrombosis owing to the time needed and technical skills required to assess calf veins (8, 12, 16, 21). Although this may be justified by the low incidence of fatal pulmonary emboli emanating from calf veins, a 20% rate of thrombus propagation has been reported (22). If duplex ultrasound is utilized for perioperative surveillance of high risk patients, then the entire deep venous system should be visualized. Evaluation of chronic venous insufficiency also requires complete superficial and deep vein assessment.

PROCEDURE

Ultrasonic examination may be started at the inguinal ligament and proceed distally or from the ankle proximally. Both transverse and longitudinal transducer orientations accurately assess the proximal venous system (8, 17). Transverse orientation appears to be less sensitive in the calf (23). The longitudinal approach facilitates rapid assessment of the venous system and transverse orientation is useful to confirm vein noncompressibility (8, 16, 17, 24–31). Additionally, longitudinal visualization of venous pathology allows differentiation of acute from chronic obstruction and is useful in identifying perforating veins and collateral channels. Evaluation of the limb for chronic venous insufficiency is extremely challenging and often technically difficult. Insonation of the deep venous system to determine the presence and location of venous valves, residual obstruction, alternate outflow channels and the presence and location of venous reflux is necessary (Fig. 3.2). Color Doppler is extremely useful in documenting venous pathology in this regard. Combined with augmentation maneuvers, color flow can determine the presence of reflux and the contribution of collateral channels and perforators to venous outflow (32). Distal augmentation can be standardized by using a rapid inflation-deflation pneumatic cuff system. Reflux at specific levels or individual veins can be determined with B-mode and Doppler ultrasound. Recently, reflux has been defined as reverse flow lasting for more than 0.5 seconds (18, 33) across a valve station.

ULTRASONIC WINDOWS

Evaluation of the superficial and, particularly, of the deep veins requires thorough anatomic knowledge of the area to be visualized. In the extremities, the deep vessels run parallel to and are contiguous with the long bones. This knowledge facilitates vessel location. Routine examination windows for the lower extremity deep venous system are noted in Figure 3.3. Regardless of which examination technique is used, scanning should begin at the location where the vein is most easily insonated. Visualization of the popliteal and proximal veins has been well described by many authors as noted earlier. Routine evaluation of the calf veins is readily accomplished and should be performed. Over half of the patients with acute DVT, particularly nonhospitalized ambulatory patients, have calf vein

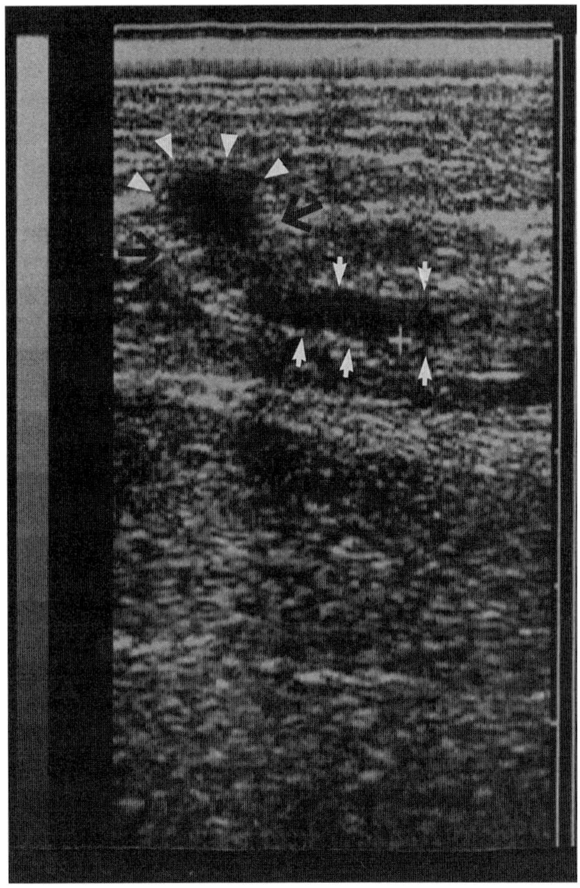

FIG. 3–2. Direct perforator (*small arrows*) to the greater saphenous vein (*arrow heads*) from an obstructed posterior tibial vein.

thrombosis alone (15). The posterior tibial veins are most easily located at the ankle region posterior to the medial malleolus and can be followed to their confluence with the peroneal vein. The anterior tibial veins are insonated by placing the transducer on the anterolateral aspect of the leg approximately 1.5 cm lateral to the tibia. These veins are almost always very small and are located directly above the interosseous membrane, which appears as a hyperechoic thick line. The peroneal vein is the deepest vein and the most difficult to visualize. It courses posterior and medial to the fibula. It can be evaluated by continuing distally from the popliteal vein using a posteromedial approach. However, this approach often becomes difficult owing to the massive gastrocnemius muscle. Therefore, a posterolateral approach just behind the fibula or an anterior approach as described for the anterior tibial veins can be used (12, 16).

Ultrasonic venography of the upper extremity and central veins is primarily indicated for detection of deep venous thrombosis. The brachial and axillary veins course with arteries of the same name and are easily insonated using a medial arm approach. The subclavian, jugular, and superior vena cava are visualized from a supraclavicular window. Color or spectral Doppler is necessary to evaluate patency because these proximal veins cannot be compressed. Flow augmentation using breath-holding and release is helpful in assessing flow; in some cases, it is possible to visualize a thrombus within the veins surrounding central venous access lines. The iliac veins and vena cava may be insonated through various well-described windows (34–36).

DIAGNOSTIC CHARACTERIZATION AND DIAGNOSTIC CRITERIA

Normal veins appear as smooth echogenically homogeneous thin tubes with elliptical valve sinuses, and long, thin valve leaflets. Blood flow may be visualized directly owing to the high acoustical impedance of red cell aggregates (37, 38). Flow in the proximal veins is spontaneous, phasic, and augmentable. Color Doppler may not visualize flow in calf and distal popliteal veins without augmentation. The saphenofemoral, saphenopopliteal, and gastrocnemius confluences with the deep veins are routinely seen. The deep femoral vein is seen in approximately one-third of scans. Perforators and other smaller tributary veins

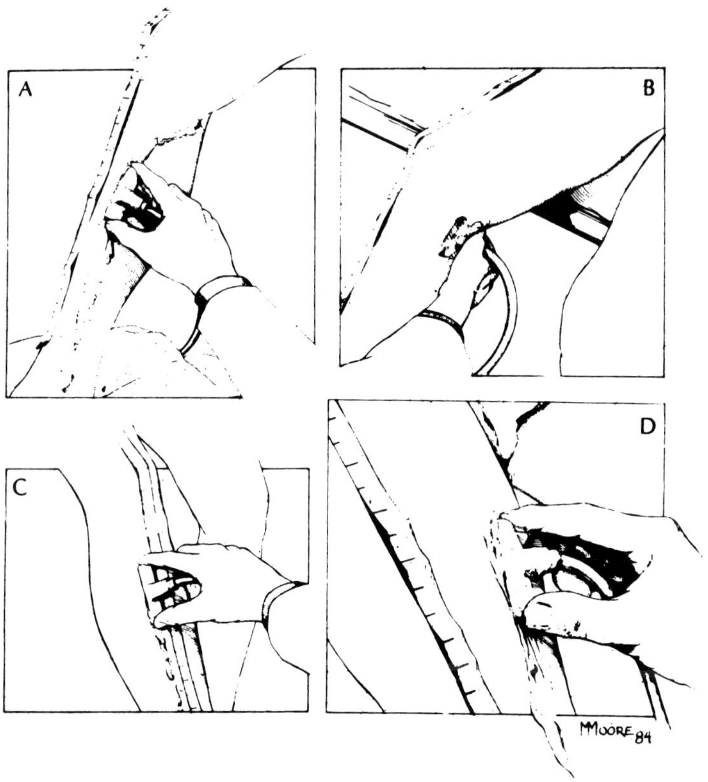

FIG. 3–3. The posterior tibial vein (**A**) is evaluated starting just superior to the medial malleolus and proceeding proximally to the popliteal vein (**B**) then distally to the peroneal veins. The anterior tibial veins (**C**) are imaged lateral to the tibia starting proximally. The superficial femoral and common femoral veins are visualized from an anterior medial approach starting in the distal thigh (**D**).

are not visualized unless abnormal flow from previous venous disease or anomalies are present.

ACUTE THROMBOSIS

Fresh thrombus has the same acoustical characteristics as flowing blood and will not be appreciated without color Doppler or compression maneuvers. Within a few hours, thrombus becomes more anechoic due to red cell compaction, fibrin deposition, and hemolysis. Approximately 24 hours after its initial formation, the thrombus is often visualized as a smooth, speckled hypoechoic mass. This acoustical appearance usually remains stable for approximately 3–5 days. As the thrombus continues to age, it becomes more organized and progressively increases in echogenicity if significant lysis has not occurred. Changes in thrombus acoustical appearance generally stabilize within 3 and 6 months after formation. Relatively fresh thrombus (7–14 days) has an elastic quality. This characteristic causes the acoustical impedance to increase when thrombus is compressed and is helpful in differentiating acute from older hypoechoic thrombus that does not increase in echogenicity with compression (7, 39).

Vein compressibility is the primary criterion utilized for detection of acute thrombosis. Total collapse of the vein when compressed by the transducer indicates patency. Acute thrombus prevents full collapse of the vessel and attenuation of the ultrasound signal, resulting in increased echogenicity of the thrombus (8, 17, 40). Color Doppler ultrasound is frequently used to confirm the presence of phasic flow in the proximal veins and to assist in locating hypoechoic luminal filling or flow defects (24, 26, 41). Absence of the color Doppler signal is an indication of total vessel obstruction.

CHRONIC THROMBUS

Patients with recent venous thrombosis have noncompressible veins with hypoechoic thrombus attached to the vessel wall that does not exhibit the acoustical compression attenuation associated with the more acute stage (8, 12, 17, 40). As thrombus ages, it becomes more hyperechoic. After several months, chronically diseased veins exhibit thick, hyperechoic walls (Fig. 3.4). Heterogeneous, hyperechoic segmental protrusions from the vein walls, which either partially or totally occlude the vein, are common (22, 42). Valve sinuses are rarely distinguishable, but when present have absent or shortened, thickened, nonfunctional valve leaflets (12). Collateral and perforating veins leading to intramuscular or superficial varicosities that are absent in normal legs are frequently observed.

CLINICAL APPLICATIONS

Over the last 10 years, ultrasonic venography has been increasingly utilized to provide precise anatomic information and measurement of physiologic parameters. As more sophisticated ultrasonic technology has evolved, it has supplanted x-ray contrast venography for the diagnosis of acute venous thrombosis.

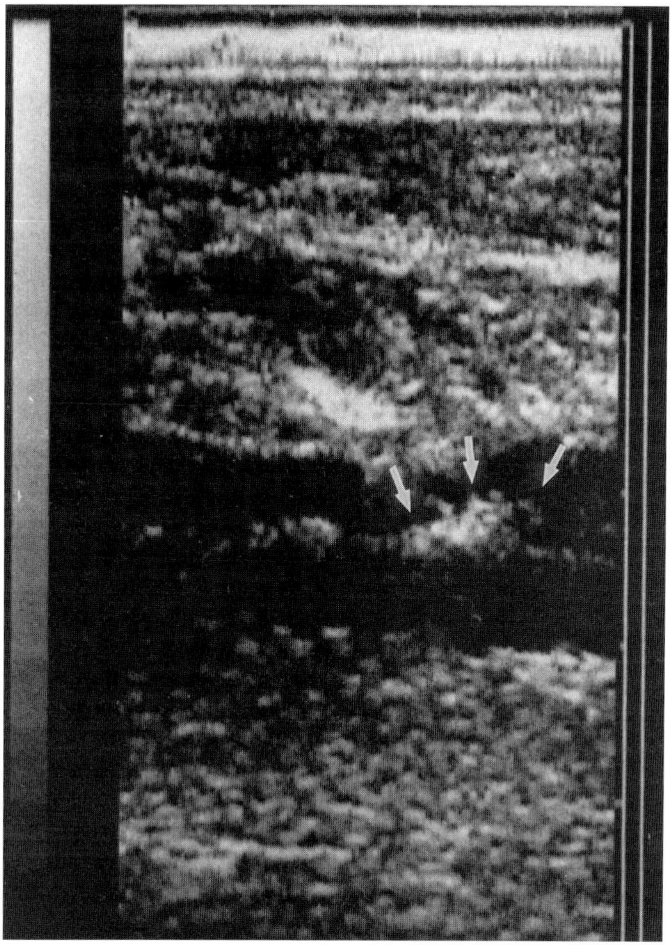

FIG. 3–4. Chronic recanalization changes that partially occlude a venous valve sinus of posterior tibial vein.

Recently, it has become the primary tool to evaluate valve function, locate and map sites of venous reflux, and differentiate between acute and chronic venous disease.

RECURRENT DEEP VEIN THROMBOSIS

Leg symptoms in patients with a previous history of deep venous thrombosis or clinical evidence of chronic venous insufficiency may be caused by recurrent thrombosis, the postphlebitic syndrome, or a variety of nonthrombotic disorders. Differentiating between these causes is important to appropriately treat the patient and avoid possible complications of unnecessary long-term anticoagulation. Duplex Doppler directly visualizes intraluminal thrombus and, as noted earlier, can readily differentiate between acute and chronic disease on the basis of clot echogenicity, venous flow patterns, and vein wall characteristics (39–41).

In a study of 38 limbs with suspected recurrent acute thrombosis, duplex Doppler was comparable to contrast venography in detecting recurrent deep vein thrombosis (12). Frequently, contrast venography was inconclusive in patients with previous venous disease owing to the masking of the venographic characteristics of acute thrombosis by abnormal flow patterns and large collateral channels. Patients with the postthrombotic syndrome frequently present with recurrent distal calf and leg pain, which is often associated with recurrent ulceration. Recurrent minor calf thrombosis is often observed in these limbs. Ultrasonic venography should be performed initially in all patients with suspected recurrent acute deep vein thrombosis. It is particularly useful in detecting suspected thrombus extension in patients with worsening symptoms and signs who are already anticoagulated (22, 41).

ORTHOPEDIC PROCEDURES

Patients with hip fracture are at high risk for the development of deep venous thrombosis. Unfortunately, only a small percentage of orthopedic surgeons use objective diagnostic tests to determine its presence (43). Recent studies have shown that acute deep venous thrombosis occurs in approximately 12% of hip fracture patients (44). Ultrasonic venography has been proven to be accurate and efficacious in assessing these patients.

Total hip and knee arthroplasty are common procedures. Despite improved methods of prophylaxis, acute deep vein thrombosis and pulmonary embolism are the leading causes of mortality and morbidity in this patient group. Even with current prophylactic regimens, the incidence of thrombosis approaches 20% in the more proximal veins (44–46). Since ultrasonic venography has excellent sensitivity in detecting asymptomatic thrombosis, it is the ideal method for perioperative screening (47). An increasing number of practitioners are performing ultrasonography on the 5th to 7th postoperative day in elective knee and hip arthroplasty patients. Several authors have reported excellent correlation between duplex scanning and contrast venography in the detection of asymptomatic postoperative thrombosis (46–48). Because of the high incidence of deep vein thrombosis ultrasound venography should be performed in all total hip and knee arthroplasty patients in the pre- and postoperative process.

UPPER EXTREMITY AND CENTRAL VENOUS THROMBOSIS

Thrombosis of the upper extremity and central veins is a frequent and important clinical problem that requires prompt diagnosis and treatment in order to decrease morbidity. From the clinical standpoint there are three major causes of upper extremity thrombosis: central venous catheters, "effort" thrombosis, and invasive tumors. Ultrasonic venography in capable hands can be as accurate as contrast venography or computed tomography in detecting both the presence and extent of central venous thrombus (49–52). Ultrasonic findings include flow attenuation, intraluminal filling defects, venous distension, and absence of flow. Color Doppler is extremely useful in insonating the jugular, innominate, and subclavian veins. Following lytic therapy or surgery for thoracic outlet syndrome, ultrasonic venography documents the results of therapy. Refinements in imaging techniques have allowed greater access to the retroclavicular, axillary and subclavian veins. Diagnosis of thoracic venous compression syndrom by Duplex ultrasound is now practical.

Internal jugular and subclavian central venous catheter insertion is often difficult. Significant complications of bleeding and pneumothorax occur when the blind technique of vein puncture is used. Color Duplex ultrasound can assess the position, size, and patency of the jugular and subclavian veins. Preoperative Duplex assessment of these vessels in patients with failed catheter placement who are high risk for complication has been found to greatly reduce the complication rate and result in easier catheter placement.

Real-time Duplex imaging during needle insertion can be used and has been found to improve the ease of catheter placement and reduce complications.

VENA CAVAL THROMBOSIS

While there are many different causes of vena caval obstruction, the primary etiologies include thrombus, extrinsic compression, and tumor. In patients with suspected caval thrombosis, ultrasonic venography can diagnose both intrinsic and extrinsic obstruction (36,53). Ultrasonic venography is useful in both the screening and follow-up of vena cava filter patients. Filter position may be better assessed when ultrasound is utilized with contrast venography (54). When tumor is the suspected cause of renal vein or caval thrombosis, ultrasound venography is an important diagnostic screening test (55).

PREOPERATIVE SUPERFICIAL VEIN ASSESSMENT

Increasing use of infrainguinal revascularization with autogenous vein has created the need for accurate preoperative assessment of vein quality. Preoperative vein quality is an important determinant of long-term bypass patency. Approximately 40% of saphenous veins will be inadequate for reverse bypass and 10–15% of veins will not be adequate for in situ bypass owing to anatomic abnormalities. If the greater saphenous vein is not adequate, then either lesser saphenous or cephalic veins must be used to accomplish autogenous reconstruction. In recent years, ultrasonic venography has been extensively used preoperatively to identify satisfactory veins for reconstruction (56–59). This procedure accurately determines size and quality of the vein preoperatively. Preoperative marking eliminates unnecessary dissection in patients without usable veins and identifies large branches and anatomic variants. Operative times are decreased and the morbidity of extensive skin flaps is avoided with preoperative scanning. Evaluation is best performed using a 7.5 MHz linear array transducer.

ARTERIOVENOUS FISTULAS AND BRIDGE GRAFTS

Arteriovenous fistulas and bridge grafts are the conduits of choice for end-stage renal failure patients undergoing dialysis. The autogenous fistula at the wrist (Brescia-Cimino) is the procedure of choice, although long-term patency may be achieved with other autogenous or synthetic grafts. Ultrasonic venography can accurately identify and map the superficial venous system of the arm and determine suitability for fistula construction (60). In obese patients or limbs with significant edema, ultrasound can determine whether adequate forearm, antecubital, or axillary veins are present. These scans are also performed using a 7.5 MHz linear array transducer with and without an arm tourniquet. Improved patient selection for construction of primary arteriovenous fistulas will result in greater initial patency rates and lessen the need for thrombectomies and revisions. This procedure should be performed in all patients in whom significant veins are not detected by physical examination. The presence of proximal venous stenosis is readily detectable. Patients with decreased dialysis efficiency calculations or increased pulsatility of the graft often have venous outflow obstruction, which is readily diagnosed and localized by Duplex. Chronic arm and shoulder swellling in these patients is usually due to proximal subclavian venous obstruction or occlusion which is easily detected by Duplex ultrasound.

DIAGNOSIS AND MANAGEMENT OF CHRONIC VENOUS INSUFFICIENCY

Important clinical and technical advances in the ultrasonic diagnosis of venous disease have sparked increasing interest in the management of venous insufficiency. As noted previously, ultrasonic venography can easily characterize deep venous abnormalities such as occluded and stenotic deep veins, and visualize incompetent collaterals and perforating veins. It is an ideal method for pretreatment assessment of all patients with primary varicose veins or patients with chronic venous insufficiency. The success of treatment is dependent upon the accurate identification of venous reflux patterns and the origin of the varicose veins. Ultrasonic scans are performed with the patient standing with the majority of weight on the contralateral limb. A color Doppler is used to locate the saphenofemoral and saphenopopliteal junctions. Compression maneuvers are performed to document the direction of flow in the saphenous and deep vessels. Incompetent greater and lesser saphenous veins are traced distally to identify incompetent perforating veins and truncal branches. Varices that do not appear to originate from the saphenous system are also scanned to identify their origin. Incompetent gastrocnemius veins are not uncommon and usually reflux into the lesser saphenous vein through the gastrocnemius point. Pretreatment mapping of varicosities and perforating veins has been shown to improve diagnostic accuracy and allow "minimal" treatment of varicose veins with excellent long-term results (33, 61).

A subpopulation of CVD patients includes those with more severe chronic problems manifested by severe pain and swelling or ulceration of the limbs. These patients are not greatly improved by varicose vein ablation and their symptoms may not be well-controlled with therapeutic stockings or attempted behavior modification. They are often candidates for venous valve reconstruction. Ultrasonic venography is used as a screening tool in these patients. Statistically, the majority of limbs have elements of both deep venous obstruction and reflux. Multilevel disease is easily identified by ultrasonic imaging. There is usually evidence of extensive calf vein segmental obstruction and multiple saphenous varicosities. The popliteal vein is variably involved with postthrombotic obstruction and reflux. The more proximal deep veins are often anatomically normal and femoral reflux is variably present. When ultrasonic venography identifies limbs with predominant venous reflux or predominant proximal venous obstruction, then more sophisticated hemodynamic tests and contrast venography may be indicated (62–64).

The high resolution capabilities of ultrasonic imaging systems today allow ready visualization of venous valves. Valve leaflets are easily seen and their function is determined using color and spectral Doppler. Ultrasonic venography can readily assess postoperative results of valvuloplasty, valve transplant, and venous bypass, thus obviating the need for contrast venography. Recently, Neglén and Raju compared descending contrast venography and Duplex imaging in patients with chronic venous insufficiency. Overall quantitative Duplex ultrasound appears to be a more sensitive method of detecting the degree and distribution of venous reflux than the "gold standard," descending contrast venography (20).

FUTURE CONSIDERATIONS

Ultrasonic venography has become the preferred tool for both venous research and clinical application. It is noninvasive, provides highly accurate anatomic information, and is uniquely suited to further elucidate pathophysiology of venous disease. New hardware and software configurations are being developed that will allow three-dimensional imaging of vessels and more accurate quantification of blood flow. Proponents of thrombolysis and surgical thrombectomy have been plagued by the inability to accurately age thrombus. This is important in order to decide which patients will benefit from lytic therapy. Results of surgical thrombectomy are poor when the thrombus is more than a week old. Fortunately, advances in imaging and computer technology are providing a method to perform tissue characterization. In the near future, exact aging of thrombus may be possible. Tissue characteristic determination may result in better patient selection and more effective lytic or surgical therapy. As ultrasound progresses into the 21st century, it will most likely complement magnetic resonance imaging and eliminate the need for the older invasive techniques.

REFERENCES

1. Anning ST. The historical aspects in the pathology and surgery of the veins of the lower extremity. Dodd H, Cockett FB, eds. London: Churchill Livingston, 1976:6–27.
2. Comerota AJ, Cranley JJ, Cook SE, Sipple P. Phleborheography—results of a 10-year experience. Surgery 1982;91:573–581.
3. Huisman MV, Buller HR, Wouter Ten Cate JV, Vreeken J. Serial impedance plethysmography for suspected deep venous thrombosis in outpatients: the Amsterdam general practitioner study. N Engl J Med 1986;314:823–828.
4. Hull RD, Hirsh J, Carter CJ, et al. Diagnostic efficacy of impedance plethysmography

for suspected deep vein thrombosis. A randomized trial. Ann Intern Med 1985;102:21–28.
5. Wheeler HB, Anderson FA Jr. The diagnosis of venous thrombosis by impedance plethysmography. In: Berstein EF, ed. Noninvasive diagnostic techniques in vascular disease. 3rd ed. St. Louis: CV Mosby Co., 1985:755.
6. Stallworth JM, Plonk GW, Horne JB. Negative phleborheography, clinical follow-up in 593 patients. Arch Surg 1981;116:795–797.
7. Flanagan LD, Sullivan ED, Cranley JJ. Venous imaging of the extremities using real-time B-mode ultrasound. In: Bergan JJ, Yao JST, eds. Surgery of the veins. Orlando, FL: Grune & Stratton, 1984:89–98.
8. Langsfeld M, Hershey FB, Thorpe L, et al. Duplex B-mode imaging for the diagnosis of deep venous thrombosis. Arch Surg 1987;122:587–591.
9. Hobbs JT. The enigma of the gastrocnemius vein. Phlebology 1988;3:19–30.
10. Neiman HL. Phlebography in the diagnosis of venous thrombosis. In: Bergan JJ, Yao JST, eds. Venous problems. Chicago: Year Book Medical Publishers, 1978;111–122.
11. Rollins DL, Semrow CM, Buchbinder D, et al. The use of ultrasonic venography in the evaluation of venous valve function. Am J Surg 1987;154:189–191.
12. Rollins DL, Semrow CM, Buchbinder D, et al. Diagnosis of recurrent deep venous thrombosis using B-mode ultrasonic imaging. Phlebology 1986;1:181–188.
13. Szendro G, Nicolaides AN, Zukowski AJ, et al. Duplex scanning in the assessment of deep venous incompetence. J Vasc Surg 1986;4:237–242.
14. Rollins DL, Semrow CM, Buchbinder D, et al. Progress in the diagnosis of deep venous thrombosis: the efficacy of real-time B-mode ultrasonic imaging. J Vasc Surg 1988;7:638–641.
15. Rollins DL, Semrow CM, Buchbinder D. The origin of deep vein thrombi in an ambulatory population. Am J Surg 1988;156:122–125.
16. Semrow CM, Friedell ML, Rollins DL. The efficacy of ultrasonic venography in the detection of calf vein thrombosis. J Vasc Tech 1988;12:240–244.
17. Semrow CM, Buchbinder D, Rollins DL, et al. Characterization of lower extremity venous disease using real-time B-mode ultrasonic imaging. J Vasc Tech 1987;6:189–191.
18. Van Bemmelen PS, Bedford G, Beach K, Strandness DE. Quantitative segmental evaluation of venous valvular reflux with duplex ultrasound scanning. J Vasc Surg 1989;10:424–431.
19. Van Bemmelen PS, Beach K, Bedford G, Strandness DE Jr. The mechanism of venous valve closure. Arch Surg 1990;125:617–619.
20. Neglén P, Raju S. A comparison between descending phlebography and duplex Doppler investigation in the evaluation of reflux in chronic venous insufficiency: a challenge to phlebography as the "gold standard." J Vasc Surg 1992;16:687–693.
21. Yucel EK, Fisher JS, Egglin TK, et al. Isolated calf vein thrombosis: diagnosis with compression US. Radiology 1991;179:443–446.
22. Krupski WC, Bass A, Dilley RB, Bernstein EF. Propagation of deep venous thrombosis identified by duplex ultrasonography. J Vasc Surg 1990;12:467–475.
23. Lensing AWA, Prandoni P, Brandjes D, et al. Detection of deep vein thrombosis by real-time B-mode ultrasonography. N Engl J Med 1989;320:342–345.
24. Persson AV, Jones C, Zide R, Jewell ER. Use of the triplex scanner in diagnosis of deep venous thrombosis. Arch Surg 1989;124:593–596.
25. Rose SC, Zwiebel WJ, Nelson BD, et al. Symptomatic lower extremity deep venous thrombosis: accuracy, limitations, and role of color duplex flow imaging in diagnosis. Radiology 1990;175:639–644.
26. Mattos MA, Londry GL, Leutz DW, et al. Color-flow duplex scanning for the surveillance and diagnosis of acute deep venous thrombosis. J Vasc Surg 1992;1:366–376.
27. Polak JF, Cutler SS, O'Leary OH. Deep veins of the calf: assessment with color Doppler flow imaging. Radiology 1989;171:481–485.

28. Manjoni M. Deep venous thrombosis: Longitudinal study with Duplex US. Radiology 1991;179:271–273.
29. Mussurakis S, Papaioannou S, Vorus D, Vrakatselis T. Compression ultrasonography as a reliable imaging monitor in deep venous thrombosis. Surg Gynec Obstet 1990;171:233–239.
30. Vaccaro JP, Cronan J, Dorfman GS. Outcome analysis of patients with normal compression US examination. Radiology 1990;175:644–649.
31. Markel A, Manzo RA, Bergelin RO, Strandness DE. Pattern and distribution of thrombus in acute venous thrombosis. Arch Surg 1991;127:305–309.
32. Semrow CS, Laborde A, Buchbinder D, Rollins DL. Preoperative mapping of varicosities and perforating veins: a preliminary report. J Vasc Tech 1990;14:72–74.
33. Sarin S, Scurr JH, Coleridge-Smith P. Medial calf perforators in venous disease: the significance of outward flow. J Vasc Surg 1992;16:40–46.
34. Taylor KJW. Ultrasonic investigation of inferior vena-caval obstruction. Br J Radiol 1975;48:1024–1026.
35. Effeny DJ, Friedman MB, Gooding GAW. Iliofemoral venous thrombosis: real-time ultrasound diagnosis, normal criteria and clinical application. Radiology 1984;150: 787–792.
36. Park HJ, Lee JB, Han MC, et al. Sonographic evaluation of inferior vena caval obstruction: correlative study with vena cavography. AJR 1985;145:757–762.
37. Sigel B, Machi J, Beitler JC, et al. Red cell aggregation as a cause of blood flow echogenicity. Radiology 1983;148:799–802.
38. Machi J, Sigel B, Beitler JC, et al. Relation of in vitro blood flow to ultrasound echogenicity. Radiology 1983;148:807–811.
39. Baxter GM, Duffy P, MacKechnie S. Colour Doppler ultrasound of the post-phlebitic limb: sounding a cautionary note. Clin Radiol 1991;43:301–304.
40. Wright DJ, Shepard AD, McPharlin M, Ernest CB. Pitfalls in lower extremity venous duplex scanning. J Vasc Surg 1990;11:675–679.
41. Killewich LA, Bedford GR, Beach KW, Strandness DE. Diagnosis of deep venous thrombosis: a prospective study comparing duplex scanning to contrast venography. Circulation 1989;79:810–814.
42. Flinn WR, Sandager GP, Cerrullo LJ, et al. Duplex venous scanning for the prospective surveillance of perioperative venous thrombosis. Arch Surg 1989;124:901–905.
43. Paiement GD, Wessinger SJ, Harris WH. Survey of prophylaxis against venous thromboembolism in adults undergoing hip surgery. Clin Orthop 1987;223:188–193.
44. Froehlich JA, Dorfman GS, Cronan JG, et al. Compression ultrasonography for the detection of deep venous thrombosis in patients who have a fracture of the hip. J Bone Joint Surg 1989;71A:249–256.
45. Stulberg BN, Insall JN, Williams GW, Ghelman B. Deep-vein thrombosis following total knee replacement. An analysis of six hundred and thirty-eight arthroplasties. J Bone Joint Surg 1984;66A:194–199.
46. Barnes CL, Nelson CL, Nix ML, Barnes RW, et al. Duplex scanning versus venography as a screening examination in total hip arthroplasty patients. Clin Orthop 1991;271:180–189.
47. Nix ML, Nelson CL, Ferris EM, Barnes RW. Duplex venous scanning: image versus Doppler accuracy. J Vasc Tech 1989;8:121–124.
48. Woolson ST, McCrory DM, Walter J, Cahill PD, et al. B-mode ultrasound scanning in the detection of proximal venous thrombosis after total hip replacement. J Bone Joint Surg 1990;72A:983–987.
49. Albertyn LE, Alcook MK. Diagnosis of internal jugular thrombosis. Radiology 1987;162:505–508.
50. Falk RL, Smith DF. Thrombosis of upper extremity thoracic inlet veins: diagnosis with duplex Doppler sonography. Am J Radiol 1989;149:677–682.

51. Wing G, Scheible W. Sonography of jugular vein thrombosis. Am J Radiol 1983;140:333–336.
52. Gooding GAW, Hightower DR, Moore EH, et al. Sonographic diagnosis of obstruction of the superior vena cava or subclavian veins. Radiology 1986;160:663–665.
53. Didier D, Racle A, Etienent JP, Weill F. Tumor thrombus of the inferior vena cava secondary to malignant abdominal neoplasms: US and CT evaluation. Radiology 1989;162:83–89.
54. Wingo JP, McDorwon-Perry JE, Nix ML, Greenfield LJ. Duplex evaluation of inferior vena cava patency: a prospective study of patients with the Greenfield filter. J Vasc Tech 1987;11:167–171.
55. Brown B, Weilemann LS, Weigand W. Ultrasonographic demonstration of renal vein thrombosis. Ultrasound 1991;14:157–159.
56. Ruoff BA, Cranley JJ, Hannan LA, et al. Real-time duplex ultrasound mapping of the greater saphenous vein before in situ infrainguinal revascularization. J Vasc Surg 1987;6:107–113.
57. Leopold PW, Shah DM, Leather RP, Karmody AM, et al. Initial experience comparing B-mode imaging and venography of the saphenous vein before in situ bypass. Am J Surg 1986;152:206–210.
58. Buchbinder DW, Semrow CM, Friedell ML, et al. B-mode ultrasonic imaging in the preoperative evaluation of the saphenous veins. Am Surgeon 1987;53:368–371.
59. Seeger JM, Schmidt JH, Flynn JC. Preoperative saphenous and cephalic vein mapping as an adjunct to reconstructive arterial surgery. Ann Surg 1987;205:733–739.
60. Katz ML, Comerota AJ, White JV, et al. B-mode imaging to determine the suitability of arm veins for primary arteriovenous fistulas. J Vasc Tech 1987;11:172–174.
61. Semrow CM, Laborde A, Buchbinder D, Rollins DL. Preoperative mapping of varicosities and perforating veins: a preliminary report. J Vasc Tech 1990;14:72–74.
62. Christopoulos D, Nicolaides AN, Irvine A, et al. Pathogenesis of venous ulceration in relation to the calf muscle pump. J Vasc Surg 1989;5:829–835.
63. Raju S, Fredericks R. Evaluation of methods for detecting venous reflux. Arch Surg 1990;125:1463–1467.
64. Raju S. New approaches to the diagnosis and treatment of venous obstruction. J Vasc Surg 1986;4:42–54.

chapter 4

Functional Duplex Evaluation of Chronic Venous Obstruction and Incompetence

Paul S. van Bemmelen

The evolution of duplex examination for chronic venous disorders is progressing from a supine to a standing position. This chapter is concerned with functional duplex tests with rapid inflation/deflation cuffs, which can only be performed in ambulatory patients who are suffering from chronic venous problems and who are suspected to harbor fresh thrombi. The test should not be performed in patients who are suspected of acute venous thrombosis. These patients are often bedridden, and inflation of pneumatic cuffs placed around a tender, swollen leg is not only painful but could carry a risk of causing pulmonary embolism.

History and physical examination remain important for the initial assessment of chronic venous patients, but it is not possible to predict the anatomic localization of obstruction or valve incompetence based on a history of deep venous thrombosis alone. In many of these patients, visible varicosities represent the tip of an iceberg, which is not amenable to clinical examination. Therefore, a complete duplex evaluation of both the deep and superficial veins is recommended.

PROCEDURE

The patient is examined in the standing position. The reflux test maneuver has been standardized with pneumatic cuffs. Rapid inflation and deflation is assured by an automatic cuff-inflator with an air source (1). Other authors have adopted this method with distal cuff deflation at multiple levels of the leg as well (2). The importance of a standing position for testing valve incompetence was reemphasized in a study comparing supine versus standing test results: approximately 71% of the incompetent areas would have been missed in the supine patient position (3).

The duplex imaging probe is directed at the confluence of the common femoral vein and greater saphenous vein in the groin. After a large cuff (24-cm width) around the thigh has been inflated to 80 mmHg for 3 seconds, reflux is measured during rapid deflation of the cuff. The sample volume is placed in the common femoral vein, the greater saphenous vein, and the proximal superficial femoral vein, respectively. Normal reflux during closure of competent valves does not exceed 0.45 seconds in duration. With the use of the color flow scanner, reflux is evident as persistent flow, depicted in the color of the retrograde flow direction instead of absence of color during cuff deflation.

The test for the evaluation of outflow obstruction is best performed at this point in the procedure. This test consists of rapid inflation, to 100 mmHg, of the large cuff applied to the calf (Fig. 4.1): if the antegrade velocity in the proximal superficial femoral vein (SFV) reaches 143 ± 29 cm/sec, a significant obstruction in the popliteal-SFV segments is unlikely (4) (Fig. 4.2). This addition to the technique takes only a few minutes to perform and helps to categorize patients with primary varicose veins versus those with secondary varicose veins. If this test shows a decreased velocity (i.e., <143 cm/sec), this usually signifies obstruction of the superficial femoral vein (Fig. 4.3).

The popliteal fossa is examined next with a cuff below the knee. After inflation of the (12-cm) cuff for 3 seconds to 100 mmHg the reflux in the popliteal vein and lesser saphenous vein are measured during deflation of the cuff. The point of entrance of an incompetent lesser saphenous vein is highly variable and must be accurately localized. Atypical termination of the lesser saphenous vein into the greater saphenous vein has been described, as well as high termination into the superficial femoral vein or profunda vein (5). Continuation of the lesser saphe-

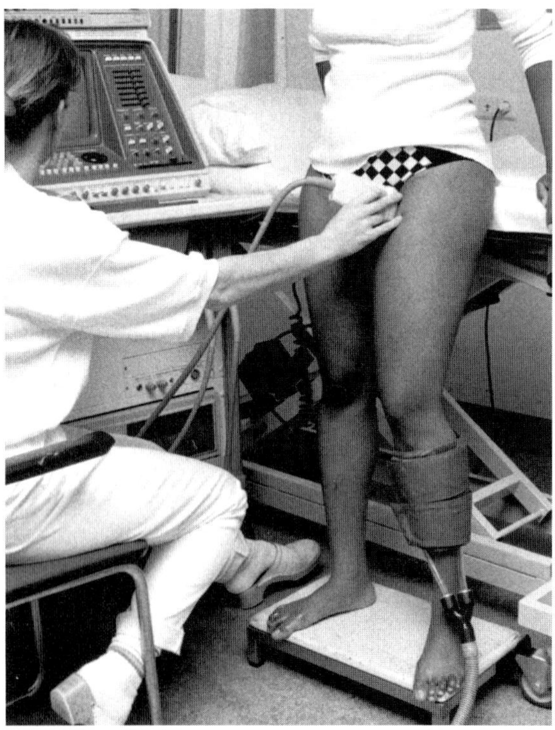

FIG. 4–1. Test for deep outflow obstruction. A large (24-cm) cuff is placed around the calf and rapidly inflated to 100 mmHg. The Doppler sample volume is placed in the proximal superficial femoral vein. Antegrade velocity is measured during cuff inflation.

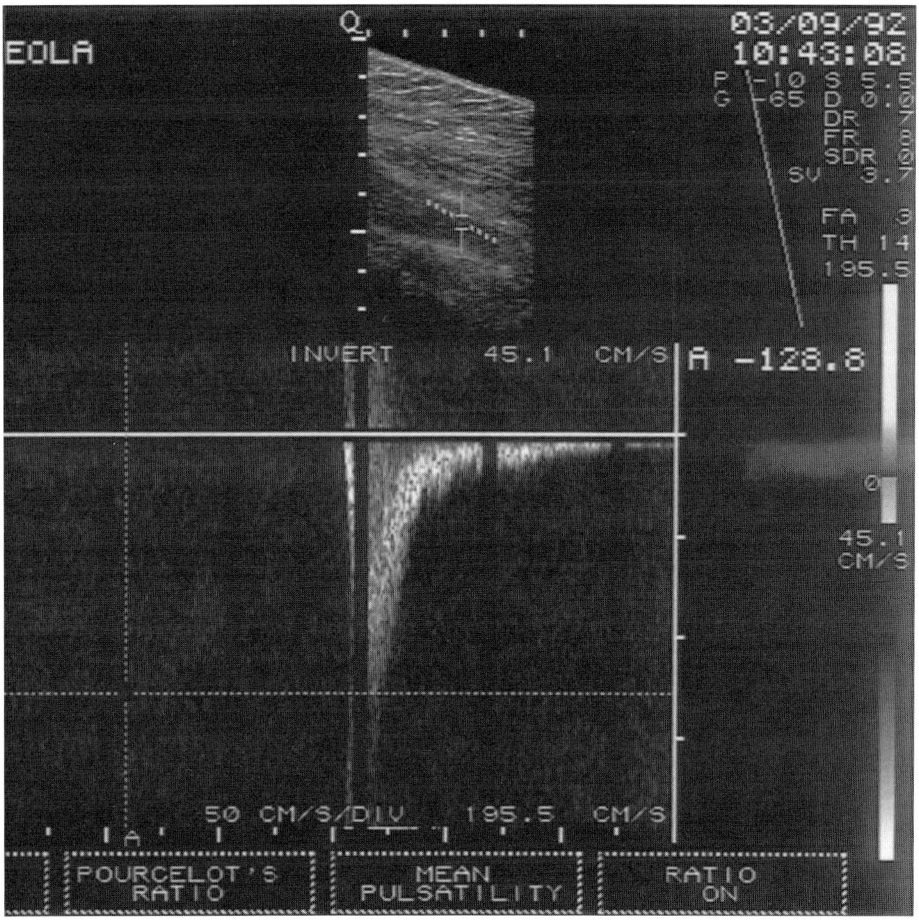

FIG. 4–2. Outflow velocity in a normal volunteer: peak velocity of 129 cm/sec flow toward the heart depicted in the negative direction.

nous vein in the thigh is common. Multiple connections of the lesser saphenous vein to both gastrocnemic and popliteal veins are possible as well. The medial side of the knee is examined for the greater saphenous vein and additional accessory veins. It is possible to calculate the reflux volume flow, using the diameter of the incompetent veins and the time averaged reflux velocity (6, 7). In spite of previous stripping operations or sclerotherapy, incompetent veins are frequently present on the medial side of the knee. After a previous stripping operation the recurrent or accessory saphenous vein can remain present as a straight vein. In other cases, the greater saphenous vein is replaced by a conglomerate of convoluted veins, in which it is impossible to identify the flow direction. The anterolateral branch of the greater saphenous vein can be identified only if significant dilatation has occurred. Scanning the anterolateral aspect of the thigh near the patella yielded incompetent anterolateral branches in 20% of 151 referred patient legs (8).

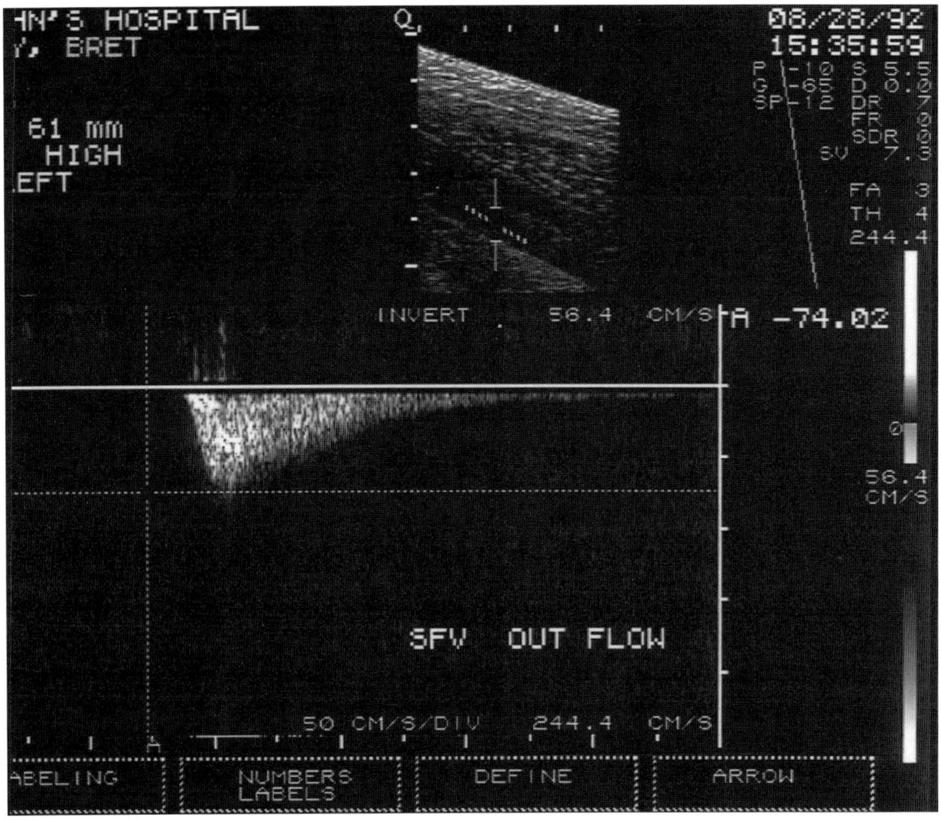

FIG. 4–3. Patient with leg ulcer and old obstruction of the superficial femoral vein. Peak velocity in proximal superficial femoral vein reaches only 74 cm/sec.

The calf level is examined with the 12-cm cuff around the ankle (100 mmHg). The greater saphenous vein often consists of two branches at this level. Evaluation of the deep calf veins including the peroneal veins is facilitated by color imaging (9). Incompetent posterior tibial veins in the calf are shown in Figure 4.4. The lesser saphenous vein can be identified at the mid calf level by its straight and deep course in the posterior midline. Reflux of this segment of the lesser saphenous vein can occur without concomitant incompetence of the proximal part of the same vein.

The ankle level is examined with a small 7-cm width cuff placed around the foot with an inflation pressure of 120 mmHg. The posterior tibial veins are easily located behind the posterior malleolus, next to the artery. The greater saphenous vein can be interrogated at its premalleolar site, unless previous surgery has been done. Ventral branches of the greater saphenous vein can be identified in the pretibial area in 13%. Further imaging of the posterior arch veins and gaiter area can be done in cases with stasis ulceration. The status of the superficial veins in association as the deep insufficiency is important in chronic venous insufficiency and ulceration (10, 11). A detailed search of the gaiter area for incompetent perforating veins has been described (12), but the hemodynamic significance of small perforating veins near the ankle is unclear.

DISTRIBUTION OF INCOMPETENT AREAS IN SYMPTOMATIC LEGS

Most veins were found to be only partially involved with incompetence. Even though the involved segment is completely afunctional with regard to valve function, the same vein can be normal at a more distal or proximal location. The distribution of superficial incompetent segments in the 140 legs that had superficial incompetence was as follows: the most frequently involved segment was the greater saphenous vein (or its recurrence after removal) at the knee level (61%). This was followed by greater saphenous incompetence at the calf level (49%). The proximal segment of the greater saphenous vein at the thigh level was incompetent in 32%, again demonstrating the occurrence of distal incompetence, while the proximal part of the same vein was competent. The anterolateral branch of the

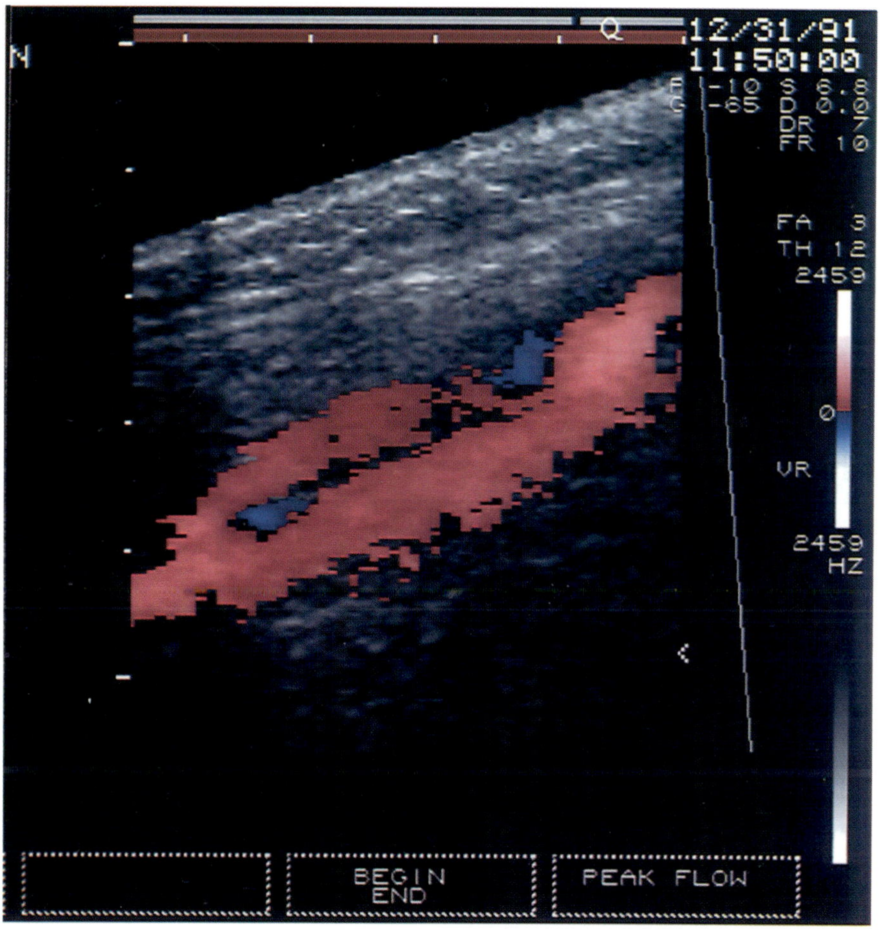

FIG. 4–4. Incompetence of deep calf veins. A 12-cm width cuff was placed around the ankle. After inflation of the cuff to 100 mmHg the cuff was rapidly deflated. Retrograde flow in posterior tibial veins is depicted in *red*. Head of the patient is to the *left*.

greater saphenous vein was incompetent in 21%, and the pretibial branches near the ankle were incompetent in 14%. The segmental involvement of the lesser and greater saphenous veins is considered next in more detail.

LESSER SAPHENOUS VEIN

Incompetence of the lesser saphenous vein is also frequently segmental: the proximal half was incompetent in 36%, while the distal half was incompetent in 31%. In 52% of affected lesser saphenous veins, the incompetence was limited to only one segment. If the distal half of the lesser saphenous remains normal (26%), the reflux from the incompetent proximal part is diverted to superficial branches. When the proximal part of the lesser saphenous is normal (21%), the reflux of the distal segment is often fed by a connecting branch from the greater saphenous system.

GREATER SAPHENOUS VEIN

The varicose greater saphenous vein shows dilatation in the thigh and upper part of the lower leg, without tortuosity, as described by previous cast studies (13). Tortuosity is usually more a feature of varicose tributaries, which can overlie the main trunk of the greater saphenous vein. When 86 cases with incompetence of the greater saphenous vein at the knee level were analyzed, less than half had contiguous incompetence from its origin in the groin down to the knee. Of those with incompetence of the distal greater saphenous vein at knee level and normal proximal segment, 34% had incompetence of deep veins (SFV-popliteal veins). In such cases, an incompetent deep to superficial perforating vein can often be identified at the upper end of the incompetent greater saphenous segment.

CLASSIFICATION

For the purpose of classification and stratification of patients, a system of levels (8) can be used: thigh, knee, calf, and ankle. The maximum number of incompetent levels is four. The numbers of incompetent levels in 151 legs referred to the vascular laboratory for evaluation (26% of the patients had undergone previous vein surgery) were as follows: 9% of the 151 legs referred with venous symptoms had a total incompetence involving all four levels of either deep or superficial veins; 35% had three-level disease; 26% had two-level disease; 23% had one-level disease; and 8% had zero levels involved. This latter finding of normal veins is to be expected when patients are selected on the basis of their complaints and have not been excluded on the basis of normal physical findings or venograms.

RELATION BETWEEN DEEP AND SUPERFICIAL INCOMPETENCE

The association of incompetence of a deep segment with the contiguous superficial segment is a frequent finding. Incompetence of the common femoral vein (CFV) in legs with incompetence of the proximal greater saphenous vein (GSV) is probably a predisposing factor, but it could be congenital and is not necessarily a result of previous thrombosis in the CFV. In several studies (10, 14), incompetence of the CFV was previously noted in approximately 70% of legs, with primary varicose veins involving the proximal greater saphenous vein. Even though saphenofemoral incompetence is frequently suspected in clinical practice, duplex confirmation is essential. Clinical impressions are frequently false. This has important implications for the chances of success with simple saphenous ligation: if there is no saphenofemoral incompetence to begin with, hemodynamics will be unchanged after simple ligation of the proximal greater saphenous vein.

In 66 cases in which either the popliteal vein or the lesser saphenous vein, or both, were affected, the distribution of incompetence was as follows: 30 cases of combined incompetence, 20 of isolated lesser saphenous incompetence, and 16 cases of isolated popliteal vein incompetence.

VEIN DIAMETER AND VALVE FUNCTION

The diameters of the incompetent veins have considerable variability: for the incompetent lesser saphenous veins, diameters ranged from 2–12 mm, mean 6.2 ± 2.8 mm. For the incompetent greater saphenous veins, diameters ranged between 2 and 19 mm measured at the knee level. Mean diameter was 5.5 ± 2.7 mm. No normal values for diameter of these veins are available in standing subjects, but considerable overlap in diameters between "normal" and incompetent veins is to be expected. This would indicate the futility of attempting to predict competence solely on the basis of a small diameter.

DISCUSSION

There is controversy in the literature regarding the importance of superficial venous incompetence in the pathophysiology of serious venous stasis problems such as ulceration. Classic studies with venous pressure measurement led to the widely accepted view that deep vein incompetence is responsible for ulceration, while superficial incompetence is related to cosmetic, minor problems. The gold standard, venous pressure, has been criticized for the use of tourniquets which are unreliable in their occlusive effect on superficial veins (15). Increasing utilization of duplex instruments will allow an accurate evaluation of the relative roles of superficial and deep incompetence in the pathophysiology of venous ulceration (10, 12).

Recognizing the clinical importance of incompetence of the lesser saphenous vein in chronic venous insufficiency is a major step toward correct treatment. Lesser saphenous vein incompetence was noted in no less than 41% of all legs referred to the vascular laboratory for venous evaluation. Previous literature regarding the anatomy of the lesser saphenous vein (16) has led to the misconception that this vein, owing to its more muscular wall and the presence of more valves, would be resistant to primary varicose degeneration. Ludbrook (17) suggested that lesser saphenous incompetence is seen only when the (deep) popliteal vein is incompetent; this is contradicted by our data. Furthermore, incompetence of the lesser saphenous was commonly seen in our material, but less than half the incompetent lesser saphenous veins were incompetent throughout. This fact has implications for reducing the extent of the operative removal of the lesser saphenous vein, which has the potential to lessen the chance of damage to the adjacent sural nerve.

Accurate localization and mapping of recurrent varicose veins after stripping of the greater saphenous vein is important for treatment. The duplex instrument is best suited for the task. When a patient presents with recurrent symptoms after previous stripping, it is necessary to investigate whether these complaints are due to deep reflux or recurrent superficial incompetence involving the knee/calf portions of the greater saphenous vein and the lesser saphenous vein. Appreciation of the frequent presence of incompetent accessory branches of the superficial system is important as well. Since the reflux in these treatable, superficial veins is probably additive to reflux existing in deep veins, their eradication is probably beneficial in the presence of deep incompetence as well, provided there is no obstruction to deep outflow.

In conclusion, functional as well as segmental duplex scanning has rapidly become the main diagnostic tool in a wide variety of venous disorders including varicose veins, recurrent varicose veins after previous surgery, ulceration of the gaiter area, and serious venous stasis complaints with or without induration of the subcutis. In these situations, segmental duplex examination provides a systematic approach to the evaluation and classification of the multiple combinations of incompetent or obstructed parts of the venous system.

REFERENCES

1. van Bemmelen PS, Bedford G, Beach K, Strandness DE. Quantitative segmental evaluation of venous valvular reflux with duplex ultrasound scanning. J Vasc Surg 1989;10:425–431.
2. Czeredarzuk M, Branas CC, Weingarten MS. Duplex imaging and distal cuff deflation to measure venous reflux time. J Vasc Tech 1991;15:196–208.
3. Foldes MS, Blackburn MC, Hogan J, et al. Standing versus supine positioning in venous reflux evaluation. J Vasc Tech 1991;15:321–324.
4. van Bemmelen PS, Bedford G, Beach K, Strandness DE. Functional status of the deep venous system after an episode of deep venous thrombosis. Ann Vasc Surg 1990;5:455–459.
5. Franco G, Nguyen Khac G, Nguyen Morere MC. Interet de l'echo-Doppler de la saphene externe. Confrontation clinique. Phlebologie 1990;43:135–145.
6. Vasdekis SN, Clarke GH, Nicolaides AN. Quantification of venous reflux by means of duplex scanning. J Vasc Surg 1989;10:670–677.
7. Bergan JJ, Beeman S, Poppiti R. Quantitative segmental evaluation of venous valve reflux: impact on clinical practice. V European-American symposium on venous diseases. Vienna, Nov. 7–10, 1990.
8. van Bemmelen PS, Mattos MA, Hodgson KJ, et al. Does air plethysmography correlate with duplex scanning in patients with chronic venous insufficiency? J Vasc Surg 1993;18:796.
9. van Bemmelen PS, Bedford G, Strandness DE. Visualization of calf veins by color flow imaging. Ultrasound Med Biol 1990;16:15–17.
10. van Bemmelen PS, Bedford G, Beach K, Strandness DE. Status of the valves in the superficial and deep venous system in chronic venous disease. Surgery 1991;109:730–734.

11. Hanrahan LM, Araki CT, Rodriguez AA, Kechejian GJ, Lamorte WW, Menzoian JO. Distribution of valvular incompetence in patients with stasis ulceration. J Vasc Surg 1991;13:805–812.
12. Hanrahan LM, Araki CT, Fisher JB, et al. Evaluation of the perforating veins of the lower extremity using high resolution duplex imaging. J Cardiovasc Surg 1991;32:87–97.
13. Cotton LT. Varicose veins, gross anatomy and development. Br J Surg 1961;48:589–598.
14. Folse R. The influence of femoral vein dynamics on the development of varicose veins. Surgery 1970;68:974–979.
15. McMullin GM, Coleridge Smith PD, Scurr JH. A study of tourniquets in the investigation of venous insufficiency. Phlebology 1991;6:133–139.
16. Marinov G. Some differences between the long and short saphenous veins as regards the structure and vascularization of the wall and location of the valves. Folia Morphol 1976;24:221–224.
17. Ludbrook J, Jamieson GG. Disorders of systemic veins. In: Sabiston DC, ed. Davis-Christopher textbook of surgery. Philadelphia: WB Saunders Co., 1977:1819–1840.

chapter 5

Air Plethysmography

D. Christopoulos and A.N. Nicolaides

The physician who is often confronted with painful, swollen, or ulcerated legs must first determine the existence of a venous problem and, secondly, must decide whether the venous disease involves the superficial or deep veins. The third task is to determine whether the problem is the result of outflow obstruction, reflux, or both. More detailed and quantitative information is required to determine the prognosis and develop a rational plan of management. Air plethysmography has become increasingly valuable in providing answers to these questions by supplementing the history and clinical examination.

Chronic swelling, lipodermatosclerosis, pigmentation, or ulceration of the lower limb due to chronic venous disease affect a considerable number of patients. In the United Kingdom, half a million people may be affected by this disease with 150,000 suffering from ulceration (1, 2). The British health service spends an estimated 100 to 200 million dollars per year on treatment. In recent years, this social problem has stimulated the evolution of surgery of superficial as well as deep veins, aiming to correct valvular incompetence and overcome venous obstruction. However, the absence of a satisfactory objective and quantitative method for the correct selection of patients and the evaluation of the results of these operations explains why surgery of the deep veins is still at an experimental stage.

Although venography and ambulatory venous pressure measurements (8) are established venous investigations, they are invasive, expensive, and time-consuming. Also, information provided is incomplete: venography shows mainly anatomy. Ambulatory pressure measurements provide a measure of the overall severity of venous disease but fail to provide enough information to determine how much of the problem is the result of venous reflux, venous obstruction, or reduction of the ejection capacity of the calf muscle pump. In recent years, noninvasive techniques have attempted to replace the above methods. Although photoplethysmography (9) has provided indirect and qualitative information to distinguish normal limbs from limbs with superficial and/or deep venous disease, venography was still necessary in serious cases because photoplethysmography could not provide a measure of the severity of deep venous disease (10) (Fig. 5.1).

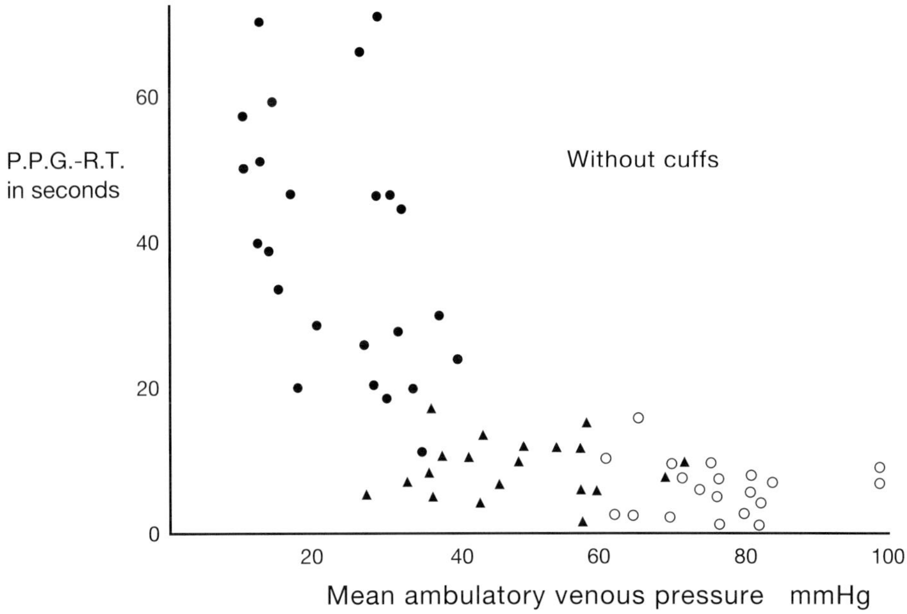

FIG. 5–1. Correlation between ambulatory venous pressure measurement (AVP) and photoplethysmography 90% recovery time (RT90). Note that for AVP ranging between 45 and 80 mmHg, the PPG 90% RT remains in the same abnormal range 1–5 sec (10).

Strain gauge plethysmography (11–13), although quantitative, provided information on a segment not necessarily representative of the whole leg (14). This test was difficult to use during changes in posture and exercise because tissue shifts interfered with the measurements (15).

Doppler ultrasound (16) and duplex scanning (17) proved to be valuable tools in the detection of reflux and obstruction in individual veins. However, the results were operator-dependent and did not provide information on the severity of outflow obstruction or the efficacy of collateral circulation.

To overcome the problems of segmental devices, air plethysmography, used experimentally in the past (18,19), has been developed recently for clinical use with the aim of replacing venography and ambulatory venous pressure measurements in the assessment of complicated cases (20). As a result, this noninvasive technique can provide quantitative information on the amount of venous reflux (21), the degree of venous obstruction (22), and the ejection capacity of the calf muscle pump (23).

AIR PLETHYSMOGRAPH AND ITS CALIBRATION

The air plethysmograph (APG) consists of a 35-cm long polyurethane air chamber (5 liters capacity) which surrounds the whole leg, connected to a pressure transducer, amplifier, and recorder (Fig. 5.2). The patient is placed in the supine position with the knee of the examined leg slightly flexed and the heel on a support; the air chamber is inflated to 6 mmHg.

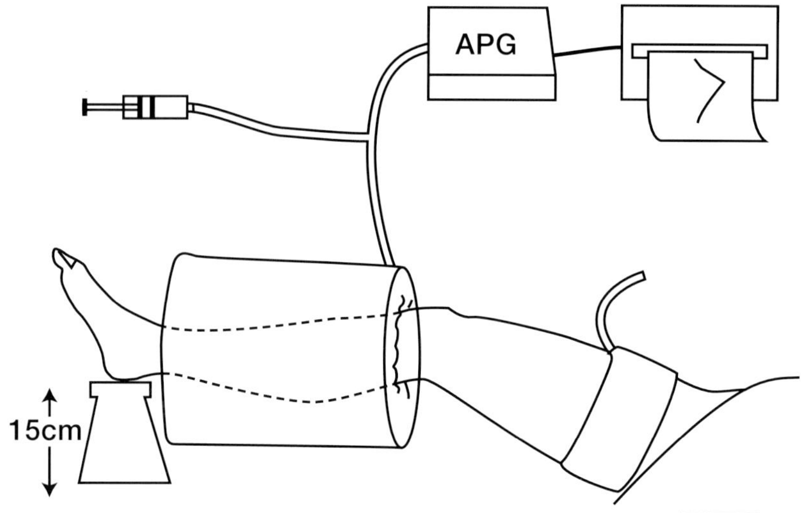

FIG. 5–2. The air-plethysmograph (*APG*) consists of an air chamber that surrounds the whole leg, the calibration syringe connected to a pressure transducer, amplifier, and recorder. Note the position of the occluding tourniquet for venous occlusion.

Calibration is performed by depressing the plunger of the syringe (Fig. 5.2), compressing the air included in the air plethysmograph (air chamber and tubing), reducing its volume by 100 ml, and observing the corresponding pressure change. After calibration the plunger is pulled back to its original position when the pressure in the air chamber returns to 6 mmHg. The pressure of 6 mmHg has been selected because it is the lowest pressure that ensures good contact between the air chamber and the limb with minimum compression of the veins. Tissue movements during changes in posture and exercise are unlikely to interfere with the measurements because the air chamber includes almost all the tissues from the knee to the ankle. The air plethysmograph is calibrated in milliliters, so that consecutive measurements in the same limb are not influenced by changes in tissue volume due to increase or decrease of edema.

EVALUATION OF VENOUS OUTFLOW

With the patient in the supine position, an 11-cm wide pneumatic tourniquet is placed around the proximal part of the thigh and inflated to 80 mmHg (Fig. 5.2). There is an increase in volume (Fig. 5.3). When a plateau is reached, the tourniquet is suddenly deflated. The observed rapid decrease in volume is a result of venous outflow. The ratio of the amount of blood that leaves the leg in the first second (V1) to the total venous volume (TVV), times 100, is the outflow fraction (OF) expressed as a percentage. The procedure is repeated with the long saphenous and/or other prominent superficial veins occluded by finger compression.

In limbs with normal deep veins, the outflow fraction is higher than 40% (range 40–70%) (22) (Fig. 5.4). Limbs with chronic deep venous obstruction on venogra-

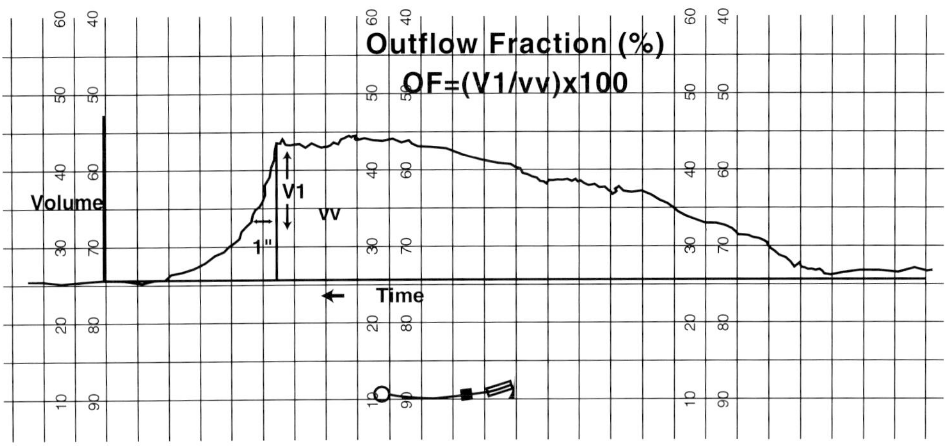

FIG. 5–3. Typical recording of venous occlusion air plethysmography. Low chart paper speed has been used during the filling phase (6 cm/min) and high during the outflow phase (60 cm/min). The outflow fraction (*OF*) is derived from OF = (V1/VV) × 100.

phy have an OF ranging from 15–38%, which is reduced further after occlusion of the superficial veins. This maneuver not only assists in the diagnosis of obstruction in borderline cases but also shows whether any dilated superficial veins are important collateral channels bypassing the obstruction, which the surgeon should not ligate.

The outflow fraction (OF) measurements correlate well with invasive quantification of the severity of venous obstruction, obtained by measuring the arm/foot pressure differential with cannulation of a vein in the arm and a vein in the foot when the patient is in the supine position (Fig. 5.5) (7,20). For practical purposes, we have considered that there is no functional venous obstruction for OF greater than 40%, moderate obstruction for OF 30–39%, and severe obstruction for OF less than 30%.

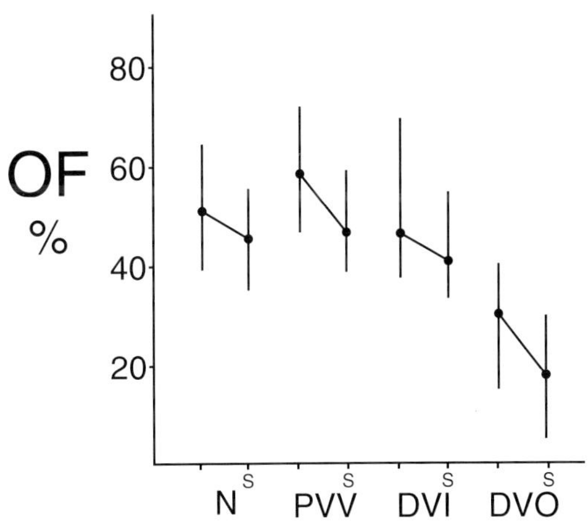

FIG. 5–4. Measurement of the outflow fraction (*OF*) in five groups of limbs, presented as median and 95% range(26) before and after occlusion of the superficial veins (S). *N* = normal limbs; *PVV* = limbs with primary varicose veins; *DVI* = limbs with deep venous incompetence, without obstruction; *DVO* = limbs with deep venous obstruction with or without incompetence.

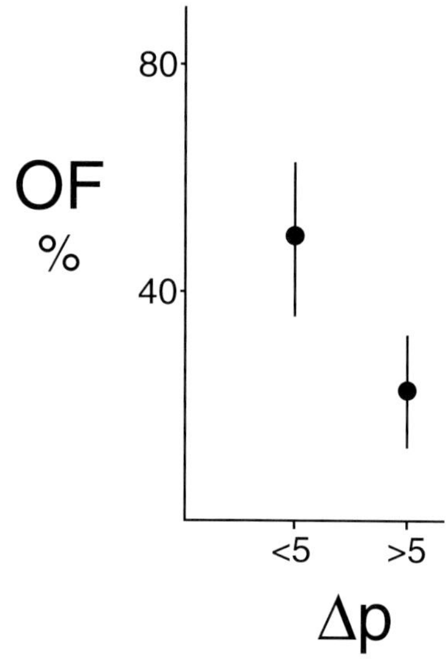

FIG. 5–5. Outflow fraction (*OF*) (median and 90% range) in 15 limbs with deep venous reflux but no obstruction (arm/foot pressure differential $p < 5$ mmHg) and eight limbs with venographic deep venous obstruction ($p > 5$ mmHg).

EVALUATION OF VENOUS REFLUX

With the patient in the supine position and the air chamber of the APG inflated to 6 mmHg, the examined limb is elevated (45°) to empty the veins. The patient is then asked to stand, with the weight mainly on the opposite limb. The observed increase in volume is a result of venous filling (Fig. 5.6). The functional venous volume (VV) ranges from 100–150 ml in normal limbs and up to 350 ml in limbs with venous diseases (Fig. 5.6**A**) (18, 21). The ratio of 90% of VV divided by the time required for 90% filling (VFT90) is defined as the venous filling index ((VFI) = 90% VV/VFT90) (Fig. 5.7). This is a measure of the average filling rate of the veins expressed in ml/sec. VFI is less than 2 ml/sec in normal limbs, which fill slowly from the arterial circulation. It is increased up to 30 ml/sec in limbs with venous reflux (Fig. 5.7). In limbs without outflow obstruction on venography, the incidence of ulceration increases with increasing values of VFI: i.e., zero for VFI less than 5 ml/sec, 46% for VFI 5–10 ml/sec, and 58% for VFI greater than 10 ml/sec, regardless of whether reflux is in superficial or deep veins (21).

The measurement of VFI can be repeated after abolition of reflux in the superficial veins at the level of the knee, by using narrow tourniquets or finger compression. VFI is reduced to less than 5 ml/sec in limbs with primary varicose veins and competent deep venous valves but not in limbs with reflux in the popliteal vein (24). Abolition of venous reflux has also been demonstrated after conventional surgery for superficial venous incompetence (25).

EVALUATION OF THE EJECTION CAPACITY OF THE CALF MUSCLE PUMP

The amount of blood ejected as a result of a single calf muscle contraction can be quantified by measuring the decrease in volume produced after a single tiptoe movement (Fig. 5.6**C**). The ejection volume (EV) is about 100 ml in

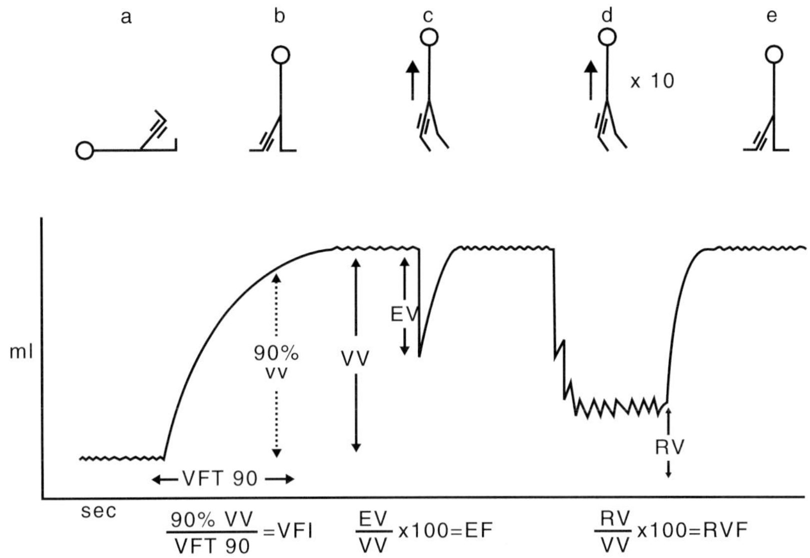

FIG. 5–6. Diagrammatic representation of a typical recording of volume changes during standard sequence of postural changes and exercise: **A.** Patient in supine position with leg elevated 45°; **B.** Patient standing with weight on nonexamined leg; **C.** Single tiptoe movement; **D.** Ten tiptoe movements; **E.** Return to resting standing position as in B. *VV* = functional venous volume; *VFT* = venous filling time; *VFI* = venous filling index; *EV* = ejected volume; *RV* = residual volume; *EF* = ejection fraction; *RVF* = residual volume fraction.

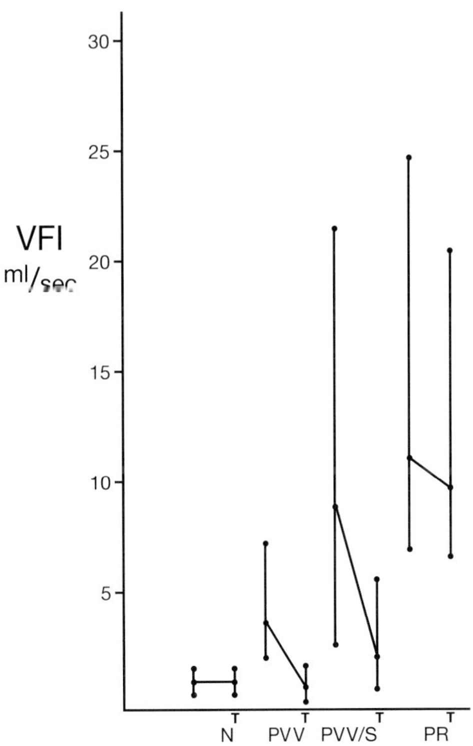

FIG. 5–7. Venous filling index (*VFI*) (median and 90% range) with and without a tourniquet (*T*) that occluded the superficial veins at the knee in normal limbs (*N*), limbs with primary varicose veins (*PVV*) and no sequelae of chronic venous disease (liposclerosis and ulceration), primary varicose veins with sequelae of chronic venous disease (*PVV/S*), and limbs with popliteal reflux (*PR*).

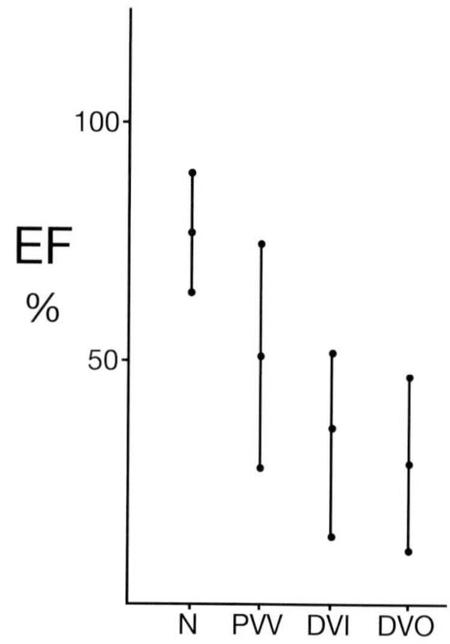

FIG. 5–8. Ejection fraction (*EF*) (median and 90% range) in normal (*N*) limbs, limbs with primary varicose veins (*PVV*), limbs with deep venous insufficiency (*DVI*), and limbs with deep venous obstruction (*DVO*).

normal limbs and also in the majority of limbs with primary varicose veins. Limbs with deep venous disease eject less (down to 20 ml) because of obstruction of the deep veins or retrograde ejection via incompetent perforating veins (20, 23).

The ejection fraction (EF) of the calf muscle pump is derived from EF = (EV/VV) × 100. The EF is more than 60% in normal limbs and down to 10% in limbs with deep venous obstruction (Fig. 5.8). The incidence of venous ulceration is also related to the EF. As shown in Figure 5.9, a poor EF was the primary cause of venous ulceration in limbs with minimal reflux. A good ejection fraction, however, significantly reduced the incidence of ulceration in limbs with marked reflux.

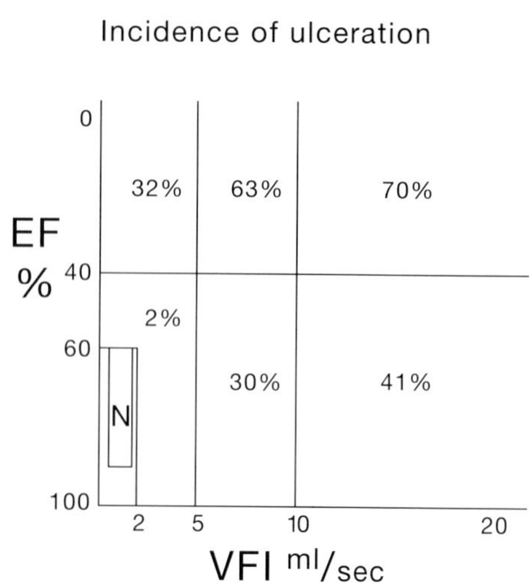

FIG. 5–9. The incidence of leg ulceration in relation to the venous filling index (*VFI*) and the ejection fraction (*EF*) of the calf muscle pump in 175 limbs with venous problems.

EVALUATION OF THE OVERALL PERFORMANCE OF THE CALF MUSCLE PUMP

The combined effect of venous reflux, obstruction and ejection capacity of the calf muscle pump is evaluated by measuring the residual volume (RV) and residual volume fraction (RVF = RV/VV × 100) after 10 tiptoe movements, at the rate of 1 per second (Fig. 5.6**D**). The measurements of RVF are shown in Figure 5.10. RVF correlates well with the measurements of ambulatory venous pressure (r = 0.81), so that the latter can be estimated noninvasively (Fig. 5.11); it also correlates well with the incidence of ulceration. The latter is zero for RVF <30% and increases gradually to 88% for RVF >80% (Table 5.1).

VALUE AND POTENTIAL OF AIR PLETHYSMOGRAPHY

The air plethysmographic (26, 27) measurements are easily performed in 10–15 minutes with excellent patient tolerance and minor practitioner training requirements. Although APG can be used as a simple screening test, it can offer a complete analysis of venous hemodynamics; it is useful in the routine clinical management of the patient as well as in research. The reproducibility of the air plethysmographic measurements is shown in Table 5.2. Limbs with edema or ulceration due to causes other than venous disease (i.e., arterial, lymphatic, cardiac, or rheumatoid) can be easily distinguished from those with venous disease (24). Also, in case of combined disease (i.e., arterial and venous), the degree of venous involvement can be precisely assessed. Limbs with primary varicose veins can be distinguished from those with deep venous disease, and in patients with combined deep and superficial disease, the pathologic contribution of each system

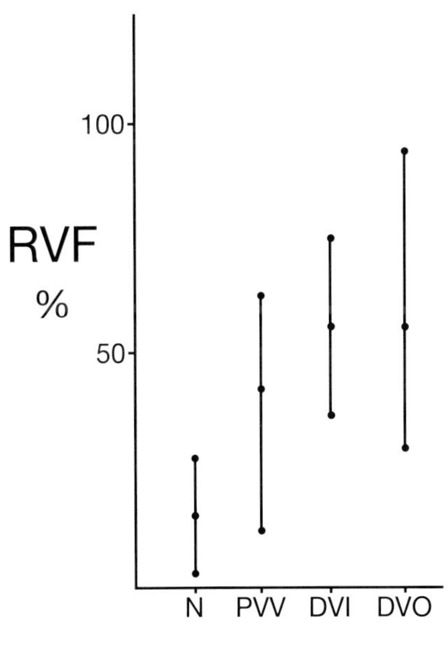

FIG. 5–10. Residual volume fraction (*RVF*) (mean and 90% range) in normal limbs (*N*), limbs with primary varicose veins (*PVV*), deep venous incompetence (*DVI*), and deep venous obstruction (*DVO*).

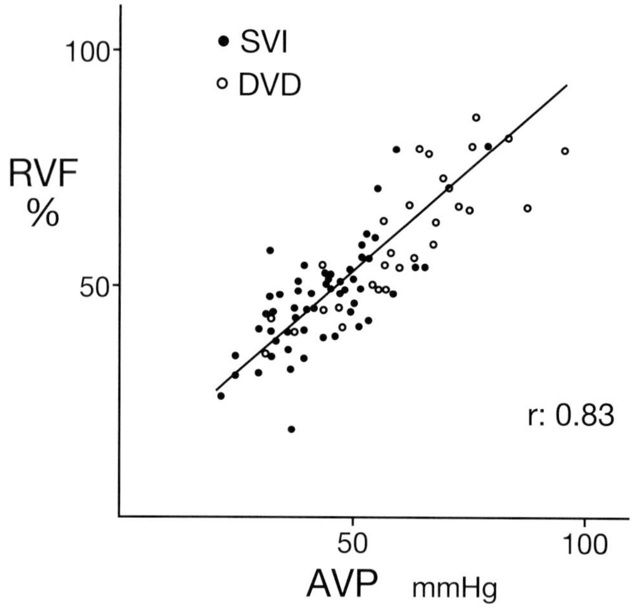

FIG. 5–11. Relationship between residual volume fraction (*RVF*) and ambulatory venous pressure (*AVP*) at the end of 10 tiptoe movements. (● = limbs with superficial venous incompetence, ○ = limbs with deep venous disease).

can be determined. Also, in limbs with prominent varicosities one can determine whether the latter are acting as outflow channels.

Deep venous disease is usually the result of the combined effect of reflux, obstruction, or poor ejection. By using air plethysmography, the contribution of each parameter can be measured and the appropriate surgical intervention can be considered for each patient. The abolition of venous reflux by conventional surgery on the superficial system has already been shown to normalize the calf muscle pump function (23).

TABLE 5-1

INCIDENCE OF LEG ULCERATION IN RELATION TO THE RESIDUAL VOLUME FRACTION (RVF) IN 175 LIMBS WITH VENOUS DISEASE

n	RVF (%)	Incidence of Ulceration (%)
20	<30	0
24	31–40	8
48	41–50	18
43	51–60	42
32	61–80	72
8	>80	88

TABLE 5-2

REPRODUCIBILITY OF AIR PLETHYSMOGRAPHIC MEASUREMENTS (ONE NORMAL LIMB, THREE LIMBS WITH PRIMARY VARICOSE VEINS, AND ONE LIMB WITH DEEP VENOUS DISEASE STUDIED ON FIVE DIFFERENT DAYS).

Measurements	Coefficient of Variation (%)
VV (ml)	10.8–12.5
VFT90 (sec)	8.0–11.5
EV (ml)	6.7–9.4
RV (ml)	6.2–12.0
VFI (ml/sec)	5.3–7.9
EF (%)	2.9–9.7
RVF (%)	4.3–8.2

One of the advantages of the APG is that it can be applied over an elastic stocking. Thus, it has been demonstrated that graduated elastic compression reduces the residual volume fraction (and consequently ambulatory venous pressure) by 20–30%, and that this is the result of a reduced venous reflux and an increased ejection fraction (20). The ability of APG to assess different kinds of compression (graduated or uniform, high or low) has opened a new avenue of investigation in this area.

Table 5.2 shows that the reproducibility of the air plethysmographic measurements would detect any change in venous hemodynamics as a result of therapy, provided it is greater than 10%. Air plethysmography is used in our hospital investigations in all cases in which the clinical and pocket Doppler examination fails to produce a clear diagnosis. This occurs in approximately 10% of all patients seen. In the past, venography was indicated in this group of patients because of a history of deep venous thrombosis, the presence of chronic swelling, liposclerosis and/or ulceration, and recurrent varicose veins. The use of air plethysmography with Doppler ultrasound or duplex scanning (if available) to localize incompetent sites (16, 17) means that venography in chronic venous disease is now indicated only in patients considered for deep venous surgery.

REFERENCES

1. Widmer LK, Stahelin HB, Nissen C, Da Silva A. Venen-Arterien-Krankheiten, koronare-Herzkrankheit bei Berufstatigen. Prospektiv-epidemiologische Untersuchung. Basler Studie I-III 1959–1978. Bern: Verlag Hans Huber, 1978:1–11.
2. Fisher H, Biland L, Da Silva A, et al. Venenleiden. Eine repräsentative-Untersuchung in der Bevölkerung der Bundesrepublik Deutschland (Tübinger studie). München: Urban und Schwarzenberg, 1981.
3. Taheri SA, Pendergast DR, Lazar E, et al. Vein valve transplantation. Am J Surg 1985;150:201–202.
4. Gruss JD. Der heutige Stand der rekonstruktiven Veneuchirurgie. Schwerpunktmed 1983;6:21.

5. Palma EC, Esperon R. Vein transplants and grafts in the surgical treatment of the postphlebitic syndrome. J Cardiovasc Surg 1960;1:94–107.
6. Husni EA. Venous reconstruction in postphlebitic disease. Circulation 1971;43(Suppl 1):147–150.
7. Raju S. New approaches to the diagnosis and treatment of venous obstruction. J Vasc Surg 1986;4:42–54.
8. Nicolaides AN, Zukowski A, Lewis P, Kyprianou P, Malouf M. The value of ambulatory venous pressure measurements. In: Bergan JJ, Yao JST, eds. Surgery of the veins. Orlando, FL: Grune & Stratton, 1985:111–119.
9. Abramowitz HB, Querel LA, Flinn WR, et al. The use of photoplethysmography in the assessment of venous insufficiency. A comparison to venous pressure measurement. Surgery 1979;86:434–441.
10. Nicolaides AN, Miles C. Photoplethysmography in the assessment of venous insufficiency. J Vasc Surg 1987;5:405–412.
11. Barnes RW, Collicott PE, Sumner DS, Strandness DE. Noninvasive quantitation of venous hemodynamics in the post-phlebitic syndrome. Arch Surg 1973;107:807–814.
12. Fernandes e Fernandes J, Horner J, Needham T, Nicolaides AN. Ambulatory calf volume plethysmography in the assessment of venous insufficiency. Br J Surg 1979;66:327–330.
13. Mason R, Giran F. Noninvasive evaluation of venous function in chronic venous disease. Surgery 1982;91:312–317.
14. Ludbrook J, Loughlin J. Regulation of the lower limb. Am Heart J 1964;67:493–507.
15. Strandness DE, Sumner DS. Hemodynamics for surgeons. New York: Grune & Stratton, 1976:404.
16. Nicolaides AN, Fernandes e Fernandes J, Zimmerman H. Doppler ultrasound in the investigation of venous insufficiency. In: Investigation of vascular disorders. New York: Churchill-Livingstone, 1981:478–487.
17. Szendro G, Nicolaides AN, Zukowski AJ, Christopoulos D, Malouf M, Christodoulou C. Duplex scanning in the assessment of deep venous incompetence. J Vasc Surg 1986;4:237–242.
18. Allan JC. Volume changes in the lower limb in response to postural alterations and muscular exercise. S Afr J Surg 1964;2:75–90.
19. Ludbrook J. The musculovenous pumps of the lower limb. Am Heart J 1966;71:635–641.
20. Christopoulos D, Nicolaides AN, Szendro G, Irvine AT, Bull ML, Eastcott HHG. Air plethysmography and the effect of elastic compression on the venous haemodynamics of the leg. J Vasc Surg 1987;5:148–159.
21. Christopoulos D, Nicolaides AN, Szendro G. Venous reflux quantification and correlation with the clinical severity of chronic venous disease. Br J Surg 1988;75:352–356.
22. Christopoulos D, Nicolaides AN, Duffy P, Georgiou I. Noninvasive quantification of outflow obstruction. J Cardiovasc Surg 1989;30:72–73.
23. Christopoulos D, Nicolaides AN, Cook A, Irvine A, Galloway GMD, Wilkinson A. Pathogenesis of venous ulceration in relation to the calf muscle pump function. Surgery 1989;106:829–835.
24. Christopoulos D, Nicolaides AN. Noninvasive diagnosis and quantitation of popliteal reflux in the swollen and ulcerated leg. J Cardiovasc Surg 1988;29:535–539.
25. Christopoulos D, Nicolaides AN, Galloway JMD, Wilkinson A. Objective noninvasive evaluation of venous surgical results. J Vasc Surg 1988;8:683–687.
26. Christopoulos D, Nicolaides AN, Duffy P. Functional diagnostic assessment of the swollen and ulcerated leg. In: Strano A, Nono S, eds. Advances in vascular pathology. New York: Excerpta Medica, 1989:185–189.
27. Comerota AJ, Harada RN, Eze AR, Katz ML. Air plethysmography: a clinical review. Int Angiol 1995;14:45–52.

chapter 6

Photoplethysmography

Richard F. Kempczinski

The lack of a simple, readily available, accurate, noninvasive technique to objectively document and quantitate venous insufficiency of the lower extremities has hindered our understanding of the pathophysiology of this common, perplexing condition. Over the years, a number of tests have been recommended, but have failed to achieve widespread acceptance because they were invasive, cumbersome, not generally available, or too complex for routine clinical use.

The introduction of photoplethysmography (PPG) (1) and the subsequent documentation that its alterations with leg exercise corresponded to similar changes in venous pressure (2) represented a major advance in the management of venous insufficiency. This technique provided the clinician with a simple, noninvasive, reliable method for studying the venous hemodynamics of patients and documenting the effect of therapy.

BASIC PRINCIPLES

To better understand the principles behind PPG, consider the example of a large reservoir filled with water. At one end, there is a small stream emptying into the reservoir; at the other end, there is a large pumping station that drains water from the reservoir and pumps it through a large pipe up a steep incline. The stream flow into the reservoir changes depending on rainfall upstream, and the volume removed by the pumping station varies with the demand for water. Normally, these two forces are in equilibrium and the level of the reservoir remains constant. If one wanted to determine whether the pumping station was allowing water to flow back into the reservoir when it was shut off for the night, one could monitor the water level in the reservoir and record how long it took to return to a certain baseline level after the pump was shut off, and compare that figure to previous similar determinations made when the pump was known to be functioning properly. For these calculations to accurately detect backflow through the pumping station, one would obviously have to normalize the stream flow and the degree to which the level in the reservoir had been lowered while the pump was operational.

Extending this analogy to the venous circulation of the lower extremities, the arterial inflow corresponds to the stream. The venous capacitance bed is the reservoir. The calf venomotor pump is the pumping station and the large pipe extending up the hill corresponds to the major venous tributaries of the legs. If we expect to accurately detect venous insufficiency by monitoring venous refilling time, we must be certain that arterial inflow into the legs is stable. We must know to what extent the venous capacitance bed was emptied by the calf venomotor pump during a standardized effort and we must be certain that the efficiency of the venomotor pump was maximized.

Venous Refilling Time

The first use of venous refilling/recovery time (VRT) to assess venous function was by Nachbur in 1971 when he reported direct venous pressure measurements before and after exercise in an attempt to differentiate normal and postphlebitic limbs (3). He noted that the VRT was much shorter in patients with chronic venous insufficiency compared to normal controls. To separate out any contribution from reflux down the superficial veins, the VRT was remeasured before and after the application of tourniquets that occluded only the superficial veins. This maneuver had been first suggested by Walker and Longland (4). If the VRT normalized following application of the tourniquet, the reflux could be presumed to be limited to the saphenous vein.

Photoplethysmograph

Because the determination of venous refilling time was based on direct venous pressure measurements that required cannulation of a foot vein, they were cumbersome, poorly accepted by patients, not amenable to repetitive determinations, and, ultimately, not widely used. When Barnes, et al., introduced what appeared to be a simple, indirect, noninvasive technique—photoplethysmography—for measuring venous refilling, there was a resurgence of interest in the principle of VRT (1).

The instrumentation consists of a transducer, a signal amplifier and a strip-chart recorder (Fig. 6.1). The transducer emits infrared light from a light-emitting diode into the underlying skin to which it has been attached with a transparent, double-backed adhesive tape. Light is reflected back from the red blood cells in proportion to the blood content of the subdermal venous plexus. This backscattered, infrared light is captured by a phototransistor receiver mounted in the transducer head next to the light-emitting diode and translated into an electrical signal, which is then filtered and amplified. When the resulting output voltage is DC-coupled and sent to a strip-chart recorder, one effectively has a continuous recording of the cutaneous blood content in the capillary microcirculation. Since the output signal is displayed as a straight line, a shift in this baseline represents a relative change in the opacity of the underlying tissue which, in turn, represents a change

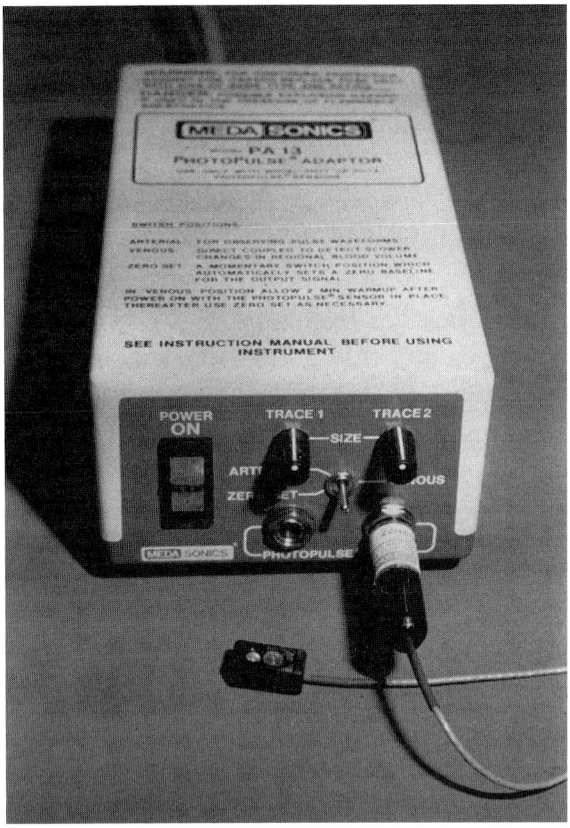

FIG. 6–1. The basic instrument consists of a photopulse adapter and the transducer which is applied to the skin.

in the blood content of the skin. The latter is governed by venous pressure, which is the product of arterial inflow and venous reflux. Thus, if arterial inflow can be normalized, dermal blood content becomes an indirect measure of venous reflux. However, since the standard PPG transducer cannot be easily and accurately calibrated, the resulting tracings, although *qualitatively* similar to direct venous pressure measurements, cannot be used to quantitate ambulatory venous pressure.

TECHNIQUE

Test Procedure

The patient is asked to sit on the edge of the examining table with his/her legs hanging over the side. Although most laboratories study patients in the sitting position, Nicolaides and Miles found poor separation between normals and patients with venous insufficiency when they performed PPG in the sitting position. They recommended that the test be performed in the standing position (5). The PPG sensor is affixed to the skin over the anteromedial aspect of each ankle above the medial malleolus with transparent, double-backed adhesive tape (Fig. 6.2). Placement directly over the saphenous vein, an obvious venous varix, or a

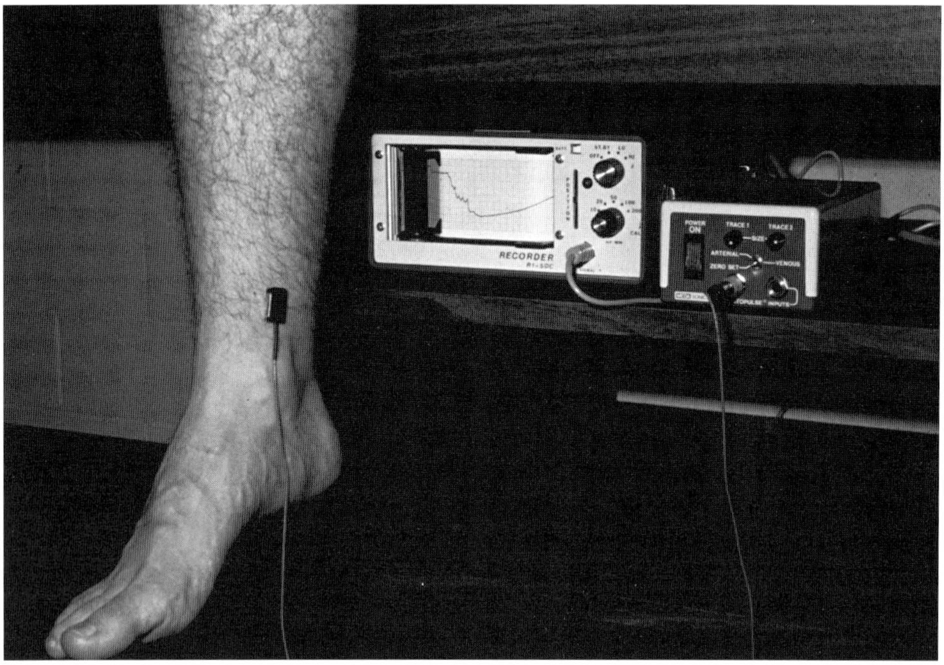

FIG. 6–2. The transducer is applied to the skin just above the medial malleolus as the patient sits on the end of a table with his/her leg hanging over the side. Note the strip-chart recorder has been positioned to be clearly visible to the examiner during calf contraction.

joint should be avoided. Although most investigators have not felt that the site of transducer placement was critical, Rosfors found that the best correlation between PPG and pressure/volume recordings made directly in the foot occurred when the transducer was placed just above the medial malleolus (6). His work suggested that PPG VRTs reflected *regional* venous hemodynamics rather than overall venous changes in the limbs and were more related to superficial than to deep venous insufficiency.

The speed of the strip-chart recorder is set to 5 mm/sec. A stable baseline is obtained and positioned near the top of the strip chart. The patient is instructed to forcefully and rapidly plantar flex the foot five times and then relax. It is useful to practice this maneuver several times before actually making any recordings in order to familiarize the patient with the test procedure and thus ensure maximum cooperation. If there is little change in the baseline, even at full gain, following active plantar flexion, the degree of patient cooperation must be evaluated. Some patients, especially those who are elderly and debilitated or who have painful, edematous limbs, are unable to generate a forceful calf contraction and effectively empty their venous capacitance bed. Failure to recognize this problem can result in a false-positive study.

In patients whose own active plantar flexion appears weak or inadequate, the examiner should sit facing the patient's lower extremities and place both hands around the fleshy part of the relaxed calf. Once the baseline stabilizes again, the calf is manually and vigorously compressed five times. If the valves of the deep venous system are competent, this invariably results in a prompt fall in dermal venous blood content (Fig. 6.3). Regardless of the method used to achieve effective venous emptying, the study should be repeated several times on each limb to ensure a consistent, reproducible tracing.

Quantitative Photoplethysmography

As previously stated, the usual technique for PPG provides only a qualitative estimate of venous refilling. Several investigators have attempted to modify the technique to provide more quantitative information. Kempczinski, et al., used a standardization device to calibrate the gain control of the PPG adaptor prior to testing (7). When the transducer was placed in this device and a button was depressed, it generated a series of sine waves of constant amplitude. The amplitude of the wave with the gain control turned to "full" was measured in millimeters. The control was then reduced until the wave was exactly one-half its previous amplitude and this position on the dial was designated "½ gain." In similar fashion, the "¼ gain" and "¾ gain" positions were determined and marked on the dial of the gain control. When these investigators rechecked the calibration of the gain control during the course of their study, they found that it had remained remarkably stable. Thus, once calibrated, the gain control of the PPG adaptor (photopulse adaptor) needed to be recalibrated only if the PPG transducer was changed. Although this calibration device permitted the PPG to be *standardized,* it was still only capable of measuring a change in dermal blood content and not absolute calf venous volume. Thus, the postexercise fall in baseline remained only a relative measure of venous emptying.

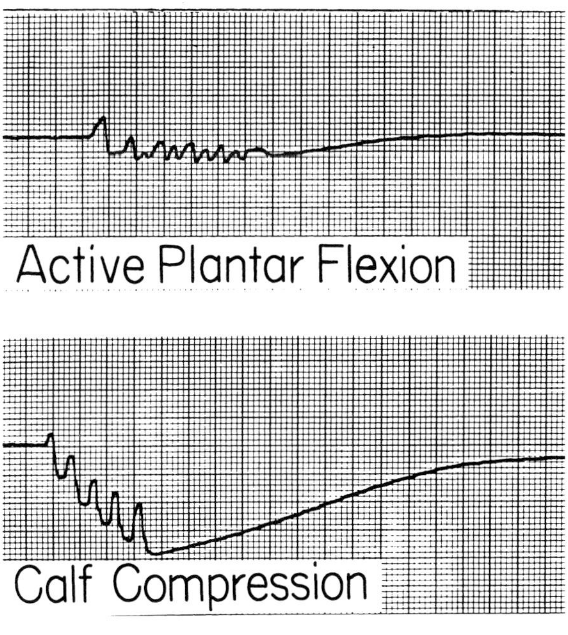

FIG. 6–3. Failure of active plantar flexion (*top*) to effectively empty the dermal venous plexus. Manual calf compression in the same patient (*bottom*) results in a normal study. (Reproduced by permission from Kempczinski RF, Berlatzky Y, Pearce WH. Semi-quantitative photoplethysmography in the diagnosis of venous insufficiency. J Cardiovasc Surg 1986;27:17–23.)

Norris, et al., attempted in vivo calibration of the PPG transducer by adjusting the gain control while asking the patient to alternately assume the supine and standing positions (8). The pen stylus of the strip-chart recorder was positioned at the lower baseline of the recording channel with the patient in the supine position. This was designated the "zero" peripheral venous pressure. The patient was then asked to stand and once the skin blood content reequilibrated (1–2 minutes), the gain control was adjusted to position the stylus toward the top of the paper at a calibrated excursion that corresponded to the measured distance between the right atrium and the position of the PPG transducer. This sequence was repeated two to three times until the calibrated excursion of the stylus accurately mirrored the estimated change in venous hydrostatic pressure. Using direct measurements of ambulatory venous pressure as their "gold standard," Norris, et al., documented a close correlation between this quantitative PPG and the estimated drop in superficial venous pressure and recovery time. Besides appearing time-consuming and cumbersome, this approach could not be validated subsequently by Nicolaides and Miles (5) and Fischer and Wuppermann found "only a poor correlation between the drop in venous blood pressure measured by invasive techniques (i.e., ambulatory venous pressure) and those estimated by transcutaneous PPG" (9). Thus, no completely satisfactory technique has been described to quantitate the degree of venous reflux measured by PPG and it remains largely a qualitative test.

Light Reflection Rheography

This photoelectric technique, which is very similar to PPG, was developed in West Germany. Unlike PPG, light reflection rheography does not require operator calibration and can quantitatively measure changes in the venous circulation. The light reflection rheograph (LRR) consists of a sensitive photoelectric sensor containing two light-emitting diodes and a thermistor probe for skin temperature measurement. Figure 6.4 compares the features of PPG and LRR. In actual use, the technique is similar to the PPG technique except the study is performed with the patient sitting with both feet on the floor. Ten foot dorsiflexions are performed over a 15-second period aided by a standardized metronome. The exam is repeated three to five times with a 2–3-minute rest period between studies to minimize the effects of exercise-induced hyperemia. If the patient is unable to perform adequate foot dorsiflexions, manual calf compression by the examiner may be substituted.

The LRR curve is the mirror image of a PPG tracing but the endpoint is virtually identical. A VRT $\geq$25 seconds is considered normal. Eighty percent of patients with severe venous insufficiency were found to have an LRR measured VRT $<$15 seconds (10). Thus, McEnroe and O'Donnell concluded that LRR was useful not only for determining the anatomic level of venous valvular insufficiency, but that it also provided important information regarding the severity of such insufficiency (10). LRR, unlike PPG, may also be used for the detection of deep venous thrombosis (11).

Tourniquet Testing

If a PPG study is abnormal, an attempt should be made to localize the site of venous valvular incompetence by the sequential application of pneumatic

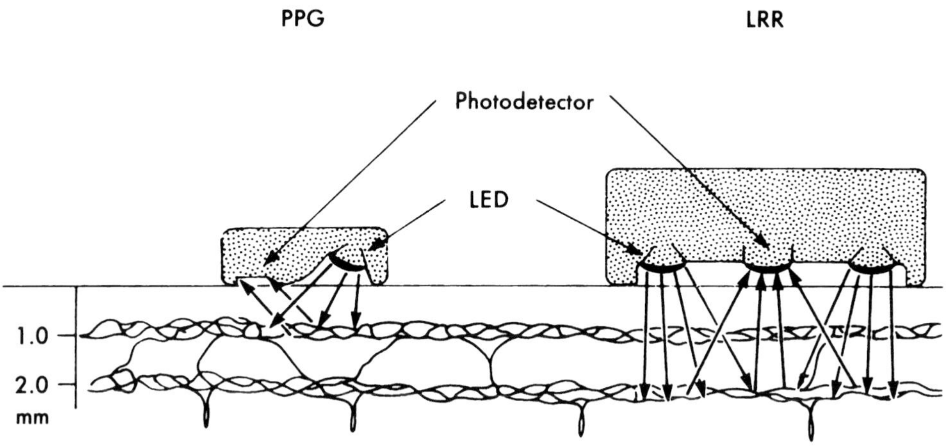

FIG. 6–4. Comparison of sensors for the photoplethysmograph (*PPG*) and the light reflection rheograph (*LRR*). Note the increased depth of penetration with LRR due to the use of two light emitting diodes versus one for PPG. (Reproduced by permission from McEnroe CS, O'Donnell TF. Noninvasive evaluation of chronic venous insufficiency. Semin Vasc Surg 1988;1:73–85.)

tourniquets. If an abnormal PPG study is corrected by the inflation of a pneumatic tourniquet above the knee to 50 mmHg, primary incompetence of the greater saphenous vein can be diagnosed. If the study remains abnormal despite the thigh tourniquet, but normalizes when a calf tourniquet is inflated, the incompetence can be presumed to be in the lesser saphenous system.

To separate calf perforator vein incompetence from deep venous insufficiency, the tourniquet should be placed at the ankle as the PPG sensor is moved down to the dorsum of the foot. If the study remains abnormal despite inflation of the ankle tourniquet, deep venous incompetence is suggested, while a normalized study indicates perforator dysfunction.

Interpretation

As seen in Figure 6.3, when the patient actively plantar flexes the foot or when manual calf compression is performed by the examiner, there is a rapid fall in the baseline. Immediately after the calf venomotor pump relaxes, the baseline begins to return to its previous level. The endpoint for determining VRT has generally been the point at which the original horizontal baseline was reached for 5 seconds or when peak overshoot of this baseline occurred. A VRT in any limb of ≥23 seconds was considered *normal*, and a VRT of ≤20 seconds was considered *abnormal* (2).

However, our initial attempts to duplicate these results were disappointing. We found that a significant number of apparently normal patients who had no clinical or physical evidence of venous insufficiency or cutaneous venous hypertension had a VRT of <20 seconds. This was seen in 30% of young, normal volunteers and 52% of our clinical patient population (7). Furthermore, we found that even minor amounts of exercise or other clinical conditions that were associated with reactive hyperemia of the lower extremity (e.g., cellulitis) invariably resulted in shortening of the VRT to ≤20 seconds and that this "abnormality" persisted for a prolonged period after cessation of exercise.

Finally, it seemed illogical to place such emphasis on the time for dermal venous refilling without measuring the antecedent venous emptying. Therefore, a new parameter called the venous recovery rate (VRR) was developed. It was better able to discriminate between normal limbs and those with angiographically confirmed venous insufficiency. It also permitted greater quantitation of the degree of venous reflux and made the technique less susceptible to the vagaries of arterial inflow. As we recall from the reservoir analogy, the time required for the baseline to return to its preexercise level not only reflects the competence of the venous valves, but also the extent of antecedent venous emptying and the arterial blood flow into the extremity (12).

Relative venous decrease (RVD) is calculated as the difference in millimeters between the original baseline and the nadir of the postexercise tracing (Fig. 6.5). Although the degree of venous emptying is largely a function of the vigor of the calf contraction or manual compression, once the patient has practiced this maneuver and understands the importance of a maximum effort, RVD is remarkably consistent on repetitive measurements. VRT, in seconds, is measured from the time exercise or manual calf compression ceased until the baseline returned to its preexercise level or stabilized at a new baseline. The slope of the recovery curve, or the VRR, can then be calculated by dividing the RVD by the VRT (Fig. 6.5).

Since the RVD is directly related to the gain setting on the photopulse adaptor, all calculations of VRR are made using the value for RVD at full gain. Thus, if the study had been performed at "$^1/_2$ gain" and the RVD measured 10 mm, it was multiplied by 2 and the resulting product, 20 mm, was then used to calculate VRR. The gain setting did not influence the VRT which, therefore, could be measured directly from the strip chart after noting the speed to which the recorder had been set during the study.

In a limited number of patients (<55%), the postexercise baseline will neither stabilize nor return to resting levels, despite repeated studies and repositioning the sensor. In such patients, the slope of the initial recovery curve should be projected to its point of intercept with the original baseline and this point then used to calculate the VRT (Fig. 6.6).

In the extremities for which complete venographic assessment was available, the mean VRR was 1.28 mm/second for normal limbs and 3.34 mm/second for those with deep venous reflux (Fig. 6.7). If 2 standard deviations are calculated around these mean values, 95% of normal limbs can be expected to have a VRR <2 mm/second (7). Therefore, the two following criteria are used in the author's laboratory for an abnormal PPG:

1. Absence of any measurable RVD, despite satisfactory calf contraction (Fig. 6.7); or
2. A VRR ≥2 mm/second.

In a group of normal volunteers, the mean preexercise VRT was 27.5 (±4.0 SEM) seconds and the VRR was 0.78 (±0.075 SEM) mm/second (Fig. 6.8). However, 30% of this group had a resting VRT of <20 seconds and would have been judged abnormal had this criterion alone been used. None had an abnormal VRR!

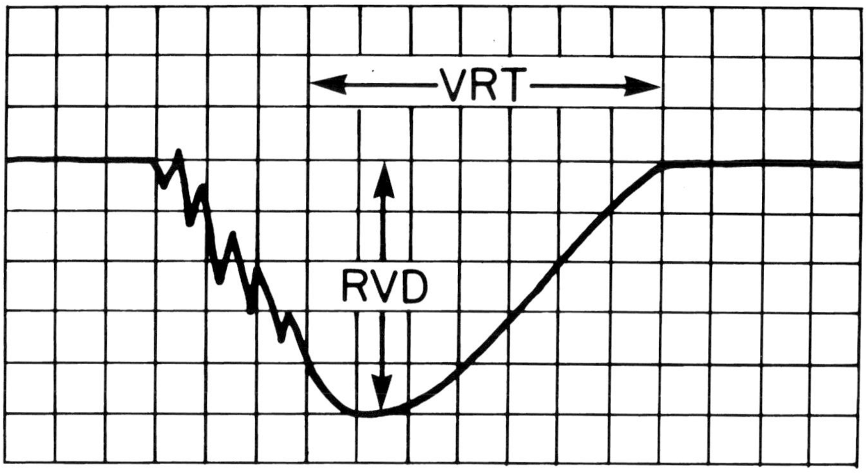

$$VRR = \frac{RVD\ (mm)}{VRT\ (sec)}$$

FIG. 6–5. Formula for calculation of venous recovery rate. *VRT* = venous recovery time; *RVD* = relative venous decrease; *VRR* = venous recovery rate. (Reproduced by permission from Kempczinski RF, Berlatzky Y, Pearce WH. Semi-quantitative photoplethysmography in the diagnosis of venous insufficiency. J Cardiovasc Surg 1986;27:17–23.)

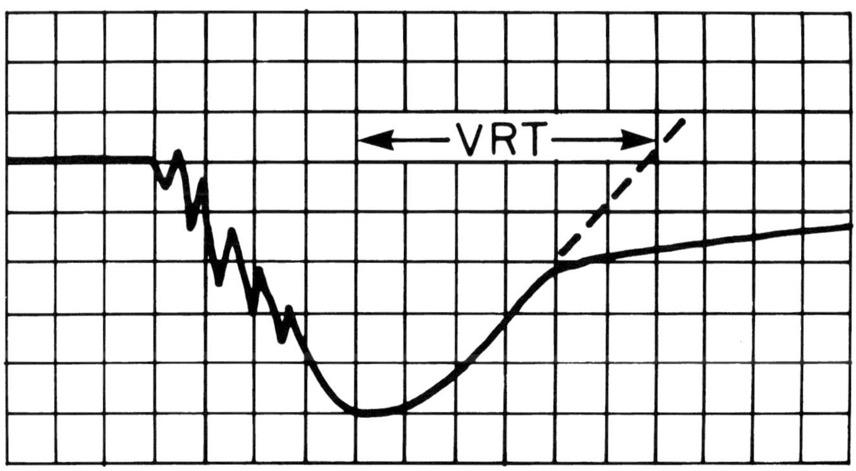

FIG. 6–6. Projection of initial slope of venous recovery curve permits calculation of venous recovery time (*VRT*) when baseline fails to stabilize or return to pre-exercise levels. (Reproduced by permission from Kempczinski RF, Berlatzky Y, Pearce WH. Semi-quantitative photoplethysmography in the diagnosis of venous insufficiency. J Cardiovasc Surg 1986;27:17–23.)

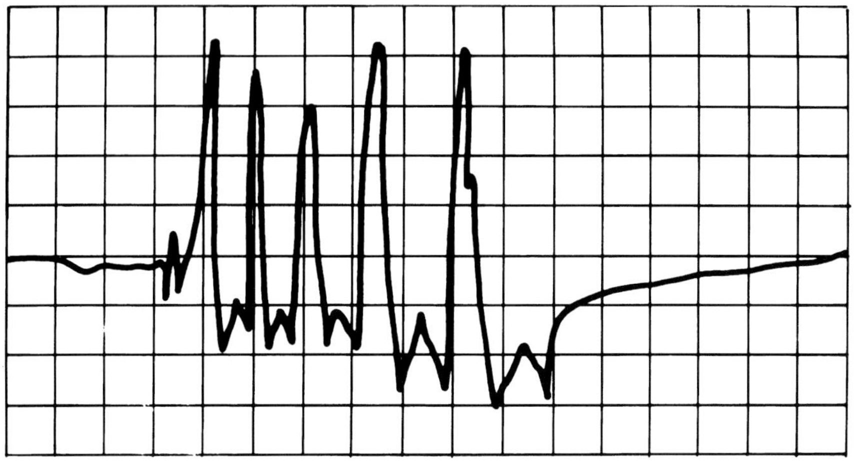

FIG. 6–7. A PPG tracing without any measurable RVD suggests complete decompensation of the calf venomotor pump. (Reproduced by permission from Kempczinski RF, Berlatzky Y, Pearce WH. Semi-quantitative photoplethysmography in the diagnosis of venous insufficiency. J Cardiovasc Surg 1986;27:17–23.)

Immediately following 5 minutes of treadmill exercise, 90% of normal volunteers had a VRT of <20 seconds and, even 5 minutes postexercise, the mean VRT for the entire group was still only 14.5 (±1.5 SEM) seconds (Fig. 6.9). In several of these subjects, measurements were repeated for up to 20 minutes postexercise and the VRT persistently remained <20 seconds. By contrast, the VRR was much less

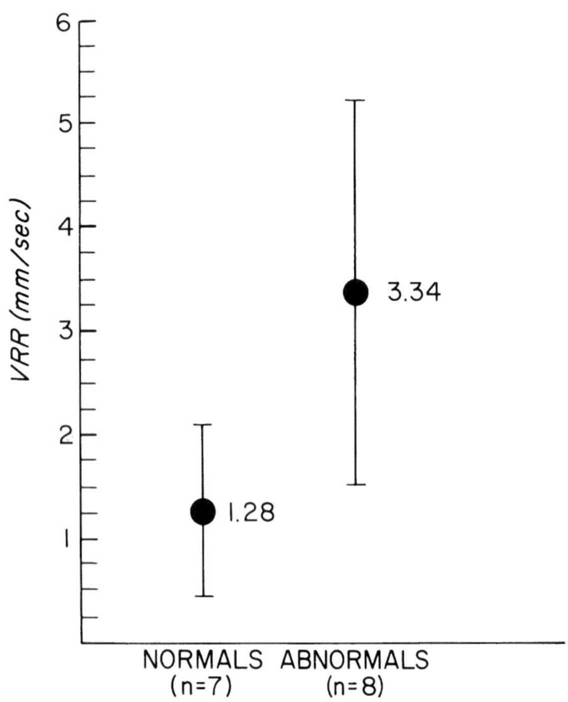

FIG. 6–8. Mean venous recovery rate (*VRR*) in limbs shown to be normal by venography compared to those with proven reflux. *Vertical bars* indicate 2 standard deviations. (Reproduced by permission from Kempczinski RF, Berlatzky Y, Pearce WH. Semi-quantitative photoplethysmography in the diagnosis of venous insufficiency. J Cardiovasc Surg 1986;27:17–23.)

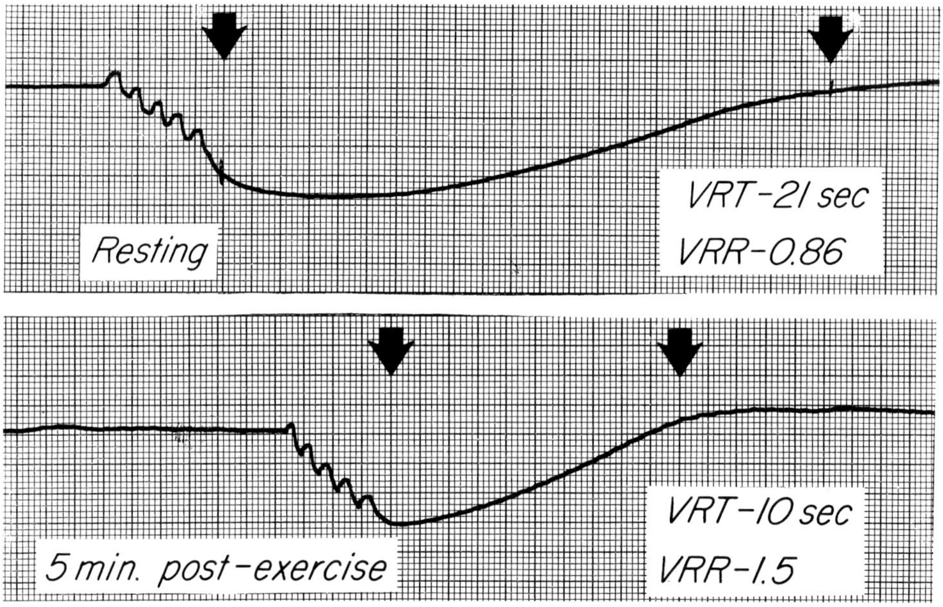

FIG. 6–9. PPG on the same patient before and 5 minutes after walking demonstrates the dramatic shortening of venous recovery time (*VRT*) while venous recovery rate (*VRR*) remains normal. (Reproduced by permission from Kempczinski RF, Berlatzky Y, Pearce WH. Semi-quantitative photoplethysmography in the diagnosis of venous insufficiency. J Cardiovasc Surg 1986;27:17–23.)

affected by exercise-induced reactive-hyperemia and remained normal in 90% of these subjects (Fig. 6.10). The mean VRR 5 minutes postexercise was 1.29 (±0.14 SEM) mm/second.

When the 151 extremities in the author's clinical series were analyzed, the PPG was normal in 88 limbs (58%) and abnormal in 63 (42%). The mean VRR for these two groups was 1.09 mm/sec and 3.12 mm/sec, respectively, which corresponded

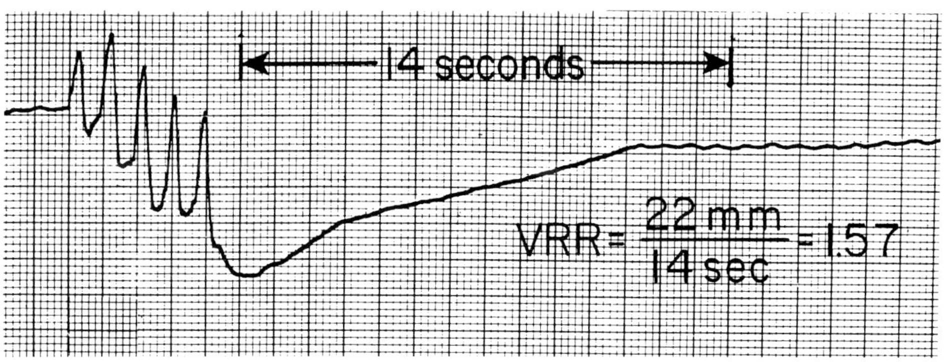

FIG. 6–10. A representative PPG tracing on an asymptomatic, young volunteer demonstrating a consistently "abnormal" venous recovery time (*14 seconds*). Note that the calculated venous recovery rate, *VRR (1.57)*, on the same tracing falls well within the "normal" range.

closely to the smaller subgroup for which venographic correlation was available. The difference between the normal and abnormal groups was highly significant ($p < 0.001$).

Other investigators have also had difficulty in determining a precise endpoint for VRT. Sarin, et al., found that a "95% Refilling Time," i.e., the time required for the PPG tracing to recover to 95% of its resting level of <15 seconds, indicated venous dysfunction with the greatest combination of sensitivity and specificity (13). This contradicted the report of Li, et al., which had suggested that the "50% Refilling Time" gave more accurate results (14).

Results

The reported accuracy for PPG depends on the gold standard against which it was compared. Unfortunately, there is no universally accepted standard for the documentation of venous reflux, and various investigators have used descending venography, ambulatory venous pressure measurements, duplex scanning, continuous-wave Doppler survey, or even clinical examination. In a study of 793 limbs with unobstructed venous reflux, Raju and Fredericks compared the results of PPG with various other parameters of venous insufficiency (15) (Table 6.1).

Compared against color duplex scans and using a 95% Refilling Time of <15 seconds as the basis for diagnosing venous insufficiency, Sarin, et al., found that PPG detected deep venous reflux with a sensitivity of 80% and a specificity of 60% (13). Welch, et al., compared the results of quantitative photoplethysmography to descending phlebography in patients with severe chronic venous insufficiency. They found that photoplethysmography could separate normal from abnormal limbs but could not distinguish the severity of reflux (16).

In a study of 20 limbs with severe venous stasis, Bays, et al., compared PPG to duplex ultrasonography (17). They also found that PPG was a sensitive method of detecting reflux, but its specificity was poor, and PPG refill times could not accurately predict the localization of reflux. Thus PPG has shown moderate sensitivity when compared with descending venograms, duplex scans, or continuous-

TABLE 6-1

ACCURACY OF PPG RELATIVE TO VARIOUS "STANDARD" TECHNIQUES TO DETECT VENOUS REFLUX*

"Gold Standard"	Sensitivity	Specificity
Descending Venography	74%	37%
CW Doppler Survey	85%	62%
Ambulatory Venous Pressure	97%	57%
Presence of Stasis Ulceration	87%	90%

*After Raju S, Fredericks R. Evaluation of methods for detecting venous reflux. Arch Surg 1990;125:1463–1467.

wave Doppler survey, and excellent sensitivity against ambulatory venous pressure measurements or the presence of stasis ulceration. However, its specificity has been uniformly poor regardless of the reference standard used.

In conclusion, although a normal PPG can safely be accepted as signifying the absence of significant venous reflux, the number of false-positive studies in limbs otherwise judged "normal" will be high. For this reason, PPG should probably not be used as the sole screening technique in patients with presumed venous insufficiency.

CLINICAL APPLICATION

We begin the evaluation of patients with symptoms of chronic venous disease by first determining the presence or absence of outflow obstruction. This initial screening can be performed using venous duplex scanning. Confirmation of a positive study and anatomic definition of the obstruction will usually mandate ascending venography. However, venograms will not be able to assess the functional significance of the obstruction, and we have adopted the *arm-foot pressure differential*, as described by Raju (18), to provide the functional information necessary for planning therapy.

If there is no evidence of significant outflow obstruction, PPG is next performed, as described earlier, to segregate patients with venous reflux from those with a nonvenous etiology for their symptoms. A normal PPG excludes significant venous reflux. If the VRR is consistently abnormal, the study is repeated following the sequential application of tourniquets as described earlier. Normalization of the VRR following tourniquets suggests superficial venous incompetence, while a persistently abnormal study suggests deep venous incompetence (Fig. 6.11). In

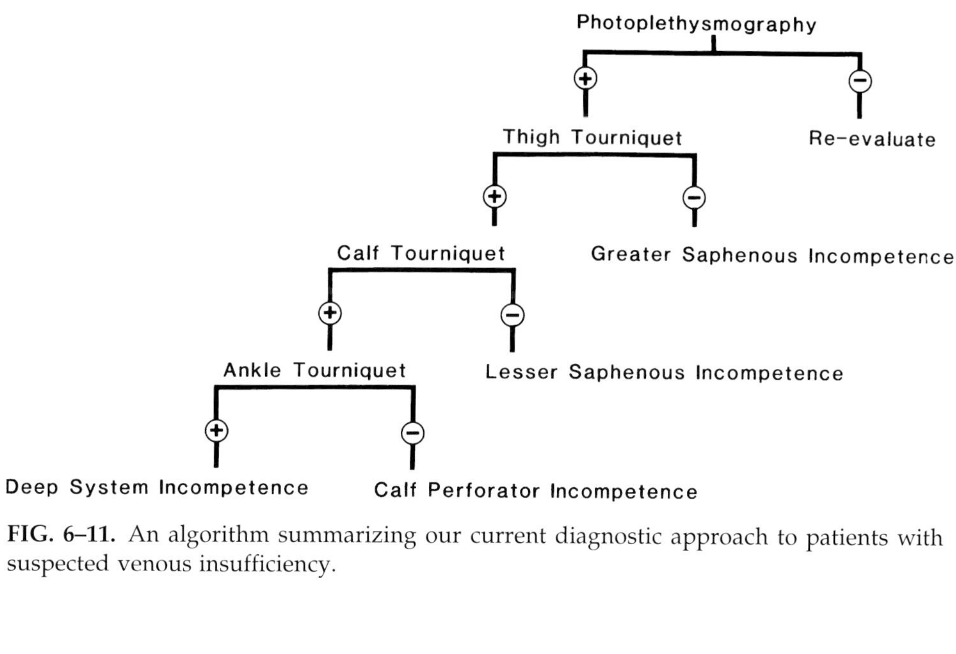

FIG. 6–11. An algorithm summarizing our current diagnostic approach to patients with suspected venous insufficiency.

those patients with chronic venous insufficiency who are not easily managed using simple measures such as elastic support, a descending venogram is then performed to document the site and extent of venous reflux and to aid in the planning of possible surgical correction.

This combination of duplex scanning, arm-foot pressure differentials, quantitative PPG, and appropriate venography is better able to gauge the relative contribution of venous outflow obstruction versus reflux in the pathogenesis of each patient's disability, and provides the clinician with a combination of objective hemodynamic and anatomic data upon which to base therapy.

REFERENCES

1. Barnes RW, Garrett WV, Hummel BA, Slaymaker EE, Maixner W, Reinertson JE. Photoplethysmographic assessment of altered cutaneous circulation in the postphlebitic syndrome. In: Proceedings of the 13th Annual Meeting of the Association for Advancement in Medical Instrumentation. Washington, DC: Mar 28–Apr 1, 1978.
2. Abramowitz HB, Queral LA, Flinn WR, et al. The use of photoplethysmography in the assessment of venous insufficiency: a comparison to venous pressure measurements. Surgery 1979;86:434–441.
3. Nachbur B. Die periphere Venendruckmessung: eine Methode zur Bestimmung der venösen Leistungreserve der unteren Extremitäten. Zentrabl Phlebol 1971;10:244–249.
4. Walker AJ, Longland C. Venous measurement in the foot in exercise as an aid to investigation of venous disease in the leg. Clin Sci 1950;9:101–107.
5. Nicolaides AN, Miles C. Photoplethysmography in the assessment of venous insufficiency. J Vasc Surg 1987;5:405–412.
6. Rosfors S. Venous photoplethysmography: relationship between transducer position and regional distribution of venous insufficiency. J Vasc Surg 1990;11:436–440.
7. Kempczinski RF, Berlatzky Y, Pearce WH. Semi-quantitative photoplethysmography in the diagnosis of venous insufficiency. J Cardiovasc Surg 1986;27:17–23.
8. Norris CS, Beyrau A, Barnes RW. Quantitative photoplethysmography in chronic venous insufficiency: a new method of noninvasive estimation of ambulatory venous pressure. Surgery 1983;94:758–764.
9. Fischer M, Wuppermann T. A new method of noninvasive estimation of ambulatory venous pressure. Surgery 1985;97:247–248.
10. McEnroe CS, O'Donnell TF. Noninvasive evaluation of chronic venous insufficiency. Semin Vasc Surg 1988;1:73–85.
11. Mitrani A, Gonzalez ML, O'Connell MT, Guerra J, Harwood RB, Gardner LB. Detection of clinically suspected deep vein thrombosis using light reflection rheography. Am J Surg 1991;161:646–650.
12. Edwards WS. The effect of altering arterial flow on ventilatory venous pressure in postphlebitic extremities. Surg Gynecol Obstet 1954;99:756–761.
13. Sarin S, Shields DA, Scurr JH, Coleridge Smith PD. Photoplethysmography: a valuable noninvasive tool in the assessment of venous dysfunction. J Vasc Surg 1992;16:154–162.
14. Li JM, Anderson FA, Wheeler HB. Non-invasive testing of venous reflux using photoplethysmography: standardization of technique and evaluation of interpretation criteria. Bruit 1983;7:25–29.
15. Raju S, Fredericks R. Evaluation of methods for detecting venous reflux. Arch Surg 1990;125:1463–1467.

16. Welch HJ, Faliakov EC, McLaughlin RL, Umphrey SE, Belkin M, O'Donnell TF Jr. Comparison of descending phlebouraphy with quantitative photoplethysmography, air plethysmography and duplex quantitative value closure time in assessing deep venous reflux. J Vasc Surg 1992;16:913–919.
17. Bays RA, Healy DA, Atnip RG, Neumyer M, Thiele BL. Validation of air plethysmography, photoplethysmography, and duplex ultrasonography in the evaluation of severe venous stasis. J Vasc Surg 1994;20:721–727.
18. Raju S. New approaches to the diagnosis and treatment of venous obstruction. J Vasc Surg 1986;4:42–54.

chapter 7

Impedance Plethysmography in the Study of Venous Disease

H. Brownell Wheeler and
Frederick A. Anderson, Jr.

Impedance plethysmography (IPG) is a simple, noninvasive bedside procedure that can measure blood volume changes in the body. It was originally developed for the evaluation of peripheral arterial disease (1) and the measurement of cardiac output (2), but its use has become widespread primarily as a reliable diagnostic method for acute deep vein thrombosis (DVT). In 1969, IPG was used to measure venous volume changes in the calf secondary to respiration, and it was observed that the amplitude of these volume changes was markedly diminished in the presence of DVT (3, 4). A diagnostic test for DVT based on these observations proved difficult to standardize in clinical practice because of variable patient respiratory effort. In 1974, a more objective and controlled IPG method for diagnosis of DVT was described, based on the venous volume response in the calf to temporary venous outflow occlusion by a pneumatic thigh cuff (5, 6). This new procedure, based on the principle of venous occlusion plethysmography (VOP) (7), was subsequently validated by several investigators and quickly became a widely used noninvasive method for the diagnosis of DVT.

An overall sensitivity and specificity of 94% for proximal DVT was reported in 11 publications with over 2400 venographic correlations (8). More recent investigators have reported lower accuracy (9–11). This probably reflects the fact that earlier validation studies usually employed venography in all patients, whereas more recent studies have obtained venographic correlations on only a small percentage of the total patient population and tend to have a higher proportion of selected, problem patients. Lower accuracies have also been reported in asymptomatic patients (9–11) in whom there is a high prevalence of nonocclusive DVT.

There has been an impressive IPG correlation with clinical outcome, which is the ultimate gold standard in healthcare (12, 13). Even if IPG fails to detect certain thrombi, it correlates well with the presence of thrombi that are clinically significant. Because of the extensive clinical validation, the low cost of the procedure, and the short time required for technician training, IPG has retained a place in the diagnostic armamentarium despite the recent advent of high resolution B-mode scanning for DVT. This chapter describes the rationale underlying the IPG/VOP procedure, the principles of testing and interpretation, the clinical application, and the cost-benefit relationship.

THEORY

IPG measures blood volume changes in the leg indirectly by recording changes in electrical resistance (impedance). Because blood is a good conductor of electricity, blood volume changes can be recorded by the measurement of electrical resistance, as defined by Ohm's Law: *Resistance = Voltage/Current*. The more blood present in a body segment, the lower the resistance to passage of electric current. The IPG instrument supplies a constant, high-frequency current, which is passed through the calf by a pair of circumferential electrodes. The low strength and high frequency of this current make it imperceptible to the patient and incapable of stimulating the heart or nervous system. A second pair of electrodes, placed inside the current electrodes, detect changes in the voltage. Since the IPG instrument maintains the current at a constant value, any voltage changes recorded are a direct reflection of changes in the electrical resistance of the calf, as predicted by Ohm's Law. Over short periods of time, changes in the electrical resistance of the calf are due solely to changes in blood volume. Thus, IPG provides a reliable, indirect means of recording changes in the blood volume of the calf between the voltage electrodes (14).

Blood volume changes in the calf during VOP are initiated by inflation of a pneumatic thigh cuff to a pressure that is above venous pressure, but below diastolic pressure. In IPG, the venous occlusion pressure has been standardized to 50 mmHg (about 70 cm H_2O). With the veins obstructed, but with arterial blood still flowing into the leg, there is a gradual increase in blood volume until the pressure in the venous system equals the occluding pressure of the tourniquet. Venous outflow is then reestablished as the IPG tracing reaches a plateau. When cuff pressure is released, there is a rapid venous outflow and a prompt return to the resting blood volume. If venous thrombosis is present, there is a much slower rate of venous emptying (Fig. 7.1). Because blood is often dammed up behind an obstructing thrombus, the initial resting blood volume may be greater than normal and the volume increase following cuff inflation may be correspondingly reduced. VOP may be thought of as a "stress test" of the ability of the leg veins to return blood to the heart. Much as a treadmill test will unmask peripheral arterial insufficiency by stressing the inflow capacity of the arterial system, VOP will reveal increased venous outflow resistance, which might not be apparent clinically.

The IPG test detects obstruction in the principal veins draining blood from the lower leg, including the popliteal, femoral, and iliac veins and the inferior vena cava. The test is not sensitive to isolated calf thrombi because of the collateral flow possible through uninvolved parallel calf veins, although the IPG result is often positive when multiple calf veins are obstructed.

The rate of venous emptying is a function of the volume of blood initially dammed up by the thigh cuff, as well as the degree of obstruction. Therefore, the

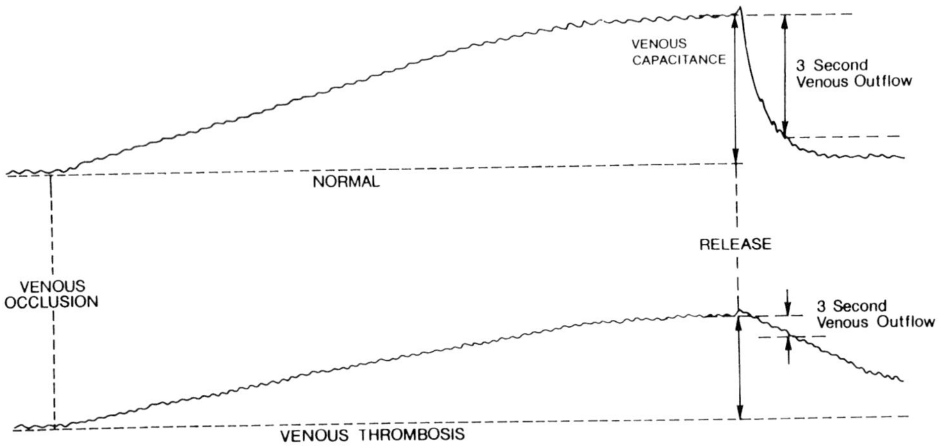

FIG. 7–1. IPG interpretation is based on (a) the increase in blood volume that follows inflation of the pneumatic cuff (venous capacitance) and (b) the decrease in blood volume that follows release of the cuff pressure (3-second venous outflow). (Reproduced by permission from Wheeler HB, Anderson FA Jr. The diagnosis of deep vein thrombosis by impedance plethysmography. In: Bernstein EF, ed. Vascular diagnosis. 4th ed. St. Louis: CV Mosby, 1993:820–829.)

accuracy of VOP interpretation can be increased by taking into consideration the volume of blood collected in the calf and the rate of subsequent venous outflow.

TEST TECHNIQUE

Patient Preparation

The patient should be physically comfortable and relaxed. Proper patient positioning (Fig. 7.2) reduces muscle tension, thereby preventing extrinsic compression of the deep veins. For best results, the test should be performed with the patient lying supine in a hospital bed, rather than on an exam table or stretcher. The foot of the bed should be elevated 20–30° so that the calf is 15–20 cm above the level of the heart. The back should be horizontal; however, a pillow may be placed under the head. The patient's weight is shifted onto the hip of the side being tested. External rotation of the leg with a slight knee bend helps avoid muscle tension and extrinsic venous compression. A pillow is placed under the calf from the heel to the knee. Positioning the heel slightly higher than the knee provides a continuous downhill plane to the heart and promotes venous drainage.

A pneumatic cuff is placed around the thigh. The cuff is applied loosely to avoid creating a continuous venous tourniquet. The cuff should be positioned as high as feasible above the knee to reduce the possibility of skin movement artifact (a large, early rise in the IPG tracing due to movement of the upper IPG electrode secondary to thigh cuff inflation). Paired circumferential electrodes are then placed around the calf. The upper electrode pair is positioned high on the calf, just below the back of the knee. The lower electrode pair is placed a hand's-breadth

(10–15 cm) below the first electrode. Because of the taper of the calf, it is usually necessary to apply the lower electrode band somewhat obliquely to ensure uniform skin contact. In applying the electrodes, the examiner should follow the natural contour of the calf and avoid excessive tension. Tight electrodes can act as venous tourniquets and cause a false-positive result, as will a tight thigh cuff.

Test Procedure

The pneumatic cuff is inflated to a pressure of 50 mmHg (about 70 cm H_2O). This pressure is maintained until the tracing reaches a plateau (usually 1–2 minutes). The cuff must be free to deflate promptly, since any mechanical delay in deflation caused by obstructed tubing might simulate a poor venous outflow from DVT. If the IPG result is clearly normal (Fig. 7.1), the test can be concluded. If the IPG result is borderline or abnormal after the first test, the venous occlusion sequence should be repeated. The technician should also quickly recheck that there is no inadvertent tourniquet effect due to a tight thigh cuff, electrodes, clothing, bandages, or tense leg muscles. An IPG test result is not accepted as conclusively abnormal until five consecutive tests are completed (15). This protocol is essential to minimize false-positive tests due to mechanical factors or to peripheral vasoconstriction. The test is easy to perform, and as little as a single day of training in a reference laboratory can be sufficient for a new IPG technician to achieve the greater than 90% accuracy rate for proximal DVT commonly reported in the literature.

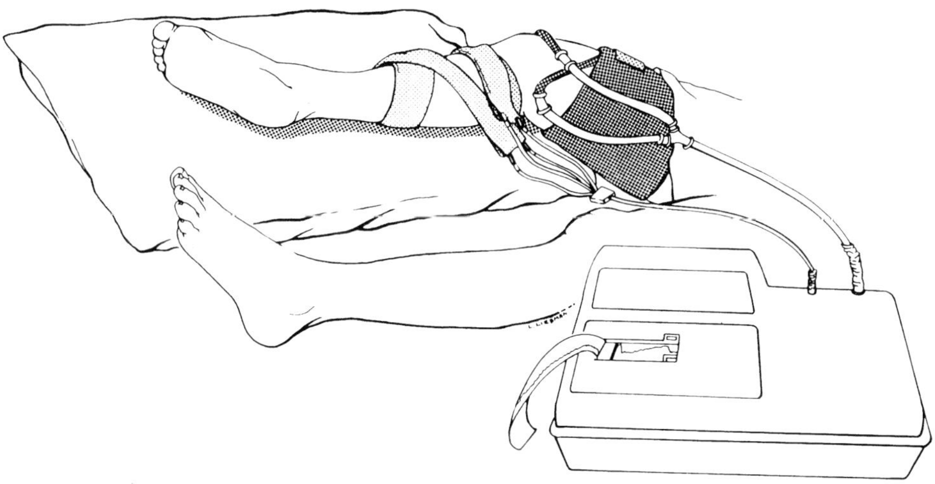

FIG. 7–2. Patient preparation for IPG testing completed. A pillow under the calf allows the patient to relax the calf muscles. Electrodes encircle the calf and the pneumatic cuff is wrapped around the thigh. The electrodes and cuff are attached to the IPG. (Reproduced by permission from Anderson FA Jr. Quantification of the degree of venous outflow obstruction from venous occlusion plethysmography [Dissertation]. Worcester, MA: Worcester Polytechnic Institute, 1984.)

SPECIAL PROBLEMS IN TESTING

Leg Wounds or Ulcers

Testing may be inadvisable in patients with bulky dressings or wounds that are draining or painful. The pneumatic cuff can be applied over light bandages and still function normally; however, the electrodes will not function unless they contact bare skin. Where sterile precautions are required, it is possible to gas sterilize IPG electrodes. They can also be cleaned with a disinfectant. It is not necessary to wash or sterilize IPG electrodes after routine patient testing. Any excess conductive paste is simply wiped off, as would be done with an ultrasound probe.

Pregnancy

In late pregnancy, compression of the mother's inferior vena cava by the fetus may cause a false-positive IPG. The IPG should first be performed with the patient in the standard position. If abnormal results are obtained, the mother's position should be modified to reduce the pressure of the fetus on the vena cava. The patient should shift her weight to the opposite side, and the leg being tested should be internally rotated. Using this maneuver, normal test results are almost always achieved in patients without DVT, even in the late stages of pregnancy (16).

Hip Surgery

Patients undergoing total hip reconstruction are often in traction during the first days following surgery and may be difficult to position for IPG testing. It is often difficult for these patients to relax the operated leg. It may also be medically inadvisable or painful to externally rotate the leg. Thus, IPG testing must occasionally be performed in these patients under less than optimal conditions (without external leg rotation). Abnormal IPG results in such patients should be viewed with caution because a positive result may be caused by poor leg position or muscle tension; however, normal IPG results are still reliable.

Massive Edema

In patients with markedly swollen, edematous legs, electrolyte-rich interstitial fluid may decrease tissue resistance below the range which the instrument has been designed to measure. In such patients, it may be necessary to increase the separation of the electrodes by moving the lower electrode several centimeters further down the calf, permitting the test to be performed by increasing the baseline tissue resistance.

Pulmonary Insufficiency

Patients in severe respiratory distress may be unable or unwilling to lie flat for more than a few minutes. These patients should be prepared for testing in whatever position they find comfortable. The back of the bed can then be lowered for the short time required to do the test.

Morbid Obesity

Markedly obese patients may be difficult to position, and the usual thigh cuff and/or electrodes may be too short. An old pair of electrodes can be used to extend the straps on the thigh cuff, and longer electrodes are available for large calves. The thigh cuff should be positioned as high above the knee as possible to avoid skin movement artifacts. With these adjustments in the usual test preparation, obese patients can be reliably tested by IPG.

INTERPRETATION

Interpretation of the IPG test is based on measurement of the blood volume dammed up in the calf following inflation of the thigh cuff (termed "venous capacitance" or VC) and the blood volume draining out of the leg within 3 seconds after tourniquet deflation (termed "3-second venous outflow" or VO_3). Venous outflow at 3 seconds has been shown to display the maximum difference between normal and abnormal IPG tracings (Fig. 7.3) (17). Because venous outflow is influenced by the initial venous volume, as well as by any venous outflow obstruction, interpretation is best expressed by plotting VO_3 as a function of VC (Fig. 7.4). Interpretation is based on a line dividing normal from abnormal IPG results, as first described at McMaster University after a comparison of over 600 IPG test results with venograms. The line was derived by a statistical method known as discriminant function analysis and is commonly referred to as the "discriminant line" (18).

The same investigators originally recommended a minimum of five test repetitions on all patients in order to reduce false-positive results (15). They observed that an occasional patient with DVT and with a low venous capacitance may have a test result marginally above the "discriminant line," until a higher VC has been achieved by repeated testing, at which point the test result will fall below the "discriminant line." However, any test that fell above a second line, somewhat above the "discriminant line," never returned to the abnormal zone on subsequent tests despite any increase in VC. Therefore, any IPG result falling above this second line has little chance of missing a clinically significant DVT. IPG testing can thus be concluded when any result falls above this second line, even if this occurs on the first test and in a patient with limited VC. Since the test can be stopped at this point, the higher line has been referred to as the "stop line" (19). However, any test results that fall between the stop line and the "discriminant line" should be considered inconclusive until the five test sequence has been completed.

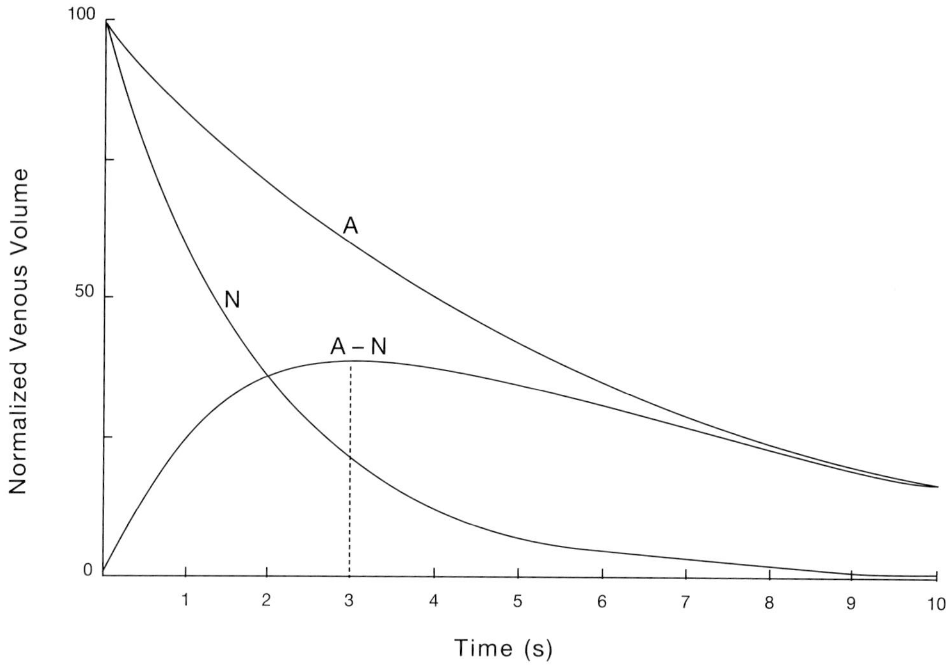

FIG. 7–3. Maximum difference between average normal (*N*) and abnormal (*A*) IPG venous outflow curves occurs at a point approximately 3 seconds from release of venous occlusion. (Reproduced by permission from Anderson FA Jr. Quantification of the degree of venous outflow obstruction from venous occlusion plethysmography [Dissertation]. Worcester, MA: Worcester Polytechnic Institute, 1984.)

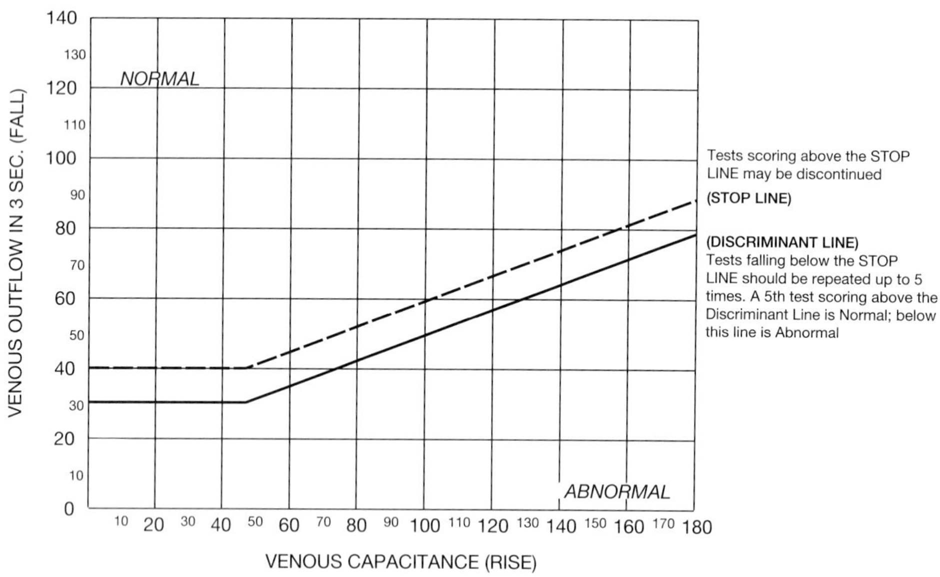

FIG. 7–4. IPG interpretation graph incorporating the discriminant line and the stop line. (Reproduced by permission from Anderson FA Jr. Quantification of the degree of venous outflow obstruction from venous occlusion plethysmography [Dissertation]. Worcester, MA: Worcester Polytechnic Institute, 1984.)

After five test repetitions, final interpretation is based on the test with the greatest VC. If this "best test" falls below the "discriminant line," the IPG result is positive, indicating the presence of venous outflow obstruction (and presumably acute DVT). Any tests during which the patient moved or which were otherwise technically unacceptable should be repeated.

This simplified "discriminant line" approach to IPG interpretation has become nearly universal and has proved highly accurate. Nevertheless, it is possible to obtain additional information and provide better quantitation by other methods of analysis. To an experienced observer, the shape of the outflow curve may reveal useful information. For example, with development of collateral circulation after DVT, an abnormal IPG test may revert to normal by discriminant line analysis; but such patients will often show a relatively flat outflow curve, as opposed to the typical concave shape observed in patients with a normal venous system. It is also possible to quantitate venous outflow by expressing the results as a percent of predicted normal, by employing the so-called "Venous Diameter Index" (VDI) (Fig. 7.5). Although beyond the scope of this chapter, quantitation of venous outflow may prove useful in future clinical applications (17, 20). At present, the principal limiting factor in validating newer methods of IPG interpretation is the difficulty of obtaining venograms on all patients with DVT.

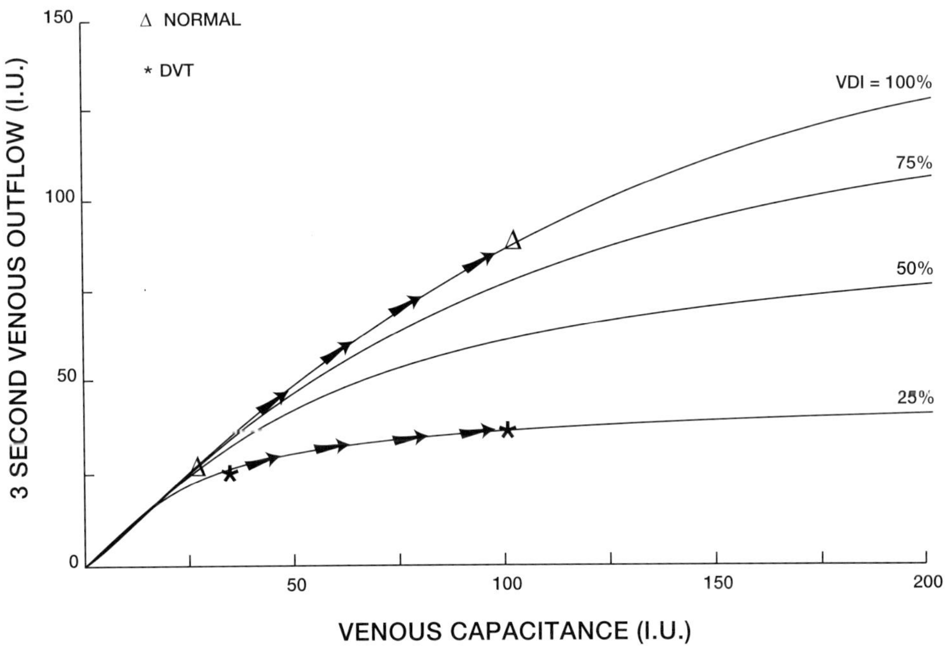

FIG. 7–5. Test points that are equivocal on initial testing are often clearly resolved by test repetition, prolonged occlusion, or other maneuvers that improve venous filling (40). The ability to increase the venous outflow rate with increases in venous capacitance depends upon the percent patency of the venous system. (Reproduced by permission from Anderson FA Jr. Quantification of the degree of venous outflow obstruction from venous occlusion plethysmography [Dissertation]. Worcester, MA: Worcester Polytechnic Institute, 1984.)

CLINICAL USES

Suspected Deep Vein Thrombosis

Patients with unilateral leg swelling and/or calf discomfort are often suspected of having DVT. The majority of these patients do not have DVT, but if the symptoms are in fact due to DVT, the disease is usually extensive. IPG is particularly useful in the initial evaluation of these symptomatic patients, since the results are usually either normal or strikingly abnormal. A negative IPG in a symptomatic patient is associated with a less than 2% incidence of acute proximal DVT (18). At the University of Massachusetts Medical Center, two-thirds of patients with clinically suspected DVT have a bilaterally negative IPG. The percentage is even higher in outpatients (21). These patients can be discharged without treatment, but should return for follow-up study. Two randomized prospective studies have shown that it is safe and highly cost-effective to withhold treatment in symptomatic patients with repeated negative IPG tests (12, 13).

Suspected Pulmonary Emboli

Over 90% of major pulmonary emboli (PE) are thought to originate from thrombi in the iliac, femoral, or popliteal veins. Thus, in patients suspected of PE, it is reasonable to use IPG to look for DVT in these vessels. A common diagnostic approach for suspected PE is to combine IPG and radionuclide lung scan. When both tests are negative, clinically significant PE is virtually ruled out. When both IPG and lung scan are positive, then the diagnosis of PE is relatively well-established. When IPG and lung scan are inconsistent, a pulmonary angiogram may be required to establish the diagnosis of PE (22). A randomized prospective study has demonstrated that it is safe to withhold anticoagulant treatment in patients with a clinical suspicion of PE and a negative IPG, even when the lung scan suggests a low probability of PE (22).

High Risk Screening

IPG screening may be useful in selected asymptomatic patients with multiple risk factors for DVT, especially when prophylaxis for DVT/PE is unavailable or contraindicated. When screening high risk patients, it is important to remember that DVT may develop relatively rapidly and that a negative IPG does not rule out the development of clinically significant DVT at a later time, perhaps even within 48 or 72 hours. Thus, once the decision has been made to undertake prospective screening for DVT, the IPG should be repeated every 2 or 3 days until the period of risk has ended. Random screening of patients who are not at high risk of DVT/PE is not cost-effective, since the prevalence of clinically significant DVT in a general hospital population is only 1–3% (23). IPG has been advocated for the screening of patients following total hip replacement in combination with the radiolabeled fibrinogen uptake test (24), but radiolabeled fibrinogen is no longer commercially available in the United States, making this recommendation obsolete. IPG is not a satisfactory endpoint by itself for screening this group of patients, since recent studies have shown that a false-negative IPG finding may occur in the presence of an asymptomatic, nonocclusive thrombus proximal to the knee (10, 25–27). Duplex scanning and/or venography may be more appropriate screening methods following total hip replacement (28).

Recurrent Deep Vein Thrombosis

Patients with a past history of DVT often present with symptoms that suggest recurrent thrombosis. It is often difficult to differentiate symptoms due to postphlebitic syndrome from symptoms due to recurrent acute DVT. If a negative IPG has previously been obtained as a baseline in such patients, a repeat IPG which has become positive confirms the diagnosis of recurrent acute DVT (29, 30). If no IPG test has been obtained previously, or if the last IPG test was abnormal, a repeat abnormal IPG is of little diagnostic assistance. After acute DVT, approximately 70% of patients will have persistently abnormal tests after 3 weeks of treatment, and approximately 40% will still be abnormal at 3 months (31). Thus, unless a previous baseline IPG has been demonstrated to be normal, one cannot assume that an acute positive IPG in these circumstances indicates recurrent DVT rather than persistent venous outflow obstruction. Even venography or ultrasonic imaging may be difficult to interpret in such patients. Use of radioactive fibrinogen uptake testing (RFUT) has been advocated to detect acute thrombosis in patients with a past history of acute DVT (29, 30), but RFUT is no longer commercially available in the United States.

Long-Term Anticoagulant Management of Deep Vein Thrombosis

Long-term oral anticoagulation poses a significant risk to some patients. Nevertheless, most physicians currently maintain patients with DVT on oral anticoagulants for at least 6 months. It may be appropriate to discontinue anticoagulation after a shorter period if the IPG test has reverted to normal and if there are no ongoing risk factors for DVT/PE, particularly if there is some reason to suspect that the patient is at greater than usual risk for bleeding from anticoagulants. However, it is potentially hazardous to discontinue anticoagulation if the IPG test continues to show significant venous outflow obstruction, since venous stasis is well-recognized as a major predisposing factor to recurrent DVT. In our experience, recurrent thrombophlebitis has not occurred in patients with normal IPG tests in whom anticoagulants were discontinued 30 days or more after the onset of treatment (21).

COST-BENEFIT CONSIDERATIONS

Because of the high cost of medical care, diagnostic tests are being carefully scrutinized with respect to their cost-benefit ratio. When employed selectively, IPG has been documented to be highly cost-effective (32, 33). The cost of an IPG test in most hospitals is equivalent to that of an electrocardiogram or a chest x-ray, usually $50 to $100. This charge compares quite favorably with the large savings made possible by elimination of unnecessary treatment or expensive alternative tests. The cost-benefit of IPG is greatest in symptomatic patients, approximately two-thirds of whom will have normal IPG results. Duplex ultrasonic scanning can also be employed for screening such patients, but is significantly more expensive. Typical hospital and professional charges for duplex venous scanning range between $300 and $600 (3 to 12 times the typical charge for IPG testing). Venography is even more expensive, as well as being invasive.

In asymptomatic patients, the cost-effectiveness of IPG depends upon the expected incidence of DVT in the patient group being studied. IPG is not cost-effective when applied randomly because of the low incidence of DVT in a general hospital population (1–3%). It has been shown to be cost-effective when applied selectively in patients at high risk, including the outpatient follow-up of patients undergoing total-hip reconstruction (9, 33).

RELATIONSHIP OF IMPEDANCE PLETHYSMOGRAPHY TO OTHER DIAGNOSTIC TESTS

IPG was first developed during the 1970s, a time when there was great interest in finding a practical noninvasive method as an alternative to either clinical diagnosis or venography for the diagnosis of DVT. Diagnostic use of a hand-held Doppler flowmeter and radioactive fibrinogen uptake were the major competitive methods employed (34, 35). Of these modalities, the Doppler flowmeter remains an inexpensive and widely available diagnostic tool, but its use for the diagnosis of DVT has become infrequent due to the subjectivity of the analysis and the expertise required on the part of the observer (8). RFUT has been invaluable in prospective studies of DVT prophylaxis, but its use for acute DVT has been limited by an inherent 24–48-hour delay in diagnosis. Other limiting factors have included its expense, lack of ready availability, and concerns about the potential risk of injecting a human blood product.

Other types of plethysmography, such as strain-gauge plethysmography and air-cuff plethysmography, were also advocated for the diagnosis of DVT. The greater acceptance of IPG was due in part to reports of greater sensitivity and specificity, particularly in the randomized prospective studies from McMaster University in which venograms were obtained in all patients (15, 18, 24, 36). IPG also benefitted from impressive documentation of clinical efficacy, particularly in randomized prospective studies (12, 13, 16, 37).

During the 1980s, high resolution B-mode scanning for study of the leg veins revolutionized the management of DVT. Like IPG, ultrasonic scanning is noninvasive and readily accepted by patients, even for repeat examinations. It also can be carried out at the bedside, if necessary. As a result, in many hospitals ultrasonography has replaced venography as the "gold standard" for anatomic diagnosis of DVT (38). In some centers, duplex scanning has become the principal diagnostic test employed for DVT. However, the high cost of ultrasonic equipment and the need for a highly skilled technologist/sonographer to insure accuracy have resulted in a continued role for IPG in many institutions. Even where duplex scanning is readily available, IPG has been used as a convenient low-cost screening method for symptomatic or high risk patients, reserving duplex scanning for patients with abnormal IPG tests. For some hospitals, venography still remains the "gold standard," but its invasive character, inconvenience, discomfort, and cost limit its widespread use. In many medical centers, a low-cost screening technique (such as IPG or hand-held Doppler flowmeter) has proved useful for initial screening or long-term follow-up, with frequent use of duplex scanning or infrequent use of venography for anatomic confirmation as desired.

SUMMARY

IPG is a convenient bedside procedure for the measurement of blood volume changes. Although widely employed for the management of DVT, it is potentially applicable for the study of other disorders of venous function as well (14, 39). A standardized IPG procedure for the diagnosis of proximal DVT has proved highly accurate in widespread application over the last two decades. The test procedure is simple to perform and interpret at the bedside. It has a high degree of accuracy, even in the hands of relatively inexperienced observers. There is a wide margin for error in test performance with a minimal loss of accuracy. Technical errors tend to be reported as false-positive results, which are less serious than false-negative findings which might leave the patient at risk for PE. Several randomized prospective studies have demonstrated the benign clinical outcome with respect to DVT/PE in patients with normal IPG tests. Patient acceptance is excellent, and no complications of the procedure have been reported. Although duplex scanning now provides an anatomic diagnosis with noninvasive methodology, it appears that the convenience, accuracy, and low cost of IPG, coupled with the extensive literature documenting its clinical utility, will result in an ongoing role. It is useful primarily as a reliable, low-cost method for initial screening and long-term follow-up, particularly in patients with physical signs or symptoms suggesting DVT.

REFERENCES

1. Nyboer J. Electrical impedance plethysmography. Springfield, IL: Charles C Thomas, 1970.
2. Kubicek WG, Kottke FJ, Ramos MU, et al. The Minnesota impedance cardiograph theory and applications. Biomed Eng 1974;9:410–416.
3. Wheeler HB, Mullick SC. Detection of venous obstruction in the leg by measurement of electrical impedance. Ann NY Acad Sci 1970;170:804–811.
4. Mullick SC, Wheeler HB, Songster GF. Diagnosis of deep vein thrombosis by measurement of electrical impedance. Am J Surg 1970;119:417–422.
5. Wheeler HB, O'Donnell JA, Anderson FA Jr, Benedict K Jr. Occlusive impedance phlebography: a diagnostic procedure for venous thrombosis and pulmonary embolism. Prog Cardiovas Dis 1974;17:199–205.
6. Wheeler HB, O'Donnell JA, Anderson FA Jr, Penney BC, Peura RA, Benedict C Jr. Bedside screening for venous thrombosis using occlusive impedance phlebography. Angiology 1975;26:199–209.

7. Dahn I, Eiriksson E. Plethysmographic diagnosis of deep vein thrombosis of the leg. Acta Chir Scand 1968;398(Suppl):33–42.
8. Wheeler HB, Anderson FA Jr. Use of noninvasive tests as the basis for treatment of deep vein thrombosis. In: Bernstein EF, ed. Vascular diagnosis. 4th ed. St. Louis: CV Mosby, 1993:862–874.
9. Mallory TH, Vaughn BK, Lombardi AV Jr, Mitchell MB. Impedance plethysmography for surveillance of deep venous thrombosis following early discharge of total joint replacement patients. Orthopedics 1990;13:1347–1351.
10. Comerota AJ, Katz ML, Grossi RJ, et al. The comparative value of noninvasive testing for diagnosis and surveillance of deep vein thrombosis. J Vasc Surg 1988;7:40–49.
11. Patterson RB, Fowl RJ, Keller JD, Schomaker W, Kempczinski RF. The limitations of impedance plethysmography in the diagnosis of acute deep venous thrombosis. J Vasc Surg 1989;9:725–730.
12. Hull RD, Hirsh J, Carter CJ, et al. Diagnostic efficacy of impedance plethysmography for clinically suspected deep-vein thrombosis: a randomized trial. Ann Intern Med 1985;102:21–28.
13. Huisman MV, Buller HR, ten Cate JW, Vreeken J. Serial impedance plethysmography for suspected deep venous thrombosis in outpatients. The Amsterdam general practitioner study. N Engl J Med 1986;314:823–828.
14. Wheeler HB, Penney BC, Anderson FA Jr. Impedance plethysmography: theoretic, experimental, and clinical considerations. In: Bernstein EF, ed. Vascular diagnosis. 4th ed. St. Louis: CV Mosby, 1993:194–204.
15. Hull R, Taylor DW, Hirsh J, et al. Impedance plethysmography: the relationship between venous filling and sensitivity and specificity for proximal vein thrombosis. Circulation 1978;58:898–902.
16. Hull RD, Raskob GE, Carter CJ. Serial impedance plethysmography in pregnant patients with clinically suspected deep-vein thrombosis. Ann Int Med 1990;112:663–667.
17. Anderson FA Jr. Quantification of the degree of venous outflow obstruction from venous occlusion plethysmography [Dissertation]. Worcester, MA: Worcester Polytechnic Institute, 1984:218.
18. Hull R, van Aken WG, Hirsh J, et al. Impedance plethysmography using the occlusive cuff technique in the diagnosis of venous thrombosis. Circulation 1976;53:696–700.
19. Taylor DW, Hull R, Sackett DL, Hirsh J. Simplification of the sequential impedance plethysmograph technique without loss of accuracy. Thromb Res 1980;17:561–565.
20. Wheeler HB, Anderson FA Jr. The diagnosis of venous thrombosis by impedance plethysmography. In: Bernstein EF, ed. Noninvasive diagnostic techniques in vascular disease. 3rd ed. St. Louis: CV Mosby, 1985:755–765.
21. Wheeler HB, Anderson FA Jr. Diagnosis of deep vein thrombosis by impedance plethysmography. In: Bernstein EF, ed. Vascular diagnosis. 4th ed. St. Louis: CV Mosby, 1993:820–829.
22. Hull RD, Raskob GE, Coates G, Panju AA, Gill GJ. A new noninvasive management strategy for patients with suspected pulmonary embolism. Arch Intern Med 1989;149:2549–2555.
23. Anderson FA Jr, Wheeler HB, Goldberg RJ, et al. A population-based perspective of the hospital incidence and case-fatality rates of venous thrombosis and pulmonary embolism: the Worcester DVT Study. Arch Intern Med 1991;151:933–938.
24. Hull R, Hirsh J, Sackett DL, Powers P, Turpie AGG, Walker I. Combined use of leg scanning and impedance plethysmography in suspected venous thrombosis. An alternative to venography. N Engl J Med 1977;296:1497–1500.
25. Paiement G, Wessinger SJ, Waltman AC, Harris WH. Surveillance of deep vein thrombosis in asymptomatic total hip replacement patients. Impedance phlebography and fibrinogen scanning versus roentgenographic phlebography. Am J Surg 1988;155:400–404.

26. Agnelli G, Cosmi B, Ranucci V, et al. Impedance plethysmography in the diagnosis of asymptomatic deep vein thrombosis in hip surgery. Arch Intern Med 1991;151: 2167–2171.
27. Cruickshank ML, Levine MN, Hirsh J, et al. An evaluation of impedance plethysmography and ^{125}I-fibrinogen leg scanning in patients following hip surgery. Thromb Haemostasis 1989;62:830–834.
28. Wheeler HB. Diagnosis of deep vein thrombosis. Using the right test for the right purpose. Arch Intern Med 1991;151:2145–2146.
29. Hull RD, Carter CJ, Jay RM, et al. The diagnosis of acute, recurrent deep-vein thrombosis: a diagnostic challenge. Circulation 1983;67:901–906.
30. Hirsh J. Clinical utility of impedance plethysmography in the diagnosis of recurrent deep-vein thrombosis. Arch Intern Med 1988;148:519–520.
31. Jay R, Hull R, Carter CJ, et al. Outcome of abnormal impedance plethysmography results in patients with proximal-vein thrombosis: frequency of return to normal. Thromb Res 1984;36:259–263.
32. Gross WS, Burney RE. Therapeutic and economic implications of emergency department evaluation for venous thrombosis. J Am Coll Emer Phys 1979;8:110–113.
33. Hull R, Hirsh J, Sackett DL, Stoddart G. Cost effectiveness of clinical diagnosis, venography and noninvasive testing in patients with symptomatic deep-vein thrombosis. N Engl J Med 1981;304:1561–1567.
34. Flanc C, Kakkar VV, Clarke MB. The detection of venous thrombosis of the legs using ^{125}I-labelled fibrinogen. Br J Surg 1968;55:742.
35. Sigel B, Felix WR, Popky GL, Ipsen J. Diagnosis of lower limb venous thrombosis by Doppler ultrasound technique. Arch Surg 1972;104:174–179.
36. Hull R, Hirsh J, Sackett DL, et al. Replacement of venography in suspected venous thrombosis by impedance plethysmography and ^{125}I-fibrinogen leg scanning: a less invasive approach. Ann Int Med 1981;94:12–15.
37. Huisman MV, Buller HR, ten Cate JW, Heijermans HSF, van der Laan J, van Maanen DJ. Management of clinically suspected acute venous thrombosis in outpatients with serial impedance plethysmography in a community hospital setting. Arch Intern Med 1989;149:511–513.
38. de Valois JC, van Schaik CC, Verzijlbergen F, van Ramshorst B, Eikelboom BC, Meuwissen OJATh. Contrast venography: from gold standard to "golden backup" in clinically suspected deep vein thrombosis. Eur J Radiol 1990;11:131–137.
39. Anderson FA Jr, Li JM, Wheeler HB. Application of impedance plethysmography to the detection of venous insufficiency. Bruit 1983;7:41–46.
40. Anderson FA Jr, Cardullo PA, Wheeler HB. Problems commonly encountered in IPG testing and their solution. Bruit 1980;4:21–24.

chapter 8

Foot Volumetry

Olav Thulesius and Anders Thurin

During quiet standing the hydrostatic pressure of the column of blood from the right atrium to the leg determines venous pressure. If upright posture is maintained, this results in an unavoidable elevation of capillary pressure and, hence, an increase in capillary filtration and edema formation. Physiologic counterregulation involves pressure reduction by foot movement and a proximal redistribution of blood in the presence of competent valves and reduction in tissue perfusion due to a venoarterial vasoconstrictor reflex.

A method for the functional evaluation of venous function in the upright position is the continuous measurement of volume changes (volumetry) in the distal part of the leg. Volumetry is a truly noninvasive technique based on the concept that measurements of venous pressure and volume in the foot rely on similar mechanisms (1–3). During quiet standing, the hydrostatic pressure in the lower extremity venous system is a function of the vertical height of the blood column from the heart to the foot. With exercise and competent venous valves, standing venous pressure at the foot is lowered (4). Reduction of venous pressure is preceded by the central dislocation of blood secondary to the compressing action of the contracting calf muscles and stretching forces of moving fascia acting on compressible vessels.

PRINCIPLE

Changes in ambulatory venous pressure as measured in a foot vein are accompanied by parallel changes of the venous volume of the distal part of the lower extremity. By the pumping action of the leg muscles blood is expelled in the cephalad direction, and this is monitored by a fall in foot volume. After exercise resting volume is slowly regained. In patients with venous insufficiency, volume reduction is reduced or absent, depending on the degree of valvular damage and/or residual venous obstruction. This technique is called foot volumetry

(1). Continuous measurement of the volume of the foot and ankle region, therefore, constitutes a simple principle for the noninvasive assessment of venous insufficiency.

Ambulatory venous pressure measurement is an invasive technique, requiring puncture of a foot vein, which may be uncomfortable and impractical particularly when repeated measurements are required. Noninvasive assessment of foot volume changes with exercise are much easier to perform and the findings correlate well with pressure measurements (2, 3). Concomitant measurement of changes of venous volume and pressure enable calculation of venous compliance (5).

APPARATUS AND PROCEDURE

The foot volumeter is an open container into which the foot is inserted. Thereafter, the container is filled with water to a level just above the malleolus. Water displacement according to the size of the foot reflects tissue volume, which includes the blood volume of the venous compartment. The water level, initially 14 cm from the bottom, is sensed by a critically damped photoelectric float-sensor, which operates an optical wedge, the output of which is continuously monitored on a strip-chart recorder.

Usually two volumeters are used to enable simultaneous measurements from both feet, and a volume recording is made on a two-channel recorder. After the feet have been placed in the volumeters, these containers are rapidly filled from a thermostated water line at a temperature of 32°C. (It is essential to keep the water temperature between 30–32°C. Higher temperatures increase arterial inflow to the foot and may give rise to false-positive readings.)

Thereafter volume calibration is performed with a water-filled syringe. When a steady baseline is achieved in the standing position, a standard exercise is performed, consisting of 20 knee bends (knee flexion about 70°) in 40 seconds, paced by a metronome. (Exercise must be standardized and should not exceed 20 knee bends in order to avoid active hyperemia.) After exercise the patient stands quietly until volume restitution has been completed. To facilitate the exercise procedure the patient grips handlebars with both hands (Fig. 8.1).

During exercise blood is expelled from the foot vessels and the water displacement is reduced in proportion to the volume of dislocated blood. During a series of knee bends the blood volume gradually declines until it reaches a steady-state level. After completion of exercise the subject stands quietly when the resting volume is again reached at varying length of time depending on the rate of arterial inflow and venous reflux. Normally, refilling flow is exclusively from the arterial side, but in cases of venous insufficiency retrograde flow (reflux) from proximally located veins occurs.

To differentiate between superficial and deep venous insufficiency repeated measurements are performed after tourniquet compression of superficial veins at different levels: above the knee, below the knee, and at the ankle, just above the volumeter. After completion of the exercise the water is sucked out of the volumeter and the total foot volume measured in a calibrated reservoir.

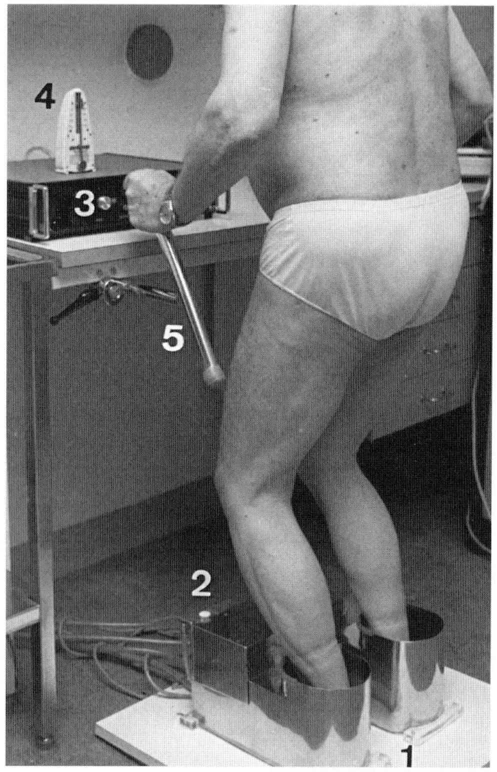

FIG. 8–1. Foot volumetry in action. *1* = Foot volumeters; *2* = Calibration syringe; *3* = Preamplifier, connected to chart-recorder; *4* = Pacing metronome; *5* = Handlebar.

INTERPRETATION

Figure 8.2 shows a recording which illustrates a case with chronic venous insufficiency with superficial and deep venous insufficiency. Quantitative evaluation is done by measuring changes of baseline and assessing the dynamic changes of the volumetric curves.

The most important parameters are the expelled volume (EV) characterizing the venous pump and the refilling flow (Q) reflecting the degree of reflux. EV is measured in absolute units (milliliters) or given in relation to foot volume (per liter of total displaced foot volume). When expressed per 100 ml tissue the result is the relative expelled volume, EVr. Refilling flow normally is equal to arterial inflow, but in patients with venous insufficiency it also reflects retrograde venous flow.

Another useful parameter is the volume restitution time (t) in seconds, or the more easily determined half refilling time (t/2). Basically, refilling time should equal expelled volume divided by refilling flow. Usually, however, the refilling time is slightly longer because of such factors as delayed compliance of the venous wall and refilling of fluid from the lymphatics. As the ratio of refilling flow, Q, and expelled volume, EVr combines two of the most important parameters of venous function.

Table 8.1 lists reference values from our laboratory. Some of the normal values decrease with age. This applies mainly to the parameter expelled volume because

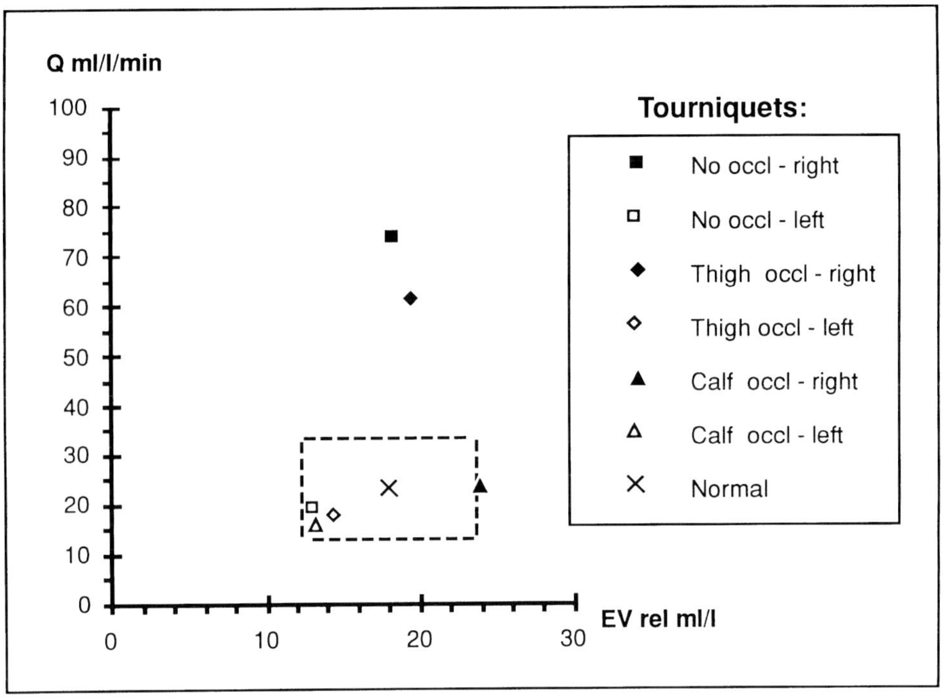

FIG. 8–2. Computer printout of the two most important volumetric parameters: expelled volume (*EV*) and refilling flow (*Q*). Normal range indicated by *square*. This chart shows an example of a patient with isolated superficial venous insufficiency in the short saphenous vein of the right leg. Application of tourniquet on thigh produces no significant benefit but application on calf lowers Q value by elimination of reflux.

muscle power and joint flexibility decline with age. Easy graphic evaluation of the results can be obtained by using our computer program which is based on a spread-sheet entry of data (compare Fig. 8.2).

CLINICAL APPLICATION

Foot volumetry evaluates the functional capacity of the peripheral venous system of the leg by assessing valvular function and the capacity of the calf-foot

TABLE 8-1

NORMAL REFERENCE VALUES FOR VOLUMETRY

Parameter	Age: 20–60	60–75 years
EV ml/l	18 (12–25)	7 (5–20)
Q ml/l/min	23 (14–34)	20 (10–30)
t sec	55 (30–80)	30 (20–70)

pump. Individual values from patients can easily be assessed using the EV/Q diagram shown in Figure 8.2.

To distinguish between superficial and deep venous insufficiency, repeat measurements are performed with tourniquet occlusion of superficial incompetent veins. Tourniquets can be applied at different levels to distinguish between insufficiency of the great and short saphenous veins, and if parameters are not normalized, deep venous insufficiency is likely to be present. Furthermore, guided compression can eliminate reflux from incompetent perforator veins.

Foot volumetry provides a quantitative estimation of the degree and location of venous insufficiency as shown by several workers (2, 3, 6). Figure 8.3 shows original volumetric records from a patient with superficial and deep venous insufficiency. Volumetry is useful for the evaluation of therapeutic interventions and can be used in follow-up studies after deep venous thrombosis to determine the incidence of postthrombotic valvular incompetence.

DISCUSSION

In the past, the "gold standard" for the evaluation of venous function was the use of ambulatory venous pressure measurement. The term "venous hypertension" has been derived from such measurements. An elevated venous pressure, however, reflects only one single aspect of the pathophysiologic disturbance

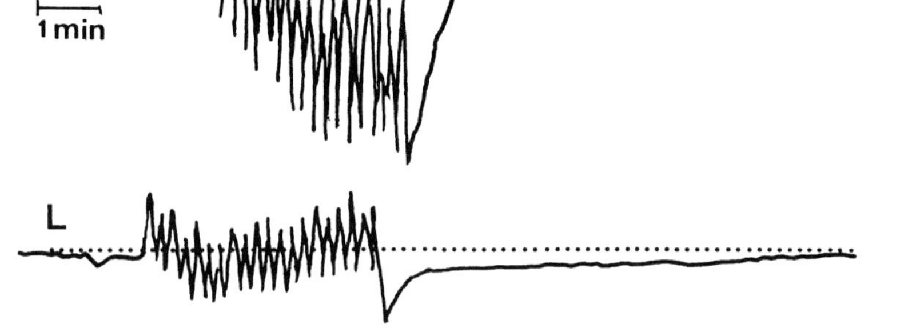

FIG. 8–3. Original recordings from a male patient, aged 55, with chronic venous insufficiency (deep venous insufficiency in popliteal vein left and superficial venous insufficiency right). *R* = Right foot volume: 1.29 l; expelled volume, EV: 15.5 ml; refilling flow, Q: 64.6 ml/l/min. *L* = Left foot volume: 1.41 l; expelled volume, EV: 3.2 ml/l; refilling flow, Q: 31.0 ml/l/min.

of chronic venous insufficiency. Equally important is the plethora of venous congestion which results in stagnation of flow, thereby facilitating trapping of white blood cells, a process that can initiate microthrombosis and tissue damage (7). Therefore, venous function is better monitored by a method that evaluates changes of volume and flow.

The assessment of distal changes of foot volume rather than changes of calf volume may be questioned. It has, however, recently been shown that this type of evaluation corresponds best to the clinical situation (8).

Foot volume at rest may be a useful parameter in itself if the effect of antiedematous therapy should be evaluated. Foot volume, V in ml, can be predicted from an equation incorporating the body surface area (BSA):

$$V = 617.3 \times BSA + 44.7$$

As shown by Norgren and collaborators (2), a useful parameter which discriminates normal individuals from patients with varicose veins and deep venous insufficiency is the ratio of refilling flow, Q to expelled volume, EVr:

$$Q/EVr$$

Exercise involving the calf-foot pump drains about 30–40% of the total blood volume contained in the vessels of the foot and mainly affects the volume of larger veins, the remaining blood being stored in venules and capillaries. (This can be shown using a plethysmograph tightly enclosing the extremity and by the application of external pressure squeezing out blood.)

Recently, we noticed that the exercise-induced mobilization (expelled volume, EV) of blood is greater in the dominant, mostly weight-bearing leg (usually the right) and, consequently, the EV values may be 10–40% higher on this side. From the combined application of volume and pressure changes calculation of venous compliance can be obtained (5). A feature commonly seen after completion of exercise is the more rapid return of the pressure rather than volume to baseline. This may be due either to delayed compliance of the venous wall or delayed filling with tissue fluid within the lymphatic system.

REFERENCES

1. Thulesius O, Norgren L, Gjöres JE. Foot volumetry: a new method for objective assessment of edema and venous function. Vasa 1973;2:325–329.
2. Norgren L, Thulesius O, Gjöres LE, Söderlundh S. Foot volumetry and simultaneous venous pressure measurements for evaluation of venous insufficiency. Vasa 1974;3:140–147.
3. Partsch H. Simultane Venendruckmessung und Plethysmography am Fuss. In: May R, Kriessmann A, eds. Periphere Venendruckmessung. Stuttgart: Georg Thieme Verlag, 1978.
4. Pollack AA, Wood EH. Venous pressure in the saphenous vein at the ankle in man during exercise and changes in position. J Appl Physiol 1949;1:649–662.
5. Norgren L, Thulesius O. Pressure-volume characteristics of foot veins in normal cases and patients with venous insufficiency. Blood Vessels 1975;12:1–12.

6. Lawrence D, Kakkar VV. Venous pressure management and foot volumetry in venous disease. In: Verstraete M, ed. Techniques in angiology. The Hague: Martinus Nijhoff, 1979.
7. Coleridge Smith PD, Thomas P, Scurr JH, Dormandy JA. Causes of venous ulceration, a new hypothesis. Br Med J 1988;296:1726–1727.
8. Rosfors S, Lamke LO, Nordström E, Bygdeman S. Severity and location of venous valvular insufficiency: the importance of distal valve function. Acta Chir Scand 1990;156:689–694.

chapter 9

Venous Hypertensive Microangiopathy: Evaluation by Laser-Doppler Flowmetry

Giovanni Belcaro

VENOUS HYPERTENSIVE MICROANGIOPATHY

The advent of laser-Doppler flowmetry (LDF) allows examination of the microcirculation in venous hypertensive microangiopathy (VHM). Venous hypertensive microangiopathy can result from either deep or superficial incompetence or a combination of the two. The result of the chronically increased venous pressure is progressively transmitted to the more distal capillary bed.

PRINCIPLES OF LASER-DOPPLER FLOWMETRY

Most commercially available instruments utilize laser light to monitor skin flow velocity utilizing the Doppler shift principle. Signal processing, however, is proprietary, based on "black box" calculations that may vary among commercial brands that are marketed. Control and test values for each particular instrument and laboratory should therefore be established.

FLOW AND FLUX

Flow indicates true skin blood flow while flux is a term used to express skin flow measurements obtained by laser-Doppler which correlate with, but are not identical to, skin blood flow. While in some situations (such as VHM) an increase in flux corresponds to an increase in skin flow, this may not be true in all conditions. Laser-Doppler measures skin flux within a depth of 0.75–1.5 mm, which is the global flow in the skin. According to some authors (1), the nutritional flow (5% of the global flow) and the thermoregulatory flow (95%) are not separately measured by laser-Doppler.

SKIN FLUX CHANGES IN VENOUS HYPERTENSION

In the skin of the perimalleolar region of subjects with venous hypertension, it is possible to observe an increase in skin flux associated with an apparent increase in the number of cutaneous capillaries that appear elongated and tortuous. There is also an increase in the average size of capillaries with thickening of the capillary wall in the presence of venous hypertension.

VENOARTERIOLAR RESPONSE

A reduction in skin flux is normally observed with change in posture from the supine to the standing position (Fig. 9.1). This phenomenon, termed the venoarteriolar response (2–5), may be decreased or altogether absent in the presence of venous hypertension (Fig. 9.2) (6). Such limbs commonly exhibit an increased skin flux, as noted earlier.

The normal venoarteriolar response is thought to be due to a sympathetic axon reflex and limits skin flow on standing (2–4). The reflex appears to control the fil-

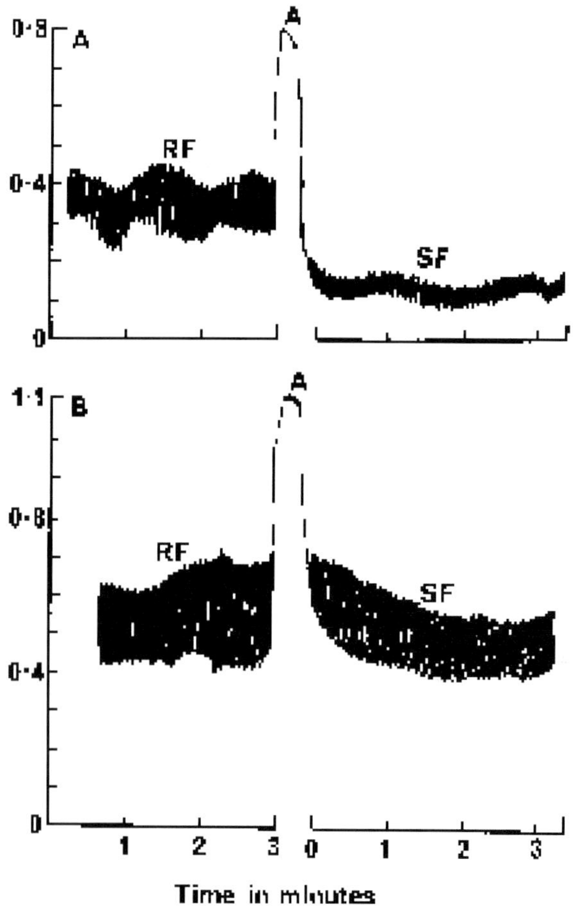

FIG. 9–1. *Top:* An example of the normal venoarteriolar response in a normal limb (perimalleolar region). Laser flux on standing (*SF*) is significantly lower than resting flux (*RF*) in the supine position. *Bottom:* The venoarteriolar response is abolished in skin with venous hypertensive microangiopathy. Also in this situation, RF is increased. (*A* indicates the motion artifact.)

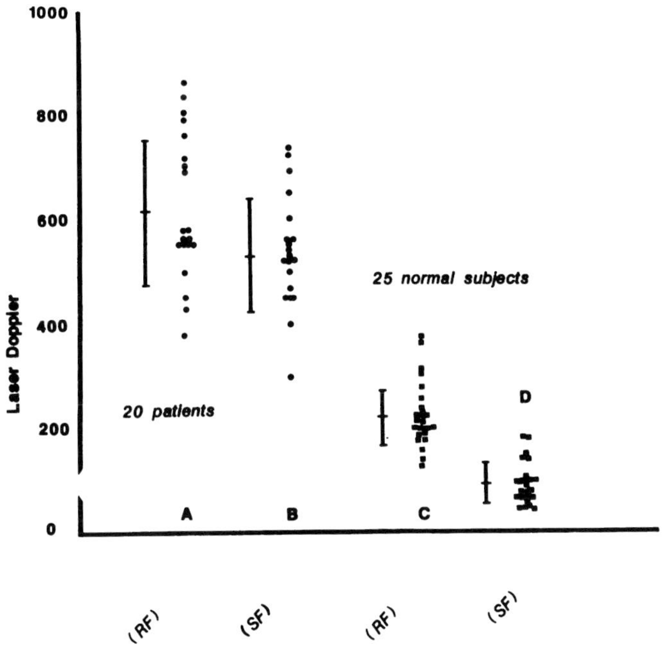

FIG. 9–2. Skin flux at supine rest (*RF*) and on standing (*SF*) in 25 normal subjects and in 20 patients with severe venous hypertension. In patients, both RF and SF are higher and the venoarteriolar response is decreased.

tration of fluid and protein into the interstitial tissue, preventing the formation of edema (5). The venoarteriolar response can be easily demonstrated by laser-Doppler instrumentation as follows: The subject is asked to rest for 30 minutes in the supine position. After this period of acclimatization, one lower limb is dropped below heart level. The lowered extremity reaches a baseline laser-Doppler flux (after a spike representing motion artifact) that is lower than before (Fig. 9.3). A greater and more reproducible skin flux decrease can be observed on standing. The venoarterial response is also observed after a change from the supine to the sitting position (Fig. 9.3). The abolition of venous reflux by application of a tourniquet in a patient with severe superficial venous insufficiency does not restore the absent venoarterial response (Fig. 9.3). This indicates that changes in the venoarterial response evolve slowly in the presence of venous hypertension and an instantaneous relationship is not present. Abolishment of reflux does not immediately restore a normal venoarterial response. The increase in skin flow and decrease in the venoarterial response appear to be related to the increased rate of capillary filtration predisposing to edema formation (3, 5).

We have also observed that the increase in skin flux in the presence of venous hypertension is related to a significant increase in transcutaneous PCO_2. A decrease in transcutaneous PO_2 (7) is not observed until very late in the evolution of microangiopathy. The cause of the increased transcutaneous PCO_2 level is not clearly understood, but it seems to be associated with conditions of high skin flux.

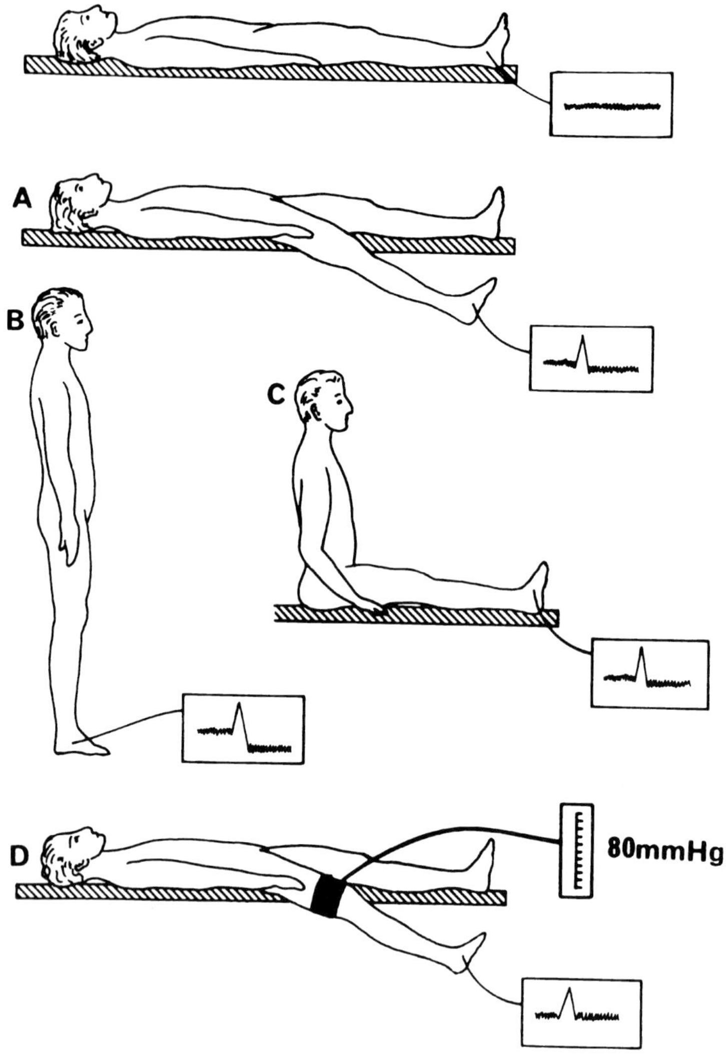

FIG. 9–3. Evaluation of the venoarteriolar response with the patient lowering the leg and foot below heart level (**A**), on standing (**B**), sitting (**C**), and with a thigh tourniquet to exclude reflux from the incompetent superficial venous system (**D**). The most evident and reproducible VAR is obtained on standing when the patient is stable holding on to a frame.

It is possible that the increase in local level of catabolic products in the presence of venous hypertension may increase tissue PCO_2 levels, leading to local vasodilatation (7). Evidence for a relationship between transcutaneous PCO_2 and microangiopathy changes in the skin was suggested by a study comparing 70 postphlebitic and 20 normal limbs. A number of parameters, including the supine resting (RF) and standing (SF) skin flux, the venoarteriolar response, transcutaneous PO_2 and PCO_2, and ambulatory venous pressure measurements (AVP), were obtained (7). Excellent correlation (r > 0.7) was observed between PCO_2 and a number of these parameters such as skin flux (supine and standing), venoarterial response (inverse relationship), and ambulatory venous pressure. In a group of 10 healthy volunteers, it was possible to reproduce many of these microcirculatory changes by 3% CO_2 inhalation for 20 minutes (Table 9.1), which increased transcutaneous skin PCO_2, with an increase in skin flux and a decrease in the venoarterial response (Fig. 9.4). An increase in the rate of ankle swelling measured by strain-gauge plethysmography was also documented with CO_2 inhalation.

LOW AND HIGH PERFUSION MICROANGIOPATHY

Two major types of microangiopathy may be observed and defined by laser-Doppler flowmetry: low perfusion microangiopathy and high perfusion microangiopathy. Low perfusion microangiopathy is present in subjects with severe peripheral vascular disease (1, 8), Raynaud's disease, and essential hypertension (9). Low perfusion microangiopathy is characterized by a decrease in skin flux and the venoarterial response as well as decreased capillary filtration and low transcutaneous PO_2 levels. However, decreased skin flux is not always present as the nutritional flow represents only 5% of the total skin flow.

In contrast, high perfusion microangiopathy is characterized by an increase in skin flux at rest, decreased venoarterial response, and a marked increase in capillary permeability and filtration (2, 5). High perfusion microangiopathy has been observed in diabetic limbs as well as in limbs with venous hypertension. A good correlation (r = 0.76) can be demonstrated between ambulatory pressure and laser-Doppler flow (Fig. 9.5). Tissue PO_2 levels are generally unaltered. Both low and high perfusion microangiopathy may lead to skin and tissue necrosis, but probably through different mechanisms. The increased capillary filtration in high

TABLE 9-1

MICROCIRCULATORY PARAMETERS IN 10 NORMAL VOLUNTEERS BEFORE AND AFTER INHALATION OF AN ATMOSPHERE WITH 3% CO_2 (20 MINUTES)

Parameter	Before	After CO_2
RF (flux units)	0.53 ± 0.01	0.87 ± 0.02*
PO_2 mmHg	68 ± 13	66 ± 12**
PCO_2 mmHg	27 ± 9	36 ± 11*
RAS ml/100 ml	1.007 ± 0.13	1.285 ± 0.15*

All measurements (MEAN ± SD) were taken at the internal perimalleolar region. *RF* = Resting Flux; *RAS* = Rate of Ankle Swelling by strain-gauge plethysmography (3).

The VAR—expressed as the percent skin flux decrease on standing—is shown in Figure 9.4.

*p = <0.05

**Not significant

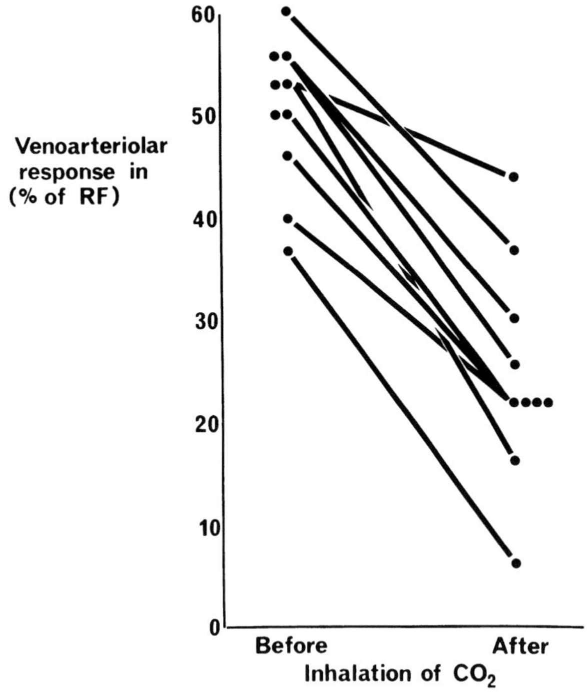

FIG. 9–4. Decrease in the efficacy of the VAR in 10 normal subjects after inhalation of an atmosphere with 3% CO_2. This finding is also associated with an increase in skin flux at rest and skin PCO_2 and capillary filtration.

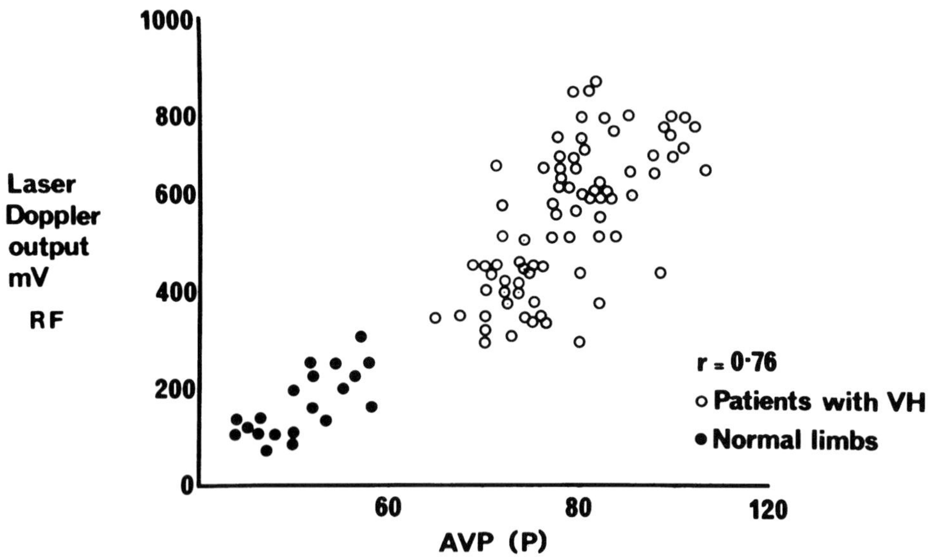

FIG. 9–5. The correlation between ambulatory venous pressure (*AVP* = pressure at the end of the 10-tiptoe exercise test) and laser-Doppler output (*RF*). The correlation between skin flux and AVP is good (r = 0.76) and there is a good separation between patients (severe postphlebitic syndrome) and normal subjects.

perfusion microangiopathy possibly leads to compression and obstruction of the nutrient capillaries. Shunting may be present and edema may slow the diffusion of nutrients and gases in the affected areas.

Bollinger has recently observed that increased capillary diffusion (Na-fluorescein) and morphologic alterations of capillaries are present even in initial stages of chronic venous insufficiency (10).

The measurement of skin flux and the venoarteriolar response may be successfully used in groups of patients to monitor the efficacy of venous treatment modalities in the presence of high perfusion microangiopathy (11). Figure 9.6 shows the dramatic effects of elastic compression below knee stockings (25 mmHg at the ankle) on skin flux before and after 4 weeks of treatment in patients with postphlebitic syndrome (11). Normal values in subjects similar in age and sex distribution are also shown for comparison. It appears that elastic compression reverses the microcirculatory abnormalities present in the postphlebitic syndrome (11). The average decrease in the size of stasis ulceration following elastic compression therapy (Δ *A* in Fig. 9.7) correlated well (r = 0.74) with the decrease in resting skin flux (Δ *RF* in Fig. 9.7).

Finally, the microcirculatory response to trauma is impaired in both diabetes and in the presence of venous hypertension (3). A hyperemic response characterized by a transient increase in skin flux is typically present after needle puncture in the vicinity of the ankle. The skin flux increase following needle injury is shown in Table 9.2. While skin flux increases 22.05 times on average in normals, the increase is significantly lower in diabetics (15.79 times) and in patients with venous hypertensive microangiopathy (13.45 times).

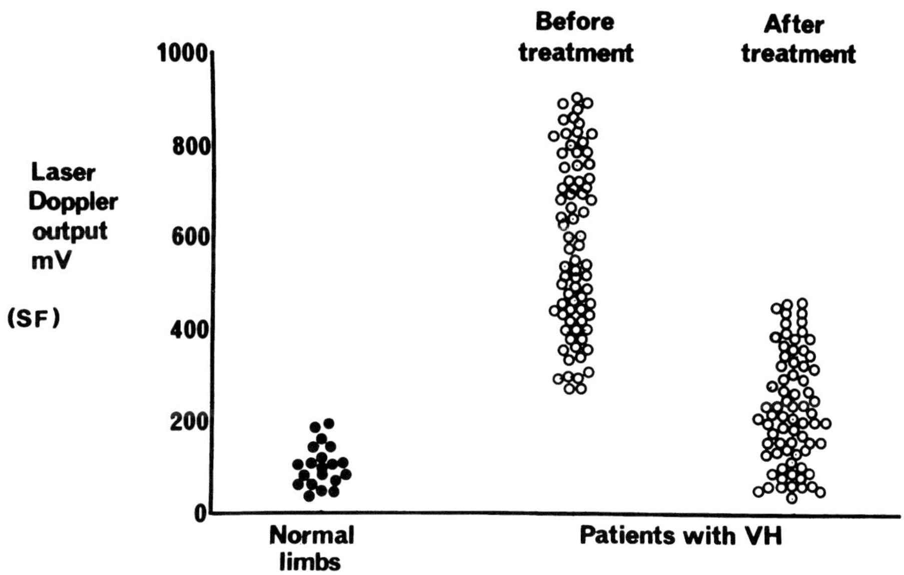

FIG. 9–6. Significant decrease in skin flux after 4 weeks of elastic compression (stockings) in patients with venous hypertension. Skin flux in normal limbs is shown for comparison.

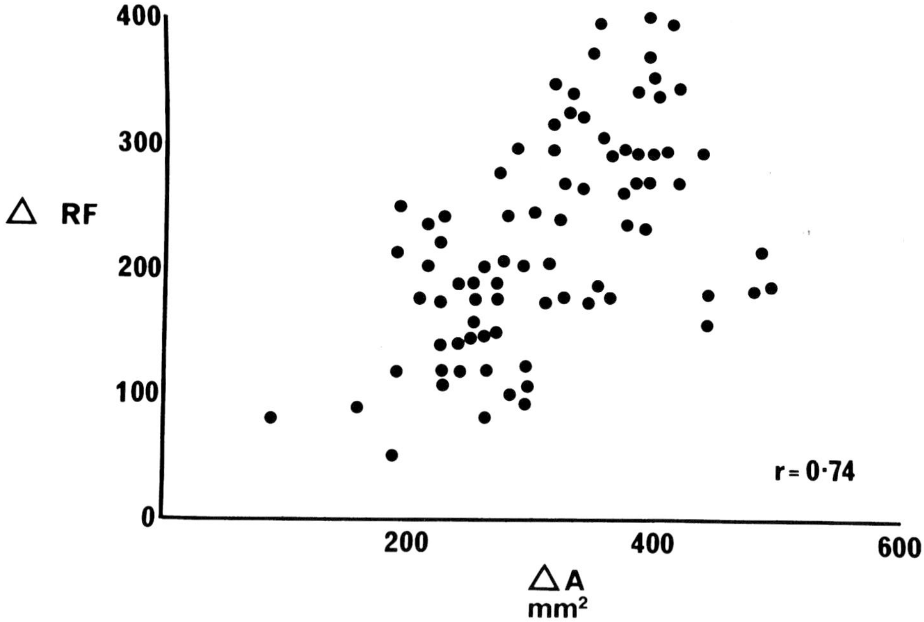

FIG. 9–7. The correlation between the decrease in skin flux at supine rest (*RF*) and the decrease in the ulcerated area in patients with postphlebitic limbs. The decrease in area (ΔAmm^2) is proportional to the decrease in RF (ΔRF) obtained with elastic compression (4 weeks).

A significant decrease in skin flux with an increase in venoarterial response has been observed in 28 patients following surgical correction of superficial incompetence. Four weeks after surgery the skin flux decreased 29% on average and the venoarterial response increased (median 34%).

TABLE 9-2

BASAL SKIN FLUX AT SUPINE REST AND AFTER NEEDLE INJURY (PERIMALLEOLAR REGION) IN THREE GROUPS OF SUBJECTS: 10 NORMALS, 8 DIABETICS, AND 10 PATIENTS WITH VENOUS HYPERTENSION DUE TO POSTPHLEBITIC SYNDROME.

	Normals n = 10	Diabetics n = 8	Patients with VHM n = 10
Basal flux	0.53	0.79*	0.88*
Peak flux	11.69	12.48*	11.84*
Times increase	22.05	13.45*	15.79*#

The three groups were comparable for age (Mean age of the three groups 43.4 ± 12) and sex distribution. Flux is expressed in units proportional to skin blood flow in ML/MIN in 100 ML of tissue.

*p = <0.05 (Difference among groups)

#p = < 0.05 (Difference between diabetics and subjects with VHM)

REFERENCES

1. Fagrell B, Intaglietta M, Tsai AG, Ostergren J. Combination of laser-Doppler flowmetry and capillary microscopy for evaluating the dynamics of skin microcirculation. In: Mahler F, Messmer K, Hammersen F, eds. Techniques in clinical capillary microscopy. Progress in applied microcirculation. Vol. 11. Basel: Karger, 1987:30–39.
2. Rayman G, Hassan A, Tooke J. Blood flow in the skin of the foot related to posture in diabetes mellitus. Br Med J 1986;292:87–90.
3. Rayman G, Williams SA, Spencer PD, Smaje LH, Wise PH, Tooke J. Impaired microvascular hyperemic response to minor skin trauma in type I diabetes. Br Med J 1986;292:1295–1298.
4. Hendricksen O. Local sympathetic reflex mechanism in regulation of blood flow in subcutaneous adipose tissue. Acta Physiol Scand 1977;(Suppl):450.
5. Belcaro G, Christopoulos D, Nicolaides AN. Skin flow and swelling in post-phlebitic limbs. VASA 1989;18:136–139.
6. Belcaro G, Grigg M, Rulo A, Nicolaides AN. Blood flow in the perimalleolar skin in relation to posture in patients with venous hypertension. Ann Vasc Surg 1989;1:5–7.
7. Belcaro G, Rulo A, Vasdekis S, Williams MA, Nicolaides AN. Combined evaluation of postphlebitic limbs by laser-Doppler flowmetry and transcutaneous $PO_2 - PCO_2$ measurements. VASA 1988;17:259–261.
8. Belcaro G, Vasdekis S, Rulo A, Nicolaides AN. Evaluation of skin blood flow and venoarteriolar response in patients with diabetes and peripheral vascular disease by laser-Doppler flowmetry. Angiology 1989;40:953–957.
9. Cesarone MR, Laurora G, Belcaro G. Microcirculation in systemic hypertension. Angiology (in press).
10. Speiser DE, Bollinger A. Microangiopathy in mild chronic venous incompetence (CVI): morphological alterations and increased transcapillary diffusion detected by fluorescence videomicroscopy. Int J Microcirc Clin Exp 1991;10:55–66.
11. Belcaro G, Grigg M, Vasdekis S, Rulo A, Christopoulos D, Nicolaides AN. Evaluation of the effects of elastic compression in patients with postphlebitic limbs by laser-Doppler flowmetry. Phlebologie 1989;41:797–802.

FURTHER READING

1. Belcaro G, Nicolaides AN, Veller M, eds. Venous disorders: a manual of diagnosis and treatment. Philadelphia: WB Saunders, 1995.
2. Nicolaides AN, Belcaro G, Chan P. Chronic deep venous insufficiency. In: Haimovici H, ed. Vascular surgery. Cambridge, MA: Blackwell Scientific, 1996:1242–1258.

chapter 10

Ascending and Descending Venography

James U. Morano

The first venograms were reported by Berberich and Hirsch in 1923 (1). Ascending venograms allow for detailed definition of the anatomy of the veins in the lower extremity. Both acute deep venous thrombosis and chronic postphlebitic changes can be detected with this study. Traumatic lesions, areas of extrinsic compression, and congenital variants and abnormalities can be studied as well. Contrast venography is generally considered the "gold standard" for evaluation of the venous system. This position is being challenged by newer modalities, particularly color coded duplex ultrasonography, which has become the technique of choice for screening of patients with possible deep venous thrombosis at many centers. Other imaging modalities that may play a role in evaluation of the venous system include nuclear medicine studies, computed tomography, and magnetic resonance imaging. However, none of these other modalities can provide as accurate a demonstration of the anatomic detail as can be obtained with a conventional ascending venogram.

RADIOLOGIC ANATOMY

The veins of the lower extremity may be classified into three major groups. These are the deep venous system, the superficial venous system, and the perforating veins. A thorough knowledge of this anatomy (2, 3), including commonly encountered variations, is essential to accurate interpretation of venograms.

The greater saphenous vein ascends along the medial aspect of the calf, passing posteromedial to the medial femoral condyle. It then continues up the medial aspect of the thigh and drains into the femoral vein below the inguinal ligament. The short saphenous vein begins in the lateral aspect of the foot, passes posterior to the lateral malleolus, and ascends in the midline of the posterior aspect of the calf. In 60% of the cases, the short saphenous vein joins the popliteal vein; variations are common.

Perforating veins allow communication between the deep veins and the superficial veins as they pass through the deep fascia. These perforating veins may be present anywhere from the foot to the thigh. The orientation of the valves within perforating veins allows for blood flow to be directed from the superficial veins into the deep venous system.

Venous valves are present in the deep veins, superficial veins, and perforating veins of the lower extremity with just a few exceptions. The perforating veins within the foot usually do not have valves (3). The larger bulbous veins draining the soleal muscles also frequently do not have valves (2). The valves in the lower extremity are oriented in such a way as to direct blood flow from the superficial venous system to the deep venous system. The valves are more frequent or located closer together in the more distal or peripheral aspect of the veins (3). More centrally, valves are less frequently seen. The common iliac veins have valves in 1.2% of cases. The inferior vena cava generally does not have valves.

ASCENDING VENOGRAPHY

Technique

Puncture Technique. Standard ascending venography technique has been described by many authors (4–9). A small-gauge butterfly needle or plastic cannula is placed into a superficial vein of the foot. The foot veins are most easily cannulated if they are adequately distended, and this is aided by performing the venipuncture with the patient in the sitting position. A superficial tourniquet may be placed above the ankle to further distend the foot veins. Frequently, however, the foot is edematous and localization of the foot veins may be difficult. In these cases, localized pressure applied with the fingers over an area on the dorsum of the foot frequently displaces the edema from this site, and makes the location of the underlying veins apparent. Alternatively, wrapping the foot in a warm towel may produce some dilatation of the veins and make the venipuncture easier. In difficult cases, cannulation of a superficial vein at the ankle or in the lower calf region may be attempted rather than that of a foot vein. This venipuncture is made in a caudad direction in these instances and surprisingly successful venograms can frequently be obtained in this fashion. When these techniques fail, the patient may be placed at bed rest with the affected foot elevated for the next 24 hours, and the foot veins can usually be cannulated with greater ease the following day.

Strictly, any superficial vein over the distal half of the dorsal region of the foot is probably suitable for performance of the study. The medial digital vein of the great toe is one of the most consistently located veins and communicates with both the superficial and deep venous systems of the foot. Local anesthesia with lidocaine is generally avoided, as this is not necessary and may obscure the position of the vein. Because of the very superficial and peripheral location of the venous punctures, ascending venograms can usually be safely performed on patients who are anticoagulated (10).

Rarely, satisfactory intravenous access into a peripheral foot vein cannot be achieved. In a study of 647 consecutive procedures, 2.3% of attempted venograms failed due to inadequate venipuncture access (11). In these cases, a venous cut-down may be required. Other authors have advocated intraosseous injections for obtaining venograms in these difficult circumstances, but potential complications from this technique include osteomyelitis and fat embolism (3, 12, 13).

Contrast Material and Injection Technique. Water-soluble contrast material should be used and the iodine concentration of the contrast material is important. If the concentration is too high, intraluminal filling defects may be obscured. If the concentration is too low, the study may not be of adequate diagnostic quality. We currently use the nonionic contrast material Opti-ray (ioversol) 240. This contrast agent provides 240 mg/ml of organically bound iodine. Each milliliter of Opti-ray 240 represents a 51% ioversol solution.

The venogram should be performed in a timely fashion so as to minimize the length of time that the contrast material remains in contact with the venous endothelium. For this reason, we prefer to perform our contrast injections by hand rather than by drip infusion as has been recommended by others (14). We prefer not to inject with power injectors, however, since the potential for significant contrast extravasation is greater.

If at all possible, the contrast injection is monitored under fluoroscopy during the hand-injected procedure. With the aid of fluoroscopic monitoring, more accurate film timing can be achieved. Additionally, the amount of contrast material used is less likely to be excessive. Our average contrast dose per leg is in the range of 75–125 ml. However, a patient with opacification of prominent superficial varicosities may require in excess of 150 ml to achieve a satisfactory study. At the completion of the procedure, the patient is placed in the horizontal position with the leg slightly elevated. Normal saline is then infused through the needle for a period of time in order to aid in clearing the leg veins of contrast material.

During the contrast injection, the venipuncture site should be kept under frequent observation. If frank extravasation occurs, the injection should be terminated immediately. If the patient complains of pain over the area but demonstrates no gross physical evidence of extravasation, fluoroscopy over the area is recommended to determine whether contrast extravasation is occurring. The ability to aspirate blood by applying suction to the syringe does not necessarily imply satisfactory needle position. Blood return can occur if the needle tip is only partially within the venous system (10). The use of a plastic cannula rather than a metal needle has been advocated to decrease complications related to extravasation (15).

Patient Positioning. Complete and homogenous opacification of the venous system of the lower extremity in the supine or horizontal position is made difficult owing to the tendency for the contrast material to layer out along the dependent surface of the vessel. Performance of ascending venography in the predominantly upright position is therefore recommended. The patient is advanced into an approximately 60° semierect position. The leg being examined should be relaxed and should be nonweight-bearing. The patient stands on a block with his/her weight supported on the contralateral leg in order to allow the leg being examined to hang freely. Even slight muscle contraction that occurs during weight-bearing may cause compression of some of the deep veins, such as the soleal veins, and prevent their opacification.

In the event that the patient cannot be placed in a semierect position, the procedure can be done in the supine position. Multiple variations in technique have been attempted in order to achieve satisfactory opacification of the venous system in the supine position. These include placement of multiple tourniquets, power injection of contrast, exercise, thigh cuffs, and manual femoral vein compression (16–19).

Filming

Performing ascending venography with fluoroscopic monitoring helps in judging the proper timing of the films as well as allowing for identification of abnormal flow patterns of the contrast. Although ascending venography can be performed with 105-mm spot films, long leg film changers, or digital subtraction angiography (20), we prefer to use 14 × 17 inch film. Anteroposterior (AP) and lateral films of the calf region are obtained with superficial tourniquets in place. We then remove the superficial tourniquets, and repeat the films without the tourniquets. While obtaining AP and lateral films of the calf region, we prefer to move the patient's leg instead of having the patient do it. This avoids the possibility of muscular contraction during the leg movement. An AP film is then obtained over the popliteal region and an additional AP film is obtained of the thigh region. The final film is obtained over the pelvis and lower inferior vena cava region. To obtain this film, the tilting table is lowered to the horizontal position as the extremity is elevated, and the exposure is then made. Improved visualization of the pelvic veins may be achieved by manual femoral vein compression, which is released just before the exposure (21).

Evaluation of Incompetent Perforating Veins

In patients with chronic venous insufficiency syndrome, evaluation of the status of the perforating veins or valves may be important. Under normal conditions the valves serve to direct blood flow from the superficial system into the deep system and prevent blood from flowing in the opposite direction. To demonstrate incompetent perforating veins, tourniquets are placed above the ankle and above the knee to occlude the superficial veins as completely as possible. When contrast is then injected in a foot vein, the contrast should be directed into the deep system. Fluoroscopic observation during the contrast injection is important to assure that any filling of the superficial veins occurs through incompetent perforators rather than filling directly when the tourniquets are not properly applied. With this technique, opacification of superficial veins occurs through incompetent perforating veins (22).

The most accurate method for demonstrating incompetent perforating veins while performing ascending venography is via an intraosseous injection (22–23). With such an intraosseous injection, contrast material flows directly into the deep veins. However, performing intraosseous injections for ascending venography presents some obvious drawbacks, such as pain and the potential for complications as previously noted.

Normal Venogram

Generally, all of the deep and superficial veins are opacified during an ascending venogram with the exception of the profunda femoral vein which opacifies in only approximately one-half of cases (24).

Pitfalls and Artifacts

Familiarity and recognition of artifacts is important since interpretation of the venogram may be compromised if they are not fully understood. Some artifacts can resemble evidence of deep venous thrombosis, and this may lead to an incorrect diagnosis (9, 25, 26).

Incomplete filling or opacification of the deep venous system represents one of the more common artifacts seen on venography. In a study of 647 consecutive procedures, 2.3% of the venograms did not achieve diagnostic opacification of the femoral and iliac veins (11). It is important to distinguish whether incomplete filling of the deep veins is secondary to artifact or due to occlusion of the vessels by thrombosis. There are numerous potential causes for incomplete filling of the deep veins in the calf region. This finding may occur when the procedure is performed in the supine position without tourniquets or when a sufficient amount of contrast material is not injected. Contraction of calf muscles can also be responsible for incomplete filling of the deep veins. Calf muscle contraction may be associated with weight-bearing (9), pain, or an uncooperative patient. The injection site may also be responsible for incomplete filling of the deep veins of the calf. If the venipuncture site is located too proximally in the foot, the contrast material may tend to bypass the deep plantar veins which are primarily responsible for opacification of the posterior tibial veins.

The use of tourniquets may also be associated with some artifacts, including incomplete opacification of the venous system. Specifically, a tourniquet placed just above the ankle may not only compress the superficial veins, but will often occlude the anterior tibial veins as well (27).

Mixing artifacts occur when the contrast material does not mix homogeneously with the blood (25, 28). The contrast material tends to gravitate to the dependent aspect of the vein. This mixing artifact is more pronounced when the patient is in a supine position. Because the contrast material tends to flow along the dependent portion of the vein, it is possible that abnormalities could be missed on the nondependent side of the vessel in the supine technique.

Inflow of unopacified blood from branches of a vein may produce streaming artifacts. Mixing defects due to inhomogeneous mixing of contrast in blood can produce a streaky appearance which can be mistaken for thrombus or postphlebitic recanalization. Both mixing and streaming artifacts tend to change in appearance and do not represent persistent defects. Fluoroscopic observation or multiple films are sometimes needed to identify these artifacts with confidence.

There may be suboptimal opacification of the veins in the regions of the valve cusps. This can be due to turbulent or sluggish flow through these areas. In these cases, the Valsalva maneuver will often minimize this artifact and is recommended for optimal evaluation of questions about the valves.

Compression artifacts are produced by extrinsic factors that produce narrowing of the veins. Hyperextension of the knee may produce narrowing of the popliteal vein, and hyperextension of the hip can produce similar findings in the femoral vein. A Baker's cyst can be responsible for compression of the popliteal vein. Another cause for a compression artifact is the presence of an arterial impression. A common site for an arterial impression on a lower extremity vein occurs in the left common iliac vein where it crosses the artery. This may cause the common iliac vein to be poorly opacified, and fibrous webs can form in this location due to chronic compression and postphlebitic changes. Webs in this location can also be congenital in origin.

Overlying shadows can be confusing and may be due to projection of veins over each other or over portions of the bones, particularly the cortex of the tibia or fibula. This pattern can simulate a thrombus, but the use of multiple projections aids in distinguishing these artifacts.

Finally, inadvertent injection of air bubbles with the contrast material can produce filling defects. These can usually be easily identified by their round or spherical configuration and their inconstant position.

Abnormal Venogram in Deep Venous Thrombosis

Ascending venography can be used to determine the presence and the extent of deep venous thrombosis. If bilateral disease is clinically suspected, the more symptomatic leg should be examined first. If no evidence of acute deep venous thrombosis is identified in that leg, then the other leg can be studied. However, if acute deep venous thrombosis is identified in the leg initially examined, it is often not necessary to examine the other leg if this will not influence the therapy which is chosen. Consequently, simultaneous bilateral ascending venograms are not attempted because the patient may be subjected to a larger contrast dose than would otherwise be the case. Another reason for not performing simultaneous bilateral venography is that it is technically more difficult, or impossible, to perform with both legs nonweight-bearing.

Most thrombus formation originates in the calf veins, although it may originate above or below this level, and may, in fact, begin at several places simultaneously (29). Thrombi often begin to form behind the valve cusps.

Direct evidence of deep venous thrombosis consists of demonstration of the actual filling defect that represents the thrombus (9, 26, 30–32). This filling defect ideally should be identifiable on at least two films obtained at differing projections (30). The filling defect may be located centrally or in an eccentric location within the vessel. Thrombus may be outlined by a thin, white line of contrast material between the clot and the vessel wall (Fig. 10.1). The upper portion of the thrombus may have a "floating tail" which may be at risk for detachment and embolization. Thrombus which has a horizontal "square cut" shape along its upper portion may indicate that a portion of the thrombus has already broken off and embolized (10).

The actual intraluminal filling defect in acute deep venous thrombosis may not always be seen, but there are other radiographic signs that represent indirect evidence for acute deep venous thrombosis and are highly suggestive of its diag-

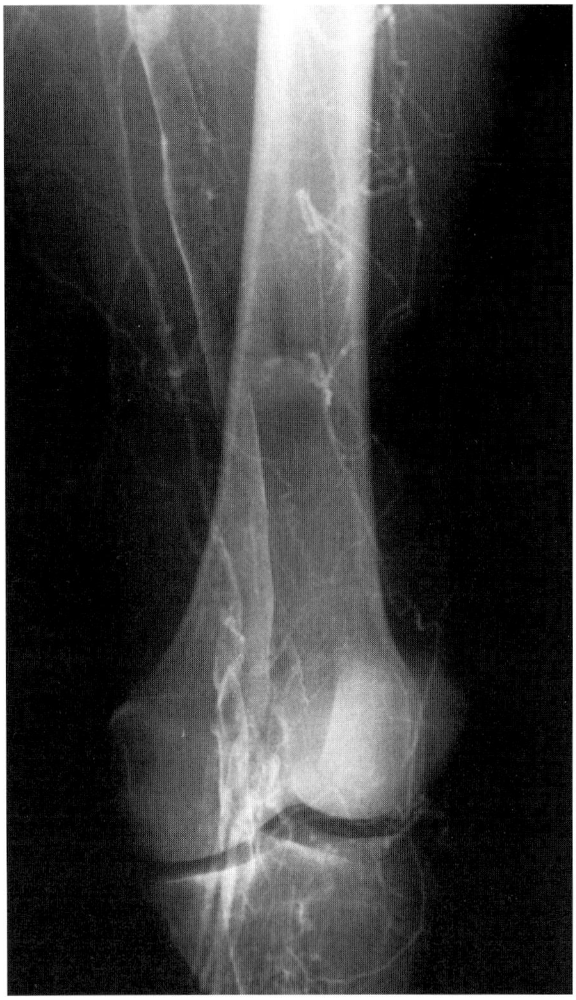

FIG. 10–1. Thrombus within popliteal vein and lower superficial femoral vein on ascending venogram. Thrombus outlined by thin streaks of contrast material between vessel wall and thrombus.

nosis. Nonopacification of portions of the deep venous system, particularly in the calf region, may indicate the presence of acute deep venous thrombosis. This lack of opacification probably occurs due to a combination of the intraluminal thrombus, as well as adjacent edema, and inflammation, which elevates pressure within the deep fascia of the calf, thus preventing the contrast material from entering the deep veins within this space. This phenomenon has been reported to occur in up to 80% of cases of extensive acute deep venous thrombosis (32). In this situation, there are abnormal flow patterns of the contrast material with shunting of flow into superficial veins which may be dilated. Enlarged collateral veins may also develop in response to an occluded segment of vein. An abrupt ending or termination of the contrast column represents an additional indirect sign of acute deep venous thrombosis. These indirect signs do not allow for a definitive diagnosis, however, as they can also be seen in other situations such as massive leg edema or poor opacification artifact.

An estimation of the potential of the thrombus to embolize can be important in management decisions. A thrombus that appears loose and nonadherent to the vein wall is more likely to embolize than one that is adherent to the vein wall. Those with a "floating tail" are also more likely to embolize (2, 10).

It may also be possible to make an estimation of the age of a thrombus based on the radiographic appearance (33). Clots less than a week old demonstrate smooth margins and tend to fill the whole vein almost completely. These fresh clots are loose, and may have only a small attachment to the vein wall, often located behind a valve. These fresh thrombi are surrounded by a very thin white line of contrast between the clot and the vessel wall. Within 48 hours to 14 days, the thrombus becomes increasingly adherent to the vein wall. Where the thrombus becomes adherent to the vein wall, the thin separating line of contrast material can no longer be seen. With additional time, the thrombus begins to lose fluid and undergoes retraction and resorption. The thrombus retracts toward the wall of the vessel where it is adherent. This allows for an increasing width of contrast material between the adherent thrombus and the non-adherent wall. The contrast column at this time is usually somewhat irregular. If the thrombus becomes adherent to the entire circumference of the vein wall, complete occlusion of the vessel may occur.

Chronic Postphlebitic Changes

When an occluded vein regains patency as a consequence of thrombus retraction, the recanalization process begins. Recanalization almost always occurs to some degree in the deep veins of the calf following thrombosis. However, the lumen of the recanalized vein often has an irregular streaky appearance, and there may actually be multiple smaller venous channels instead (Fig. 10.2). During the recanalization process, the valves are frequently damaged and thus become incompetent (34). The valve sites may appear damaged on the venogram or may no longer be seen at all. Occasionally, a vein may regain a normal radiographic appearance after recanalization.

Recanalization changes do not always occur following a thrombotic occlusion. The vein may remain permanently occluded if this process does not occur. However, dilated collateral venous channels develop in this situation and adequate venous return is regained in most instances (2). The collateral veins that develop in response to an obstructed vein enlarge almost immediately, unlike the development of collateral arteries around an arterial obstruction (2). Consequently, the extent of collateral vein visualization is often not an accurate means of establishing the duration of a venous obstruction.

Any of the veins in the deep venous system may remain permanently obstructed after thrombosis. However, some veins are more prone to this complication. These include the left common iliac vein, the superficial femoral vein near the level of the adductor canal, and the inferior vena cava (2). Although difficult to prove conclusively, it has been suggested that the increased incidence of thrombotic occlusion of the left common iliac vein may be related to "normal" compression of this vein by the right common iliac artery (35, 36).

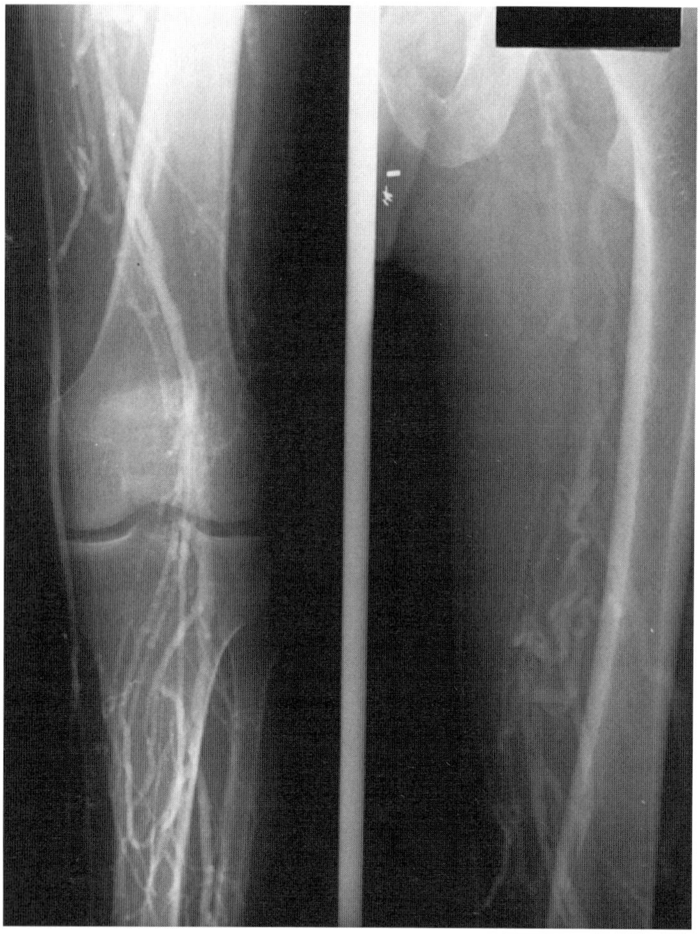

FIG. 10–2. Chronic postphlebitic changes demonstrated on ascending venogram. Streaky, irregular contour of popliteal vein and multiple irregular venous channels replacing superficial femoral vein.

Varicose Veins

Varicose veins are dilated, elongated, and tortuous veins. They can be classified as primary or secondary varicose veins. In primary varicose veins, the deep venous system of the lower extremity is normal and patent, and the superficial varicosities represent a primary abnormality. The deep system is often incompetent to varying degrees in the presence of superficial varices. Secondary varicose veins generally occur as a response to other abnormalities, most commonly due to previous deep vein thrombosis. In secondary varicose veins, the deep venous system has a postphlebitic appearance, as well as demonstrating superficial varicosities on the venogram. Incompetent perforating veins are also seen, and can be recognized on the ascending venogram (22). The incompetent communicating veins demonstrate abnormal flow patterns with contrast flowing from the deep venous system to the superficial system where they often enter a varicose vein. These incompetent perforating veins appear as dilated channels with no valves seen, and they typically narrow as they pass through the fascia to enter the superficial system (10).

Demonstration of superficial varicosities can best be achieved by doing ascending venography without superficial tourniquets. Some varicose veins that are particularly large and obvious on clinical examination may not opacify during ascending venography. This is because they represent relatively large volume spaces with slow mixing and exchange of the contrast material with blood (3). However, nonopacification of these large varices may not be critical since ascending venography is generally performed on these patients to evaluate the deep venous system and perforating veins so as to distinguish primary from secondary varicosities. In this situation, ascending venography is best performed with a superficial tourniquet above the ankle and with close fluoroscopic observation. Utilizing this technique, the contrast material should remain in the deep venous system, and opacification of the superficial veins should occur only through incompetent perforating veins. When an incompetent perforating vein is located, the tourniquet can be moved progressively higher, looking for additional incompetent perforating veins at higher levels. Direct puncture and opacification of varices of interest ("varicography") can be accomplished if anatomic detail is required for surgical intervention (2).

Complications

Systemic reactions to contrast material can occur with venography as well as any other radiologic studies which use these contrast agents. Fortunately, serious reactions are uncommon (37).

Contrast material is irritating to the endothelium of the vessel walls. This can be responsible for the development of venous thrombosis subsequent to the venogram (38–43). However, the incidence of clinically significant thrombophlebitis is relatively low (2, 10). The incidence of thrombophlebitis following venography can be reduced in several ways. Minimizing the amount of time that the contrast material remains in contact with the vessel wall helps in preventing thrombosis, and elevation of the leg at the end of the examination aids in accomplishing this. Supine venography and early ambulation have been associated with fewer instances of thrombosis (37). Infusion of heparinized saline following the contrast injection is also advocated to clear the contrast material from the veins (43). Use of nonionic or low osmolarity contrast agents is also associated with reductions in this complication (39, 41, 44), as is dilution of standard ionic contrast agents (42).

The irritating nature of contrast material on the venous endothelium is also responsible for some pain or discomfort that is often encountered during venography, particularly with the older ionic contrast materials. However, the pain is apparently related in part to the sodium content of the contrast agent, and thus agents such as meglumine diatrizoate or meglumine iothalamate may be preferable. The discomfort for the patient can be further reduced by dilution of these ionic contrast materials (40). Adding lidocaine to the contrast material may also minimize the pain (45). However, the nonionic contrast materials provide much less discomfort to the patient and may be painless on injection (46–48). For these reasons, the contrast material of choice for venography is the new generation of low osmolarity contrast materials.

Pulmonary embolization can theoretically occur as a complication of venography. Pulmonary emboli can arise from venous thrombosis that occurs secondary to the venogram, but this is very rare (49). It is also possible that the venogram itself can be responsible for dislodging preexisting thrombi, but this is also rare (3, 10).

Contrast extravasation at the venipuncture site may occur, usually associated with needle-tip dislodgement, but clinically significant extravasation of contrast material is rare. Nonetheless, serious complications from contrast extravasation can occur (37, 49, 50). In these patients, a chemical cellulitis can progress to ulceration, skin necrosis and even gangrene. Patients with peripheral vascular arterial disease or chronic venous insufficiency are at increased risk of these local complications (3, 10). To best avoid these problems, the venipuncture site should be inspected frequently during the contrast injection. Often, when the extravasation begins, the patient complains of pain at the injection site and this should prompt careful examination of the area. Contrast injection should not be made if significant extravasation is occurring.

Other Methods

There are numerous noninvasive means for evaluating for deep venous thrombosis in the lower extremities (51–58). These are covered in detail elsewhere in this volume.

A number of nuclear medicine isotope scans have been developed which can be used in the detection of venous thrombosis. The use of iodine-125 fibrinogen, indium-111 platelet, and technetium-99m red blood cell scans have all been described for this purpose (59–61).

Computed tomography (CT) scanning is also sometimes useful. In our experience, filling defects in the femoral veins are often detected incidentally on the lower slices of routine abdominal/pelvic CT scans after administration of intravenous contrast. Magnetic resonance imaging (MRI) may also play a role in detection of venous thrombus. Early reports indicate some promise in this area (62).

DESCENDING VENOGRAPHY

Descending venography provides important information in patients with chronic venous insufficiency (63, 64). Anatomic and functional evaluation of the venous valves in the lower extremities of these patients has become crucial with recent advances in surgical treatment of this disorder. Descending venography delineates the exact location of the valves in the leg veins and provides an assessment of the competence of these valves. The information obtained from these examinations allows for more knowledgeable treatment decisions.

Our method for performing descending venography has been previously described (65). Using standard angiographic technique, a 5-French endhole catheter with one or two distal sideholes is positioned at the junction of the external iliac vein and the common femoral vein. The fluoroscopic table and patient are then rotated into a 60° semierect position. The patient bears weight on a block placed under the contralateral foot so that the leg being examined will be relaxed and bear no weight. The patient is then instructed to perform a Valsalva maneuver. Because some patients seem to have difficulty in understanding the instructions to bear down, we employ a technique that hopefully provides a more standardized or controlled Valsalva maneuver. This is done by connecting the barrel of a 10-ml syringe to the tubing on a mercury column blood pressure manometer. The patient is instructed to blow into this syringe hub so as to elevate the mercury column to the 40-mm mark and maintain it at this level. Contrast material is then injected by hand under fluoroscopic observation. Both spot films and videotape are used to provide permanent documentation of the findings (Fig. 10.3).

Some reports in the literature support the performance of descending venography with the patient in the supine position rather than in the semierect posi-

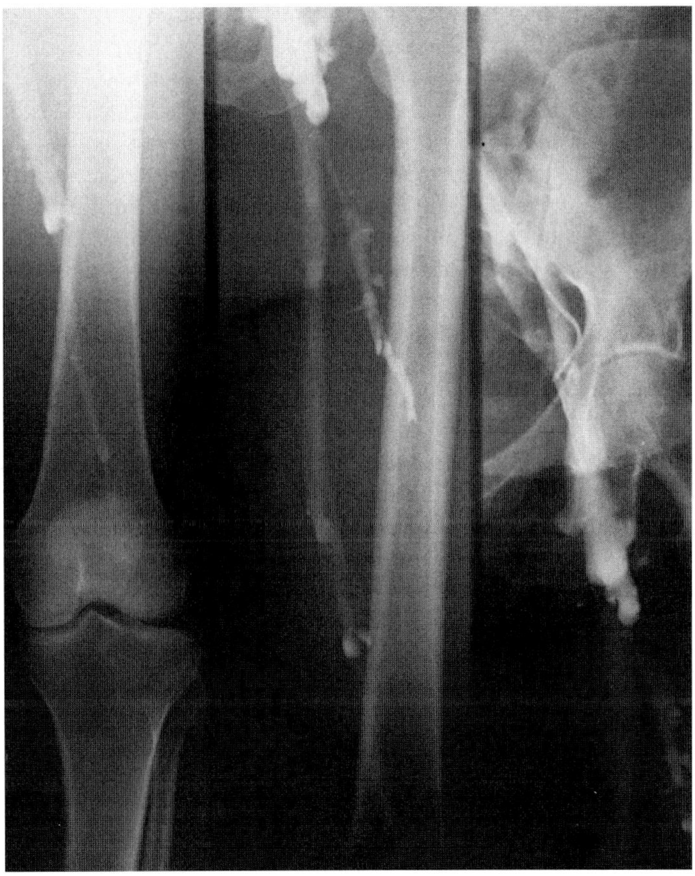

FIG. 10–3. Descending venogram. Reflux of contrast material down superficial femoral vein to popliteal vein and some reflux into profunda femoral vein as well.

tion (66–69). The stated rationale for supine descending venography is that the higher specific gravity or density of the contrast material as compared to blood will cause the contrast material to pass slowly downward while the patient is in the semierect position, exaggerating or falsely increasing the degree of reflux. However, we have not found this to be a significant problem. While it is true that in the semierect position a small amount of contrast material may settle and pass through normal open venous valves during quiet or normal breathing, this has been accepted as normal (63, 66). Most of the contrast material flows superiorly toward the heart during quiet breathing. However, when the Valsalva maneuver is performed and the valve stations are stressed, the valve cusps should close tightly and be competent, whether or not the contrast material is heavier than blood.

All of our descending venography is now performed with the standardized Valsalva maneuver described above. In a series of descending venograms, 475 legs were examined, both during normal respiration and the Valsalva maneuver (65). Although 54% of these extremities demonstrated a similar degree of reflux during both normal respiration and the Valsalva maneuver, 45% of the extremities showed substantially more reflux with the Valsalva maneuver. In only 1% of the legs was there a significant increase in reflux seen with normal respiration, compared with reflux during the Valsalva maneuver. As alluded to earlier, this may have been due to normally functioning valves that are open most of the time during normal respiration, but this part of the examination would not seem appropriate for determining the competence of a valve at closure. Consequently, we perform our studies exclusively with the Valsalva maneuver.

The interpretation of descending venograms involves identification of valvular incompetence within veins of the lower extremity. Specifically, one must determine whether reflux occurred into the superficial femoral vein, profunda femoral vein, saphenous vein, and/or popliteal vein. Additionally, the inferior extent of the contrast material reflux is noted. We grade the extent of reflux according to these classification systems: (a) KISTNER Classification (Grade 0 indicates valvular competence with no significant reflux below the common femoral vein. Grade 1 indicates minimal valvular incompetence with reflux beyond the uppermost valves but not below the upper thigh. Grade 2, mild incompetence, signifies reflux to the distal or lower thigh level, but above the knee. Grade 3, moderate incompetence, indicates reflux to the level of the knee or just below the knee. Grade 4, severe incompetence, signifies reflux into the calf veins.) and (b) RASV Classification. Alternatively, reflux has been classified as single level/single system, single level/multisystem, or multilevel/multisystem. In a series of symptomatic patients, multivalvular insufficiency or multisystem reflux appeared necessary to produce symptoms in most instances (70). The latter classification appears to correlate better with patient symptomatology and hemodynamics than the KISTNER classification (71).

Deep venous reflux, either alone or in combination with superficial venous reflux, is the primary basis of the clinical presentation of chronic venous insufficiency disease (65, 70). In a series of positive descending venograms on 485 legs, reflux into the deep venous system occurred in 98% (65). Isolated reflux into the superficial venous system (saphenous vein) occurred in only 2% of those extremities that showed reflux. In 82% of the legs that demonstrated reflux, all of the reflux occurred into the deep venous system alone.

Modern surgical techniques can help the surgeon to repair and alleviate some of the problems related to venous valvular insufficiency (70). The need for accurate identification of valvular anatomy and valvular competence becomes obvious, and descending venography can play a crucial role in evaluating these patients so that a proper course of treatment may be planned.

REFERENCES

1. Berberich J, Hirsch S. Die roentgenographische Darstellung der Arterien und Venen am lebenden Menschen. Klin Wochenschr 1923;2:2226.
2. Almen T, Nylander G. Serial phlebography of the normal lower leg during muscular contraction and relaxation. Acta Radiol 1962;57:264–272.
3. DeWeese JA, Rogoff SM. Functional ascending phlebography of the lower extremity by serial long film technique. AJR 1959;81:841–854.
4. Greitz T. The technique of ascending phlebography of the lower extremity. Acta Radiol 1954;42:421–441.
5. Greitz T. Ascending phlebography in venous insufficiency. Acta Radiol 1955;44:145–162.
6. Gullmo A. On the technique of phlebography of the lower limb. Acta Radiol 1956;46:603–620.
7. Rabinov K, Paulin S. Roentgen diagnosis of venous thrombosis in the leg. Arch Surg 1972;104:134–144.
8. Kadir S. Diagnostic angiography. Philadelphia: WB Saunders, 1986:536–583.
9. Naidich JB, Feinberg AW, Karp-Harman H, Karmel MI, Tyma CG, Stein HL. Contrast venography: reassessment of its role. Radiology 1988;168:97–100.
10. Rabinov K, Paulin S. Venography of the lower extremities. In: Abrams HL, ed. Abrams angiography. Boston: Little, Brown and Company, 1983:1877–1921.
11. Halliday P. Phlebography of the lower limb. Br J Surg 1968;55:220–226.
12. Thomas ML, Fletcher EWL. The techniques of pelvic phlebography. Clin Radiol 1967;18:399–402.
13. Kirschner LP, Twigg H, Farkas J. Drip infusion venography. Radiology 1970;96:413–415.
14. Gothlin J. The comparative frequency of extravasal injection at phlebography with steel and plastic cannula. Clin Radiol 1972;23:183–184.
15. Coel MN. Adequacy of lower limb venous opacification: comparison of supine and upright phlebography. AJR 1980;134:163–165.
16. Nicolaides AN, Kakkar VV, Field ES, Renny JTG. The origin of deep vein thrombosis: a venographic study. Br J Radiol 1971;44:653–663.
17. Pavlov H, MacMoran JW, Funch RB, Bernhard RA, D'Orazio EA. Simplified outpatient lower extremity venography. Radiology 1978;126:525–527.
18. Smith TP, Cardella JF, Darcy MD, Hunter DW, Castaneda-Zuniga WR, Amplatz K. Lower-extremity venography: value of femoral-vein compression. AJR 1986;147:1025–1026.
19. Lee KR, Templeton AW, Cox GG, Dwyer SJ, McClure CB. Digital venography of the lower extremity. AJR 189;153:413–417.
20. Dure-Smith P, Tison JB. Ilio-femoral segment and inferior vena cava visualization using a non-catheter technique: an adjunct of leg phlebography. Radiology 1984;153:251–252.
21. Thomas ML, McAllister V, Rose DH, Tonge K. A simplified technique of phlebography for the localization of incompetent perforating veins of the legs. Clin Radiol 1972;23:486–491.

22. Halliday P. Intra-osseous phlebography of the lower limb. Br J Surg 1967;54:248–257.
23. Redman HC. Deep venous thrombosis: is contrast venography still the diagnostic "gold standard"? Radiology 1988;168:277–278.
24. Almen T, Nylander G. False signs of thrombosis in lower leg phlebography. Acta Radiol 1964;2:345–352.
25. Thomas ML, McAllister V, Tonge K. The radiological appearances of deep venous thrombus. Clin Radiol 1971;22:495–501.
26. Greitz T. Phlebography of the normal leg. Acta Radiol 1955;44:1–20.
27. Thomas ML, Carty H. The appearances of artefacts on lower limb phlebograms. Clin Radiol 1975;26:527–533.
28. Browse NL, Thomas ML. Source of non-lethal pulmonary emboli. Lancet 1974;1:258–259.
29. DeWeese JA, Rogoff SM. Phlebographic patterns of acute deep venous thrombosis of the leg. Surgery 1963;53:99–107.
30. Borgstrom S, Greitz T, Linden W, Molin J, Rudies I. Ascending phlebography in fresh thrombosis of the lower limb. AJR 1965;94:207–212.
31. Brodelius A, Lorinc P, Nylander G. Phlebographic techniques in the diagnosis of acute deep venous thrombosis of the lower limb. AJR 1971;III:794–801.
32. Thomas ML, Browse NL. Venography of the lower extremity. In: Neiman HL, Yao JST, eds. Angiography of vascular disease. New York: Churchill Livingstone, 1985:421–480.
33. Thomas ML, McAllister V. The radiological progression of deep venous thrombus. Radiology 1971;99:37–40.
34. Edwards EA, Edwards JE. The effect of thrombophlebitis on the venous valve. Surg Gynecol Obstet 1937;65:310–320.
35. Cockett FB, Thomas ML. The iliac compression syndrome. Br J Surg 1965;52:816–821.
36. May R, Thurner J. The cause of the predominantly sinistral occurrence of thrombosis of the pelvic veins. Angiology 1975;8:419–427.
37. Coel MN, Dodge W. Complication rate with supine phlebography. AJR 1978;131:821–822.
38. Albrechtsson U, Olsson CG. Thrombotic side-effects of lower-limb phlebography. Lancet 1976;1:723–724.
39. Thomas ML, Briggs GM, Kuan BB. Contrast agent-induced thrombophlebitis following leg phlebography: meglumine ioxaglate versus meglumine iothalamate. Radiology 1983;147:399–400.
40. Bettman MA, Paulin S. Leg phlebography: the incidence, nature and modification of undesirable side effects. Radiology 1977;122:101–104.
41. Walters HL, Clemenson J, Browse NL, Thomas ML. ^{125}I-fibrinogen uptake following phlebography of the leg. Radiology 1980;135:619–621.
42. Bettmann MA, Salzman EW, Rosenthal D, et al. Reduction of venous thrombosis complicating phlebography. AJR 1980;134:1169–1172.
43. Arndt RD, Grollman JH, Gomes AS, Bos CJ. The heparin flush: an aid in preventing post-venography thrombophlebitis. Radiology 1979;130:249–250.
44. Laerum F, Holm HA. Postphlebographic thrombosis. Radiology 1981;140:651–654.
45. Silverbach S. The use of xylocaine to diminish leg cramps in venography. Radiology 1979;133:788–789.
46. Thomas ML, Walters HL. Metrizamide in venography. Br Med J 1979;2:1036.
47. Bettman MA, Robbins A, Braun SD, Wetzner S, Dunnick NR, Finkelstein J. Contrast venography of the leg: diagnostic efficacy, tolerance, and complication rates with ionic and nonionic contrast media. Radiology 1987;165:113–116.
48. Hall-Craggs MA, Hine AL. Ascending lower-limb phlebography: a comparative study of Hexabrix 320, iohexol 300 and iohexol 240. Br J Radiol 1986;59:685–687.
49. Gordon IJ. Evaluation of suspected deep venous thrombosis in the arteriosclerotic patient. AJR 1978;131:531–533.

50. Spigos DG, Thane TT, Capek V. Skin necrosis following extravasation during peripheral phlebography. Radiology 1977;123:605–606.
51. Vogel P, Laing FC, Jeffrey RB, Wing VW. Deep venous thrombosis of the lower extremity: US evaluation. Radiology 1987;163:747–751.
52. Appelman PT, DeJong TE, Lampmann LE. Deep venous thrombosis of the leg: US findings. Radiology 1987;163:743–746.
53. Raghavendra BN, Horii SC, Hilton S, Subramanyam BR, Rosen RJ, Lam S. Deep venous thrombosis: detection by probe compression of veins. J Ultrasound Med 1986;5:89–95.
54. Cronan JJ, Dorfman GS, Scola FH, Schepps B, Alexander J. Deep venous thrombosis: US assessment using vein compression. Radiology 1987;162:191–194.
55. Cronan JJ, Dorfman GS, Grusmark J. Lower-extremity deep venous thrombosis: further experience with and refinement of US assessment. Radiology 1988;168:101–107.
56. Aitken AGF, Godden DJ. Real-time ultrasound diagnosis of deep vein thrombosis: a comparison with venography. Clin Radiol 1987;38:309–313.
57. Benedict KT, Wheeler HB, Patwardhan NA. Impedance plethysmography: correlation with contrast venography. Radiology 1977;125:695–699.
58. Ramchandani P, Soulen RL, Fedullo LM, Gaines VD. Deep vein thrombosis: significant limitations of noninvasive tests. Radiology 1985;156:47–49.
59. Harris WH, Salzman EW, Athanasoulis C, et al. Comparison of 125-I fibrinogen count scanning with phlebography for detection of venous thrombi after elective hip surgery. N Engl J Med 1957;292:665–667.
60. Seabold JE, Conrad GR, Ponto JA, et al. Deep venous thrombophlebitis: detection with 4-hour versus 24-hour platelet scintigraphy. Radiology 1987;165:355–360.
61. Leclerc JR, Wolfson C, Arzoumanian A, Blake GP, Rosenthall L. Technetium-99m red blood cell venography in patients with clinically suspected deep vein thrombosis: a prospective study. J Nucl Med 1988;29:1498–1506.
62. Spritzer CE, Sussman SK, Blinder RA, Saeed M, Herfkens RJ. Deep venous thrombosis evaluation with limited-flip-angle, gradient-refocused MR imaging: preliminary experience. Radiology 1988;166:371–375.
63. Kistner RL, Ferris EB, Randhawa G, Kamida C. A method of performing descending venography. J Vasc Surg 1986;4:464–468.
64. Herman RJ, Neiman HL, Yao JST, Egan TJ, Bergan JJ, Malave SR. Descending venography: a method of evaluating lower extremity venous valvular function. Radiology 1980;137:63–69.
65. Morano JU, Raju S. Chronic venous insufficiency: assessment with descending venography. Radiology 1990;174:441–444.
66. Thomas ML, Keeling FP, Ackroyd JS. Descending phlebography: a comparison of three methods and an assessment of the normal range of deep vein reflux. J Cardiovasc Surg 1986;27:27–30.
67. Muth TJ. Venography of the lower extremities. Postgrad Med 1966;A69–A72.
68. Ackroyd JS, Thomas ML, Browse NL. Deep vein reflux: an assessment by descending phlebography. Br J Surg 1986;73:31–33.
69. Thomas ML, Bowles JN. Descending phlebography in the assessment of long saphenous vein incompetence. AJR 1985;145:1255–1257.
70. Raju S, Fredericks R. Valve reconstruction procedures for nonobstructive venous insufficiency: rationale, techniques, and results in 107 procedures with two- and eight-year follow-up. J Vasc Surg 1988;7:301–310.
71. Raju S, Fredericks R. Evaluation of methods for detecting venous reflux: perspectives in venous insufficiency with descending venography. Arch Surg 1990;125:1463.

chapter 11

Lymphedema

J. Leonel Villavicencio and Emmanouil Pikoulis

HISTORIC NOTE*

Lymphatic vessels were first recognized by Gasparo Asellius, Professor of Anatomy at Pavia University in Italy. On July 23, 1622, while performing observations on the recurrent nerve in a live, well-fed dog, he noted the presence of many small white vessels along the intestine. Initially, he thought that they were nerves, but when he incised one, he noted white fluid. He later repeated the experiment on animals which had not been fed and noticed that the white vessels were not present. The little white vessels were designated vasa lactea (1). Pecquet, in 1651, noticed that the intestinal lymphatics drained into a dilated area that he called receptaculum chyli. It was Bartholin, in 1653, who used the term "lymphatics" for the first time. A better understanding of the role of the lymphatics came during the latter part of the 19th century from the work of Starling (2). Starling clarified the relationship between the hydrostatic pressure of the blood and the colloid osmotic pressure of the plasma proteins at the microcirculatory level. Drinker (3) measured protein flow from the capillaries to the interstitial tissues and strengthened the concept that the capillary vessels are an important physiologic mechanism to return the large protein molecules to the central circulation. The merit of quantifying the magnitude of the capillary exchanges was addressed by Landis (4). Mayerson (5) contributed greatly to clarifying the role of the lymphatic system, stating that it cleared the tissue spaces of protein and other large molecules that could not be reabsorbed directly into the bloodstream. Depending on the specific tissue, approximately 90% of the interstitial fluid is drained through venous capillary reabsorption and the remaining 10% through the lymphatic system. This system performs multiple functions: it eliminates

*The opinions or assertions contained herein are those of the authors and are not to be construed as official or as reflecting the view of the Department of Defense, Department of the Army, or the Uniformed Services University of the Health Sciences.

macromolecules and toxic substances from the tissues; assists in clearing injured tissue debris; and regulates tissue fluid volume, protecting the circulating blood volume against hypovolemia. Lymphocytes and other cells enter the circulation via the lymphatic system along with protein and other large molecules. The different types of lymphatic cells are now identified by surface markers. The concept that lymphocytes derive from specialized structures which are closely related to the immunologic system is supported by Moretta and Mingari (6).

Along with proteins, lipoproteins and chylomicrons enter the circulation through the lymphatic system, contributing to form the stream of a system which handles large volumes of fluid, fat, protein, and cells. The intestinal lymphatics absorb cholesterol, fatty acids, and triglycerides, which give chyle its whitish aspect. The exudate from the peritoneal cavity is continuously absorbed by the lymphatics, and this function is the basis of peritoneal dialysis.

The embryologic development of the lymphatic system was studied by Savin (7) and Huntington (8). These investigators observed that the lymphatics generally course along the major veins, and when obstructed, several forms of communications between the lymphatics and the venous system will develop (lymphovenous anastomosis) (9).

ANATOMIC AND PHYSIOLOGIC CONCEPTS

The network of lymphatic capillaries which absorb lymph from the interstitial space have been called "initial lymphatics" by Casley-Smith (10). These lymphatics are made up of a single layer of flat endothelial cells varying in diameter from 10–60 μm. The lymph capillaries end blindly in rounded ends and are absent in the cornea and central nervous system deep to the meninges, cartilage, and tendon. The lymphatic capillaries drain into the larger valved channels of the deeper layers of the dermis and the subcutaneous tissue. The valved lymphatic trunks course along the veins superficial to the muscular fascia and pass through a small number of popliteal and epitrochlear nodes in the upper and lower extremities, respectively. From 8–11 lymphatic channels are present in the lower extremity along the course of the saphenous vein. The number of trunks increase in number as they become more proximal. The number and size of the lymph nodes are important because they may be, in some cases, the site of chronic inflammation and obstruction to the lymph flow. Along the course of the lesser saphenous vein, there is an important lymphatic pathway which drains into the popliteal nodes of the deep system.

In the adult male, approximately 60% of the body weight consists of water. There are three anatomically separable compartments. Two-thirds of the total body water is found as intracellular fluid and one-third is in the extracellular compartment. One-fifth of the extracellular compartment fluid is plasma and the remainder is interstitial fluid (ISF). A 70-kg man has 42 liters of body water, of which 14 liters are extracellular fluid and 11.3 liters are interstitial fluid. The transportation of fluid from blood to tissue is very important for the viability of the living cell. For this reason, it is important to understand the mechanisms that determine fluid exchange across the capillary endothelium. Starling (2) stated that "the two processes of lymph production and absorption are exactly proportional."

The forces that promote filtration out of the capillary into the interstitial fluid are the hydrostatic pressure within the capillaries, and the interstitial oncotic pressure given by the small amounts of protein present in the interstitial fluid. On the other hand, the forces that regulate filtration from the interstitium into the capillaries include the plasma oncotic pressure, which is originated by the concentration of the plasma protein, and the pressure secondary to turgidity of the interstitium.

The plasma oncotic pressure averages 24 mmHg (11). This pressure corresponds to an approximate concentration of plasma protein of 7%. The hydrostatic capillary pressure averages 32 mmHg in the arterial system and 15 mmHg in the venous capillary. The capillary flow is governed by the differences in the hydrostatic and colloid osmotic pressures of plasma; in this manner, fluid is filtered from the capillaries into the tissues in the arterial end of the capillary and is reabsorbed from the tissues through the venous end of the capillary network (12).

It is accepted that lymph formation and flow depend greatly upon tissue movement or activity related to muscle contractions. For this reason, the rate of lymph formation and flow can be quantified by measuring the disappearance of isotope-labeled albumin from the subcutis (13, 14). Pressures within the lymphatic system range from slightly negative in the initial lymphatics, up to 30 mm or higher in large collecting vessels (200–300 μm). Depending on the contractions of an initial lymphatic vessel, intraluminal pressures are negative (about -1 mmHg) or positive (about $+1$ mmHg) as determined by direct puncture (15).

In the collecting lymphatic, a valvular system helps in maintaining ascending, proximal lymphatic drainage. The large efferent trunks arising from the inguinal and axillary nodes continue their course in close relationship with the major vessels. There is a separate deep lymphatic system which communicates with the superficial network under special circumstances. The thoracic duct carries large amounts of lymph from the distal parts of the body and drains into the left subclavian vein. A separate right component of the thoracic duct ends on the right subclavian vein. The amount of lymph returned to the circulation in a 24-hour period approximates the plasma volume (5).

LYMPHATIC VISUALIZATION AND IMAGING

The lymphatic system is the "poor relative" of the well-to-do family of arterial and venous systems. The last four decades have witnessed an unprecedented progress in the management of diseases of the arterial and venous systems. In contrast, study of the disorders of the lymphatic system lags behind and still poses a great challenge for the medical profession. One of the major obstacles to study of the lymphatic system is the difficulty in visualizing these small structures. Following the pioneer work of Hudack and McMaster, who demonstrated the small vessels of the skin after injecting patent blue dye intradermally in man (16), Servelle in 1944 (17) and Kinmonth in 1952 (18) described the clinical use of lymphangiography. The classification of Kinmonth was a great step forward in the understanding of the pathology and etiology of lymphatic diseases. From the visualization of the lymphatics in different clinical subsets arose a classification of lymphedema that has proved very useful for the better understanding of the pathophysiology of the disease and, at the same time, establishing guidelines for prognosis and treatment of the different types of lymphedema encountered in clinical practice.

Kinmonth established his classification based on clinical, lymphangiographic, and histopathologic studies. From the lymphangiographic studies, Kinmonth recognized the following types of patterns: a normal lymphatic system, hypoplasia of the lymphatic trunks, aplasia of the trunks and lymph nodes, and hyperplasia or varicose dilatations of the lymphatics. The primary lymphedemas have one or several of the described patterns. Patients with secondary lymphedemas develop abnormal patterns of lymphatic transport due to damage to the trunks or the lymph nodes.

The technique for direct lymphangiography, as described by Kinmonth, involved the injection of patent blue dye into the interdigital spaces of the foot or hand (Fig. 11.1). Vigorous massage and movements of the extremity were recommended to facilitate the progression of the dye toward the proximal lymphatics. Often, the injection of the vital dye could readily demonstrate an obstructive pattern to the lymphatic flow by staining the cutaneous lymphatics in areas several inches away from the injection site. This pattern, termed "dermal backflow," is easily recognized during the injection of the dye. The technique requires a small incision, which may be transverse or longitudinal, on the dorsum

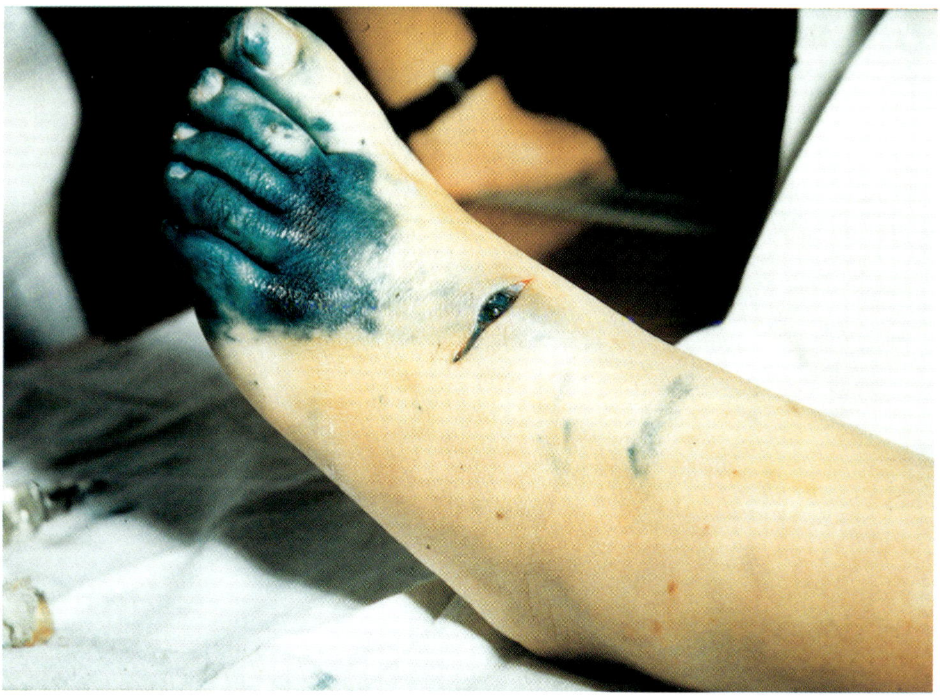

FIG. 11–1. Injection of patent blue into the interdigital spaces of the foot. A transverse incision has been made. The lymphatic vessels selectively take up the blue vital dye and can easily be seen against the yellowish background of the subcutaneous tissue.

of the foot. Dissection continues carefully through the epidermis and dermis. One can readily see lymphatic trunks using 4× magnification or a microscope. The lymphatic trunk appears in a beautiful blue against the yellowish background of the subcutaneous fat. Cannulation of the lymphatic with a fine plastic tube and injection of an oil contrast material (ethiodol) is accomplished utilizing an infusion pump. The contrast material should be injected slowly, at an approximate rate of 0.10–0.20 ml/min until 5–10 ml have been injected. Most of the contrast material is observed in the lymph nodes and filling the lymphatic trunks, which can be usually seen increasing in number as the contrast reaches the inguinal or pelvic regions. In normal individuals, 8–11 trunks can be easily seen in the upper third of the thigh (Fig. 11.2). The lymphangiogram should be evaluated immediately after the injection of the contrast media and 24 hours later, to observe the distribution and concentration of the dye in the lymph nodes. Lymphangiography was performed extensively by Kinmonth and his group and served as the basis for the study of large numbers of patients with various anomalies of the lymphatic system (19). Absence of lymph nodes and abnormal collection of contrast are observed in secondary lymphedema after surgery for malignancy (Fig. 11.3). Dermal backflow (Fig. 11.4) is observed in obstructive lymphedema, either primary or secondary. Lymphangiography has been important to identify the nature and extent of the lymphatic system damage after vein stripping or saphenous vein harvesting for coronary bypass surgery (Fig. 11.5). Because of its invasive nature, tedious technique, and the exquisite skills necessary for its performance, this method is now rarely used.

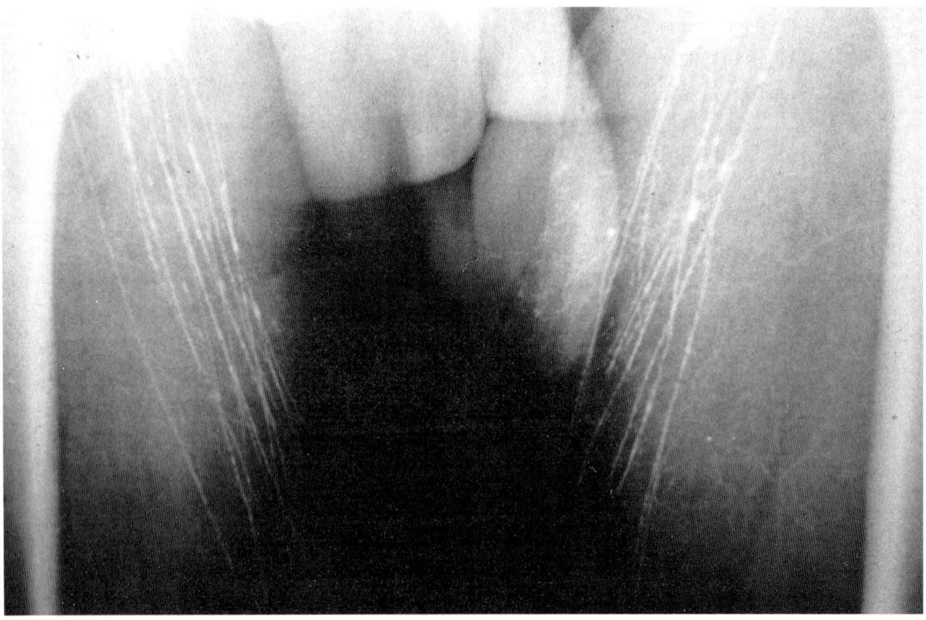

FIG. 11–2. Between 8 and 11 lymphatic trunks can be seen in the upper third of the thigh. The lymphatic valves appear as small dilatations along the course of the trunk. This is a normal lymphangiographic pattern.

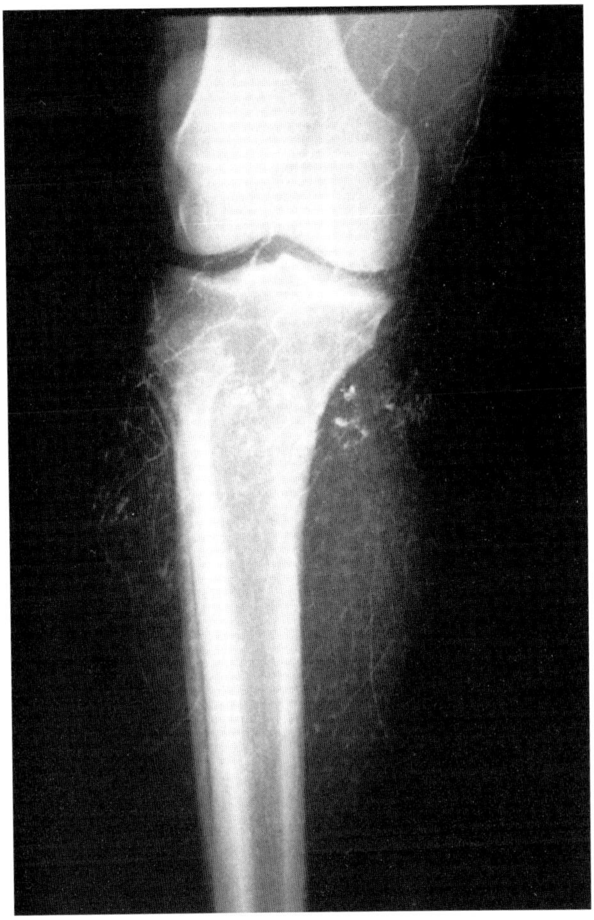

FIG. 11–3. Absence of lymphatic trunks and lymph nodes. Patient had a radical inguinal node dissection for malignancy 3 years earlier. The radiologic contrast is scattered along the course of the saphenous vein. This is a pattern of obstruction.

Other methods utilized to evaluate the lymphatic system include the intravenous injection of fluorescein dyes as described by Bollinger, et al. (20). The method has been used to differentiate edema secondary to chronic venous insufficiency and swelling from lymphedema. Patients suffering from venous disease have larger pericapillary "halos" (21).

The Kinmonth technique was a cornerstone in the understanding of the lymphatic system. However, it offers only a morphologic aspect of the lymphatic system, and provides little or no information on the hemodynamics of the lymph flow. Lymphoscintigraphy was introduced by Sherman and Ter-Porgassian (22). Colloidal gold was initially utilized to visualize the lymphatics. The radiation dose proved excessive owing to the large size of the particles. Antimony trisulfide colloid labeled with technetium has been used to evaluate disorders of the swollen extremity. The introduction of small particle-sized colloids such as antimony trisulfide allows better visualization of lymphatic trunks and flow dynamics (23–25). Since its introduction, lymphoscintigraphy has been utilized extensively in several centers (26, 27). The lymphoscintigraphy technique as described by our group at Walter Reed Army Medical Center (28) requires the injection of the colloid subcutaneously into three interdigital web spaces of each foot. One millicurie

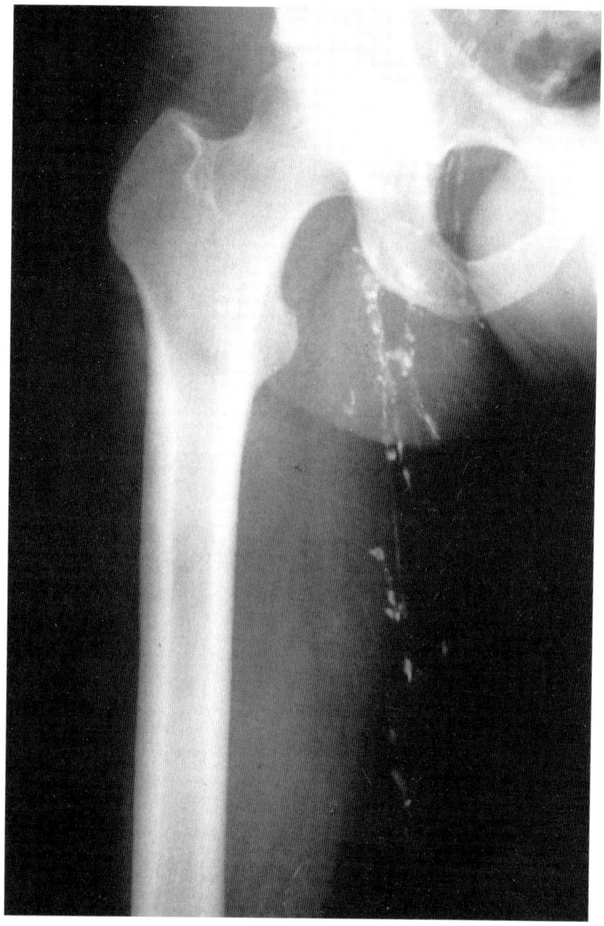

FIG. 11–4. Lymphangiographic pattern of dermal backflow. Small, scattered lymph vessels are observed in the upper leg and lower thigh. Small collections of contrast material are observed in the upper part of the leg. This is a pattern of obstruction in a patient with congenital lymphedema.

of Tc-Sb_2S_3 is mixed with 0.3–0.5 ml of normal saline for each foot injection. Before the injection of the isotope, the patient is exercised either by ambulating or performing stationary foot presses. Utilizing a gamma camera, images are obtained at 10-minute intervals with a large field of view. Three consecutive images over the pelvis are obtained immediately after the injection at 10-minute intervals. If inguinal nodes are not seen within 30 minutes, pelvic imaging is repeated at 1 hour and repeated at the second and fourth hours after the injection if there is still no visualization at that time. If additional images are needed after 1 hour as a result of delayed visualization of the inguinal nodes, the patient ambulates again before repeating the films. Assessment of lymphoscintigraphy involves three components: (a) an interpretation of the drainage pattern; (b) the degree of visualization of the tracer in the inguinal nodes; and (c) the rate of flow. Abnormal lymphoscintigraphic patterns include dermal backflow, complete obstruction, lymphoceles, reflux, and lateral channels. Visualization is considered normal when there is a bilateral symmetric transit of the tracer to the inguinal nodes within 1 hour (Fig. 11.6). Abnormal visualization will show either a decreased or enhanced visualization of the isotope at the inguinal nodes. Flow is considered

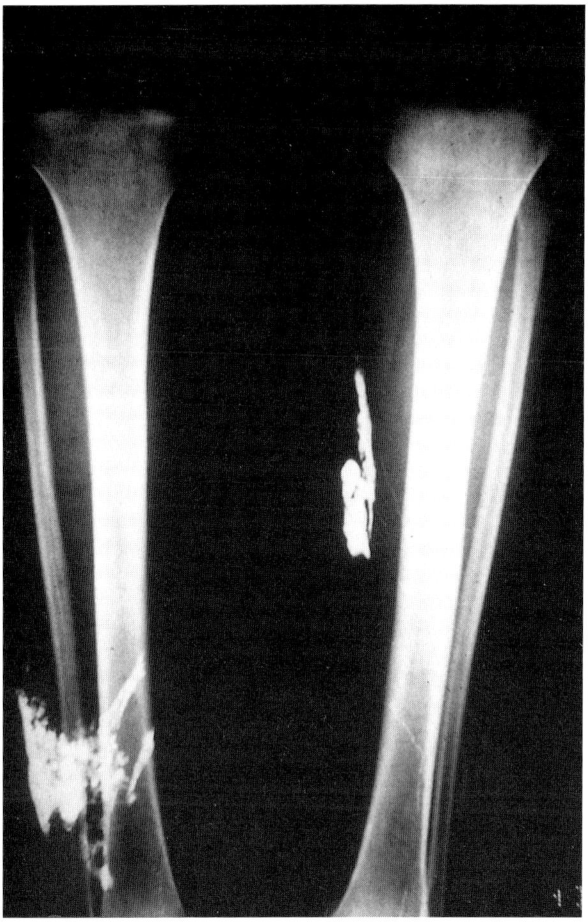

FIG. 11–5. The extensive damage to the lymphatic system produced during vein stripping is clearly demonstrated in this patient. The procedure was performed 1 month after surgery. (Courtesy of J.L. Villavicencio. Reproduced by permission from Hammond SL, Gomez ER, Coffey JA, et al. Involvement of the lymphatic system in chronic venous insufficiency. In: Bergan JJ, Yao JST, eds. Venous disorders. Philadelphia: WB Saunders, 1991:336.)

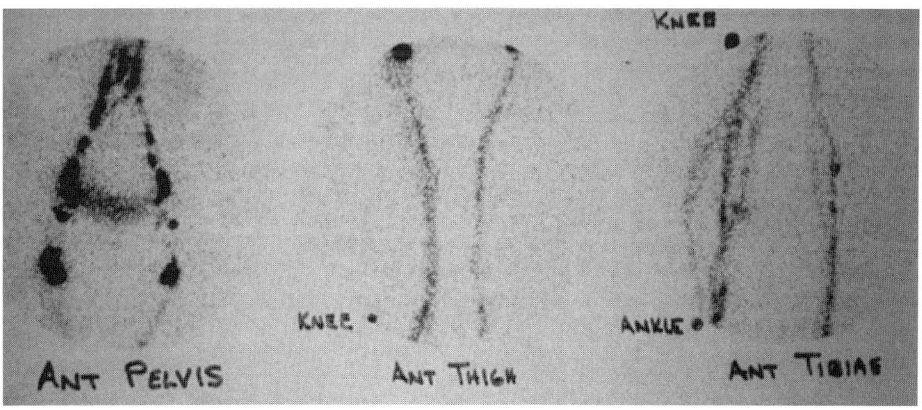

FIG. 11–6. Lymphoscintigraphy. Normal pattern. There is bilateral symmetric transit of the tracer to the inguinal nodes within 1 hour. (Reproduced by permission from Collins PS, Villavicencio JL, Abreu SH, et al. Abnormalities of lymphatic drainage in lower extremities. A lymphoscintigraphic study. J Vasc Surg 1989;9:146.)

normal if there is activity of the tracer at the groin within 30 minutes. Accelerated flow is described when visualization occurs on the initial 10-minute image, and delayed flow is considered when there is no visualization of the inguinal nodes after 60 minutes (Fig. 11.7).

Dermal backflow represents an alternative pathway of lymphatic collateral circulation and it may be present in any type of lymphatic obstruction (29). In some severe cases of total obstruction of the lymphatic flow, crossover of the tracer from one side to the other may be observed.

Abnormal patterns of lymphatic flow by lymphoscintigraphy or other methods may be observed in patients in whom the lymphatic circulation is secondarily affected. Such is the case in patients with chronic venous insufficiency. Collins, et al. (30), studied a group of patients with chronic venous disease in whom lymphatic patterns of flow were evaluated prospectively by lymphoscintigraphy. Most patients in the study had a postphlebitic syndrome. All had an abnormal lymphoscintigraphic flow pattern. Nine had evidence of lymphatic obstruction and one had an enhanced flow pattern. Severe abnormalities of lymphatic flow were observed in patients with the Klippel-Trenaunay syndrome, as well as in patients who were submitted to arterial reconstruction using the saphenous vein (Fig. 11.5).

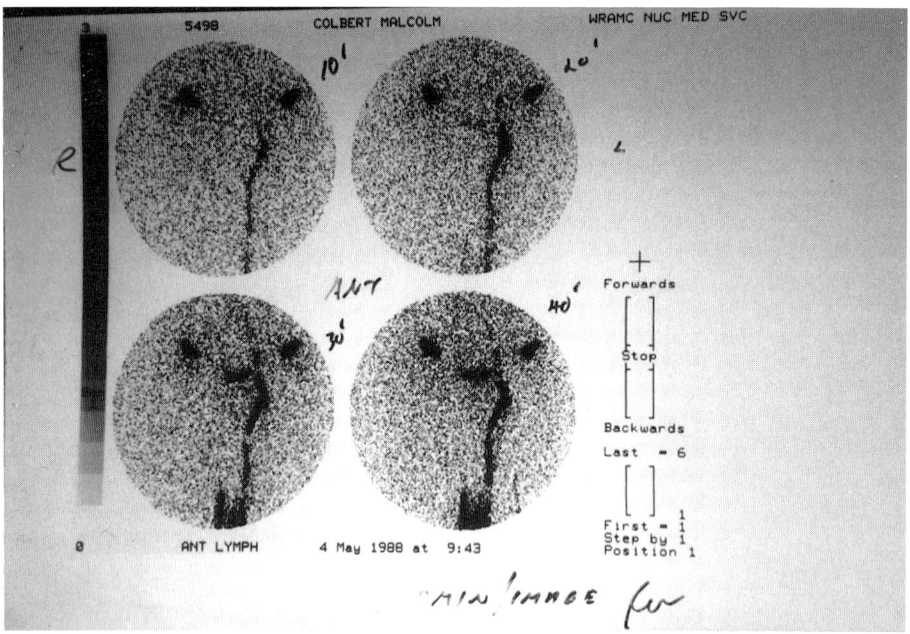

FIG. 11–7. Abnormal lymphoscintigraphy in a patient with lymphedema tarda of the right lower extremity. The isotope appears in the left groin at 10 minutes and its concentration is normal in the films taken at 20, 30, and 40 minutes. The right lower extremity has a pattern of obstruction. There was no visualization of lymphatic trunks at 40 minutes. (Reproduced by permission from Collins PS, Villavicencio JL, Abreu SH, et al. Abnormalities of lymphatic drainage in lower extremities. A lymphoscintigraphic study. J Vasc Surg 1989;9:146.)

Witte (31) summarized the advantages and drawbacks of lymphoscintigraphy thusly:

> "[I]n the upper limbs which have been notoriously difficult to study even with oil contrast lymphography, lymphoscintigraphy (LS) provides excellent images of para-axillary nodal anatomy. Preliminary experience with LS suggests that disruption of axillary truncal continuity is quite variable from patient to patient. Therefore, LS seems to be a promising indicator as to whether lymphedema is likely to appear (or progress) and whether prophylactic or therapeutic remedies are appropriate. In the lower extremities, visualization of truncal anatomy and regional nodes ('hot spots') is also excellent. Para-iliac collectors are usually seen, and sometimes even the thoracic duct is imaged. However, once the isotope reaches the bloodstream, it is rapidly picked up by the lungs, heart, liver and spleen, the images of which tend to obscure the upper abdominal and mediastinal lymphatics. Unlike oil contrast which delineates characteristic intranodal architectural patterns (as in Hodgkin and non-Hodgkin lymphoma) LS only displays node size as dense radioactive 'spots.' Accordingly, at this stage, use of LS for illustrating lymph nodal abnormalities is limited to either their presence or absence. Another potential advantage of LS is that it is now possible to examine the peripheral lymphatics in a wide variety of poorly understood disorders characterized by edema."

With the introduction of technetium-99m human serum albumin (32–34), and with the technologic advances in the digital gamma camera, it is now possible to obtain whole-body imaging of the peripheral lymphatic system with improved resolution. McNeill, et al., have utilized whole-body lymphoscintigraphy as a method for the initial assessment of the peripheral lymphatic system (35). Using whole-body lymphangioscintigraphy, they studied 20 patients with congenital and acquired lymphedema and concluded that it is the method of choice for the initial assessment of congenital or acquired lymphedema. They found three major scintigraphic patterns: obstruction, hypoplasia, and aplasia. Because the tracer enters the lymphatics by diffusion rather than by direct injection, lymphoscintigraphy accurately and reliably delineates the anatomy and the physiologic status of the peripheral lymphatic system.

Magnetic resonance imaging (MRI) has demonstrated value in the investigation of congenital vascular malformations, as well as in disorders of the lymphatic system. MRI has been used to differentiate lipedema from chronic venous edema and lymphedema. Lymphedema appears clinically as deposition of fat behind the malleoli and below the knee. MRI has shown an increased amount of subcutaneous fat without increase in the vascular imaging or in the characteristic images of water accumulation. Characteristically, the ratio between the superficial and deep tissues was found to be increased. On the other hand, in venous edema and lymphedema, there is no change in the superficial/deep compartment ratio. All patients with lymphedema show the typical honey-comb pattern in the subcutaneous tissue. A distinct advantage of the method is the visualization of the lymphatic trunks or nodes proximal to lymphatic obstructions which cannot be visualized by lymphoscintigraphy. The ability of MRI as an adjunct to visualize lymphatic trunks and nodes should be of great value in the understanding of other disorders of the lymphatic system and their response to treatment (36).

Future refinements in resolution and magnification of the MRI images, including use of superparamagnetic contrast agents (37), may place MRI, together with lymphoscintigraphy, as the preferred techniques in the investigation of a wide variety of vascular and lymphatic disorders.

CLINICAL MANIFESTATIONS AND MANAGEMENT OF LYMPHEDEMA

Primary Lymphedema

Primary lymphedema includes the following conditions:

Milroy or familial lymphedema.
Gonadal dysgenesis.
Turner syndrome, which is associated with webbing of the neck, short stature, cubitus valgus, and genital anomalies.
Lymphedema precox, a form of lymphedema which appears between birth and puberty.
Lymphedema tarda, which is the clinical manifestation of lymphedema appearing after the age of 35.

A characteristic of the primary lymphedemas is that there is one or more of the following anomalies of the imaging of the lymphatic system: megalymphatics or hyperplastic trunks with valveless, refluxing vessels; hypoplasia; or aplasia, in which there is an absence of reduction in the number of lymphatic trunks and/or lymph nodes. An important differentiation should be made between congenital lymphedema and Milroy's disease. Congenital lymphedema appears at birth with no history of lymphedema in the family (Fig. 11.8). On the other hand, Milroy's disease (38) is a congenital form of lymphedema which predominantly affects males. In individuals with some form of primary lymphedema, swelling appears at any time from birth to puberty. Often, there is a history of trauma, infection, or surgical intervention. Sprains or orthopedic procedures may precipitate the appearance of progressive swelling in an apparently healthy extremity. Young women with frequent vaginal infections secondary to trichomoniasis or moniliasis may complain of distal edema on the dorsum of the foot which gradually progresses towards the knee. In these cases, ilioinguinal lymph nodes may be affected by the episodes of chronic inflammation and become fibrotic and present an obstacle to the lymph flow. As happens with all forms of lymphedema, episodes of lymphangitis and cellulitis worsen the disease. These episodes are usually secondary to streptococcus and have a tendency to occur frequently if the swelling is not controlled. Anomalies in the development of the intestinal lymphatics with hypoplasia or aplasia may produce chyloascites. In these cases, chyle exudes from the intestinal wall and is not reabsorbed adequately. In other cases, a chylous fistula has been described as a cause of intraperitoneal lymph collection. In these cases, lymph can leak through the inguinal spaces and produce chyledema of the lower extremity, as we have observed in some of our young patients. Congenital anomalies of the thoracic duct, such as absence, hypoplasia, or hyperplasia, produce chylothorax which may be of severe consequences in the development of the child.

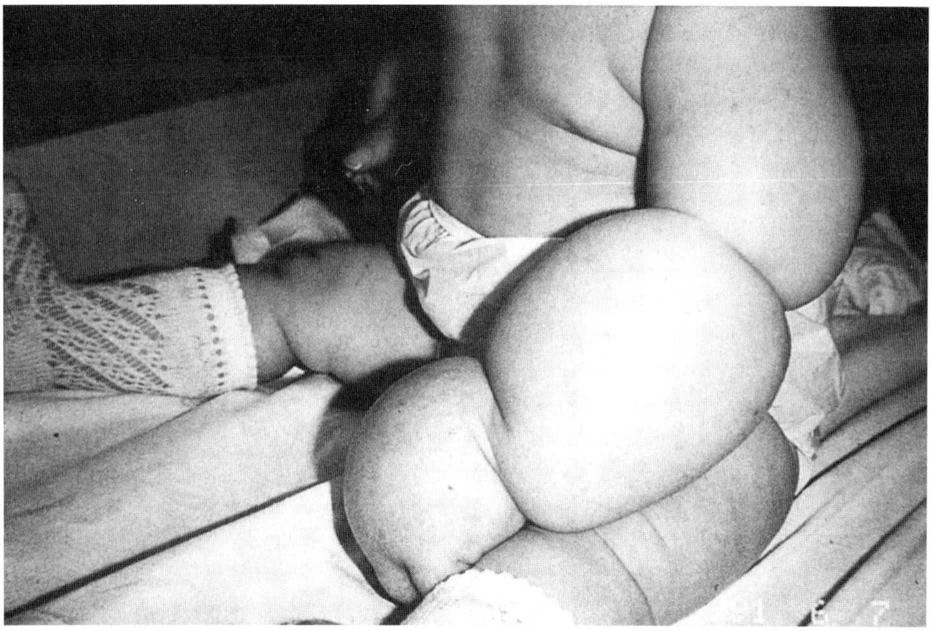

FIG. 11–8. Congenital lymphedema of the left upper extremity in a child. (Courtesy of Professor C. Papendieck, Buenos Aires, Argentina.)

Secondary Lymphedema

The normal lymphatic system may be damaged in the course of trauma, infections, surgery, radiation, neoplasias, burns, animal bites, filariasis, tuberculosis, and other diseases that may involve the lymphatic channels or the lymph nodes. As described earlier, lymphatic disorders may occur in the course of chronic venous edema, such as the postthrombotic syndrome with or without ulceration. A severe case of lymphatic obstruction occurs after infection by *Wuchereria bancrofti*, a disease which is transmitted by mosquitos. The microfilaria lodge in the regional nodes and the main lymphatic trunks, producing gross swelling of the scrotum and the lower extremities (Fig. 11.9).

A common cause of lymphedema is radical mastectomy. This was particularly severe in those cases followed by radiation of the axilla. The incidence of lymphedema has decreased following the modifications in the surgical technique for the treatment of breast carcinoma.

Treatment

Conservative Measures. Intensive efforts should be directed to reduce induration and edema as much as possible. To accomplish this, the following recommendations should be made: the patient should sleep with the foot of the bed elevated 15–20 cm, which is best accomplished by placing bricks or wooden blocks between the foot of the bed and the floor. The extremity should be carefully washed each day with soap and water and lubricated with lanolin or other good

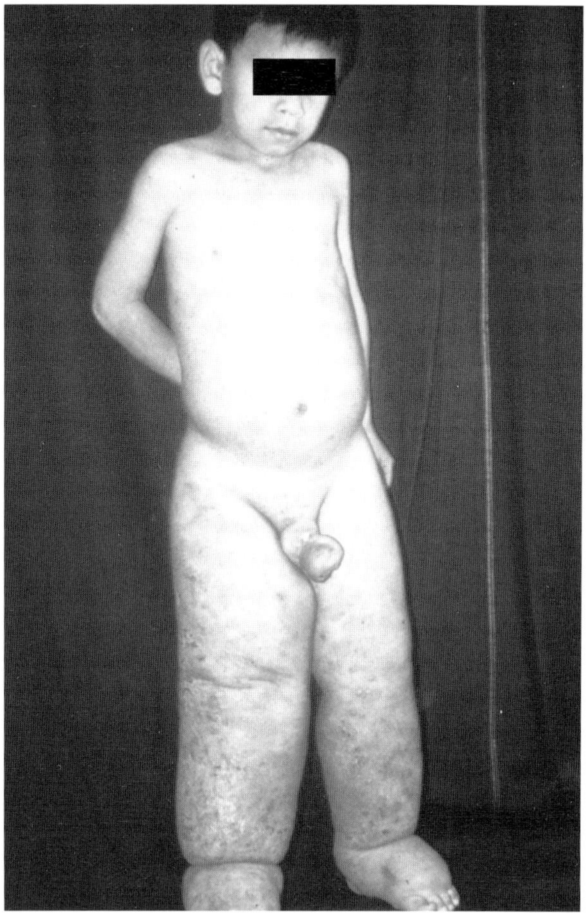

FIG. 11–9. Young boy showing the classic scrotal and lower extremity swelling seen in filariasis. The patient came from a tropical zone of Mexico. (Courtesy of Dr. M. Valdez.)

skin softener. Gentle massage from foot to thigh or from hand to shoulder for 30 minutes twice a day should be recommended. Emphasis should be placed upon the areas where induration is most severe; any skin condition or fungus infection should be treated immediately. The use of prophylactic antibiotics (penicillin or wide-spectrum antibiotics) should be recommended whenever an infectious process is discovered, or when the patient is going to be submitted to a dental procedure or any other examination that may result in the release of bacteria into the circulation. An acute episode of lymphangitis may occur in the course of an ear, tooth, or paranasal sinus infection. Reduction in salt intake and judicious use of diuretics should be recommended. In general, diuretics are not routinely used and should be employed only when the accumulation of fluid in the extremities seems to be larger than usual; trauma to the affected extremity should be avoided. The use of protective clothing and insect repellents, and avoidance of scratches or any other type of injury, such as small cuts while cutting toenails or fingernails, should be advised.

External compression in the form of elastic stockings, elastic bandages, and intermittent pneumatic compression is the mainstay of the nonoperative management of lymphedema. Elastic stockings control swelling and maintain limb size, but do not usually reduce the lymphedematous tissue. CircAid, a nonelastic, custom-fitted garment made of a series of velcro bands, has proven very effective to control swelling in lymphedema and other conditions where edema is a prevalent sign. Sequential, high-pressure intermittent pneumatic compression in our clinic has been able to control most forms of lymphedema. Most cases of so-called intractable lymphedema respond to a period of 2–3 days in bed with a program of 3 hours on, 1 hour off intermittent pneumatic compression using a multichambered compression device. With these measures, the degree of subcutaneous fibrosis (fibredema) may be prevented to a greater extent. Those patients with grossly enlarged extremities, or with a severe degree of fibrosis, are candidates for surgical management (39).

Surgical Management. The great majority of patients with lymphedema will respond to conservative measures. However, there is a group of approximately 10% of all patients with lymphedema in whom some form of surgical treatment is indicated. The surgical procedures designed to treat lymphatic disorders are classified into two main categories: excisional and physiologic. Excisional operations are indicated in patients with minimal or absent response to a well-designed conservative treatment. Among the multiple excisional procedures described, there are two that deserve mention. The procedure described by Charles (40) consists of the excision of skin, subcutaneous tissue, and fascia followed by free skin grafts. This operation is particularly useful in patients with severely damaged skin. The second excisional procedure, which we have used almost exclusively, is Kinmonth's modification of Homan's procedure (41). In 1975, Chilvers and Kinmonth reviewed a series of 108 excisional operations, classifying their results as poor in 19 patients, moderate in 60 patients, and good in 29 patients. In general, it can be stated that the results of the modified Homan's procedure are quite satisfactory in properly selected patients. The patient must be informed that these operations are palliative rather than curative. Table 11.1 is a summary of the results of some reported series.

TABLE 11-1

SURGERY FOR LYMPHEDEMA: EXCISIONAL PROCEDURES FOR LYMPHEDEMA

		Results (%)		
Author	No.	Good	Fair	Follow-up (Yrs)
Miller	21	0	100	1–4
Bunchman	5	100	0	1
Fonkalsrud	6	100	0	>1
Bunchman	14	100	0	5
Dellon	12	100	—	10
Thompson	50	58	42	1–10
Kinmonth	108	27	56	1–5

The physiologic operations attempt to bridge the obstructed areas with segments of lymphatics, either free or attached, or with tissues such as omentum or small bowel. Lymphangiographic proof of patency of these bridges has been demonstrated by Kinmonth.

Anastomosis between the lymphatics distal to the obstruction and the venous system has been performed by Degni (42), O'Brien (43), and others (Fig. 11.10). O'Brien reported 52 patients who had microlymphatic surgery in whom 42% had at least a 10% reduction in limb volume. Baumeister reported 55 patients in whom he performed a microsurgical lymphatic grafting. He transplanted autogenous lymphatic grafts from the patient's thigh to different areas depending on the site of the lymphatic blockade. In his study of 55 patients, only 30 had postoperative lymphoscintigraphy to evaluate graft patency and changes in lymph transport capacity (44). Gloviczki performed lymphovenous anastomosis in 34 dogs, using cinelymphangiography to prove patency of the anastomosis. He reported that four of six anastomoses were patent at 3 months and two of six at 8 months (45). The problem of direct reconstructions in the lymphatic system, either by direct lymphovenous anastomosis or by lymphatic transplantation, has been the difficulty in obtaining objective evidence of patency of the procedure. Postoperative lymphography, which has been attempted by some investigators, has been accom-

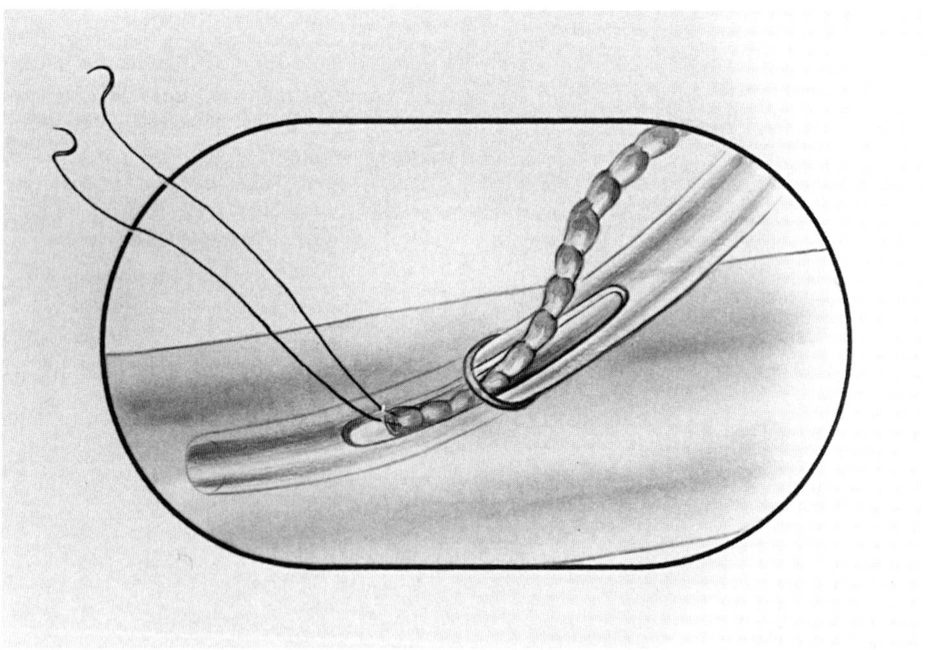

FIG. 11–10. Lymphovenous insertion. The lymphatic trunk has been dissected and divided at its proximal end. A "mattress" suture with a double arm 10–0 monofilament suture is passed through one side of the lymphatic mouth. The lymphatic trunk is inserted in the groove of a specially designed plastic cannula. The two needles exit 2 mm distal to the point of entrance in the vein. Four or five lymphatic trunks can be accommodated along a 4- or 5-cm length of saphenous or femoral vein.

TABLE 11-2

SURGERY FOR LYMPHEDEMA: LYMPHOVENOUS ANASTOMOSIS

Author	Year	No. Pts.	Results % Good to Excellent	Follow-up (Yrs)
Cordeiro	1980	123	70	10
Degni	1980	52	75	6
Krylov	1982	50	30	?
Nieuborg	1982	47	68	1
Gong-Kang	1985	91	79	2**
Zu, et al.	1987	48	33	
Zu, et al.		185	73	
Villavicencio	1987	44	s53/p40	2–10
Gloviczki	1988	14	50	4**
			25	
O'Brien	1990	90*	83*	5**

*Available for follow-up (total of 134 patients); 52 patients had lymphovenous shunts alone; 38 had combined procedures.
**Mean
s = secondary
p = primary

panied by lymphangitis, which obstructs the recently created anastomosis. There are reports that lymphoscintigraphy, which has little effect on the lymphatic endothelium, has demonstrated patency of the lymphaticovenous anastomosis in some patients. Table 11.2 is a summary of the clinical results of surgery on the lymphatics.

With the availability of new lymphatic imaging techniques, the patency of the reconstructive procedures on the lymphatic system needs to be demonstrated objectively. Microvascular anastomosis utilizing 10–0 or 11–0 nylon and 70-micron needles will undoubtedly be reevaluated in the future.

Suction lipectomy has recently been introduced as a form of treatment, especially in mild lymphedema without fibrosis and skin changes. Improvement in function and appearance has been reported, but the improvement seems to be temporary and of relatively short duration (12–24 months) (46).

REFERENCES

1. Asellius G. De Lattibus Sine Lacteis Venis. Mediolani, Apud Io B Bidellium, 1627.
2. Starling EH. On the absorption of fluids from the connective tissue spaces. J Physiol (Lond) 1896;19:312.
3. Drinker CK, Field ME. The protein content of mammalian lymph and the relation of lymph to tissue fluid. Am J Physiol 1931;97:32.
4. Landis EM. Capillary permeability and the factors affecting the composition of the capillary filtrate. Ann NY Acad Sci 1946;46:713.

5. Mayerson HS. The physiologic importance of lymph. In: Hammington WF, ed. Handbook of physiology. Vol. II. Washington, DC: American Physiological Society, 1963:1035–1073.
6. Moretta L, Mingari MC, Moretta A, Fauci AS. Human lymphocyte surface markers. Hematology 1982;19:273.
7. Sabin FR. The origin and development of the lymphatic system. Baltimore: The Johns Hopkins Press, 1912:7–24.
8. Huntington GS. The anatomy and development of the systemic lymphatics in the domestic cat. Philadelphia: Wistar Institute Press, 1911.
9. Blalock A, Robinson CS, Cunningham RS, Gray ME. Experimental studies of lymphatic blockage. Arch Surg 1937;34:1049.
10. Casley-Smith JR. The fine structure and functioning of tissue channels and lymphatics. Lymphology 1980;12:177.
11. Landis EM. Capillary pressure and capillary permeability. Physiol Rev 1934;14:408–481.
12. Landis EM, Popheimer JM. Exchange of substances through the capillary walls. In: Handbook of physiology. Vol. II. Sect. 2. Washington, DC: American Physiological Society, 1963:961–1054.
13. Reed RK, Johansen NS, Noddeland H. Turnover rate of interstitial albumin in rat skin and skeletal muscle. Effects of lymph movement and motor activity. Acta Physiol Scand 1985;125:711.
14. Schmid-Schonbein GW, Zweifach BW. Fluid pump mechanisms in initial lymphatics. News Physiol Sci 1994;9:67.
15. Hargens AR, Zweifach BW. Contractile stimuli in collecting lymph vessels. Am J Physiol 1977;233:H57.
16. Hudack SS, McMaster PD. The lymphatic participation in human cutaneous phenomena. J Exb Med 1933;57:751.
17. Servelle M. A propos de la lymphographie experimentale et clinique. J Radiol Electro Med Nucl 1944.;26:165.
18. Kinmonth JB. Lymphangiography in man. Clin Sci 1952;II:13.
19. Kinmonth JB. Methods of lymphography. In: Kinmonth JB, ed. The lymphatics. Surgery, lymphography and disease of the chyle and lymph systems. 2nd ed. London: Edward Arnold, 1982:1–17.
20. Bollinger A, Jager K, Siger F, et al. Fluorescence microlymphography. Circulation 1981;64;1195–1200.
21. Saner H, Boss C, Mahler F. Demonstration of the peri-capillary space after intravenous administration of sodium fluorescein. In: Bollinger A, Partsch H, Wolfe JHN, eds. The initial lymphatics: new methods and findings. International symposium. Zurich. 1st ed. New York: Thiem Stratton, 1985:94–97.
22. Sherman AI, Ter-Porgassian M. Lymph node concentration of radioactive colloidal gold following interstitial injection. Cancer 1953;6:1238–1240.
23. Ege GN, Clark RM. Internal mammary lymphoscintigraphy in the conservative surgical management of breast carcinoma. Clin Radiol 1980;31:559–63.
24. Kaplan WD. Iliopelvic lymphoscintigraphy. Semin Nucl Med 1983;13:42–53.
25. Bennett LR, Lago G. Cutaneous lymphoscintigraphy in malignant melanoma. Semin Nucl Med 1983;13:70–74.
26. Cambria RA, Bender CE, Hauser MF, et al. Lymphoscintigraphy and lymphangiography. In: Gloviczki P, Yao JST, eds. Handbook of venous disorders. Guidelines of the American Venous Forum. New York: Chapman & Hall Medical, 1996:580–599.
27. Cambria RA, Gloviczki P, Naessens JM, et al. Non-invasive evaluation of the swollen extremity with lymphoscintigraphy: a prospective semi-quantitative analysis in 386 extremities. J Vasc Surg 1985;18:773–782.

28. Hammond SL, Gomez ER, Coffey JA, et al. Involvement of the lymphatic system in chronic venous insufficiency. In: Bergan JJ, Yao JST, eds. Venous disorders. Philadelphia: WB Saunders, 1991:333–343.
29. Sty JR, Boedecker RA, Scanlon JT, Babbitt DP. Radionuclide "dermal backflow" in lymphatic obstruction. J Nucl Med 1979;20:905–906.
30. Collins PS, Villavicencio JL, Abreu SH, et al. Abnormalities of lymphatic drainage in lower extremities. A lymphoscintigraphic study. J Vasc Surg 1989;9:145–152.
31. Witte CL. Lymphatic imaging. Lymphology 1993;26:109–111.
32. Ohtake E, Matsui K. Lymphoscintigraphy in patients with lymphedema: a new approach using intradermal injections of technetium-99m human serum albumin. Clin Nucl Med 1986;11:474–478.
33. Nawaz K, Hamad MM, Sadek S, et al. Dynamic lymph flow imaging in lymphedema: normal and abnormal patterns. Clin Nucl Med 1986;11:653–658.
34. Weissleder H, Weissleder R. Lymphedema: evaluation of qualitative and quantitative lymphoscintigraphy in 238 patients. Radiology 1988;167:729–735.
35. McNeill GC, Witte MH, Witte CH, et al. Whole-body lymphangioscintigraphy: preferred method for initial assessment of the peripheral lymphatic system. Radiology 1989;172:495–502.
36. Case TC, Unger EE, Bernas MJ, et al. Lymphatic imaging in experimental filariasis using magnetic resonance. Invest Radiol 1992;27:293–297.
37. Weissleder R, Elizondo G, Wittenburg J, et al. Ultra small superparamagnetic iron oxide: an intravenous contrast agent for assessing lymph nodes with MR imaging. Radiology 1990;175:494–498.
38. Milroy WF. Chronic hereditary edema. JAMA 1928;91:1172.
39. Pappas CJ, O'Donnell TF. Long-term results of compression treatment for lymphedema. J Vasc Surg 1992;16:555–564.
40. Charles H. Radical excision of hypertrophied skin and subcutaneous tissue of the leg in the treatment of lymphadema. In: Latham A, English JC, eds. A system of treatment. Vol. 3. London: Churchill, 1912.
41. Kinmonth JB. The lymphatics. 2nd ed. London: Edward Arnold, 1982:173–178.
42. Degni M. New technique of lymphatic-venous anastomosis for the treatment of lymphedema. Vasa 1974;3:479.
43. O'Brien BMC, Mellow CG, Khaancanchi RK, et al. Long-term results after microlymphaticovenous anastomosis for the treatment of obstructive lymphedema. Plast Reconstruc Surg 1990;85:562–572.
44. Baumeister RG, Siuda S. Treatment of lymphedemas by microsurgical lymphatic grafting. What is proved? Plast Reconstruc Surg 1990;85:64–74.
45. Gloviczki P, Hollier LH, Nora SE, Kage MP. The natural history of microsurgical lymphovenous anastomoses: an experimental study. J Vasc Surg 1986;4:148–156.
46. Sando WC, Nahai F. Suction lipectomy in the management of limb lymphedema. Clin Plast Surg 1989;16:369–373.

chapter 12

Ambulatory Venous Pressure Regulation and Pressure Measurements

Seshadri Raju

AMBULATORY VENOUS PRESSURE

Ambulatory venous pressure changes have traditionally been explained on the basis of hydrostatic column segmentation due to valve closure with calf exercise. However, a detailed consideration of the pressure changes that occur with calf muscle exercise makes it clear that compliance pressure generated by the venous segment below the valve plays a significant role in ambulatory venous pressure regulation (Fig. 12.1) (1).

The tibial valve is normally located approximately 30 cm above foot level. In the resting state, the valve is open and pressures (in centimeters of blood) at the foot level and immediately above and below the valve are as shown in Figure 12.1. With calf muscle exercise, the venous segment below the valve is emptied of the ejected volume of blood and partially collapses (Fig. 12.1**B**). The pressure immediately above the closed tibial valve would be 90 cm of blood, representing the column height from the valve level to the heart. The pressure at the top of the residual column of blood below the closed valve will be zero. As this column grows in height from arterial input to touch the valve, the pressure relationships around the closed valve will be as shown in Figure 12.1**C**. Although the blood column below the valve has been restored to its full potential height, column pressure just below the closed valve is still zero and is inadequate to overcome the high pressure above the valve to open it.

To open the valve, distension of the venous segment below the closed valve by continued arterial input with generation of additional compliance pressure is necessary. At an intermediate point of distension, a pressure of 30 cm may be recorded below the closed valve and a pressure of 60 cm of blood would be recorded at the foot level (Fig. 12.1**D**). Since the valve is still closed, the physical column height is only 30 cm, which represents a hydrostatic column pressure component of 30 cm of blood at the foot level. The additional 30 cm (60 cm − 30 cm) represents

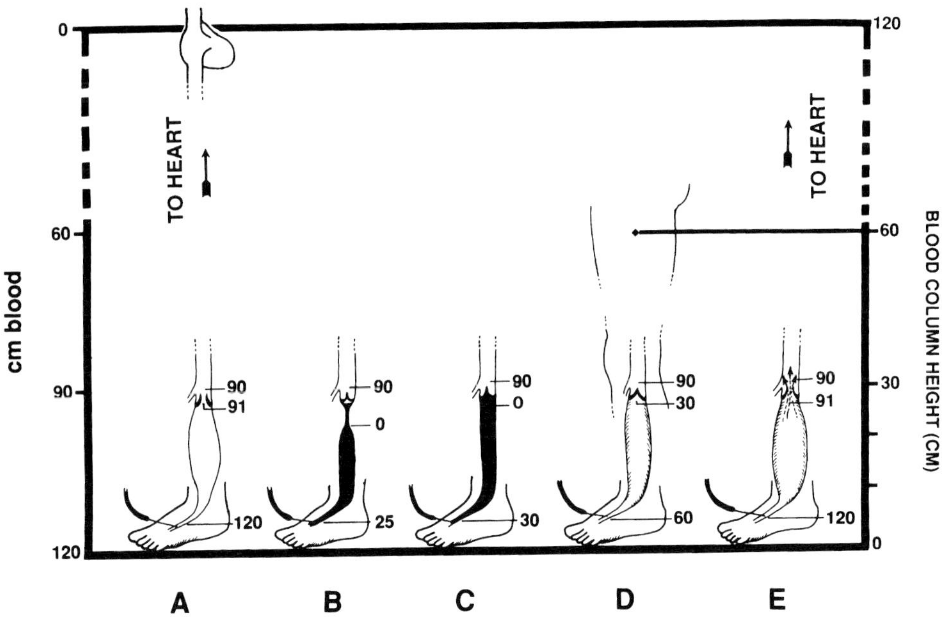

FIG. 12–1. Scheme of nominal pressure relationships related to tibial valve closure after calf muscle contraction. Hydrostatic pressure forces alone will be insufficient to open the closed tibial valve. Generation of compliance pressure by distension of tibial vein segment by arterial input is necessary for valve opening. By permission of J Vasc Surg (1).

compliance pressure generated by the distended venous tube below the valve. The entire 60 cm clearly cannot be due to hydrostatic column pressure alone because the column height would have to be 60 cm, a much higher pressure than could be allowed by the closed tibial valve. With continued distension of the venous tube by arterial input and increasing compliance pressure, the tibial valve finally opens when the pressure below the valve reaches 91 cms, overcoming the pressure above the valve (Fig. 12.1E).

The fact that veins are collapsible tubes introduces additional complexities in ambulatory foot venous pressure regulation. The volume pressure relationship in collapsible tubes, such as latex, is nonlinear (Fig. 12.2). In experimental settings the latex tube is often used as a proxy to mimic the collapsible properties of veins (2), although the latter differ from the latex in some aspects of the pressure volume relationship (3). The similarities, however, are such that the use of latex to explore the behavior of veins in the experimental setting is generally accepted. Volume pressure curves generated in a mechanical model of "calf venous pump" utilizing a graduated valve and a latex tube are shown in Figure 12.3. The pressure remains relatively low and constant as the tube fills up to about 70% of its potential volume capacity. This stage of volume filling is called the bending regimen of a collapsible tube because the volume is accommodated as the tube simply abandons its collapsed shape and assumes a circular shape in cross-section without stretching its walls. The perimeter of the circular tube at this stage is equal to the perimeter of the dumbbell-shaped collapsed tube in cross-section. Roughly

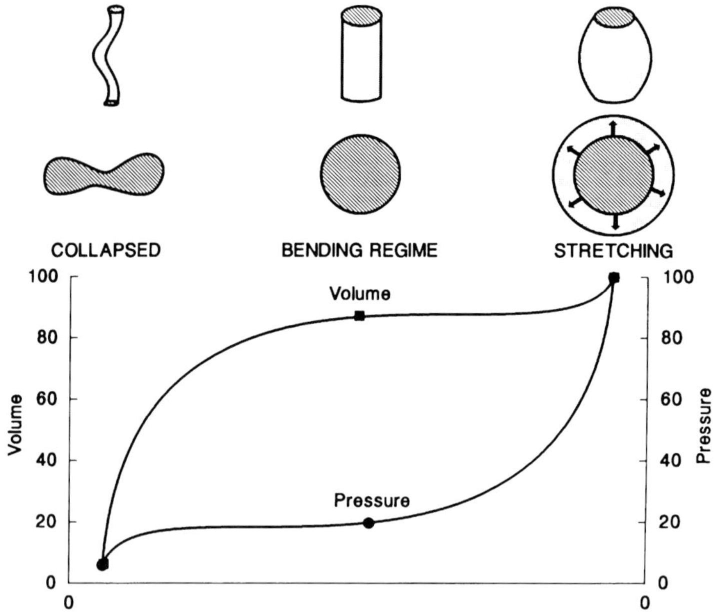

FIG. 12–2. Nominal volume pressure relationship in a collapsible tube; *upper* panel represents degree of collapse at various points of interest.

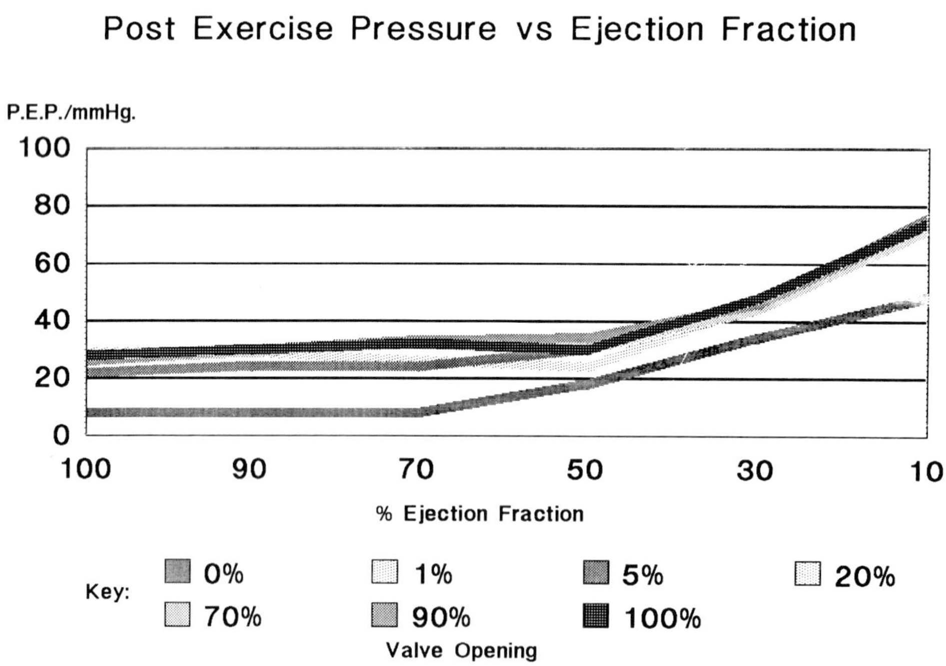

FIG. 12–3. Volume pressure relationships generated in a mechanical model of calf venous pump. The pressure remains constant for a wide range of ejection volumes and reflux valve settings. (By permission of J Vasc Surg [1].)

an additional 30% volume can be accommodated in the tube as it distends by stretching its wall (stretching regimen), increasing the perimeter of the tube in cross-section from the previous stage. A marked pressure increase is noted during the stretching regimen; the volume increment is relatively small in comparison to the filling during the bending regimen.

The nonlinear volume pressure relationship evident of collapsible tubes confers interesting properties that may be significant in foot venous pressure regulation. Most of the pressure drop with calf exercise occurs during ejection of the initial 30–40% of volume in the pump. Increasing the ejection fraction beyond this point results in relatively little additional pressure reduction; the residual pressure remains fairly constant even as the tube is emptied further. Even as the graduated valve is set at different open positions to mimic varying degrees of "reflux," there is little difference in the generated pressure curves. These curves are roughly similar, remaining at a relatively constant low pressure level.

Thus, the fluid mechanics in the collapsible tube appear to confer significant buffering qualities that tend to retain constant low "postexercise" pressure in the pump for a wide range of ejection fractions and valve reflux. This inherent compensatory mechanism for deficiencies of the calf venous pump and valve function may have obvious physiologic importance.

Using the mechanical model described earlier, "ambulatory venous pressure" reduction can be shown to be due primarily to tube collapse rather than valve closure (Fig. 12.4). When the valve is closed after the tube is fully distended, reach-

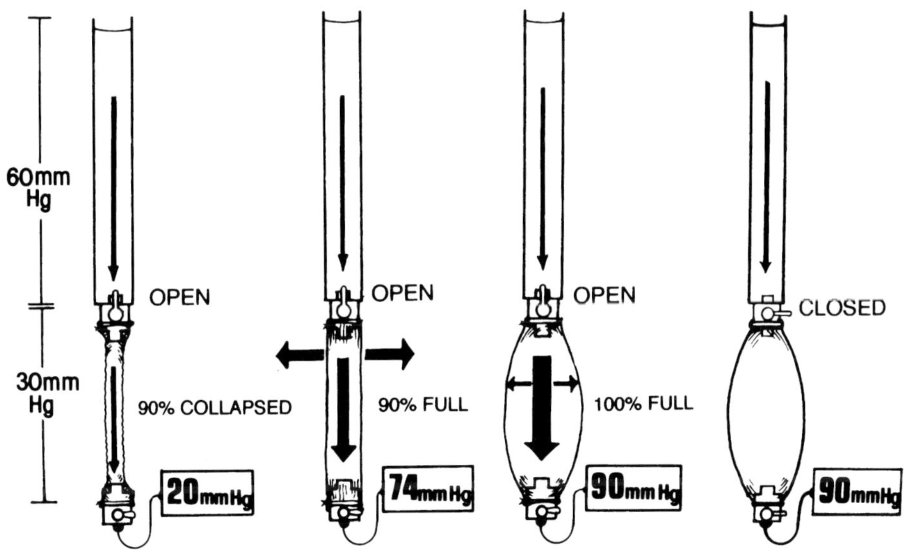

FIG. 12–4. Pressure reduction in a tube is primarily due to tube collapse and *not* due to valve closure. This can be demonstrated with use of a mechanical model consisting of a collapsible tube and a valve. With the tube collapsed and valve open (**A**) the tube pressure is low even though a full hydrostatic column is present. As the tube fills and distends, tube pressure gradually increases (**B**) reaching a maximum of 90 mmHg (**C**), corresponding to the hydrostatic column height. When the valve is closed at this point, segmenting the column, there is no immediate reduction in the tube pressure which remains unchanged at 90 mmHg (**D**). (By permission of J Vasc Surg [1]).

ing a recorded pressure of 90 mmHg at the bottom, little pressure changes are noted immediately after valve closure although the fluid column has been physically segmented. The crucial role of tube collapse and compliance in venous pressure regulation suggests that wall property changes in the venous wall, such as may occur in postthrombotic syndrome, may result in significant alterations in the buffer function of the calf venous pump; ambulatory venous hypertension from decreased wall compliance may result from decreased wall compliance independent of capacitance reduction and valve reflux abnormalities that may occur after a bout of deep venous thrombosis.

The volume pressure relationship in venous tubes, although generally similar to that obtained in latex tubes, is less nonlinear (3). Stretch relaxation is also evident. Tube collapse clearly occurs, however, in the physiologic setting. Dynamic venography shows a significant reduction in the caliber of tibial veins and soleal sinusoids after calf exercise (4), although it is not known whether veins collapse to a dumbbell shape in cross-section.

In the physiologic setting, dissipation of the stretching regimen probably occurs during ambulatory venous pressure changes. In the latex model, an ejection fraction of 30–40% is adequate to carry the tube from the stretching to the bending regimen. Such fractional volume changes are well within the physiologic range. In the single-tube single-valve mechanical model, "postexercise pressure" changes primarily occur with ejection fraction increments (1); reflux valve settings exert little influence on this parameter. With increasing reflux, however, recovery times are progressively shorter. With a 10% valve opening in this model, reflux filling of the latex tube occurs almost instantaneously with a recorded recovery time of a second or less. Increasing the valve opening beyond this point does not measurably affect the already very short recovery time. A more complex calf pump model consisting of an upper pump and a conduit below reveals less pressure buffering in the conduit. An interesting observation in the latter model was the active role of the conduit in overall pump function and pressure regulation due to the elastic properties of the conduit wall. Studies with this model now in progress indicate that conduit elasticity has a far greater impact on postejection conduit pressure and recovery time than pump wall properties. While the complex human calf pump cannot be accurately duplicated in a mechanical model, such experiments help to clarify general fluid dynamic principles that are likely important in vivo. This is particularly true for collapsible tubes where mathematical resolution of their complex behaviors has been difficult and actual behavior often deviates from the predicted.

The nonlinear volume pressure relationship in collapsible tubes may result in interesting volume reflux behavior. For example, consider a pair of venous segments of equal capacitance with an intervening incompetent valve (Fig. 12.5). If the upper tube is full and the lower one is empty, a significant reflux gradient will be present and reflux will occur across the valve. Because of the nonlinear volume pressure relationship a reflux gradient across the valve will largely disappear (except for gravity gradient) with as little as 30–40% of upper tube volume refluxing into the lower tube. Even though the upper tube would contain substantially more volume than the lower tube at this stage, both tubes would be in the bending regimen with similar pressures. Thus, high gradient reflux tends to be limited due to the nonlinear volume pressure relationship. If the upper tube

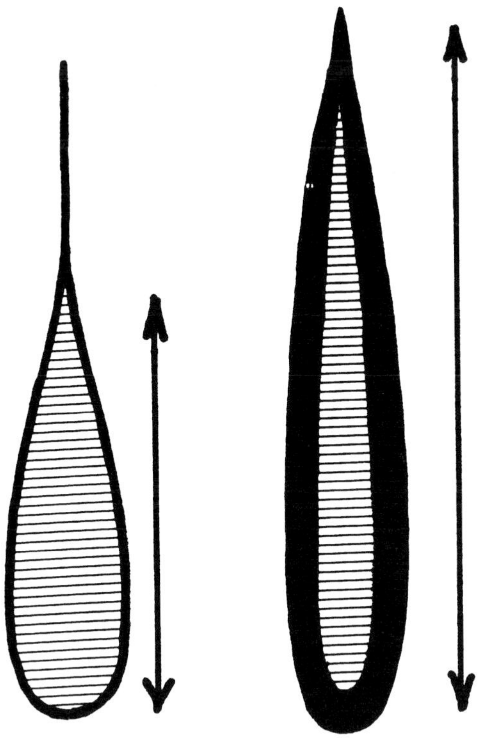

FIG. 12–5. Wall thickening will increase residual fluid column height in a collapsible tube (after Johnson HD, Pflug J. The swollen leg. London: Heinemann, 1975). Reflux across an incompetent valve between an upper and lower venous tube segment of equal capacitance is governed by the nonlinear volume pressure relationship that prevails in collapsible tubes.

was full and lower tube 70% full, substantial pressure equalization (except for gravity differences) across the valve will occur with as little as 15% of upper tube volume refluxing into the lower tube. In clinical measurement of ambulatory venous pressure, the monitoring site is the dorsal foot vein, which is separated from the calf venous pump by a number of unidirectional valves. Although rapid equilibration of pressure between the monitoring site and the calf venous pump takes place, identical pressures and wave forms may not be obtained, especially when there is an up-slope in the pressure curve. When recovery times are extremely short owing to massive reflux, there may not be adequate time for equilibration of pressure between the calf venous pump and the monitoring site. Thus, the relationship between ejection fraction and postexercise pressure on the one hand, and reflux and recovery times on the other, may be different in the clinical setting than demonstrated in the single tube mechanical model. The nonlinear volume pressure relationship seen in the mechanical model is strikingly similar to simultaneous volume and pressure data obtained by plethysmographic and foot venous pressure recordings in healthy volunteers (Fig. 12.6**A** and **B**). In both instances, most of the volume filling appears to have occurred during the bending regimen. The great part of "recovery time" appears to represent the stretching regimen as the full tube further distends. Volume addition to the tube during this phase is relatively minor. Massive reflux can shorten recovery times by abbreviating both the bending and stretching phases of volume recovery. Because most of the recovery time represents the stretching phase, changes in wall property that limit stretching (i.e., decreased compliance due to deep vein thrombosis [DVT])

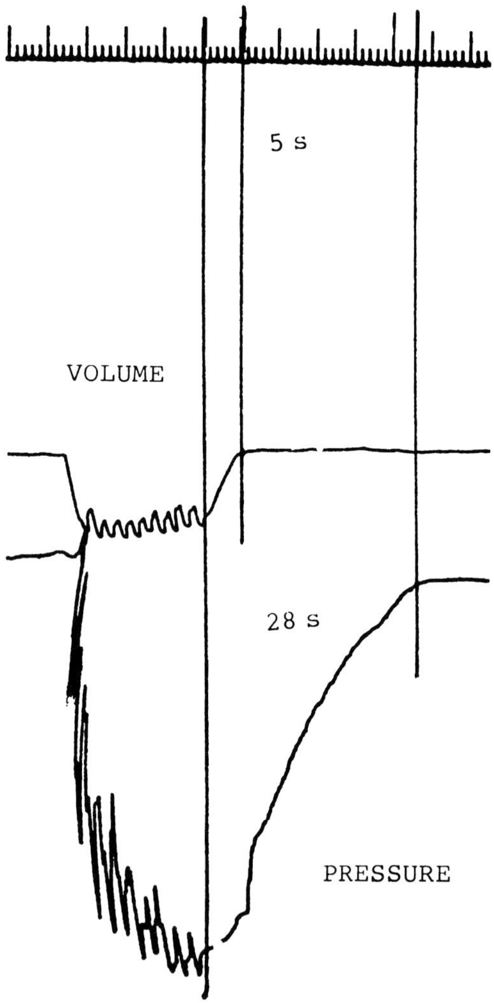

FIG. 12–6. **A.** Simultaneous plethysmographic and ambulatory venous pressure tracings in a healthy limb. Note that 90% of ejected volume has been recovered in 5 seconds, with ambulatory venous pressure still close to its nadir. Recovery time for ambulatory venous pressure is 28 seconds. **B.** Similar relationship between volume and pressure is noted in mechanical model. After ejection, 75% of volume recovery takes place, whereas postejection pressure is still at or near its nadir. (By permission of J Vasc Surg [1].)

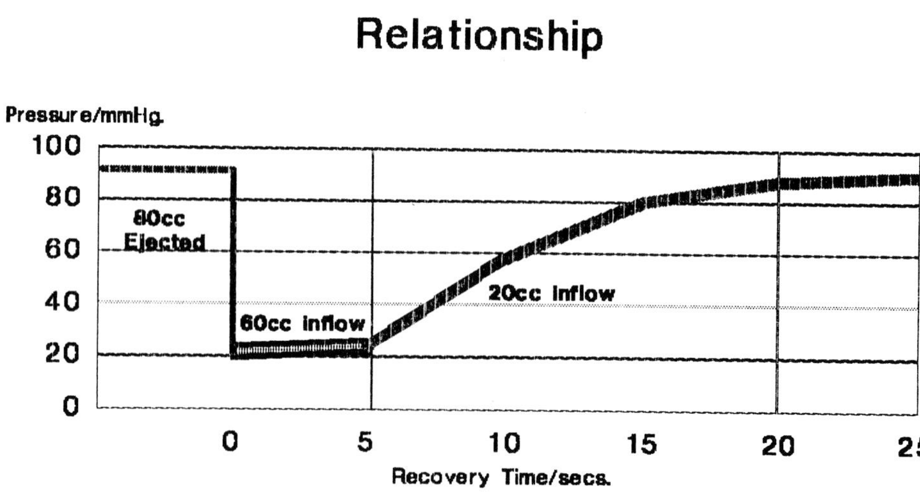

can shorten recovery time even in the absence of reflux. The influence of arterial inflow on ambulatory venous pressure measurements has been little appreciated. Arterial inflow does not remain static but increases with increasing ejection fraction as the arteriovenous (AV) differences widen (1). Increased arterial inflow also increases residual pressure in the collapsible tube after ejection. Increased arterial inflow also decreases recovery times. Plethysmographic studies indicate that arterial inflow in the adult human limb averages approximately 2–3 ml per second. In patients with Klippel-Trenaunay syndrome, the arterial inflow may be as high as 10–20 ml per second, because of abnormal AV connections that often are not seen on arteriography. It can be appreciated that ambulatory venous pressure recovery times can be shortened with an increase in postexercise pressure by such increased arterial inflow. A reduction in the calf venous pump capacitance after deep venous thrombosis due to clot retention, loss of compliance volume and fibrous contraction, or disappearance of capacitance veins can also shorten recovery times. In most laboratories, a shortened recovery time is usually interpreted as synonymous with the presence of reflux. As detailed earlier, many other factors should be considered in interpreting shortened recovery times. Ambulatory venous pressure has long been considered the "gold standard" in assessing the hemodynamic effects of reflux. As the foregoing discussion suggests, postexercise pressure and recovery times are influenced by a multitude of factors and reflux is but one of many such variables. The incidence of stasis ulceration increases as postexercise pressure rises (Table 12.1). The correlation is not absolute, however, because many patients with ambulatory venous hypertension remain free of ulcers and some with *normal* postexercise pressure develop stasis ulceration (5). The precise relationship between ambulatory venous pressure and the development of a stasis ulcer is not known. A time lag undoubtedly exists between the development of ambulatory hypertension and the development of an epithelial ulcer. Comerota and colleagues have shown that there is no difference in the ambulatory venous pressure of clinical Class 3 patients without stasis ulceration and patients with ulcer (6). Most patients with ambulatory venous hypertension present with both—a short recovery time and an elevated postexercise pressure—but, in some, only one of these parameters is abnormal with the other in the

TABLE 12-1

THE INCIDENCE OF LEG ULCERATION (ACTIVE OR HEALED) IN RELATION TO AMBULATORY VENOUS PRESSURE *P* IN 251 LIMBS

n	P (mmHg)	Incidence of Ulceration (%)
34	<30	0
44	31–40	12
51	41–50	22
45	51–60	38
34	61–70	57
28	71–80	68
15	>80	73

"normal" range. The relative importance of time and pressure as represented by these indices in the generation of venous stasis pathology is not known. Postexercise pressure is an extreme measurement reached at the end of forced calf muscle exercise. Most normal adults in the course of normal activities probably attain a mean pressure much higher than the nadir seen in the ambulatory venous pressure tests. Such data are not available for obvious reasons. Calf muscle dysfunction can contribute to ambulatory hypertension in the absence of other abnormalities already discussed. Patients with venous stasis ulceration often exhibit poor calf muscle function as measured by plethysmography (7).

VALSALVA VENOUS PRESSURE

There is a measurable increase in foot venous pressure in the recumbent patient with exertion of the Valsalva effort. In adult, healthy individuals without reflux, Valsalva foot venous pressure elevation is less than 4 mmHg (5). When valve reflux is present, much higher pressures are recorded (Table 12.2). The test is highly reproducible.

After successful valve reconstruction this parameter normalizes or significantly decreases, correlating well with clinical improvement. In comparing this test of reflux with ambulatory venous pressure measurement, it was noted that approximately 20–25% of patients with stasis ulceration have postexercise pressure values considered in the normal range (5). Similarly, approximately 15% of patients with stasis ulceration show "normal" Valsalva-induced foot venous pres-

TABLE 12-2

VALSALVA FOOT VENOUS PRESSURE ELEVATION IN NORMAL REFLUXIVE AND VALVE RECONSTRUCTED LIMBS

	Normal Limbs	Refluxive Limbs	Valve Reconstructed Limbs Surgical Success: Preoperative	Valve Reconstructed Limbs Surgical Success: Postoperative
Valsalva foot venous pressure mmHg (mean ± SD)	1.8 = 0.7	7.9 = 5.1	9.2 = 5.3	4.2 = 2.5
	n = 18	*n* = 63	*n* = 41	*n* = 41
	p <0.001		*p* <0.004	

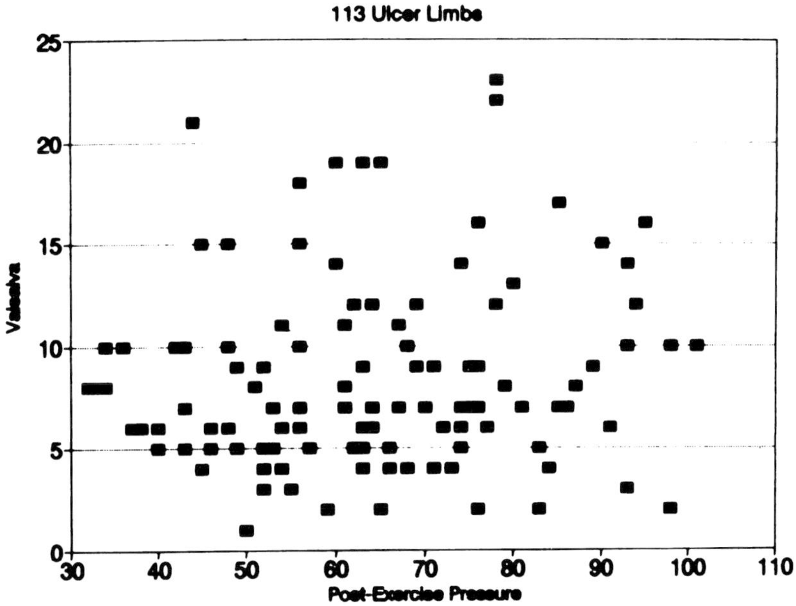

FIG. 12–7. Relationship between Valsalva-induced foot venous pressure elevation and ambulatory venous pressure in 113 ulcerated limbs. Twenty-five limbs have ambulatory pressures of 50 mmHg or less. Seventeen limbs are shown to have Valsalva-induced foot venous pressure elevation of 4 mmHg or less. (By permission of J Vasc Surg [5].)

sure elevation, i.e., less than 4 mmHg. It was also noted that when one value was normal, the other was invariably abnormal. In a series of 113 patients with stasis ulceration, 25 limbs had postexercise pressure of less than 50 mmHg, of which 23 had abnormal Valsalva foot venous pressures. In the same series, 17 limbs had normal Valsalva-induced foot venous pressure values, but 16 of these had abnormal postexercise pressures, i.e., greater than 50 mmHg. Approximately 60% of the group had abnormal values for both tests. Only 3 of 113 patients had *normal* values for both tests. The Valsalva foot venous pressure test may be used in documenting hemodynamic reflux in 20–25% of patients who develop a stasis ulcer without demonstrable ambulatory venous hypertension (Fig. 12.7).

REFERENCES

1. Raju S, Fredericks R, Lishman P, Neglén P, Morano J. Observations on the calf venous pump mechanism: determinants of postexercise pressure. J Vasc Surg 1993;17:459–469.
2. Attinger EO. Wall properties of veins. IEEE Trans Biomed Eng 1969;16:253–261.
3. Moreno AH, Katz AI, Gold LD, Reddy RV. Mechanics of distension of dog veins and other very thin-walled tubular structures. Circ Res 1970;27:1069–1080.
4. Almen T, Nylander G. Serial phlebography of the normal lower leg during muscular contraction and relaxation. Acta Radiol 1972;57:264.

5. Raju S, Fredericks R. Hemodynamic basis of stasis ulceration: a hypothesis. J Vasc Surg 1991;13:491–495.
6. Welkie JF, Comerota AJ, Katz ML, Aldridge SC, Kerr RP, White JV. Hemodynamic deterioration in chronic venous disease. J Vasc Surg 1992;16:733–740.
7. Araki CT, Back TL, Padberg FT, et al. The significance of calf muscle pump function in venous ulceration. J Vasc Surg 1994;20:872–879.

chapter 13

Rational Approach to Diagnosis of Venous Insufficiency

Peter Neglén and Clarence M. Jabs

Acute venous insufficiency is caused by sudden obstruction of the venous outflow, usually by an acute venous thrombosis or, very rarely, by extrinsic compression. Chronic venous insufficiency is a far more complex disorder. It involves to varying extent the large veins with pathologic changes of wall, lumen, and valves, in addition to the microcirculation of the subcutaneous tissue and skin.

Venous function is dependent on several factors including outflow obstruction, reflux, calf muscle pump function, venous volume, and vein wall compliance and geometry. To direct treatment, it is not only important to measure the global venous hemodynamic impact of a venous disease, but also to apply investigative methods to identify anatomic sites of dysfunction and to discriminate between pathophysiologic factors.

A test should be identified as whether it measures anatomic or functional aspects of venous insufficiency. Each test should be assessed for sensitivity, specificity, positive and negative predictive values, and accuracy. These calculations may be hampered by the difficulty of finding tests for reference. Many tests, e.g., ambulatory dorsal vein pressure measurements and descending phlebography, which have for decades been considered "gold standards," are now being challenged for that position.

The various available methods of investigation are described here with their advantages and disadvantages.

DORSAL FOOT VEIN PRESSURE

The only way to ascertain venous pressure is to measure it directly. Usually a vein of the dorsum of the foot is cannulated, but the pressure can be measured at any site that lends itself to cannulation or catheterization.

Ambulatory Venous Pressure

In the 1940s Pollack and Wood observed a decrease in venous pressure in the foot during walking and a gradual recovery when walking stopped (1). This led to the development of the ambulatory venous pressure (AVP) measurement. Together with phlebography, it became widely used to describe venous function.

To measure venous pressure at the foot level, a scalp needle can be introduced at the foot level and the pressure measured at rest and after exercise or compression of the calf muscles. From the resulting curve, the percent drop of pressure and the venous filling time can be calculated (Fig. 13.1).

The result of the ambulatory venous pressure measurement is difficult to interpret. It has been shown that a lesser drop of dorsal vein pressure on exercise is directly correlated to a higher frequency of venous ulcer (2). However, severe chronic venous insufficiency with venous ulcer may occur with normal AVP values. In approximately 20% of patients with venous ulceration, the AVP is less than 50 mmHg (2, 3).

Fundamental to the result of the AVP drop is the function of the calf muscle pump. This pump is dependent on normal calf mechanics, i.e., ankle movement, muscle mass, venous volume, degree of reflux or obstruction of the outflow venous channels (i.e., saphenous, popliteal, femoral, and iliac veins), competency of

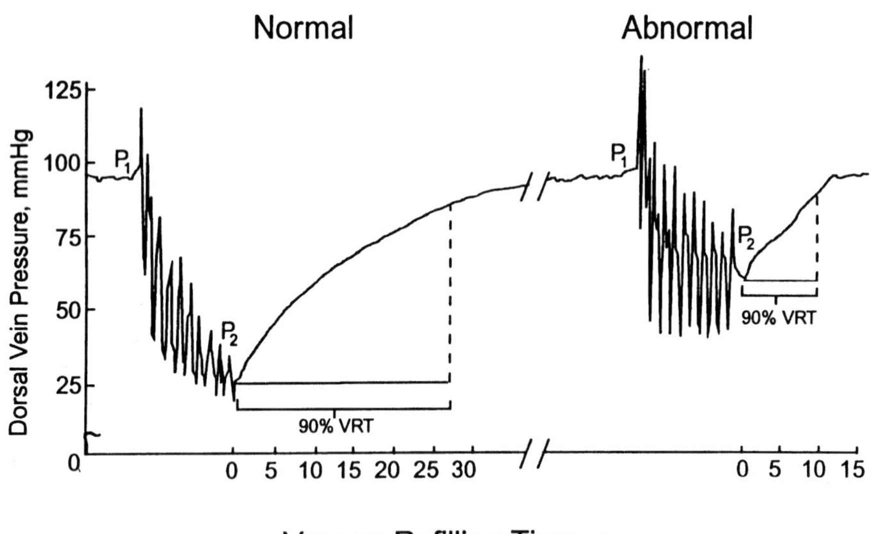

FIG. 13–1. Foot vein pressure curve obtained in a normal limb and a limb with prominent venous reflux. The pressure was recorded at rest and during 10 tiptoe movements until it returned to baseline level. The percent drop of pressure ($P_1 - P_2/P_1 \times 100$, %) is markedly less in the abnormal limb and the venous refilling time (VRT, seconds) is shorter.

the perforators connecting the deep and superficial leg compartments, and vein wall compliance and geometry. The result of AVP measurement reflects the global venous hemodynamic situation taking all these factors into account.

Improvement of refilling time using a tourniquet was assumed to indicate isolated long saphenous or short saphenous vein incompetence (4). However, tourniquets have been shown to give inconsistent compression of superficial veins and also to affect reflux in the deep veins. It has been shown that the pressure to occlude a competent long saphenous vein is extremely variable (40–300 mmHg) (5). Therefore, AVP measurement cannot consistently separate deep from superficial valve dysfunction.

The invasiveness of the technique used to obtain the pressure is the main disadvantage. Noninvasive techniques were developed later and quickly replaced the AVP. However, many still consider the AVP test the "gold standard" of venous function tests and maintain that all noninvasive tests should be compared to it.

Arm-Foot Venous Pressure Differential and Reactive Hyperemia Foot Vein Pressure Elevation

Raju has described a method using vein pressure measurements to assess the degree of hemodynamically significant obstruction (6). With the patient in the supine position, venous pressures in the dorsum of the foot and hand are simultaneously measured through venous transducers and recorded. In normal patients, the foot pressure is not more than 4 mmHg above the arm pressure.

Through the same venipuncture in the foot used for the arm-foot differential pressure measurement, foot pressure can be continuously recorded on a strip chart. The arterial inflow may be occluded by inflating a thigh cuff to 200–300 mmHg and maintaining the pressure for 3 minutes, followed by a sudden release of the thigh cuff. The resulting ischemia during cuff inflation leads to reactive hyperemia at release and increase of the venous pressure, which is monitored on the recorder. The difference between the maximal level reached and the resting value should not exceed 6 mmHg in normal limbs.

The two tests are performed and evaluated in conjunction with each other. A grading system has been constructed based on the degree of hemodynamic compensation by development of collateral flow in chronic venous obstruction. Limbs with phlebographic evidence of obstruction, a difference of arm and foot pressure $\leq$4 mmHg at rest, and an increment of less than 6 mmHg during reactive hyperemia are considered to be fully compensated (grade 1). Using these pressure measurements limbs with obstruction have been classified in four grades (Table 13.1).

The accuracy of this classification is difficult to validate since no "gold standard" exists. However, logic correlation to findings of obstruction and degree of collateralization on ascending and transfemoral phlebography has been described (6–8). Resistance to venous outflow has been determined by simultaneous volume-pressure measurement of the calf and found to relate to the grading of obstruction according to Raju (9, 10).

TABLE 13-1

GRADING OF OBSTRUCTION IN PATIENTS WITH CHRONIC VENOUS INSUFFICIENCY FOLLOWING PREVIOUS DEEP VEIN THROMBOSIS*

		Arm/Foot Venous Pressure Differential (Normal <4 mmHg)	Reactive Hyperemia Foot Venous Pressure Elevation (Normal <6 mmHg)
Grade 1	Fully compensated	≤4 mmHg	≤6 mmHg
Grade 2	Partially compensated	≤4 mmHg	>6 mmHg
Grade 3	Partially decompensated	>4 mmHg	>6 mmHg
Grade 4	Fully decompensated	>4 mmHg	≤6 mmHg

*Based on Raju S. New approaches to the diagnosis and treatment of venous obstruction. J Vasc Surg 1986;14:42–54.

PHOTOPLETHYSMOGRAPHY

Photoplethysmography (PPG) and light reflection rheography measure the reflection of infrared light by red blood cells in dermal capillaries. The detector is usually placed above the medial malleolus. Following dorsal or plantar flexion of the foot, blood content in the skin is pumped out and light reflection decreased. When the exercise ends, the blood is replaced. The recorded curve is very similar in shape to the one obtained by ambulatory venous pressure measurement (Fig. 13.2). However, the PPG signal cannot be adequately calibrated and the only part of the curve that can be used for quantification is the postexercise refilling time (normal value <15–20 seconds).

After its introduction, PPG rapidly replaced ambulatory vein pressure measurements, mainly because it was a simple noninvasive and inexpensive method. A significant linear correlation of venous refilling time between PPG results and direct pressure measurements has been found ($r = 0.86–0.90$) (11–13).

Photoplethysmography was early claimed and widely accepted to diagnose long and short saphenous vein incompetence. The reflux was thought to be limited to the superficial veins when the refilling time was normalized by a tourniquet applied above the ankle or on the thigh. This assumption has been shown to be wrong. There is a great variability in the cuff pressure necessary to occlude the superficial system (5). When using standard tourniquet occlusion of the superficial system, the correlation between PPG results and direct pressure measurement has been shown to be poor (14). Recently, refilling times as measured by PPG and reflux detected by segmental duplex scanning were compared in 151 symptomatic legs (15). No agreement was found between refilling time as measured by PPG and the presence of main stem superficial incompetence as evaluated by placement of tourniquets. PPG recordings of different areas of the same leg have also been shown to give different results (14). It appears that PPG refilling time in some situations may reflect the local hemodynamics and the status of dermal vein valves rather than the venous circulation of the whole leg.

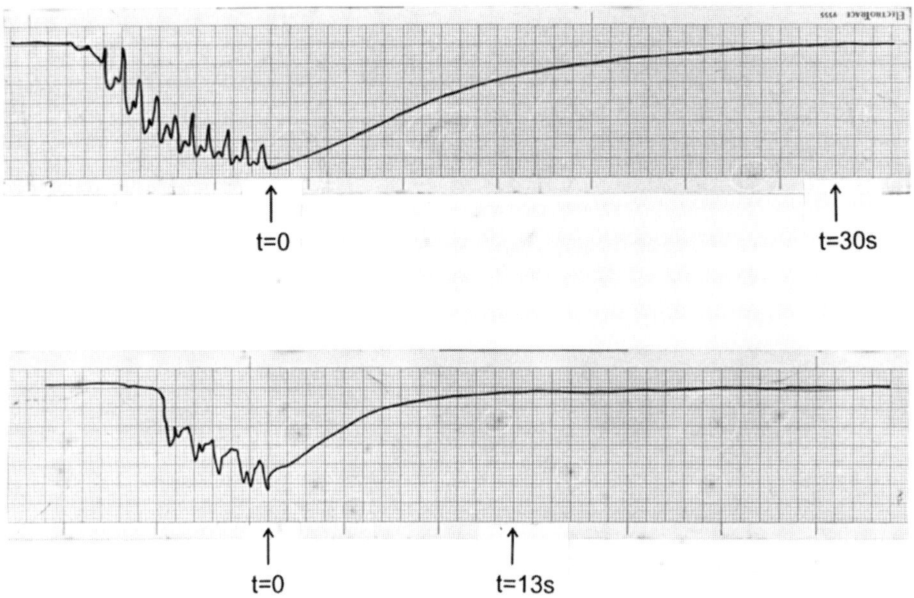

FIG. 13–2. Photoplethysmographic recording (PPG) during several dorsiflexions of the foot and the recovery phase in a normal lower limb (*top*) and a limb with reflux (*bottom*). Since the volume calibration of the PPG is inadequate, the magnitude of drop is not reliable. However, the time lapse of return to the original level accurately reflects the venous refilling time. The normal value is >20 seconds.

Therefore, the tourniquets, together with any kind of plethysmographic method, are not useful in identifying anatomic sites of venous incompetence.

PLETHYSMOGRAPHY

Plethysmography was among the earliest methods applied to the measurement of blood flow in the lower extremities and has provided much information regarding the venous circulation. The Greek origin of the word is *plethysmos* (increase) and *graphein* (to write). Regardless of which technique is used (air, water, impedance, or strain-gauge plethysmography), they all measure changes of volume of a certain portion of the body.

Strain-Gauge Plethysmography

The development of electronics in the 1940s made the development of the mercury-in-silastic strain-gauge possible. The resistance of the mercury-filled tube is directly proportional to its length. Thus, as the calf expands, when the outflow is obstructed, the tube wrapped around a leg is stretched and the resistance increased. Since the length-resistance relationship is known by electrical calibration, the volume of the slice of the calf under the strain-gauge loop can be measured.

Strain-gauge plethysmography has been mainly used in the vascular laboratory to assess venous outflow obstruction in chronic or acute venous disease. Despite refinement of the calculations for calf volume expansion and maximal venous outflow during venous occlusion plethysmography (16, 17), this test, like all plethysmographic tests, mainly reveals obstruction of the axial outflow veins. Often such major involvement is already obvious from the clinical condition (18). Moderate and mild obstruction is not consistently detected by this method. The accuracy in detecting deep vein thrombosis in the calf veins was only approximately 50%.

The strain-gauge can also be used to evaluate reflux by calculating the venous refilling time after erect exercise in a similar way as with photoplethysmography, foot vein pressure, and foot volumetry. The value of this test is discussed below.

Impedance Plethysmography and Phleborrheography

Blood is a good conductor of electricity. Impedance plethysmography (IPG) measures a change of blood volume in a part of the body. A decrease of tissue electrical resistance to passage of an electric current indicates blood volume expansion (19). When the electrodes are placed on the leg, calf volume changes can be measured during and after proximal venous occlusion by cuff inflation. The retainment of blood displaced from the calf within 3 seconds after release of thigh compression determines proximal venous occlusion.

Phleborrheography (PRG) is a whole-leg plethysmography using multiple air filled cuffs to detect volume changes in different segments of the leg with distal compression (20). The loss of propagating volume wave detects proximal occlusion. Both methods have been shown to detect acute large proximal axial vein thrombosis with high accuracy. As is the case for strain-gauge plethysmography, the sensitivity and specificity to detect calf vein thrombosis are low. Neither of the tests has been shown to have a place in the determination of outflow obstruction in chronic venous insufficiency. In more than half the patients, the tests normalize 3–6 weeks following acute thrombosis.

Air Plethysmography

Air plethysmography (APG) was used by Allan (21) in the 1960s to study volume changes of the calf in response to posture and exercise and Cranley developed the phleborrheograph in the 1970s. In 1987, Christopoulos, et al. (22), described a new air plethysmograph, consisting of a plastic air chamber that surrounded the leg from ankle to knee, which could be calibrated in milliliters, thus allowing the results to be obtained in absolute units.

Volume change measured by strain-gauge plethysmography represents only the segment under the strain-gauge loop and not necessarily the whole leg. With the new APG, with the lightweight plastic air bag, exercises such as toe stands or walking can be performed, increasing the possibilities of testing venous function. Tissue shifts of the leg due to the effect of gravity in different positions is theoretically less likely to affect the APG result compared to strain-gauge plethysmography because the air bag includes all tissue between knee and ankle.

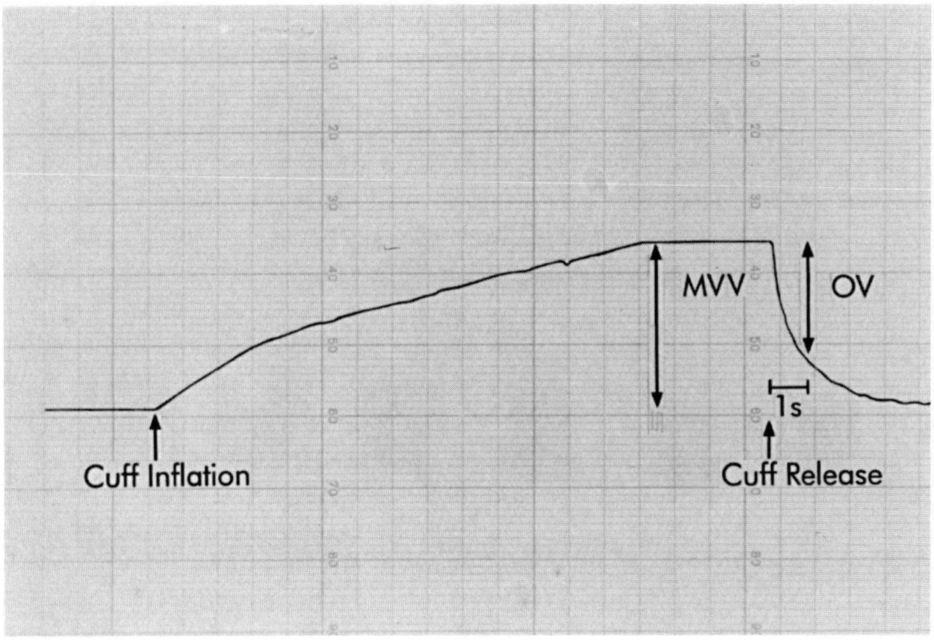

FIG. 13–3. Volume curve obtained using an air plethysmograph during venous occlusion induced by cuff inflation to 70 mmHg (*MVV* = maximal venous volume reached during occlusion, ml). On cuff release, the decrease in volume during the first second (*OV*, ml) can be measured and the outflow fraction (OF_1s) calculated ($OF_1s = OV/MVV \times 100$, %).

Reproducibility variance with air plethysmography is on the order of 10%, a result which could not be obtained by strain-gauge plethysmography (23).

Since the air bag allows the patient to stand up from the supine position and perform ankle movement, a number of potentially important qualities of venous function can be measured. When measuring outflow obstruction for detection of deep vein thrombosis, for example, the air bag is fitted with the patient in supine position and the lower limb raised 30°. A standard venous occlusion plethysmography can be performed by inflation of a thigh cuff to 70 mmHg, occluding venous outflow. Upon release of the cuff the decrease of volume can be measured during the initial 3 seconds and an outflow fraction calculated (Fig. 13.3). This test appears to have the same flaws in measuring outflow obstruction in acute, as well as chronic, obstruction, as other plethysmographic methods (24).

To assess reflux and calf pump function, the patient is asked to stand up from the supine position and the venous filling time can be measured. Since the volume change is obtained in absolute units, the actual reflux (venous filling index, VFI), measured as ml/sec, is possible to calculate. Christopoulos, et al. (25), found that a VFI below 2 ml/sec indicated absence of significant reflux and that the veins are filling slowly from the arterial circulation. With VFI above 3 ml/sec the incidence of severe clinical symptoms and ulcer was shown to rise. Above 7 ml/sec the incidence of ulcers is approximately 50% or more.

By asking the patient to do one tiptoe movement with the weight on both legs and then return to the original position, the ejected volume and the ejection fraction of one calf muscle contraction can be measured. Also, by asking the patient to do 10 tiptoe movements, the calf is emptied and the residual venous volume and residual volume fraction can be calculated. The residual volume fraction (RVF) has been stated to be "the most useful single noninvasive index of the overall efficacy of the calf muscle pump" (26, 27) and has been demonstrated to have a good linear correlation with AVP at the end of exercise (r = 0.83) and has been suggested to replace AVP (22). Several other investigators have not been able to produce this correlation (28–31).

The new air plethysmography is certainly a valuable research tool since it gives volume changes in absolute values, allows exercise, and in combination with simultaneous vein pressure measurements provides an opportunity to analyze the pressure/volume relationship of the calf. The value and validity of the different parameters must be further elucidated and interpretations should be made cautiously.

Foot Volumetry

This foot plethysmograph was introduced by Thulesius, et al., in 1973 (32). The foot volumeter measures alterations of foot volume by displacement of water in a temperature-controlled water bath during exercise and at rest. The resulting curve is closely related to venous pressure changes (33–35) and is an overall estimation of the calf muscle pump function. It can give quantitative values of expelled venous volume and refilling flow. Calf pump function measured this way has been shown to improve after varicose vein surgery (33) and the test seems to differentiate degrees of chronic venous insufficiency, but its accuracy has not been evaluated against modern reflux assessment with the duplex scanner.

CONTINUOUS-WAVE DOPPLER ULTRASOUND

The portable, hand held continuous-wave Doppler (CWD) device is a valuable clinical tool. The simple ultrasound probe can detect blood flow by a frequency change of a sound wave bouncing off the moving red blood cells, which is directly proportional to the speed of the cells. The 5-MHz probe is the most commonly used because of its practical frequency for adequate depth to study both the arterial and venous systems. It can be used for all veins in the limbs, as well as the iliac veins in the lower abdomen. The regular pulsatile blood flow of the arteries is relatively easier to analyze than the phasic flow of the venous system, which is heavily influenced by intrathoracic and abdominal pressures and skeletal muscle contraction.

The CWD has been used to assess patency and competency of the deep veins, long and short saphenous veins, and the connection of varicose veins with the saphenous system.

Patency Detection by Continuous-Wave Doppler

Patency of the deep veins is examined with the patient in supine position, the trunk of the body elevated 30° to fill the veins. To examine the popliteal vein it is sometimes necessary to turn the patient to the prone position. The veins are most easily localized by finding the accompanying artery, identifying the typical low pitched venous sound in phase with the breathing. Contrary to the arterial flow sound, the venous sound disappears when the breathing stops. This technique can be applied for the common femoral, superficial femoral, popliteal, and posterior tibial veins. Normally, the femoral vein blood flow in this position varies with the breathing, stops with a deep breath or Valsalva maneuver, and suddenly increases when the Valsalva is released (Fig. 13.4). Usually the vein blood flow is augmented through any segment by distal compression. In case of obstruction, no sound may be detected or a continuous background sound insensitive to respiratory changes may be heard from collateral flow.

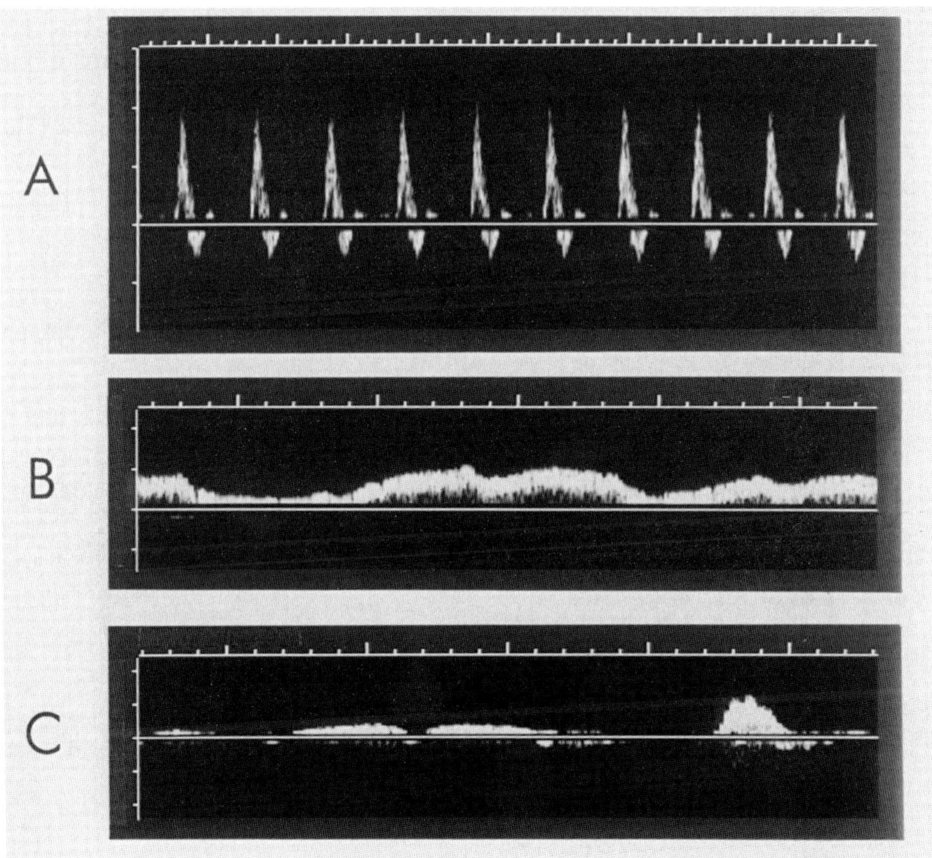

FIG. 13–4. Graphic representation of Doppler ultrasound flow of the femoral vessels. **A.** Arterial triphasic pulsatile flow; **(B)** venous flow phasic with breathing; and **(C)** venous flow increase after Valsalva maneuver, which temporarily halts the flow.

The accuracy of the CWD in detecting venous occlusion is 88% in the main axial veins above the knee, but in most hands the test is unreliable below the knee with false-positive rates of 20–50% (36, 38). The test often fails even in the axial veins if the thrombus is only partially occlusive. Additionally, CWD does not identify the cause of obstruction, which may not be intraluminal from deep vein thrombosis, but extraluminal compression from hematoma, enlarged lymph nodes, or other pathology.

Reflux Detection by Continuous-Wave Doppler

To test for reflux, the patient should be in a standing position so that when the venous reservoir is maximally filled, distal compression will give a sufficient forward pulse wave and reflux can be accentuated by full gravity. Absence of detectable retrograde flow after cough or Valsalva maneuver or sudden release of distal compression indicates competent veins under the CWD probe. In contrast, if a retrograde flow of more than 0.5 seconds duration is demonstrated, there is venous reflux (39, 44). Of greatest interest has been examination of the region of the junction between the long and short saphenous veins and common femoral and popliteal veins, respectively. The objective has been to delineate the presence of reflux per se and to attempt to localize it to the deep or superficial system. The abolishment of reflux after application of tourniquet compression has been used to indicate superficial reflux only.

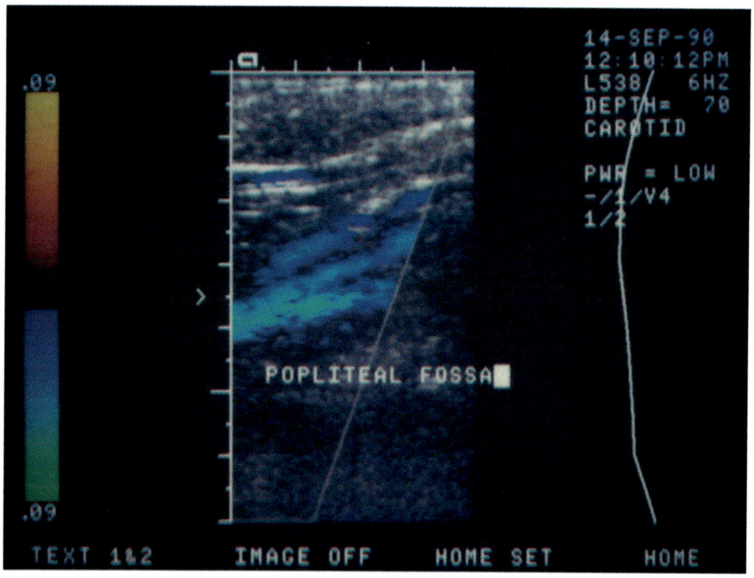

FIG. 13–5. Color duplex Doppler image of the popliteal fossa showing the short saphenous, two gastrocnemius, and the popliteal veins in same field (*top* to *bottom*). It is easy to understand that a continuous-wave Doppler ultrasound of the popliteal fossa can give a false-positive indication of popliteal vein incompetence.

However, the CWD method for detecting reflux has limitations. The use of tourniquets has been shown to introduce error in the discrimination of superficial and deep reflux (5, 15) as discussed earlier. It is important to realize that contrary to the pulsed-wave Doppler ultrasound, the continuous-wave Doppler detects all flow in any artery or vein within the path of the ultrasonic beam. Thus, when refluxive superficial veins overlie the deep veins, CWD can give false-positive indications of deep incompetence. In the groin, it cannot differentiate between reflux in the common femoral vein, long saphenous vein, or a tributary vein at the junction. In the popliteal fossa, an incompetent gastrocnemius, Giacomini, or short saphenous vein may mimic findings of deep reflux although the popliteal vein is competent (Fig. 13.5). Superficial varicosities above the saphenous veins may false-positively indicate stem insufficiency.

The use of CWD to detect perforator incompetence has been suggested (39, 40). With a tourniquet occluding the superficial system, blood can be squeezed through the perforator by proximal compression and reflux may be detected by listening to the flow over the perforator. This method has been shown to have poor accuracy (41). Obviously, it is flawed by the fact that one is uncertain whether all blood flow in the superficial compartment has been obstructed and the correct site of the perforator identified. With the introduction of duplex Doppler scanning this method has become obsolete.

DUPLEX SCANNING AND COLOR-FLOW IMAGING

Duplex Doppler ultrasound scanning is an investigation combining B-mode echographic imaging and pulsed-wave Doppler ultrasound (45). In contrast to the continuous-wave Doppler, which analyzes the frequency change of ultrasound as the sound wave is reflected by the red blood cells, the B-mode scan analyzes the amplitude of the reflected ultrasound and the time of transmittance through tissue, providing a measure of density. Depth is determined by echo arrival time, and brightness is determined by echo amplitude. The different tissue densities can be presented in grayscale and a picture provided. When a pulsed Doppler signal is used in conjunction with the B-mode image, the site of the sample velocity of flow can be accurately identified. Therefore, the limitation of the continuous-wave Doppler to define the precise site of insonation is set aside.

In the latest duplex Doppler machines, the Doppler signals may be depicted as colored pixels in the B-mode image. Different color can be given to different velocities and directions, often facilitating detection of turbulence and identification of arteries and veins.

Patency Detection by Duplex Doppler

The development of real-time B-mode scanning made it possible to image the deep venous system. The venous flow and valve cusp movement can be visualized and chronicity of thrombotic obstruction is suggested by clot echogenicity and vein wall changes (Fig. 13.6) (46, 47). The addition of pulse-wave

Doppler made it possible to combine the criteria of Doppler ultrasound and imaging, increasing the accuracy to the level of phlebography.

The patient is initially examined in the supine position with the trunk raised 30°, and with the hip slightly flexed and externally rotated. The common and superficial femoral veins can be examined in this position. The popliteal and proximal calf veins are best visualized in the prone position, while the peroneal and tibial veins are best shown when the patient is sitting on the edge of the couch with the leg resting on a stool.

One of the most discriminating signs of deep vein thrombosis in the axial vein is the inability to compress the vessel, since the lumen is partially or completely full of thrombus (48, 49). The compression is performed with the probe producing a cross-sectional image rather than longitudinal (Fig. 13.7). Other imaging criteria are lack of movement of red cell aggregates and valve cusps, and a direct visualization of the thrombus itself. The indirect criteria of continuous-wave Doppler as described earlier (augmentation by distal compression and absence of spontaneous phasic flow with respiration) are applicable for duplex scanning as well, in the longitudinal plane. The major difference is the knowledge from which

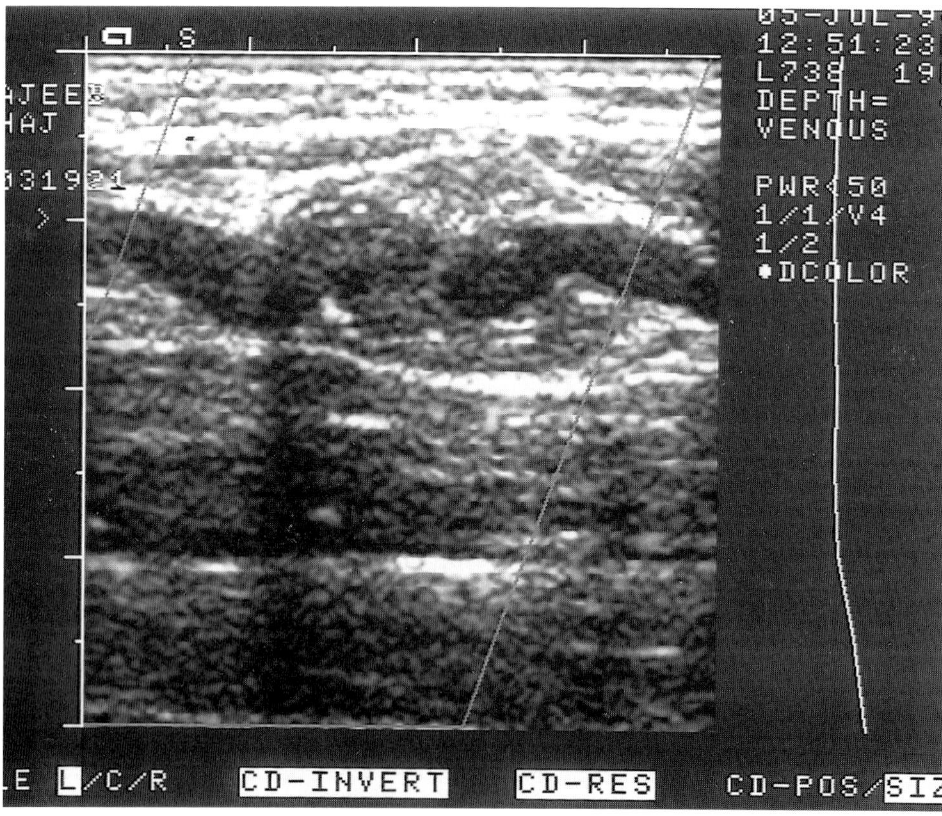

FIG. 13–6. A real-time B-mode scan image of a deep venous thrombosis of the femoral vein. The valve sinus is partially filled with thrombosis of higher echogenicity.

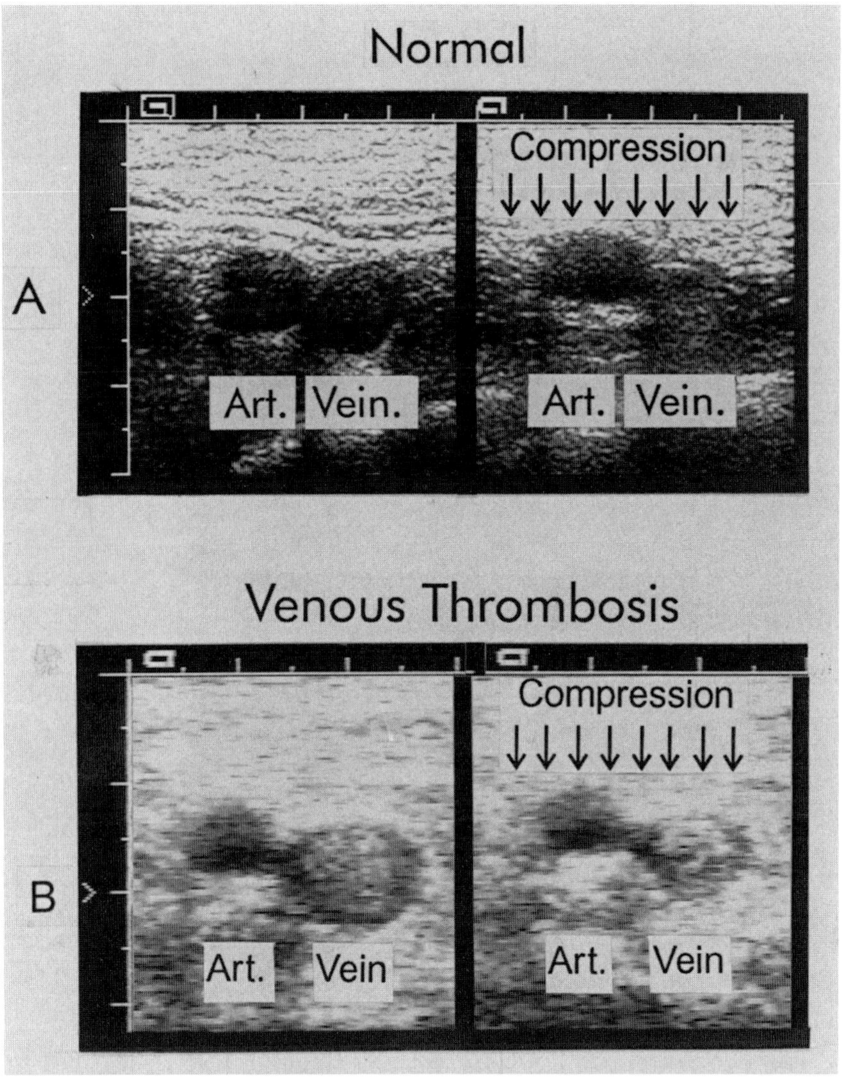

FIG. 13–7. Cross-sectional image of the femoral vessels with and without probe compression. **A.** Normal vessels with total collapse of the vein on compression. **B.** Inability to compress a vein full of thrombus. A higher echogenicity can be seen in the vein. The artery is largely unaffected by compression.

vessel the flow sound arises. It is recommended that several criteria be used to diagnose deep vein thrombosis to improve accuracy (50, 51).

Often it is not possible to directly image the iliac vein segment and indirect assessment with audible Doppler examination of the common femoral vein must be performed (52). When it is necessary to delineate the top of an iliofemoral thrombus with duplex scanning, the results are disappointing because a fresh thrombus can have the same acoustic appearance as flowing blood, and inaccurate indirect Doppler methods may be required (53).

Color-flow imaging and development of "slow flow" mode allowing detection of flow velocities as low as 0.3 cm/sec have facilitated diagnosis of thrombus, especially in the calf veins (54, 55). Spontaneous venous flow can be easily seen in the femoropopliteal segment. Augmentation by compression of the foot or distal calf is usually necessary to view the tibioperoneal veins (56). Using color-flow greatly facilitates the identification of these veins, distinguishing artery from vein, and reduces the need to use the audible Doppler.

Diagnosis of recurrent clot in patients with a previous history of deep vein thrombosis may be difficult. Many of the duplex scan criteria for acute and chronic venous abnormalities are similar (57). The role of duplex scanning to detect chronic venous obstruction is still evolving. Duplex ultrasonogram, like ascending phlebography, can only give the anatomic localization of obstructed vein segments, but does not provide information about their hemodynamic significance.

Diagnosis of Reflux by Duplex Doppler

When the veins of the lower limbs are being evaluated for reflux, the patient is standing with the weight on the nonexamined leg, preferably holding on to a support to avoid instability and contraction of the leg muscles. The saphenofemoral junction and the leg veins are examined with the patient facing the investigator, and the popliteal region with the patient facing away. By compression of the limb distal to the placement of the probe, the blood is forced antegrade and on sudden release a retrograde flow can be graphically and audibly shown if the valves below the position of the probe are incompetent (Fig. 13.8). If no retrograde flow occurs, the valve is competent. If color-flow imaging is available, sampling of flow using the pulsed Doppler is unnecessary. Commonly, flow toward the heart is usually depicted in blue and away from the heart in red. On release of the compression, the color-flow will change from blue to red if reflux is present (Fig. 13.9). This examination can be performed on a number of segments within the superficial and deep venous systems, providing a map of the venous system of the lower limb (Fig. 13.10).

There are controversies regarding the optimal technique to induce reflux using the duplex instrument. The best position of the patient for examination is contested. The standing position has been feared to be less sensitive to test valve incompetence. The supine position, in contrast, is not considered physiologic by some, since gravity is a major contributor to venous pressure. Although arguments have been raised for the supine position (58), most investigators favor examining the patient standing; the results correlate well with clinical severity (59).

Imaging of the popliteal and femoral valves with the patient in the supine position and in erect position with no weight-bearing shows that the valves are open or seem to float or flutter in a semiopen position (60, 61). The valve movement is passive and the valve does not close on cessation of flow, but requires a retrograde flow. It is doubtful if proximal or distal manual compression, especially in the upper part of the limb, consistently produces sufficient retrograde flow velocity to close the valve (more than 30–35 cm/sec) in a supine subject (62, 63). On the other hand, a standardized Valsalva maneuver can produce adequate retrograde flow, but usually only in the iliofemoral segment. Distally, in the superfi-

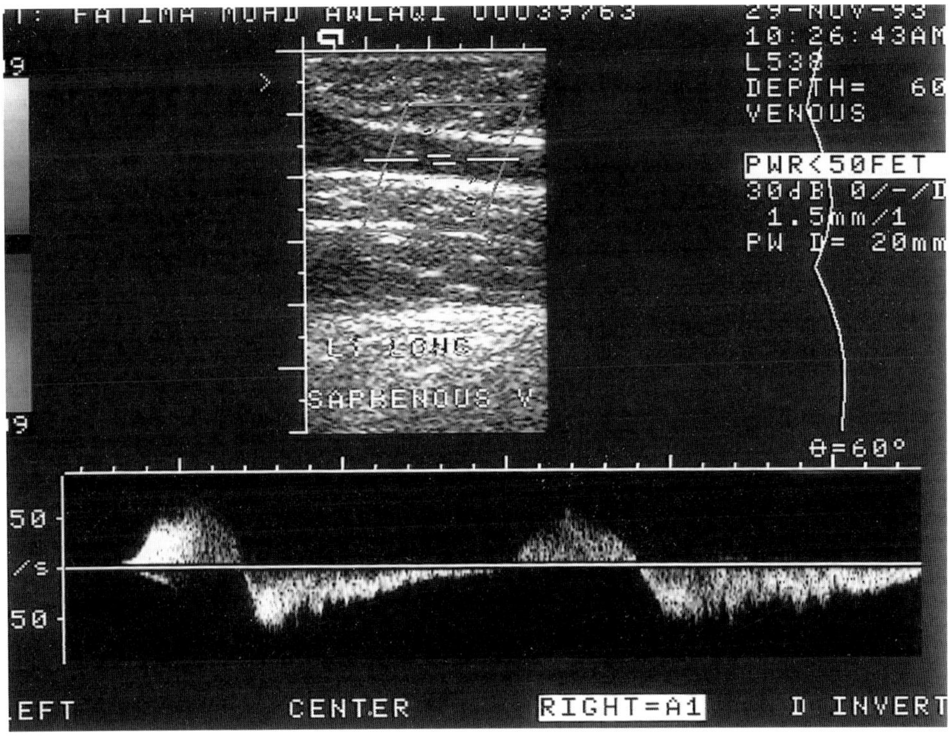

FIG. 13–8. Duplex Doppler image of long saphenous vein incompetence. The velocity obtained by the pulsed Doppler is graphically shown in the *bottom* part. On distal compression, the flow is forced antegrade (*above white line*) and on sudden release of compression reflux is indicated by retrograde flow (*below white line*).

cial femoral and popliteal veins, the maneuver often does not increase the velocity enough to close the valve. This is especially inhibited by proximal competency. Therefore, there is an argument for standardization of the induced compression (64, 65). It is necessary to use an automatic cuff inflator. This makes it possible to inflate and deflate the cuffs rapidly (in less than 0.3 second). The cuffs are placed on the thigh (inflation pressure 80 mmHg; width 24 cm), calf (100 mmHg; 12 cm), and foot (120 mmHg; 7 cm). Reflux is considered significant if the duration of retrograde flow is more than 0.5 second (65). Other measurements (66) are possible through the software of the duplex scanner, e.g., peak flow velocity and diameter. Since the vein is considered to be circular when distended, the cross-section area can be calculated. Thus, the volume flow in ml/sec can be obtained. The importance of these measurements to describe reflux needs to be further assessed.

PHLEBOGRAPHY

Phlebography is an investigation visualizing the venous system by injecting contrast medium into the veins. It is an invasive study with certain risks of causing pain, thrombosis, or necrosis following extravasation (66–68). With the

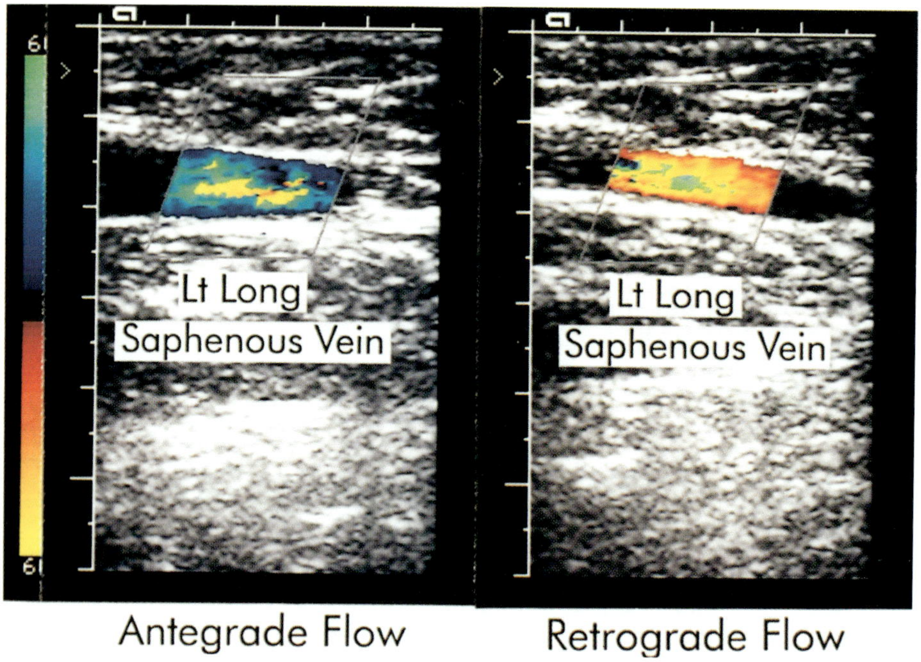

FIG. 13–9. Color-flow imaging of long saphenous vein incompetence. Antegrade flow during compression is depicted as blue, and retrograde flow at the release of compression due to reflux is shown as yellow-red. Sampling of pulsed Doppler flow is not necessary to detect reflux, which shortens the time of investigation.

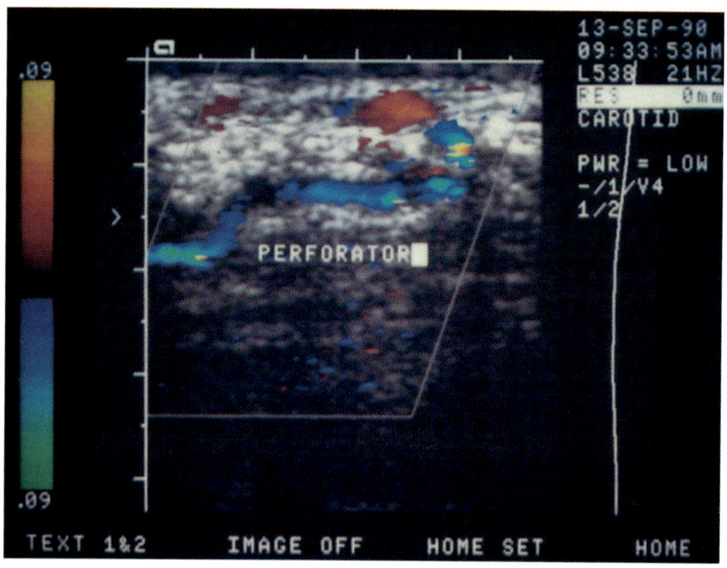

FIG. 13–10. Color-flow image of a perforator. Color duplex scanning is probably the best method to delineate incompetent perforators, but the investigation is very time-consuming if the whole limb is to be meticulously scanned.

introduction of low osmolar contrast media, these complications have considerably decreased (69, 70).

Ascending Phlebography

Ascending phlebography is an investigation in which contrast medium is injected into a foot vein and followed proximally. The technique is described in detail elsewhere (71). It is important to use a tourniquet at the ankle during injection to force contrast into the deep veins and avoid early filling of the superficial system, which will give confusing images, mixing the deep and superficial systems at the same time. The upper limit of any obstruction should always be displayed. If the contrast filling is inadequate to evaluate the patency of the common femoral and iliac veins and the inferior vena cava, a transfemoral injection should be performed for adequate visualization of these veins.

Ascending phlebography is used to test patency of the veins, i.e., identify and localize any obstruction present (Fig. 13.11). It is the time-honored method for diagnosing acute deep vein thrombosis, although it has recently been replaced in most centers by duplex Doppler ultrasound scanning. The accuracy is approximately 95%, approaching 100% for large thrombi in the major veins (71). It is considered important to attempt to outline the thrombus itself rather than rely on nonfilling of veins. Misinterpretation due to poor technique can occur with ascending phlebography: the profunda and internal iliac veins are rarely visualized, the iliac system is often not opacified adequately, and it is common not to be able to visualize all deep veins of the calf.

In patients with chronic venous insufficiency of the lower limb, vein segments may be totally occluded or have a narrowed irregular lumen with thickened vein wall. Valves may have been deformed or destroyed in the recanalization process. It is important to understand that the presence of occluded veins on phlebography is a morphologic finding and does not necessarily mean that there is a functional obstacle to the total outflow from the leg. Collaterals may compensate adequately for the obstruction. Neither anatomic site nor extent of obstruction by phlebography has been shown to determine hemodynamic severity (72).

Descending Phlebography

Descending phlebography is performed by injecting a bolus of contrast medium through a cannula or catheter introduced by puncturing the common femoral vein at the groin level. With the patient in a 60° erect tilt and performing a Valsalva maneuver simultaneously with the injection, reflux will be indicated by contrast flowing distally (Fig. 13.12).

With regard to descending venography, two main technical details have been debated: type of breathing and proper positioning of the patient. In some aspects, these issues also apply to the technique of reflux detection by duplex Doppler scanning. The importance of the Valsalva maneuver has been stressed in several studies (73–75). Since it is important to create a sufficiently high retrograde flow velocity to close the valve (63), a standardized Valsalva maneuver is executed by

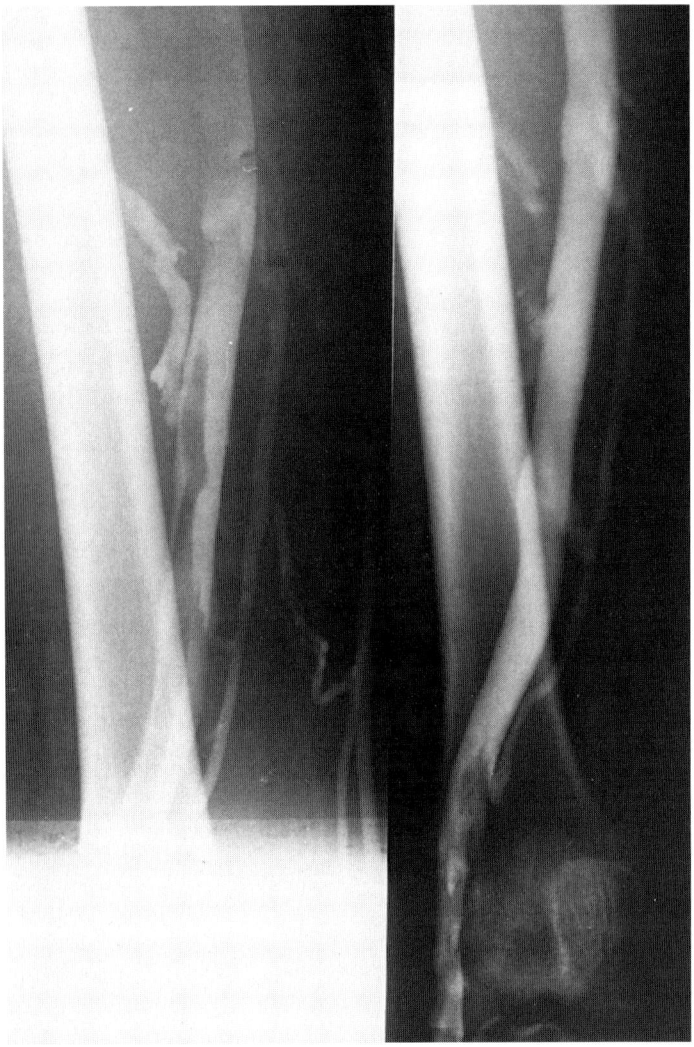

FIG. 13–11. Detail of an ascending phlebogram revealing a "floating tail" of a deep vein thrombus in the lower thigh (*left*). Subsequently, the patient had a verified pulmonary embolism and a repeat phlebogram (*right*) showed disappearance of the "floating tail."

having the patient blow into a manometer and generate a pressure of 30–40 mmHg. More controversial is the position of the patient, i.e., supine or semierect. Some investigators favor the supine position because it may minimize overdiagnosis from trickling down of contrast medium, which has a higher specific gravity than blood (74, 76). By contrast, others fear an underdiagnosis of reflux unless a semierect (60°) position is used (75) and believe the semiupright position more adequately represents the clinical situation and is pathophysiologically more correct (73). False-negatives appear to be less with the semierect technique (75) using duplex Doppler as the reference standard.

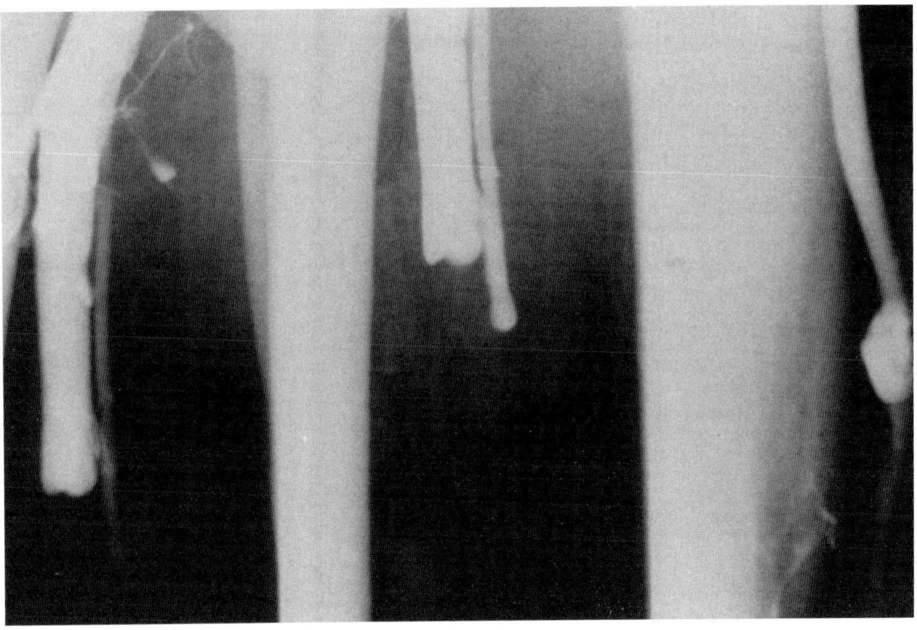

A

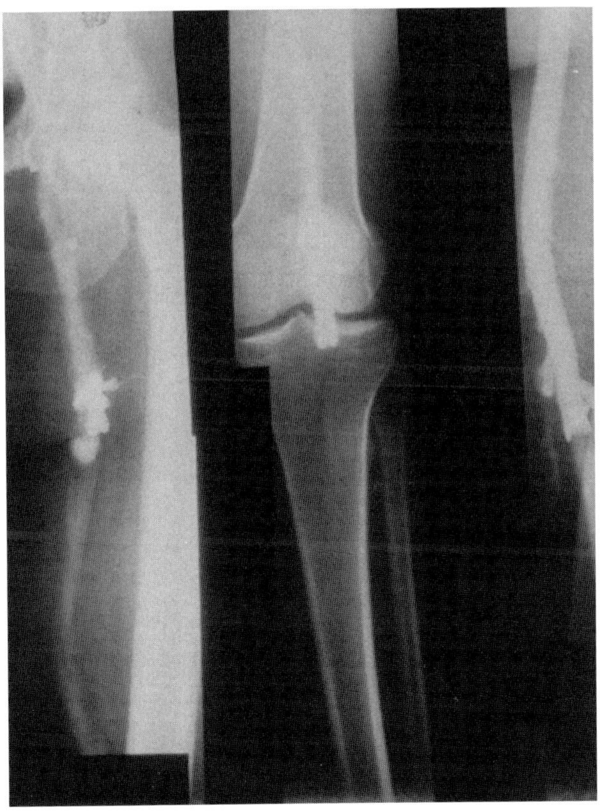

B

FIG. 13–12. Descending phlebography showing varying degrees of axial deep incompetence according to Kistner's classification (107, 108): (**A**) reflux to upper thigh (grade 1); (**B**) reflux to the popliteal level (grade 2); and (**C**) reflux into the upper calf (grade 3).

C

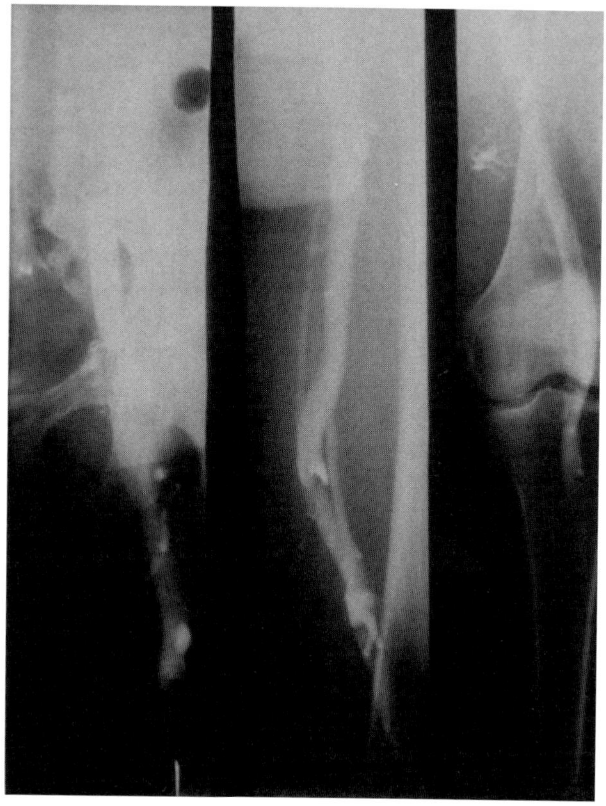

FIG. 13–12. Continued

TESTS MEASURING OBSTRUCTION

Acute Venous Obstruction

The most common cause of acute venous obstruction is deep vein thrombosis. Symptoms and signs of deep venous thrombosis are highly variable from asymptomatic to severely symptomatic. Other pathology, e.g., myositis, Baker's cyst rupture, tendonitis, etc., may produce similar symptoms and signs. Therefore, attempts have been made to identify a noninvasive test with high sensitivity for screening purposes.

Strain-gauge and impedance occlusion plethysmography and phleborrhaphy are poorly reliable for detecting thrombosis of small peripheral calf veins, deep femoral, and internal iliac veins, and, for that matter, any nonocclusive, nonobstructing thrombus. Several studies comparing these tests to ascending phlebography have shown a high specificity (90–93%) to detect femoral or iliac vein occlusion, but the accuracy to detect calf vein thrombosis is 50% or less (77–81). Taking into account all types of acute venous thrombosis, including calf vein thromboses (which are the majority), these tests are only approximately 60% accurate and the negative predictive value is only 60–70%. The value of these tests for surveillance is debatable (82). A more detailed discussion of this issue appears elsewhere in this book.

Duplex Doppler scanning and impedance plethysmography were compared to ascending phlebography in 25 patients with femoropopliteal thrombosis (83). Both noninvasive methods had high sensitivity (90–100%), but specificity was 100% for scanning while only 63% for the plethysmography. Thus, duplex scanning for detection of above knee thrombus was accurate in 97% and the impedance plethysmography in only 72%. Venous duplex imaging has been shown to be significantly more sensitive than rheophlebography for detecting both above and below knee thrombi and has a better negative predictive value (84). Duplex scanning is superior to the traditional plethysmographic methods and lacks some of their diagnostic limitations. It has largely replaced other noninvasive screening techniques.

Ascending phlebography is the time-honored diagnostic standard to detect deep vein thrombosis in symptomatic patients. Its role as such is now challenged by color-flow imaging. Comparison of these two investigative tools in several studies has proven color-flow imaging in symptomatic patients to have a sensitivity of 90–100% and specificity of 93–98% to detect thrombus in the iliofemoropopliteal vein segment, with lower values for veins of the leg (73–94% and 75–93%, respectively) (85–87). Color duplex flow scanning may have difficulty visualizing the calf veins in up to 40% of symptomatic limbs mainly because of prominent calf swelling, obscuration by multiple collateral veins, obesity, or any other situation that will give poor sound penetration. It is especially difficult to detect short, nonocclusive thrombi. The accuracy is as high as 98% if the examination is technically adequate, but otherwise falls to 57% (87). The examination is strongly investigator-dependent and adequate accuracy can be obtained only by skilled personnel. Under optimal circumstances, color Doppler scanning can be used as the primary test in patients with symptoms suggestive of deep venous thrombosis. However, ascending phlebography should still be used when there is no sonographic clot above the knee and the calf veins cannot be adequately visualized. In patients with a previous history of deep venous thrombosis, it might be difficult to assess whether the thrombosis is new or old with ultrasound scan; phlebography may be somewhat better (57, 87).

In patients with suspected deep venous thrombosis, there may be causes other than venous obstruction. Ultrasound scanning may be beneficial in revealing extravascular masses. As ultrasound has become more extensively used for screening intramuscular hematomas, Baker's cysts and other cystic structures, intramuscular lipomas, aneurysms, and neoplasms have been shown to cause compression of the deep veins to mimic the symptoms and signs of deep venous thrombosis (88, 89).

When color-flow scanning is used for surveillance, the sensitivity in detection of below knee thrombi decreases to 56–78%; however, the negative predictive value is still 94–96% (84, 85, 87). In the asymptomatic patient being screened to rule out deep vein thrombosis, or when pulmonary embolism is suspected, it is important to detect small thrombi. In this situation, phlebography is currently superior to color-flow imaging.

Chronic Venous Obstruction

A reliable quantitative measurement of outflow obstruction in chronic venous insufficiency is needed for research purposes and to evaluate methods of treatment. When significant venous obstruction is suspected in limbs with chronic venous insufficiency, ascending phlebography and duplex Doppler scanning will delineate only anatomic sites of obstruction and cannot be used to evaluate the hemodynamic significance. Attempts to compare pressure measurement with site and extent of obstruction have failed to find any reliable correlation with morphologic changes revealed by ascending phlebography (72).

Nicolaides and Sumner (90) found that plethysmographic outflow fraction at 1 second could discriminate between limbs with arm/foot pressure difference below or above 5 mmHg. In contrast, others have found poor accuracy of maximal venous outflow and outflow fraction to detect postthrombotic obstructions (10, 91, 92). Outflow plethysmography was unable to discriminate between patients with and without symptomatic venous claudication (92). Comparison of assessment by plethysmographic outflow fraction and Raju's test of arm-foot venous pressure differential (combined with the reactive hyperemia test), and calculation of resistance by simultaneous pressure/volume measurement during plethysmographic outflow (10) suggested that the pressure measurements using Raju's classification (6, 7) were the most adequate. It appears that plethysmographic methods using cuffs for occlusion are flawed. Varicose superficial collaterals commonly seen in postthrombotic limbs may have great capacitance. Sudden release of the thigh cuff that emptied them could result in a high mean volume outflow initially or larger 1 second outflow fraction obscuring any deep vein obstruction (93).

It is difficult to compare tests for obstruction since no reliable reference method exists. Lacking an accepted "gold standard," it seems that the combination of arm-foot venous pressure differential and foot venous pressure elevation after reactive hyperemia (Raju's test) is the most reliable test currently available for detecting and grading the global hemodynamic impact of chronic venous obstruction. If bypass surgery is planned, an ascending phlebography is necessary to delineate the anatomic distribution of narrowed and occluded segments.

TESTS MEASURING REFLUX

Postthrombotic chronic venous insufficiency is most often due to combined valve reflux and obstruction. Methods to test reflux may be performed for different purposes: (a) for screening; (b) for quantitation of reflux; and (c) for localization of anatomic site of reflux if present.

Continuous-Wave Doppler Examination

A screening test for identifying the presence of reflux should be noninvasive and fairly simple. The handheld, continuous-wave Doppler examination has been found to be a reliable screening tool with excellent sensitivity (>90%) but poor specificity (around 70%) (94). It will reveal any reflux, but is unable to identify the exact site and accurately quantify the reflux.

Venous Refilling Time

There is a good correlation between the venous refilling time measured by invasive pressure in the dorsal foot vein and by noninvasive photoplethysmography or strain-gauge plethysmography after calf exercise (11–13). The venous refilling time determination per se has been shown to be directly related to the number of refluxing venous segments. However, a similar relation exists between the number of incompetent vein segments identified by duplex Doppler and increasing severity of clinical signs of swelling, pigmentation, and ulceration (14, 15, 31, 95). On one hand, the use of refilling time may not add any more information in evaluation of the severity of venous disease than clinical examination; on the other, a normal PPG result will exclude major venous reflux in limbs of patients with ambiguous symptoms and signs (sensitivity 90%). The inaccuracy in using tourniquets with plethysmographic methods to determine involvement of superficial or deep system was addressed earlier. Since refilling time is related to involved venous segments, it is still valuable to evaluate the result of surgical correction of reflux (96, 97). A shorter refilling time, although not normalized, probably indicates less reflux after surgical correction, e.g., after removal of the long saphenous vein.

Venous Filling Index

Venous reflux measured as venous filling index by air plethysmography was shown to correlate directly to the ulcer frequency (25). Several other reports have not been able to duplicate this initial report by Christopoulos, et al., which showed excellent differentiation between different clinical severity stages (15, 28, 98–100). Although venous filling index has shown a significant correlation to the number of involved segments ($r = 0.96$) and phlebographic reflux, the ability to distinguish between patients with swollen pigmented leg and those with ulcerated limbs was poor. A possible explanation is that the clinical deterioration is not caused by increase of venous hypertension but by ongoing changes of the microcirculation of the skin. However, similar to venous refilling time by photoplethysmography, venous filling index is valuable to exclude significant venous incompetence, but cannot be used to locate the site of reflux. It has been shown to be a valuable test to assess the result of surgical correction of venous reflux (101).

Duplex Doppler and Color-Flow Imaging

Using the software in the duplex Doppler scanner, several parameters, such as reflux duration, peak flow velocity, vessel cross area, and volume flow, can be measured or calculated. The importance of these measurements in individual segments is not known and needs further assessment.

Several attempts have been made to describe the total contribution of reflux in the whole limb with chronic venous insufficiency. Total valve closure time has been calculated by adding the duration of reflux in the superficial femoral and popliteal veins. A value of more than 4 seconds of reflux has been shown to correlate well with severe axial incompetence phlebographically (102). This value does not include the contribution of reflux in the superficial system, the importance of which has previously been underestimated but recently pointed out in a number of studies (31, 103–106). Total reflux exceeding 10 ml/sec (adding the retrograde volume flow in the long saphenous, short saphenous, and popliteal veins) has been shown to be associated with a high incidence of pigmentation and ulceration (66%) of the legs, while limbs with reflux flow below 10 ml/sec had no skin changes (64). A multisegment score based on measurements of significant duration of reflux in the segments of both superficial and deep systems has been shown to correlate well with the clinical severity (59). Although reflux can be described in different ways for each individual segment, the significance of the reflux detected in different veins and its individual contribution to the clinical condition needs further study (106).

Quantification of reflux may be less important than the ability of the duplex scanning to identify the anatomic distribution of reflux. The use of duplex scanning has certainly revealed that many patients with chronic venous insufficiency have only partial or segmental involvement of the superficial or deep venous systems, and not continuous axial incompetence as previously thought. It is also the method of choice for identifying sites of incompetent perforators at the junction between the short saphenous and popliteal veins. Although difficult to image each valve station in detail, the duplex scanning has made possible noninvasive identification of diseased vein segments with high accuracy in order to direct the treatment.

Descending Phlebography

Descending phlebography is an invasive study with potential complications and discomfort for the patient. The degree of radiologic reflux has been graded in different ways (107–109). The most commonly used is Kistner's classification (107, 108). This denotes axial incompetence in the deep system, i.e., 0 = no reflux, 1 = reflux of only the upper thigh, 2 = reflux reaching the lower thigh to the popliteal level, 3 = reflux reaching below the popliteal level into the upper calf, and 4 = reflux to the ankle along the entire deep vein system (Fig. 13.12). This classification does not consider the contribution of the superficial system to chronic venous insufficiency, which may be important. Therefore, a different assessment based on the number and level of venous system involved has been suggested (109). One point each is given to reflux in the long saphenous, superficial femoral, profunda femoral, and popliteal veins. This method of scoring reflux on descending venography (94) or duplex scanning (31) appears to correlate somewhat better than the Kistner scoring system with other measures of venous reflux.

The potential disadvantages of the descending phlebogram include: (a) A proximal competent valve will prevent the evaluation of reflux of distal veins; (b) the result is influenced by the heavy contrast medium; (c) all valves are in the open position in the relaxed horizontal and vertical leg; and (d) proximal obstruction may catch the push of the Valsalva maneuver, thus giving a false-negative finding (110).

Descending phlebography is superior to duplex scanning to provide anatomic detail of valve stations and valve structure. The deep femoral vein incompetence is more accurately delineated by this test than any other. Therefore this technique will continue to be used in patients undergoing valve reconstruction surgery.

TESTS FOR EVALUATION OF CALF MUSCLE PUMP FUNCTION

It has been suggested that ambulatory vein pressure can be replaced by the residual volume fraction obtained with air plethysmography as a measure of calf pump function (22, 26, 27). A good correlation with the lowest ambulatory venous pressure ($r = 0.83$) was described. However, Welkie, et al. (28), have shown a slightly lower correlation in 56 patients ($r = 0.76$). They found that patients with outflow obstruction had a poor correlation ($r = 0.40$); if these patients were excluded, the correlation improved to 0.86. Some laboratories, including ours, have not found any good correlation between AVP and RVF (29). Payne, et al. (30), found the correlation extremely poor in 103 limbs with different grades of venous insufficiency ($r = 0.03$). It is too early to accept the residual venous volume fraction as a replacement for ambulatory venous pressure and more studies are needed to further assess the relationship. Theoretically, it would be surprising if the calf pressure would be directly correlated to the volume only, since pressure is also influenced by vein wall compliance, resting venous volume, and outflow obstruction, which are greatly changed in chronic venous disease (60, 111).

The value and validity of ejection fraction obtained with air plethysmography is yet to be fully elucidated. It has been shown that APG's differentiation between reflux (VFI, ml/sec) and calf muscle pump ejection fraction (EF, %) might be helpful (27). On theoretic grounds, it can be said that surgery to eliminate reflux is more likely to succeed in the presence of a normal or near normal ejection fraction and major reflux abnormality. A sufficient ejection fraction seems to be able to compensate for a certain amount of reflux (60).

SUMMARY

The duplex Doppler has largely replaced other techniques as the initial method of choice to delineate both obstruction and reflux. It is primarily a qualitative method even though attempts to utilize this tool in a quantitative fashion are underway. If obstruction is suspected, duplex scanning combined with Raju's test of arm/foot venous pressure differential (with reactive hyperemia component) provides the necessary physiologic configuration to address treatment. If reflux is detected on duplex scanning, additional physiologic configuration may be obtained by APG. There is, as yet, no substitute for ambulatory venous pressure measurement as a global index of abnormal pathophysiology caused by obstruction, reflux, or combined obstruction/reflux pathology.

Major surgical intervention to correct these pathologies requires preoperative contrast venography (ascending to delineate obstruction and descending to delineate reflux). For postoperative follow-up, duplex scanning aided by the arm/foot differential test, if indicated, is recommended.

REFERENCES

1. Pollack AA, Wood EH. Venous pressure in the saphenous vein in ankle in man during exercise and changes in posture. J Appl Physiol 1949;1:649–653.
2. Nicolaides AN, Hussein MK, Szendro G, Christopoulos D, Vasdekis S, Clarke H. The relation of venous ulceration with ambulatory venous pressure measurements. J Vasc Surg 1993;17:414–419.
3. Raju S, Fredericks R. Hemodynamic basis of stasis ulceration—a hypothesis. J Vasc Surg 1991;13:491–495.
4. Nicolaides AN, Zukowski AJ. The value of dynamic venous pressure measurements. World J Surg 1986;10:919–924.
5. McMullin GM, Coleridge Smith PD, Scurr JH. A study of tourniquets in the investigation of venous insufficiency. Phlebology 1991;6:133–139.
6. Raju S. New approaches to the diagnosis and treatment of venous obstruction. J Vasc Surg 1986;14:42–54.
7. Raju S. A pressure-based technique for the detection of acute and chronic venous obstruction. Phlebology 1988;3:207–216.
8. Raju S, Fredericks R. Venous obstruction: an analysis of one hundred thirty-seven cases with hemodynamic, venographic, and clinical correlations. J Vasc Surg 1991;14:305–313.
9. Nicolaides AN, Sumner DS. Investigations of patients with deep vein thrombosis and chronic venous insufficiency. Los Angeles: Med-Orion Publishing Company, 1991:56–62.
10. Neglén P, Raju S. Detection of outflow obstruction in chronic venous insufficiency. J Vasc Surg 1993;17:583–589.
11. Abramowitz HB, Queral LA, Flinn WR, et al. The use of photoplethysmography in the assessment of venous insufficiency: a comparison to venous pressure measurements. Surgery 1979;86:434–441.
12. Nicolaides AN, Miles C. Photoplethysmography in the assessment of venous insufficiency. J Vasc Surg 1987;5:405–412.
13. van den Broek TAA, Rauwerda JA, Kuijper CF, van Rij GL, Bakker FC. Failure of quantitative venous photoplethysmography to assess venous insufficiency: a prospective clinical study. Netherlands J Surg 1989;41:104–107.
14. Rosfors S. Venous photoplethysmography: relationship between transducer position and regional distribution of venous insufficiency. J Vasc Surg 1990;11:436–440.
15. Van Bemmelen PS, van Ramhorst B, Eikelboom BC. Photoplethysmography reexamined: the lack of correlation with duplex in venous insufficiency. Surgery 1992;112:544–548.
16. Bygdeman S, Aschberg S, Hindmarsh T. Venous plethysmography in the diagnosis of chronic venous insufficiency. Acta Chir Scand 1971;137:423–428.
17. Dahn I, Eiriksson E. Plethysmographic diagnosis of deep venous thrombosis of the leg. Acta Chir Scand 1968;398(Suppl):33–42.
18. Hallböök T, Ling T. Pitfalls in plethysmographic diagnosis of deep vein thrombosis. J Cardiovasc Surg 1973;14:427–430.
19. Wheeler HB, Anderson FA Jr. The diagnosis of venous thrombosis by impedance plethysmography. In: Bernstein EF, ed. Non-invasive diagnostic techniques in vascular disease. St Louis: CV Mosby, 1985:755–765.

20. Cranley JJ, Flanagan LD, Sullivan ED. Diagnosis of deep vein thrombosis by phleborrheography. In: Bernstein EF, ed. Non-invasive diagnostic techniques in vascular disease. St Louis: CV Mosby, 1985:730–741.
21. Allan JC. Volume changes in the lower limb in response to postural alterations and muscle exercise. South African J Surg 1964;2:75–90.
22. Christopoulos DC, Nicolaides AN, Szendro G, Irvine AT, Bull M, Eastcott HHG. Air-plethysmography and the effect of elastic compression on venous hemodynamics of the leg. J Vasc Surg 1987;5:148–159.
23. Fernandes e Fernandes J, Horner J, Needham T, Nicolaides AN. Ambulatory calf volume plethysmography in the assessment of venous insufficiency. Br J Surg 1979; 66:327–330.
24. Neglén P, Raju S. Detection of outflow obstruction in chronic venous insufficiency. J Vasc Surg 1993;17:583–589.
25. Christopoulos DC, Nicolaides AN, Szendro G. Venous reflux: quantitation and correlation with the clinical severity of chronic venous disease. Br J Surg 1988;75:352–356.
26. Nicolaides AN, Sumner DS. Investigations of patients with deep vein thrombosis and chronic venous insufficiency. Los Angeles: Med-Orion Publishing Company, 1991:46.
27. Christopoulos D, Nicolaides AN, Cook A, Irvine A, Galloway JMD, Wilkinson A. Pathogenesis of venous ulceration in relation to the calf muscle pump function. Surgery 1989;106:829–835.
28. Welkie JF, Comerota AJ, Katz ML, Aldridge SC, Kerr RP, White JV. Hemodynamic deterioration in chronic venous disease. J Vasc Surg 1992;16:733–40.
29. Gillespie DL. Letter to the editor. J Vasc Surg 1993;18:140.
30. Payne SPK, Thrush AJ, London NJM, Bell PRF, Barrie WW. Venous assessment using air-plethysmography; a comparison with clinical examination, ambulatory venous pressure and duplex assessment. Br J Surg 1993:967–970.
31. Neglén P, Raju S. A rational approach to detection of significant reflux with duplex Doppler scanning and air plethysmography. J Vasc Surg 1993;17:590–595.
32. Thulesius O, Norgren L, Gjöres JE. Foot volumetry, a new method for objective assessment of oedema and venous function. Vasa 1973;2:325–329.
33. Norgren L, Thulesius O, Gjöres JE, Söderlundh S. Foot-volumetry and simultaneous venous pressure measurements for evaluation of venous insufficiency. Vasa 1974;3:140–147.
34. Partsch H. Simultane Venendruckmessung und Plethysmographie am Fub. In: May R, Kriessmann A, eds. Periphere Venendruckmessung. Stuttgart: Georg Thieme, 1978:147–156.
35. Lawrence D, Kakkar VV. Venous pressure measurement and foot volumetry in venous disease. In: Verstraete M, ed. Techniques in angiology. The Hague: Martinus Nijhoff, 1979.
36. Nicolaides AN, Fernandes e Fernandes J, Zimmerman H. Doppler ultrasound in the investigation of venous insufficiency. In: Nicolaides AN, Yao JST, eds. Investigation of vascular disorders. New York: Churchill Livingstone, 1981:478–487.
37. Sigel B, Felix WR, Popky GL, Ipsen J. Diagnosis of lower limb venous thrombosis by Doppler ultrasound technique. Arch Surg 1971;104:174–179.
38. Milne RM, Gunn A, Griffiths JMT, Ruckley CV. Postoperative deep vein thrombosis, a comparison of diagnostic techniques. Lancet 1971;2:445–447.
39. Folse R, Alexander RH. Directional flow detection for localizing venous valvular incompetence. Surgery 1970;67:114–121.
40. Miller SS, Foote AV. The ultrasonic detection of incompetent perforating veins. Br J Surg 1974;61:653–656.
41. O'Donnell J, Burnand KG, Clemenson G, Lea Thomas M, Browse NL. Doppler ex-

amination vs. clinical and phlebographic detection of the location of incompetent perforating veins. Arch Surg 1977;112:31–35.
42. Hoare MC, Royle JP. Doppler ultrasound detection of saphenofemoral and saphenopopliteal incompetence and operative venography to ensure precise sapheno-popliteal ligation. Aust NZ J Surg 1984;54:49–52.
43. Nicolaides AN, Sumner DS. Investigations of patients with deep vein thrombosis and chronic venous insufficiency. Los Angeles: Med-Orion Publishing Company, 1991:5–9.
44. van Bemmelen PS, Bedford G, Beach K, Strandness DE. Quantitative segmental evaluation of venous valvular reflux with duplex ultrasound scanning. J Vasc Surg 1989;10:424–431.
45. Kremkau FW. Principles of color flow imaging. J Vasc Tech 1991;15:104–111.
46. Roghavendra BN, Rosen R, Lam S, Riles T, Horii SC. Deep venous thrombosis: detection by high resolution real-time ultrasonography. Radiology 1984;152:789–793.
47. Hannan LJ, Stedje KJ, Skorez MJ, Karkow WS, Flanigan LD, Cranley JJ. Venous imaging of the extremities: our twenty-five hundred cases. Bruit 1986;10:29–33.
48. Roghavendra BN, Horii SC, Hilton S, Subramanyam BS, Rosen RJ, Lam S. Deep venous thrombosis: detection by probe compression of veins. J Ultrasound Med 1986;5:89–95.
49. Cronan JJ, Dorfman GS, Scola FH, Schepps B, Alexander J. Deep venous thrombosis: US assessment using vein compression. Radiology 1987;162:191–194.
50. Killewich LA, Bedford BS, Beach KW, Strandness DE Jr. Diagnosis of deep venous thrombosis. A prospective study comparing duplex scanning to contrast venography. Circulation 1989;79:810–814.
51. Wester JPJ, Holtkamp M, Linnebank ERM, et al. Non-invasive detection of deep venous thrombosis: ultrasonography versus duplex scanning. Eur J Vasc Surg 1994;8:357–361.
52. Sarpa MS, Messina LM, Smith M, Chang L, Greenfield LJ. Reliability of venous duplex scanning to image the iliac veins and to diagnose iliac vein thrombosis in patients suspected of having acute deep vein thrombosis. J Vasc Tech 1991;15:299–302.
53. Levén HO, Al-Hassan H. Ultrasonic diagnosis of iliofemoral venous thrombosis: merits and disadvantages. Phlebography 1990;5:107–112.
54. van Bemmelen PS, Bedford G, Strandness DE. Visualization of calf veins by color flow imaging. Ultrasound Med Biol 1990;16:15–17.
55. Council on Scientific Affairs, American Medical Association. Doppler sonographic imaging of the vascular system. JAMA 1991;265:2382–2387.
56. Foley WD, Middleton WD, Lawson TL, Erickson S, Quiroz FA, Macrander S. Color Doppler ultrasound imaging of lower extremity venous disease. AJR 1989;152:371–376.
57. Cronan JJ, Leen V. Recurrent deep venous thombosis. Limitations of US. Radiology 1989;170:739–742.
58. Masuda EM, Kistner RL. Prospective comparison of duplex scanning and descending venography in the assessment of venous insufficiency. Am J Surg 1992;164:254–259.
59. Neglén P, Raju S. A comparison between descending phlebography and duplex Doppler investigation in the evaluation of reflux in chronic venous insufficiency: a challenge to phlebography as the "gold standard." J Vasc Surg 1992;16:687–693.
60. Raju S, Fredericks R, Lishman P, Neglén P, Morano J. Observation on the calf venous pump mechanism: determinants of postexercise pressure. J Vasc Surg 1993;17:459–469.
61. Sigel B, Machi J, Bierler JC, et al. Red cell aggregation as a cause of blood flow echogenicity. Radiology 1983;148:799–806.
62. Timmons MJ. William Harvey revisited: reverse flow through the valves of forearm veins. Lancet 1984;2:394–395.

63. van Bemmelen PS, Beach K, Strandness DE. The mechanism of valve closure. Arch Surg 1990;125:617–618.
64. Vasdekis SN, Clarke GH, Nicolaides AN. Quantification of venous reflux by means of duplex scanning. J Vasc Surg 1989;10:670–677.
65. van Bemmelen PS, Bedford G, Beach K, Strandness DE. Quantitative segmental evaluation of venous valvular reflux with duplex ultrasound scanning. J Vasc Surg 1989;10:424–431.
66. Beckwith TC, Richardson GD, Sheldon M, Clarke GH. A correlation between blood flow volume and ultrasonic Doppler wave forms in the study of valve insufficiency. Phlebology 1993:8:12–16.
67. Lea Thomas M, MacDonald LM. Complications of ascending phlebography of the leg. Br Med J 1978;2:317–318.
68. Berge T, Bergquist D, Efsing HO, Hallböök T. Local complications of ascending phlebography. Clin Radiol 1978;29:691–696.
69. Almén T. Contrast agent designs: some aspects of the synthesis of water soluble contrast agents of low osmolarity. J Theor Biol 1969;24:216–226.
70. Albrechtsson U, Olsson CG. Thrombosis after phlebography: a comparison of two contrast media. Cardiovasc Radiol 1979;2:9–18.
71. Browse NL, Burnand KG, Lea Thomas M. Diseases of the veins. Pathology, diagnosis and treatment. 1st ed. London: Edward Arnold, 1988:103–106.
72. Raju S, Fredericks R. Venous obstruction: an analysis of one hundred thirty-seven cases with hemodynamic, venographic, and clinical correlations. J Vasc Surg 1991;14:305–313.
73. Kistner RL, Ferris EB, Randhawa G, Kamida C. A method of performing descending venography. J Vasc Surg 1986;4:464–468.
74. Lea Thomas M, Keeling FP, Ackroyd JS. Descending phlebography: a comparison of three methods and an assessment of the normal range of deep vein reflux. J Cardiovasc Surg 1986;27:27–30.
75. Morano JU, Raju S. Chronic venous insufficiency: assessment with descending venography. Radiology 1990;174:441–444.
76. Gullmo AL. The phlebographic Trendelenburg test. Br J Radiol 1963;24:375–379.
77. Barnes RW, Hokanson DE, Wu KK, Hoak JC. Detection of deep vein thrombosis with an automatic electrically calibrated strain gauge plethysmograph. Surgery 1977;82:219–223.
78. Hallböök T, Ling L. Plethysmography in the diagnosis of acute deep vein thrombosis. Vasa 1974;3:263–268.
79. Cooperman M, Martin EW Jr, Satiani B, Clark M, Evans WE. Detection of deep venous thrombosis by impedance plethysmography. Am J Surg 1979;137:252–254.
80. Hull R, Taylor DW, Hirsh J, Sackett DL, Powers P, Turpie AG. Impedance plethysmography: the relationship between venous filling and sensitivity and specificity for proximal vein thrombosis. Circulation 1977;58:898–902.
81. Comerota AJ, Cranley JJ, Cook SE, Sipple A. Phleborrheography: results of a ten-year experience. Surgery 1982;91:573–581.
82. Huisman MV, Buller HR, ten Cate JW, Vreeken J. Serial impedance plethysmography for suspected deep venous thrombosis in outpatients. N Engl J Med 1986;314:823–828.
83. Rosner NH, Doris PE. Diagnosis of femoropopliteal venous thrombosis: comparison of duplex sonography and plethysmography. AJR 1988;150:623–627.
84. Comerota AJ, Katz ML, Greenwald LL, Leefmans E, Czeredarczuk M, White JV. Venous duplex imaging: should it replace hemodynamic tests for deep venous thrombosis? J Vasc Surg 1990;11:53–61.
85. Mattos MA, Londrey GL, et al. Color-flow duplex scanning for the surveillance and diagnosis of acute venous thrombosis. J Vasc Surg 1992;15:366–376.

86. Nicolaides AN, Sumner DS. Investigations of patients with deep vein thrombosis and chronic venous insufficiency. Los Angeles: Med-Orion Publishing Company, 1991:18–21.
87. Rose SC, Zwiebel WJ, Nelson BD, et al. Symptomatic lower extremity deep venous thrombosis: accuracy, limitations, and role of color duplex flow imaging in diagnosis. Radiology 1990;175:639–644.
88. Buchbinder D, McCullough GM, Melick CF. Patients evaluated for venous disease may have other pathologic conditions contributing to symptomatology. Am J Surg 1993;166:211–215.
89. Thulesius O, Thurin A. Extravascular masses masquerading as deep venous thrombosis. Phlebology 1993;8:158–161.
90. Nicolaides AN, Sumner DS. Investigations of patients with deep vein thrombosis and chronic venous insufficiency. Los Angeles: Med-Orion Publishing Company, 1991:48–62.
91. Åkesson H, Brudin L, Jensen R, Ohlin P, Plate G. Physiological evaluation of venous obstruction in the post-thrombotic leg. Phlebology 1989;4:3–14.
92. Baumgartner I, Franzcek UK, Bollinger A. Venous claudication evaluated by ambulatory plethysmography. Phlebology 1992;7:2–6.
93. Eriksson E. Plethysmographic studies of venous disease of the legs [Thesis]. Department of Physiology and Radiology, University of Lund, Sweden, 1968. Acta Chir Scand 1968;(Suppl): 398.
94. Raju S, Fredericks R. Evaluation of methods for detecting venous reflux. Arch Surg 1990;125:1463–1467.
95. Iafrati MD, Welch H, O'Donnell TF, Belkin M, Umphrey S, McLaughlin R. Correlation of venous noninvasive tests with the Society for Vascular Surgery/International Society for Cardiovascular Surgery clinical classification of chronic venous insufficiency. J Vasc Surg 1994;19:1001–1007.
96. Pearce WH, Riccoe J-B, Queral LA, Flinn WR, Yao JST. Haemodynamic assessment of venous problems. Surgery 1983;93:715–721.
97. Sarin S, Shields DA, Scurr JH, Coleridge Smith PD. Photoplethysmography: a valuable noninvasive tool in the assessment of venous function? J Vasc Surg 1992;16:154–162.
98. van Bemmelen PS, Maltos MA, Hougson KJ, et al. Does air plethysmography correlate with duplex scanning in patients with chronic venous insufficiency? J Vasc Surg 1993;18:796–807.
99. Welch HJ, Faliakou EC, McLaughlin RL, Umphrey SE, Belkin M, O'Donnell TF Jr. Comparison of descending phlebography with quantitative photoplethysmography, air plethysmography, and duplex quantitative valve closure time in assessing deep venous reflux. J Vasc Surg 1992;16:913–920.
100. Cordts PR, Hartono C, LaMorte WW, Menzoian JO. Physiologic similarities between extremities with varicose veins and with chronic venous insufficiency by utilizing air plethysmography. Am J Surg 1992;164:260–264.
101. Christopoulos D, Nicolaides AN, Galloway JMD, Wilkinson A. Objective noninvasive evaluation of venous surgical results. J Vasc Surg 1988;8:683–687.
102. Welch HJ, Faliakou EC, McLaughlin RL, Umphrey SE, Belkin M, O'Donnell TF Jr. Comparison of descending phlebography with quantitative photoplethysmography, air plethysmography, and duplex quantitative valve closure time in assessing deep venous reflux. J Vasc Surg 1992;16:913–920.
103. Gooley NA, Sumner DS. Relationship of venous reflux to the site of venous valvular incompetence: implications for venous reconstructive surgery. J Vasc Surg 1988; 7:50–59.

104. van Bemmelen PS, Bedford GB, Beach K, Strandness DE Jr. Status of the valves in the superficial and deep venous system in chronic venous disease. Surgery 1991;109:730–734.
105. Hanrahan LM, Araki CT, Rodriguez AA, Kechejian GJ, LaMorte WW, Menzoian JO. Distribution of valvular incompetence in patients with venous stasis ulceration. J Vasc Surg 1991;13:805–812.
106. Payne SPK, London NJM, Jagger C, Newland CJ, Barrie WW, Bell PRF. Clinical significance of venous reflux detected by duplex scanning. Br J Surg 1994;81:39–41.
107. Kistner RL. Transvenous repair of the incompetent femoral vein valve. In: Bergan JJ, Yao JST, eds. Venous problems. London: Year Book Medical Publishers, 1978:493–509.
108. Herman RJ, Neiman HL, Yao JST, Egan TJ, Bergan JJ, Malave SR. Descending venography: a method of evaluating lower extremity venous valve function. Radiology 1980;137:63–69.
109. Raju S. Valve reconstruction procedures for chronic venous insufficiency. Semin Vasc Surg 1986;27:27–30.
110. Athanasoulis CA, Yucel EK. Venous reflux: assessing the level of incompetence. Radiology 1990;170:326–327.
111. Neglén P, Raju S. Compliance of the normal and post-thrombotic calf. J Cardiovasc Surg (Torino) 1995;36:225–231.

section III

Techniques

chapter 14

Sclerotherapy for Varicose Veins: Guidelines and Procedures

J. Leonel Villavicencio, Richard K. Spence, John R. Pfeifer, Joann M. Lohr, Robert Cranley, Mitchel P. Goldman, and Emmanouil Pikoulis

HISTORICAL REVIEW

It is generally recognized that the operation introduced by Trendelenburg in 1860, and published in 1890, was the beginning of modern surgery for varicose veins (1). Intraluminal stripping as a surgical procedure was first reported by Keller in the United States in 1905 (2), even though Charles Mayo had performed an operation for varicose veins in Rochester, Minnesota, in 1888, and reported the results of his operation with an external stripper in 1904 and 1906 (3, 4). Babcock, in 1907 (5), reported stripping of the saphenous vein with an instrument that was the prototype of all intraluminal strippers currently used. The Mayo and Babcock operations were extensively utilized by American surgeons for more than two decades. Surgery had been accompanied by considerable morbidity. Sepsis and pulmonary embolism were frequent in the preantibiotic era when bed rest for 8–10 days was recommended for patients. Sclerotherapy was received with great expectations after many years of experience in Europe and replaced surgery as the treatment of choice. It was introduced in 1927 by McPheeters and Dixon (6–8) of the Mayo Clinic, using a solution of quinine and urethane. Sodium morrhuate was introduced in 1931, and was extensively used in the United States during the next two decades. Failure of the injection treatment of varicose veins was recognized early by McPheeters and De Takats (8, 9), and later by Smith (10), who published one of the first large clinical series emphasizing the poor long-term results obtained with the method.

The reports of these investigators were confirmed and expanded in the publications by Ochsner (11) and Waugh (12). The latter reported a recurrence rate of nearly 60% at 5 years using sclerotherapy either alone or in combination with high ligation. These experiences were later confirmed by Hobbs (13) and Einarsson, et al. (14), in randomized controlled studies. The failure of sclerotherapy rekindled the interest in the surgical procedures when, in 1957, Myers reported the excellent results obtained by an extensive operation for varicose veins utilizing new instrumentation (15).

With the advent of new sclerosing agents that are less toxic and highly effective, there has been a wave of enthusiasm for sclerotherapy in the United States that has made it necessary to reassess our knowledge of this form of treatment and establish guidelines for the training and practice of sclerotherapy for physicians.

The physician should be familiar with the following aspects of sclerotherapy: indications, contraindications, diagnostic methods to identify the etiology of the varices, its distribution, and the points of reflux. The physician should also become familiar with the available sclerosing agents, their modes of action, materials, techniques, compression methods, complications, and long-term results.

TRAINING OF THE PHYSICIAN

Optimally, during his or her training the physician should have received instruction in the nonoperative and operative management of venous diseases, including stasis dermatitis, venous ulceration, varicose veins, and telangiectasias, and, preferably, have had exposure to sclerotherapy procedures either during training or by attending sclerotherapy courses which may include videotape and live demonstrations. Additionally, it is desirable that the training be complemented by specific instruction in centers of sclerotherapy recommended by recognized professional societies. Sclerotherapy is taught to residents and vascular fellows at the Venous and Lymphatic Teaching Clinics at Walter Reed Army and National Naval Medical Centers in Washington, DC.

DIAGNOSIS

A complete clinical history and physical examination should be performed during the initial visit. Symptoms relative to menses, activity, presence of pain, edema, heaviness, and type of work should be investigated. During the initial visit, it is determined whether the patient is a candidate for sclerotherapy or for surgery or for both. After the interview, the physical examination will confirm the clinical impression. Noninvasive vascular examination and/or invasive testing (Doppler ultrasound, duplex scanning, air plethysmography, photoplethysmography, phlebography) should be judiciously employed to obtain information about the etiology of the varicose veins and the hemodynamic assessment of the superficial and deep systems. This is important because if there is severe reflux, sclerotherapy will be only temporarily successful. On the other hand, if the varicosities are secondary to arteriovenous fistula, sclerotherapy is not indicated because there is the risk of the sclerosing agent passing into the arterial system, producing serious complications.

INFORMED CONSENT

Patients considered for sclerotherapy should be informed of the nature of the treatment that they will receive, the results that may be expected, and the anticipated side effects that may reasonably be expected from the treatment (e.g., skin necrosis, pigmentation, thrombophlebitis). All patients should sign an Informed Consent Form. Preinjection photography is strongly recommended. Patient's consent should be obtained.

HISTORY

The etiology of the varicose veins should be determined. Each of the following four groups of varicosities has a different etiology, pathophysiology, and treatment: (a) familial or primary (telangiectasias are considered in this group); (b) postthrombotic or secondary; (c) congenital malformations of venous predominance; and (d) posttraumatic or acquired arteriovenous fistula. In most patients, the diagnosis can be made during the initial interview. Special emphasis should be placed on obtaining a history of diseases which may modify the therapeutic approach, such as asthma, allergic diseases, tendency to keloids or pigmentation, bleeding diathesis, history of deep venous thrombosis, and hypercoagulable states.

The intake of medications that may interfere with the clotting mechanism, such as aspirin, anticoagulants, and certain anti-inflammatory agents, should be investigated. The use of oral contraceptives, estrogens, and other hormonal agents whose role in the coagulation mechanisms is well-known should also be investigated.

PHYSICAL EXAMINATION

The patient should be examined in the upright position under good illumination. Tangential lighting is excellent for demonstration of the bulging varicose veins. The distribution of the varicosities should be carefully noted. The physician should be familiar with the indications for and use of the noninvasive vascular instrumentation techniques.

Primary varicose veins appear early in life and are usually present in one or more members of the family. "Venous spiders" (telangiectasia), venous lakes, and other skin blemishes appear, especially in women, on the medial, posterior, and lateral aspects of the thigh and less often in the lower leg and calf. These blemishes have a striking familial tendency (Fig. 14.1).

Varicose veins may appear in the extremities as a sequelae of postthrombotic syndrome. In these cases, edema, pigmentation, eczema, and venous ulcers may also be present (Fig. 14.2). Even though less common, primary deep and superficial venous insufficiency may produce similar manifestations. Patients with congenital malformations of venous predominance may have varicose veins, "portwine stains," hypertrophy of soft tissues, and bone overgrowth of the ex-

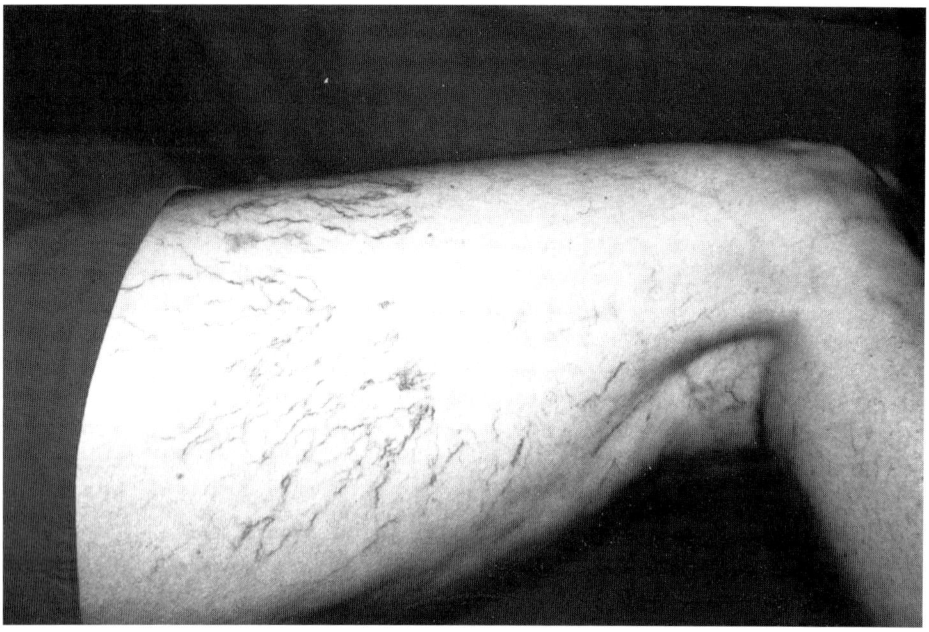

FIG. 14–1. Extensive telangiectasia and branch varicosities in a young woman. Venous lakes and other skin blemishes appear especially on the lateral aspects of the thigh and often in the lower leg and calf. These blemishes have a striking familial tendency.

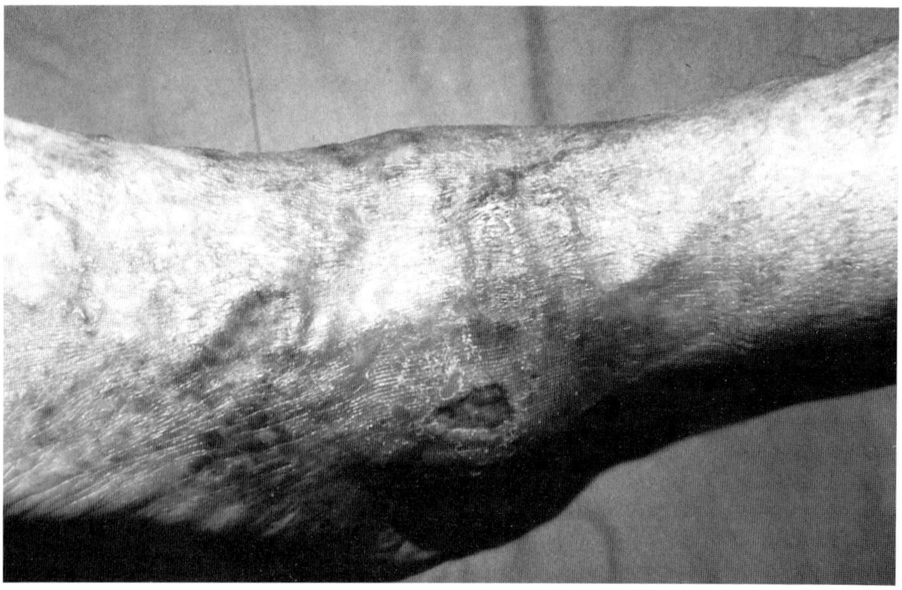

FIG. 14–2. Large varices surrounding a leg ulcer. Sclerotherapy, in these cases, enhances the ulcer healing by eliminating temporarily the venous hypertension present in the ulcer area. Sclerotherapy followed by a 1–2 week period of compression is highly effective in this condition.

tremity. In these patients, the presence of congenital arteriovenous fistula should be ruled out. Patients with predominantly venous malformations may benefit from sclerotherapy (Fig. 14.3). The presence of AV fistulae is a contraindication for sclerotherapy.

Varicose veins may also be a manifestation of traumatic arteriovenous fistula. The hemodynamic effects on the venous system will depend on the location, size and duration of the fistula. Acquired AV fistulae are treated surgically or by endovascular techniques. Sclerotherapy may be used only after the arteriovenous shunt has been corrected.

The venous tributaries of the internal iliac vein may be a source of varicose veins. The internal pudendal, obturator, and gluteal veins are tributaries of the internal iliac vein and drain the venous areas of the buttocks, upper and medial aspects of the thigh, and perineum. An intrapelvic source of varicose veins must be recognized. Sclerotherapy is useful in mild cases of vulvar varices.

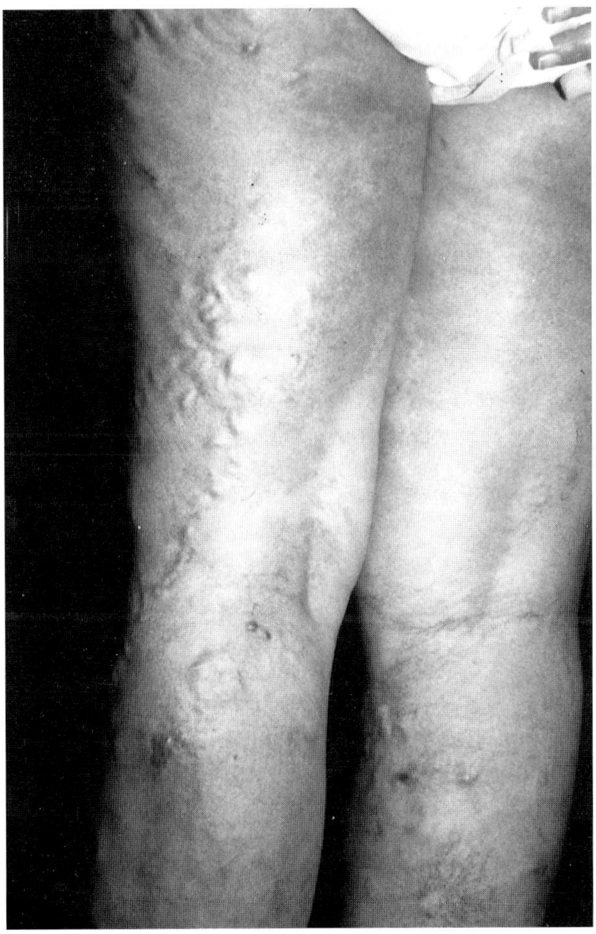

FIG. 14–3. Varicose veins in a patient with Klippel-Trenaunay syndrome. When surgery is not feasible because of deep venous anomalies, sclerotherapy and external compression are the main forms of treatment for this disease.

LABORATORY EXAMINATION

The clinical history and the physical examination should be supplemented by laboratory data on an individual basis. Appropriate blood tests should be performed in patients with hypercoagulability or other manifestations of systemic disease. These include, but are not limited to: protein S, protein C, antithrombin III, and lupus anticoagulant.

NONINVASIVE VASCULAR EXAMINATION

Doppler ultrasound examination is valuable to assess reflux at the saphenofemoral and saphenopopliteal junctions and other areas of perforators (Fig. 14.4). Air plethysmography, photoplethysmography, and color duplex scanning are the most widely used noninvasive tests. Noninvasive vascular testing should be utilized to assess the hemodynamics of the superficial and deep venous systems, to detect incompetent perforators and to rule out venous thrombosis. These tests are rarely indicated in cases of telangiectasia. In general, the routine use of these expensive vascular examinations in sclerotherapy patients should be discouraged.

Invasive studies such as ascending or descending phlebography are indicated in complex cases of venous disorders such as congenital malformations, pelvic varices, and recurrent varicose veins to guide the physician in selecting a therapeutic option.

In all patients with venous disease, a complete examination of the arterial system is essential. Assessment of peripheral pulses should be done in all patients. Ankle/brachial index determinations should be done when clinically appropriate.

INDICATIONS FOR SCLEROTHERAPY

Surgical techniques carefully tailored for each type of venous problem have provided lasting relief to a large number of patients. Sclerotherapy is an excellent method of treatment, but it has very definite indications. The judicious combination of selective venous surgery and sclerotherapy constitutes the best management for most types of varicose veins. The following are the indications for sclerotherapy:

Superficial venules, "venous spiders" (veins under 1 mm), venous lakes, and other small venous blemishes. The treatment of these superficial varicosities is mainly cosmetic, even though some of them may be symptomatic (Fig. 14.1).

Varicosities of 1–3 mm in diameter in the absence of detectable valvular reflux.

Postoperative residual veins. These are veins under 3 mm in diameter that the surgeon chose not to excise in order to limit the number of incisions. They may be treated by sclerotherapy when the superficial ecchymoses have disappeared and the incisions are healed.

Varicosities 3–4 mm in diameter observed during the postoperative follow-up period. These veins should be treated by sclerotherapy when they are not secondary to a missed incompetent perforator. Residual and/or recurrent incom-

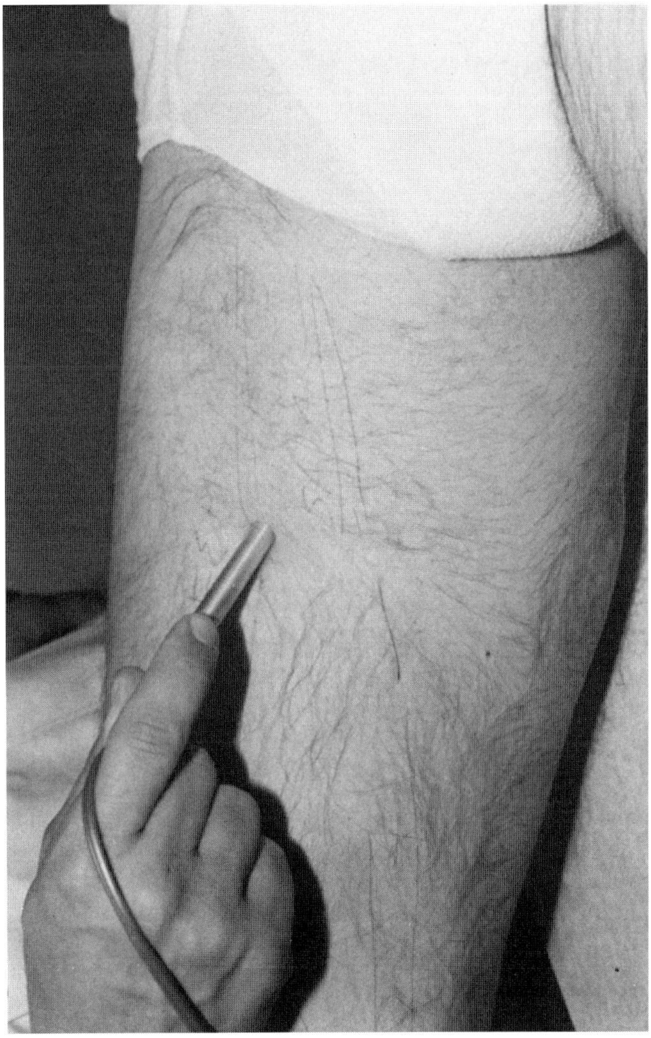

FIG. 14–4. Doppler ultrasound examination is valuable to assess reflux at the saphenofemoral and saphenopopliteal junctions and other areas of perforators. Duplex color-flow and Doppler are the most widely used noninvasive examinations.

petent perforators 4 mm or larger should be surgically divided under local anesthesia, although sometimes they can also be sclerosed with varying degree of success. Once the reflux is eliminated, remaining varicosities may be treated by sclerotherapy.

Small congenital vascular malformations of venous predominance, such as cavernous hemangiomas, may be successfully eliminated by sclerotherapy (Fig. 14.5). In extensive venous malformations where surgery is not indicated, sclerotherapy may offer palliative relief. Such is the case in certain variants of the Klippel-Trenaunay syndrome in which there is hypoplasia or aplasia of the deep venous system (Fig. 14.6).

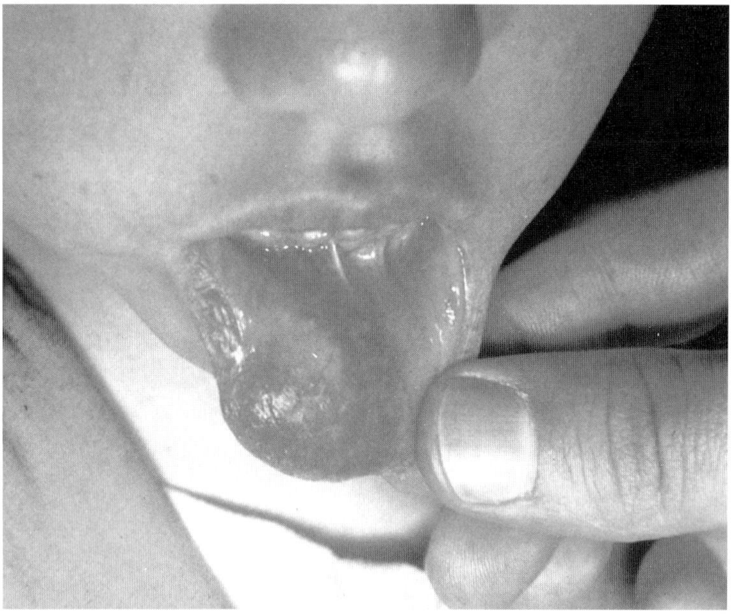

FIG. 14–5. Cavernous hemangioma of the lip in a young boy. Small congenital vascular malformations such as this may be successfully treated by sclerotherapy. Several sessions with 0.5% Polidocanol or 0.25% Sotradecol are very effective.

Bleeding varicosities can be effectively controlled by the injection of a concentrated sclerosing agent. The agent should be injected following the empty vein technique. Adequate compression is used for 1 week or longer. This treatment produces immediate thrombosis of the vein and temporarily controls the problem.

Incompetent Perforators

Sclerotherapy of incompetent perforators requires a special expertise. According to most reports, it is accompanied by a high incidence of recurrence, and may lead to deep venous thrombosis. Injection of "duplex-guided" sclerosing agents at the saphenofemoral or saphenopopliteal junctions is not recommended (Fig. 14.7). In most published series, the recurrence rate is unacceptably high and the risks involved should not be considered lightly (16). Incompetent large perforators (>4 mm), properly identified, are best treated surgically.

In the case of large varices surrounding a leg ulcer, sclerotherapy enhances the ulcer healing by eliminating temporarily the venous hypertension present in the ulcer area (Fig. 14.2).

Contraindications

The list of contraindications for sclerotherapy varies in different countries and in different medical specialties. In several European countries, it is common to inject large varicose veins and perforators. In France, Switzerland, Germany, and the United Kingdom, there are phlebologists who practice the injection of large varicose veins, disregarding the presence of reflux points. There are several randomized prospective studies which have demonstrated that sclerotherapy as a single form of treatment for all forms of varicose veins has a high incidence of recurrence. For this reason, most vascular surgeons will not inject large varicose

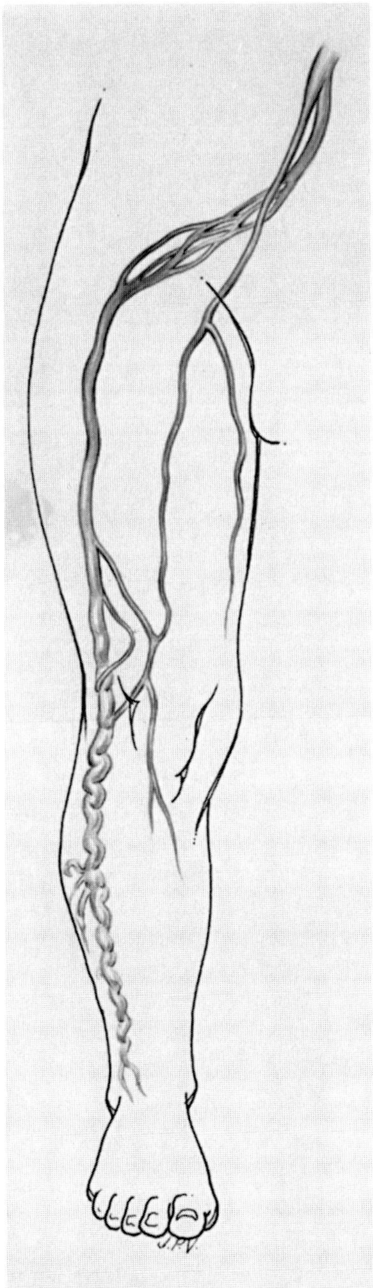

FIG. 14–6. Diffuse congenital malformation of venous predominance, where sclerotherapy may offer palliative relief. Four to six sessions with high concentrations of a sclerotherapy agent, followed by 1 or 2 weeks of compression, may bring relief to patients with deep venous anomalies.

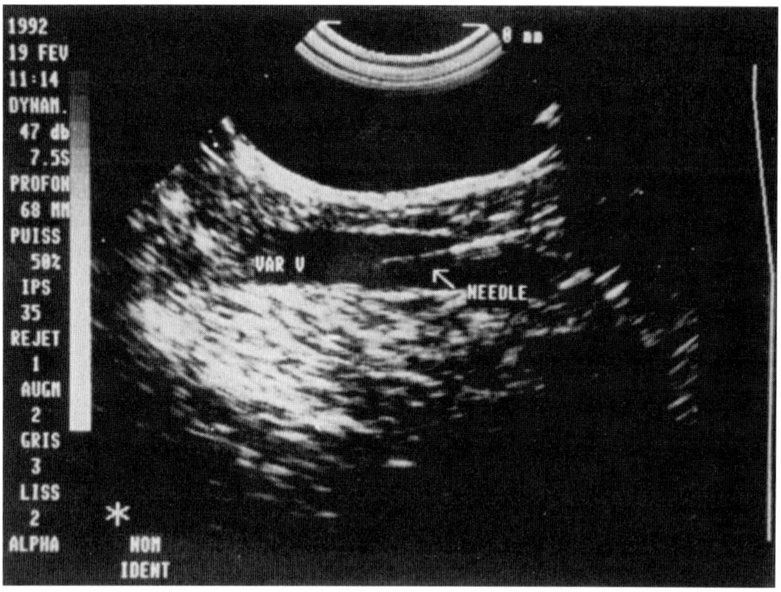

FIG. 14–7. "Duplex-guided" or echosclerotherapy has been used to deliver sclerosing agent to the saphenofemoral or saphenopopliteal junctions. In most published series, the recurrence rate is unacceptably high and the risks involved should not be considered lightly. This procedure is not recommended. (Reproduced by permission from Bergan JJ, Goldman MP. Varicose veins and telangiectasiae. St. Louis: Quality Medical Publishing Company, 1993:226–258.)

veins connected to an important source of reflux. These patients are best treated by surgery. Contraindications include:

Pregnant women should not be injected. In cases of vulvar varices, threatening rupture, or large varicose veins in the neighborhood of a leg ulcer, a localized injection can be performed in a pregnant woman to temporarily solve an important clinical problem.

Sclerotherapy in elderly and sedentary patients should be individualized. There are some elderly individuals with normal skin and good physical condition who may be submitted to sclerotherapy without problems. On the other hand, there are elderly and debilitated patients who are not good candidates for sclerotherapy owing to their lack of mobility and increased risk for deep venous thrombosis.

Generalized, severe systemic disease (diabetes; cardiac, renal, hepatic, pulmonary, and collagen diseases; and malignancies).

Advanced rheumatic disease, osteoarthritis or any disease of the musculoskeletal system that interferes with the patient's mobility.

Arterial insufficiency of the lower extremities as evidenced by intermittent claudication, coldness, skin atrophy, and weak or absent pulses, is a contraindication. In questionable cases, ankle-brachial index should be determined. Patients with ankle-brachial index below 0.8 should not be injected.

Patients with a history of severe allergic disease or bronchial asthma should be carefully evaluated. Even with the newer sclerotherapy agents, serious anaphylactic reactions have been reported on rare occasions. In cases of history of severe allergic disease, the safest sclerosing agents are 65% dextrose and 11.7–23.4% hypertonic saline.

Acute febrile illnesses as manifested by fever (38°C or higher) with signs and symptoms of acute systemic disease.

Acute superficial or deep thrombophlebitis.

Obesity. Mobility is restricted in obese individuals and external compression is difficult to apply. Treatment under these conditions should be individualized and the risk benefit of the procedure should be carefully considered.

Varicose veins in communication with a source of venous reflux demonstrated by bidirectional Doppler ultrasound and/or duplex scanning studies have an unacceptable high incidence of recurrences.

Patients on anticoagulants. Because of the risk of extensive ecchymosis secondary to the venipuncture, patients on anticoagulants, aspirin, or anti-inflammatory drugs should stop treatment 2 weeks before the injections.

Treatment

General Measures. Patients with chronic venous insufficiency will benefit with the following measures.

Elevation. If there are no contraindications of elevation of the extremity, the patient should be advised to sleep with the foot of the bed elevated 6–8 inches, placing wooden blocks between the floor and foot of the bed.

External Compression. This may be in the form of elastic bandages, elastic stockings or nonelastic compression systems. It is recognized that compression is the mainstay in the treatment of venous disease.

Hygiene of the Extremity. Cleansing and lubrication of the extremity should be recommended to every patient.

Treatment by Injection of Sclerosing Agents

General. All currently employed sclerosing agents produce a similar histologic effect. The endothelial cells swell and become disrupted immediately after the injection. The acute inflammatory reaction forms a red thrombus. The reaction may range from a complete lack of effect to a strong periphlebitic reaction. According to their mode of action, the sclerosing agents may be classified as (a) osmotic, (b) detergent, or (c) corrosive. Examples of osmotic agents are sodium chloride (23.4%), glucose (65%), and sodium salicylate. The detergent agents are Sotradecol (sodium tetradecyl sulfate), aethoxysklerol (Polidocanol), and sodium morrhuate. Corrosive agents are sodium and potassium iodide with the addition of benzyl alcohol and Chromglycerin (Scleremo).

Selection of the Sclerotherapy Agent. Each sclerotherapy agent has a unique safety and efficacy profile. The agent, concentration, and quantity of the solution injected is determined by the type, size, and site of the varicose vein to be injected. The Food and Drug Administration has approved Sotradecol, sodium morrhuate, and ethanolamine oleate. A Phase III multicenter trial of Polidocanol is underway to provide the basis for approval of this sclerosing agent, which is widely used in other parts of the world. Hypertonic saline is not approved by the FDA as a sclerosant agent.

Concentration of Agent for Different Vein Sizes. See Table 14.1 for guidelines.

Telangiectasias (Venous Spiders). Veins measuring 1 mm or less in diameter are best treated with a concentration of 0.125–0.250% Sotradecol or 0.5% Polidocanol. Hypertonic saline in strengths of 11.7–23.4%, mixed with a small amount of lidocaine to decrease the burning sensation, has been extensively used in the treatment of small venous blemishes and telangiectasias. It should be noted that some of the telangiectatic webs appear to be connected to larger feeding veins. The presence of these communications makes it necessary to treat the larger veins first, as recommended by the French School of Sclerotherapy. Polidocanol (0.5%) may, on occasion, be injected paravascularly without producing necrosis.

Veins Measuring 1–3 mm in Diameter. In these veins, concentrations of 23.4% hypertonic saline, 0.5–0.75% Sotradecol, or 0.75%-1% Polidocanol are usually successful in achieving sclerosis. The lower concentration (0.5%) should be used for the smaller vein size. As the vein approaches 3 mm in diameter, the higher concentration (0.75%) may be utilized.

TABLE 14-1

GUIDELINES FOR SURGERY AND SCLEROTHERAPY

	Concentration of Sclerosant		
Vein Size	**Hypertonic Saline**	**Sodium Tetradecyl Sulfate (Sotradecol)**	**Polidocanol (Aethoxysklerol)**
Telangiectasiae (under 1 mm)	11.7–23.4%* + lidocaine	0.125–0.25%	0.5%
Veins 1–3 mm	15–23.4% + lidocaine	0.5–0.75%	0.75–1%
Veins 3–6 mm	—	1–3%*	2–3%*
Veins >6 mm		Surgical treatment	
Saphenofemoral & saphenopopliteal junctions		Surgical treatment	

*Smaller concentrations are used for smaller caliber veins.

Varicose Veins 3–6 mm in Diameter. These veins are best treated with concentrations of 1–3% Sotradecol or 2–3% Polidocanol. These concentrations are also useful in some small congenital vascular lesions of venous predominance with vessels ranging from 3–4 mm in diameter. Again, the lower concentrations should be used for the veins of smaller size.

Large Veins Surrounding Ulcers of the Legs. Sclerosis of these veins with 3% Sotradecol or 3–4% Polidocanol is successful in inducing thrombosis of the varix and is especially useful in controlling an episode of bleeding. This method enhances healing of the ulcer while definitive measures for its treatment are considered (Fig. 14.2).

Varicosities Associated with Congenital Vascular Anomalies. Small hemangiomas or varicosities accompanying malformations such as the Klippel-Trenaunay syndrome may be treated with high concentrations of sclerotherapy agents such as 3% Sotradecol or 4% Polidocanol. Sclerotherapy in these cases is performed either as a supplement to surgery, or as a sole form of treatment when surgery cannot be performed and the patient needs some form of palliation (Fig. 14.6).

Materials. The following materials should be available:

Disposable 1–3 ml syringes (non-Luer-Lok).
Fine hypodermic needles $^1/_2$ inch in length, short bevel, 27-, 30-, or 33-gauge.
Skin antiseptic agent.
Sterile gauze (4" × 4"), and other agents for local compression such as dental rolls, foam rubber cushions, felt pad, etc.
Sclerosing agent. The syringes should be properly labeled with the concentration and nature of the material utilized.
Clear light source.
Magnifying loops (magnification +2–3×).
Caliper for vessel diameter measurement.
External compression material. This may be in the form of elastic stockings (20–30 mm of pressure), elastic bandages, or nonelastic material.
No. 65 Beaver surgical blades with handle (for microthrombectomy).
An emergency kit should be available in every room where sclerotherapy is performed. It should contain epinephrine solution 1:1000, injectable corticoids (Solu-Cortef, Solu-Medrol), heparin, benadryl, alupent inhaler, and oxygen.
A photographic camera with synchronized flash. A photo should be taken before and at least 16 weeks after the treatment. Patients often forget the pretreatment appearance. The photographic documentation may clear any misunderstandings.

TECHNIQUES OF SCLEROTHERAPY

General Principles

Successful sclerotherapy is based first on the elimination of the reflux points. Often, this is best accomplished surgically. Once the reflux points have been controlled, the treatment should proceed as follows:

(a) Large varices should be treated first and the small ones last.
(b) From the most proximal varices to the most distal ones.

The small caliber veins should always be injected with minimal concentration of the sclerotherapy agent. Large veins are best treated with higher concentrations of the agent. The use of sclerosing solutions that are too strong for the size of the vein is still one of the most common errors and a potential source of complications.

Techniques for Small Veins (Telangiectasia or Spider Veins). Good lighting and magnification (+2–3×) are essential (Fig. 14.8). Patients should be injected in the recumbent position, beginning with injections on the area that the patient considers the "worst area." The technique of the "air block" is useful in small veins and telangiectasia (Fig. 14.9). The tiny air bubbles will produce immediate blanching of the vein when the needle is correctly placed. The technique of air block may be abandoned when enough experience has been acquired. Small volumes of the agent minimize patient discomfort and prevent complications. Each injection should deliver from 0.25–0.5 ml. Immediately after the injection, the veins appear reddish and swollen as a consequence of local inflammation. A total volume of 2–4 ml of sclerosing agent may be injected during the first session, distributed among different areas. The total volume of hypertonic saline may be up to 10 ml. The injected area is compressed with a thick piece of gauze, foam rubber cushions, or dental rolls. Firm external compression is applied over the

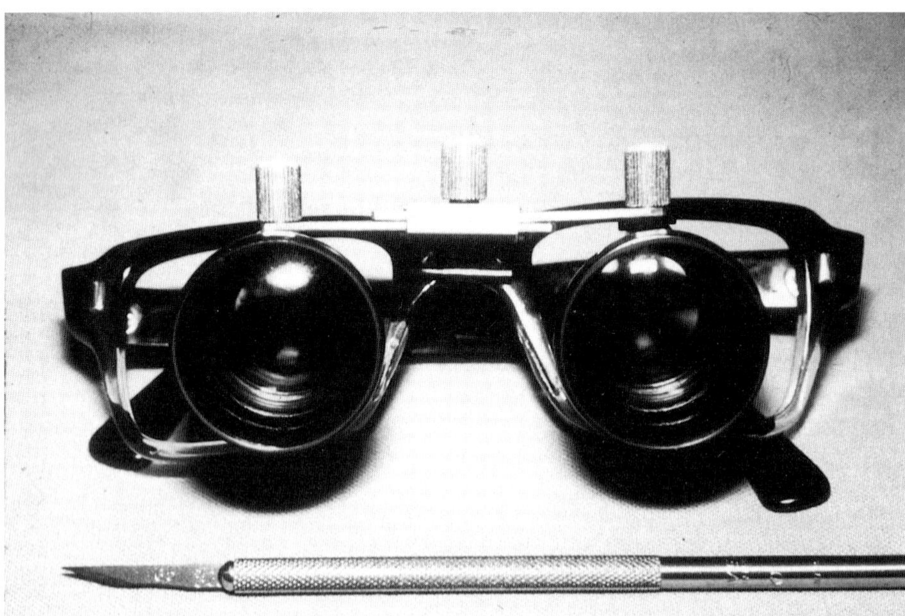

FIG. 14–8. Good lighting and 2−3× magnification are essential for visualization of small veins. A Beaver blade, which is used for microthrombectomy, is shown at the bottom of the photograph.

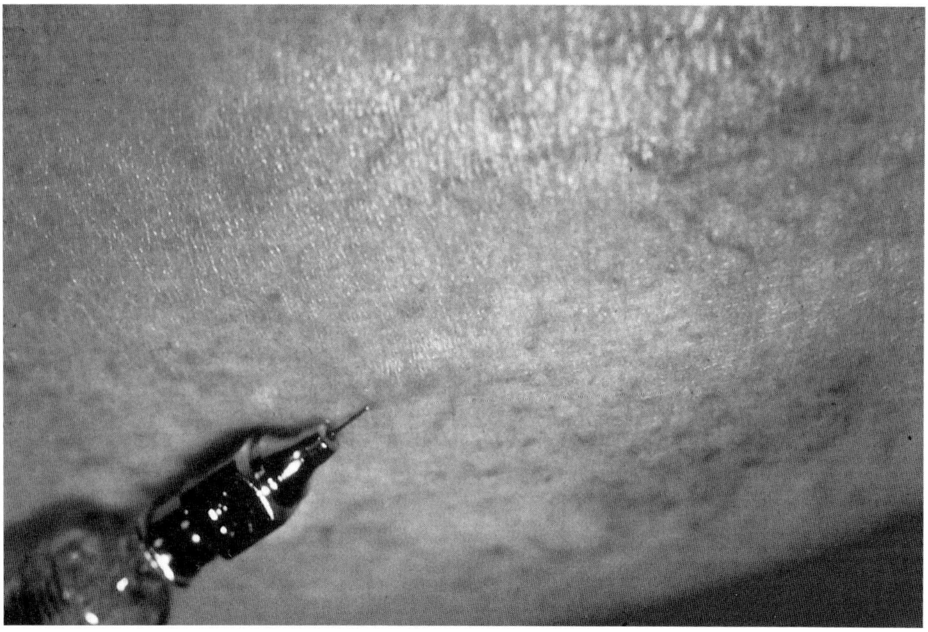

FIG. 14–9. The technique of "air block" is shown here. A very small amount of air is mixed with a sclerosing agent and the syringe is shaken vigorously to produce a froth. The tiny air bubbles will produce immediate blanching of the vein when the needle is correctly placed. In this photograph, a 30-gauge needle has been introduced into an area of spider veins and blanching is clearly observed.

entire leg, care being taken to protect the flexion areas of the ankle and behind the knee. Thigh-high elastic stockings are more comfortable than elastic bandages, which tend to dislodge with patient activity. The compression is kept in place for a minimum of 3 days. One week later, the leg is examined and any thrombus is evacuated with a No. 65 Beaver blade. In small veins, a 22-gauge needle is also effective. External compression is applied again for 3 days and the extremity is reexamined 1 week later. Patients are instructed to ambulate as much as possible and avoid prolonged standing or sitting positions.

Injection of Veins from 3–6 mm in Diameter. The veins should be examined with the patient in the upright position. Injection is performed in the recumbent position. A tilting table is ideal for sclerotherapy. For larger veins, a $^1/_4$ inch, 25–27-gauge needle is best. In this technique, the vein is punctured, the tilted table elevated, and the injection performed into an empty vein. Aspiration of blood confirms the intravascular position of the needle. The volume injected depends on the caliber of the vessel. An amount of 0.5 ml is usually sufficient per vein site. Several sites along the course of the same vein may need to be injected. The total volume injected in different sites will depend on the sclerosing agent used and the manufacturer's specifications. After the injection has been completed, pressure is applied over the injected veins with a thick piece of gauze or a foam rubber cushion. Compression (20–35 mm pressure) should be applied for at least 1 week and should not be removed at all during this period.

Postsclerotherapy Compression

External compression may be applied by several methods including the use of elastic bandages, local padding, and elastic stockings. Graduated compression is highly recommended, applying the strongest pressures at the ankle and the lowest at the knee. Compression can be applied by bandages of the elastic or nonelastic type. For sclerotherapy, the most commonly used bandages are elastic. The patient must be instructed to apply the bandage correctly and to identify any source of problems secondary to the improper application of the bandage. The correct application of an elastic bandage is an art and must be taught to the health professional. Additional compression may be applied in special areas by using rubber cushions or folded gauze. The aim is to produce apposition of the inflamed vein walls and avoid thrombus formation.

Compression Stockings. Graduated compression stockings are available in below the knee, above the knee, mid-thigh, thigh-high, and other styles. The type of stocking to be recommended is determined by the anatomy of the extremity, as well as by the type of varicosity injected. Compression stockings are available as Class I (10–20 mmHg), Class II (20–30 mmHg), Class III (30–40 mmHg), and Class IV (40–50 mmHg). The stockings should be worn during the entire period of treatment.

Postinjection Thrombectomy

Following the injection of a sclerosing agent into veins of any size, it is common that a thrombus forms within the injected veins despite adequate compression. When left in situ, the thrombus organizes and the blood turns into hemosiderin, transforming the blue vein into a brownish cord. This is an undesirable effect called pigmentation. It occurs in approximately 20% of all injected veins and usually fades away in 80% of the patients within 2 years.

The thrombus or intravascular hematoma, as it is also known, may be easily evacuated during the first 2–3 weeks after the injection, thus diminishing the amount of trapped blood and, consequently, the amount of hemosiderin. It has been the experience of many investigators that the early evacuation of the thrombus leads to decreased incidence and severity of pigmentation. There has been, however, no randomized study proving or disproving this observation. Even though the ideal time to evacuate the thrombus is during the first 2–3 weeks when the material has not become organized, evacuation of thrombus has been successful in some cases even after 8 weeks postinjection.

Technique

Veins 1 mm or Less. Thrombectomy of veins of this size can be successfully performed using loop magnification and a 22-gauge needle or the tip of a No. 65 Beaver blade. The latter is an extremely sharp instrument, superior to the No. 11 blade. After skin asepsis, a quick needle puncture or ministab incision (1.5 mm) is performed. Anesthesia is not necessary because the procedure is usually painless. A good rule of thumb is to make one puncture or ministab incision every 3 mm along the entire length of the thrombosed vein (4 punctures in a 1 cm vein) (Fig. 14.10). Once the incision has been made, gentle extrusion of the thrombus can be performed between two "Q-tips." Efforts to extrude the trapped blood through two or three ministab incisions or needle punctures in a long segment of vein usually result in incomplete evacuation of the thrombus.

Veins Larger Than 1 mm. Larger veins should be thrombectomized through 2-mm ministab incisions placed 3 mm apart along the axis of the vein. Incisions should be made with the No. 65 Beaver blade (Fig. 14.8). Satisfactory thrombus extrusion cannot be obtained through needle punctures. In large veins (3–5 mm in diameter), gentle extrusion of the thrombus is performed between the

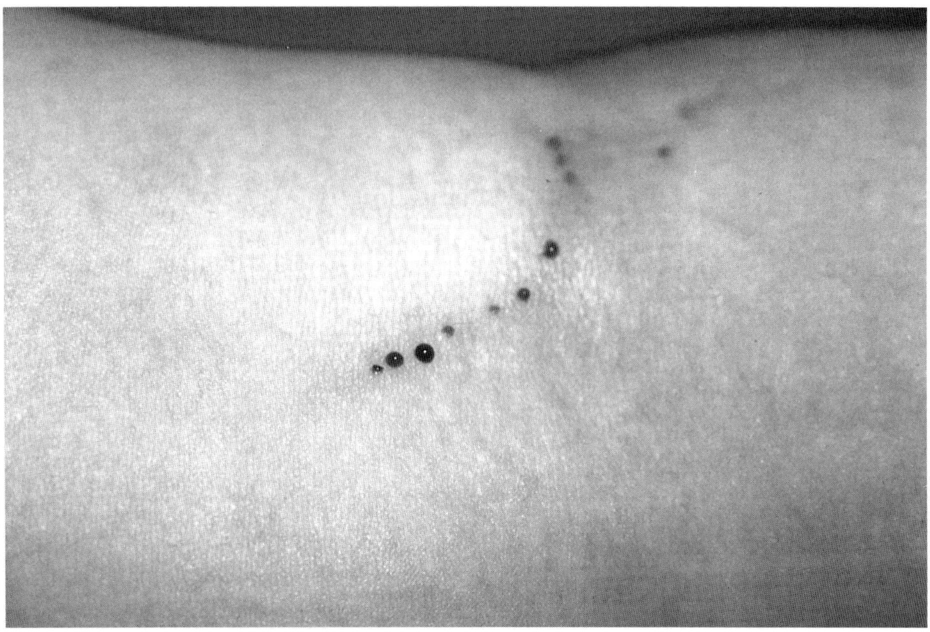

FIG. 14–10. Microthrombectomy. Following sclerosing therapy, it is common for a thrombus to form within the injected veins. When left in situ, the thrombus organizes and the blood turns into hemosiderin, transforming the blue vein into a brownish cord. To prevent this, microthrombectomy should be performed. In veins of 1 mm or less, the thrombus can be extruded using a 22-gauge needle or a No. 65 Beaver blade.

tips of the gloved fingers. Gloves should be utilized in all microthrombectomy procedures.

At the end of the procedure, compression is applied with a folded, sterile 4" × 4" gauze. A Kerlix gauze bandage secures the compression pads in place. External compression is applied with an elastic stocking or elastic bandage. In the case of veins under 1 mm, compression is used for only 24 hours. In larger veins, it is recommended that compression be maintained for a minimum of 3 days. A follow-up "retouch" visit to clear any remaining thrombus should be scheduled for 1 week later. Photographs of the treated areas should be obtained before and 12–16 weeks after the procedure.

Complications

Every sclerosing agent may have undesirable reactions. Table 14.2 illustrates the incidence of complications and side effects observed among the most commonly used sclerosing agents in the United States.

The most common complications and side effects of sclerotherapy are the following:

Pigmentation. Brown streaks develop in 10–30% of all patients treated for essential telangiectasia; in 80% of the cases, they resolve spontaneously between 6–24 months (Fig. 14.11). Pigmentation can be observed with any of the sclerotherapy agents described, including saline. Microthrombectomy, by removing the thrombus that contains the mixture of red cells and sclerosing agent, may diminish the incidence of pigmentation.

Transient Edema and Swelling. This complication occurs in almost every patient and begins shortly after injection. This is an inflammatory reaction that produces mild discomfort during the first 10–30 minutes postinjection.

Ecchymosis. Ecchymosis occurs in about 20% of the patients, especially in older individuals with fragile skin. It usually disappears after the second or third week.

TABLE 14-2

SCLEROSING AGENTS' COMPLICATIONS

Agent	Pigmentation	Allergic Reaction	Necrosis	Pain
Sodium tetradecyl sulfate	++	+	++*	+
Polidocanol	+	+	+*	0
Hypertonic saline	+	0	+++*	+++

+, Minimal; ++, moderate; +++, significant

*Concentration dependent

(Reproduced by permission from Goldman MP. Sclerotherapy. 2nd ed. St Louis: Mosby-Yearbook, 1995:336.)

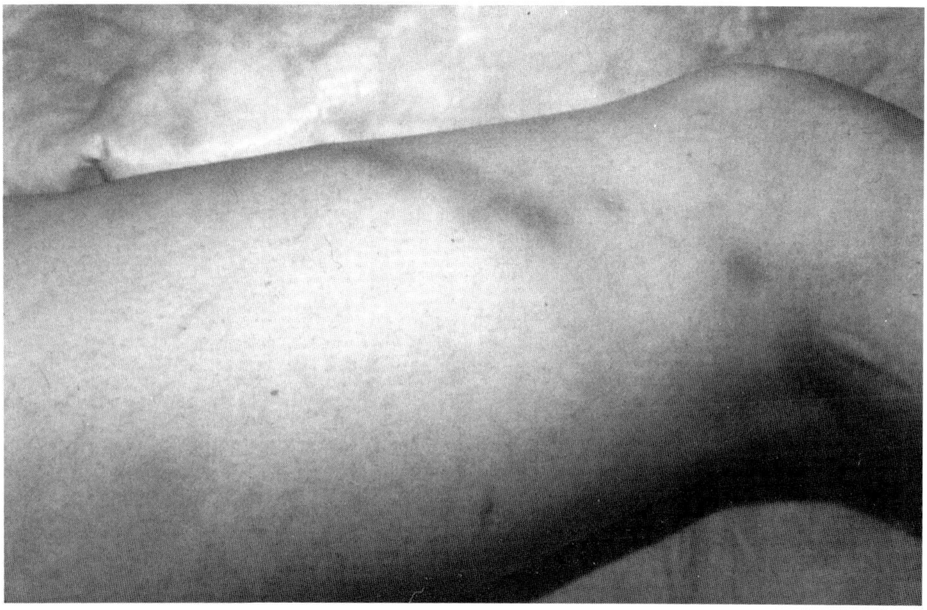

FIG. 14–11. Pigmentation. Brown streaks develop in 10–30% of all patients treated with a sclerosing agent. In 80% of the cases, they resolve spontaneously between 6–24 months. Microthrombectomy may diminish the incidence of pigmentation.

Pain, Tenderness, and Discomfort. The injection of most sclerosing agents produces a certain degree of pain and discomfort, which gradually disappears and is greatly relieved by compression.

Thrombophlebitis. The injection of a sclerosing agent produces acute inflammation of the vein. Often a thrombus is formed at the injected site and may involve veins located several inches away from the site of the injection. To prevent this occurrence, the amount of substance injected should be small (usually 0.5 ml or less) and compression should be applied on the injected vein immediately after the injection.

Skin Necrosis. Skin necrosis (Figs. 14.12 and 14.13) is usually the result of the following:

(a) Too high concentration of a sclerosing agent for the size of selected vein.
(b) Extravasation.
(c) Excessive pressure in the syringe.
(d) Fast injection.
(e) Injection into a skin arteriole (red spider veins).

Ineffective Injection. This is usually the result of an inadequate concentration of the sclerosing agent for the size of the vein chosen. The physician observes that the vein persists at the injected site. A second injection with a higher concentration is usually effective.

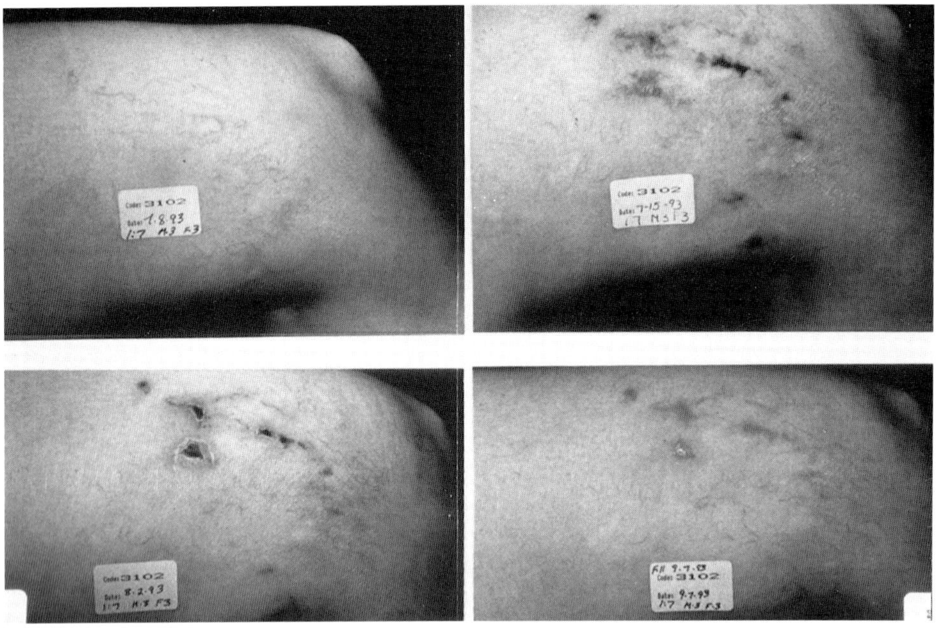

FIG. 14–12. Skin necrosis in the course of sclerotherapy for spider veins. In this case, higher than desirable concentration of the sclerosing agent for the size of the selected vein was responsible for the complication. Slow healing is apparent in the right lower quadrant.

Deep Venous Thrombosis. This complication is rare. However, it has been reported by several authors and is associated with injections into large segments of varicose veins ranging in size from 8 mm or more, using high concentration agents. Difficulty in mobilization of the patient, bed rest, or sitting for prolonged periods of time contribute to increase the incidence of this complication. If unusual swelling or pain develops after the injection, examine the deep system with duplex scanning as soon as possible.

Anaphylactic Reactions. This complication has been greatly reduced with the use of the modern and more purified sclerotherapy agents. However, any physician performing sclerotherapy should be prepared to manage a major anaphylactic reaction. A kit containing oxygen, epinephrine, and injectable steroids should be available at all times.

Matting. Matting is the development of a reddish area of very fine vessels that appear in the surroundings of the injected vein. It occurs in 10–30% of all patients treated for telangiectasia and in about 15% of all patients treated for varicosities of larger vessels. Matting often resolves spontaneously within a year. Sometimes the problem may be permanent. Hormone therapy and obesity contribute to a higher incidence of matting (Fig. 14.14).

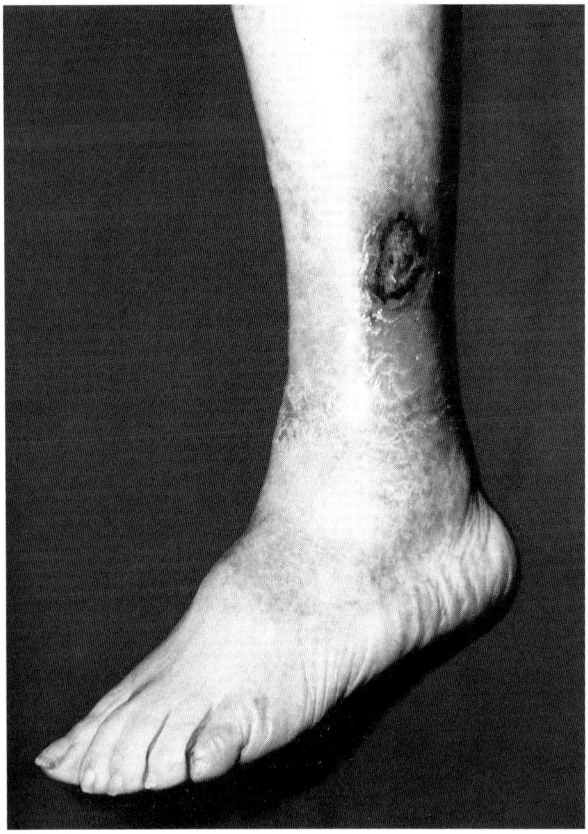

FIG. 14–13. Extravasation of a highly concentrated sclerosing agent. Deep tissue necrosis may require skin grafting.

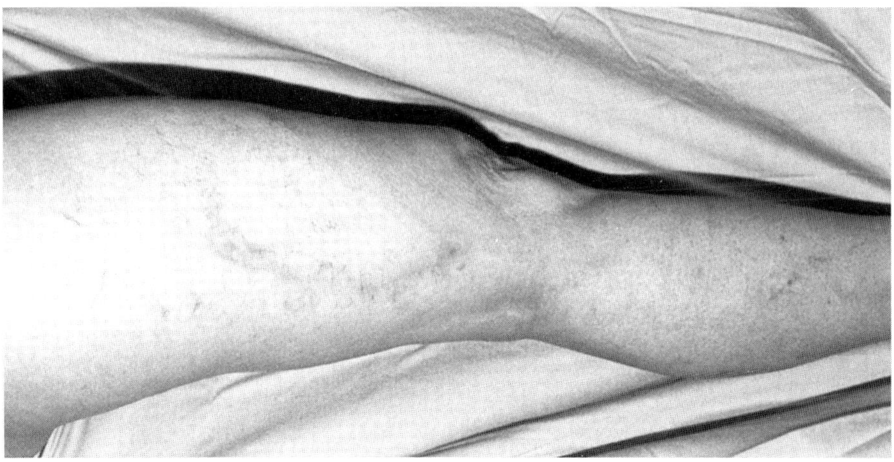

FIG. 14–14. Neovascularization or "matting" consists of a reddish area of very fine vessels that appear in the surroundings of the injected vein. In this case, a 4-mm diameter vein had been injected 4 weeks earlier. Matting occurs in 10–30% of all patients treated for telangiectasia and in about 15% of patients treated for varicosities of larger veins.

Visual Manifestation. Bright lights, migraine headaches, dizziness, and hypotension are rare manifestations, but the physician should be aware of their occurrence.

Intra-arterial Injection. This complication is serious and often leads to gangrene. There are certain dangerous areas that should be avoided. The posterior tibial artery is susceptible to this complication because of its superficial position. The saphenofemoral and saphenopopliteal junctions are high risk areas and should always be approached surgically.

Compression after Sclerotherapy

Although there are physicians who do not use compression after a session of sclerotherapy, there are reasons to suggest that compression is useful even in vessels of a small diameter:

(a) A more effective fibrosis of the vessel can be obtained when there is direct apposition of the vessel walls.
(b) Compression will decrease the extent of thrombus formation in the injected vessel. When the thrombus is minimized, there is a lesser degree of pigmentation.
(c) Good compression will improve the efficiency of the calf muscle pump and will prevent the extension of the thrombus into the deep system.
(d) Compression decreases the amount of discomfort secondary to the injection. The duration of compression for veins other than telangiectasia must be for a minimum of 1 week. In most European centers that follow the schools of Sigg and Fegan, compression is applied for 3 weeks.

Results

Excellent results can be obtained when the principles and guidelines of sclerotherapy are followed. Complete disappearance of the varicosities may be observed as soon as a month after a single treatment (Fig. 14.15**A** and **B**). Most often, several sessions are necessary to eliminate the unsightly venules and telangiectasia (Fig. 14.16**A** and **B**).

LASER AND ELECTRODESICCATION IN THE MANAGEMENT OF TELANGIECTASIA

Electrodesiccation was used extensively by our group from 1968 to 1982 in the management of telangiectasia and other venous blemishes 1 mm or less. Even though we used specially designed apparatuses to vary the intensity of the electrical current necessary to destroy the tiny cutaneous vessels, the procedure produced varying degrees of pain and small hypopigmented scars. In an effort to decrease or prevent the dermal necrosis induced by electrodesiccation, special

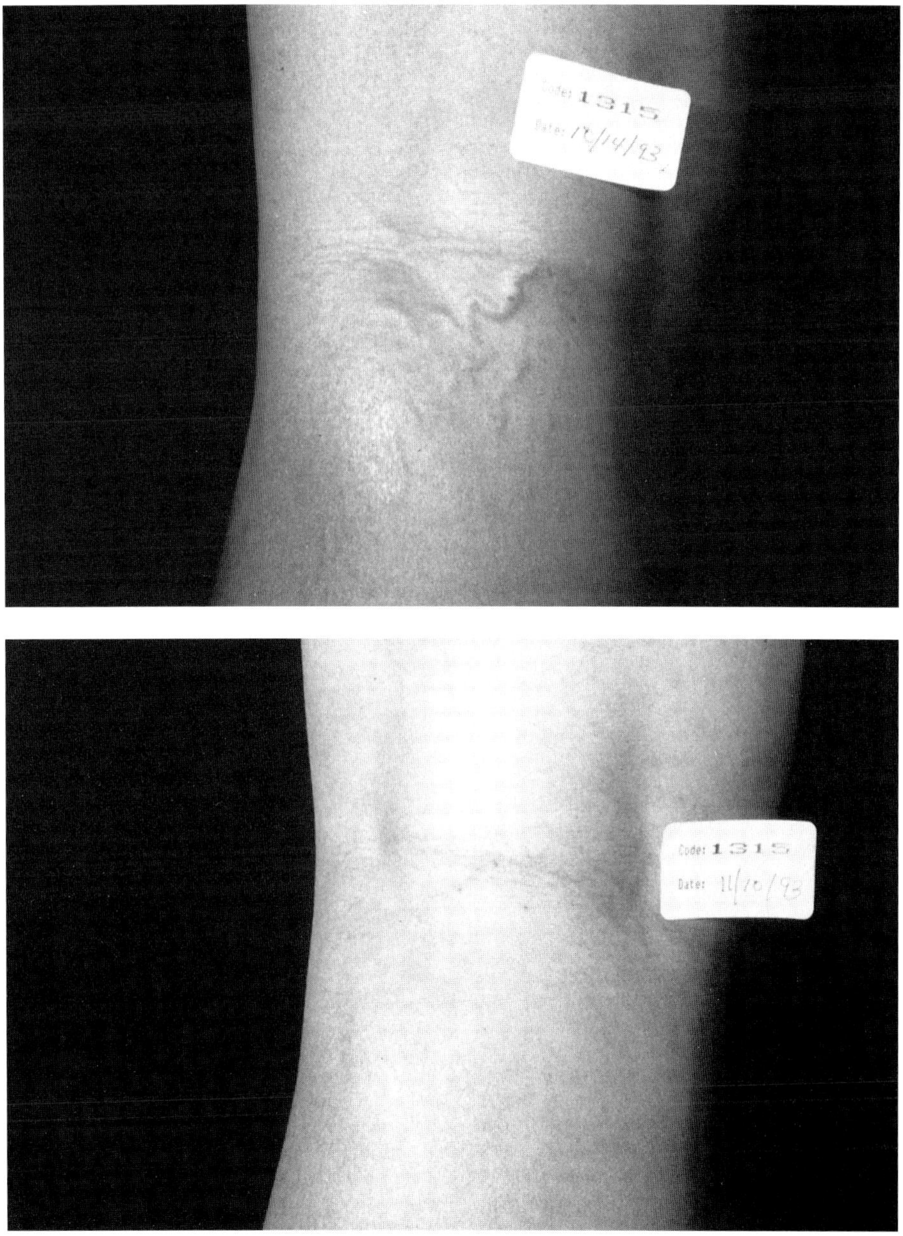

A

B

FIG. 14–15. A. A 3.5-mm vein before treatment. **B.** Complete disappearance of the varicosities is observed as soon as 4 weeks after a single treatment.

insulated super-fine needles have been developed by the electro-medical industry. The needles have an insulated shaft which leaves 1 mm bare at the tip. This allows the needle to be introduced producing minimal dermal scarring. Since the procedure produces varying degrees of pain, and patients have different toler-

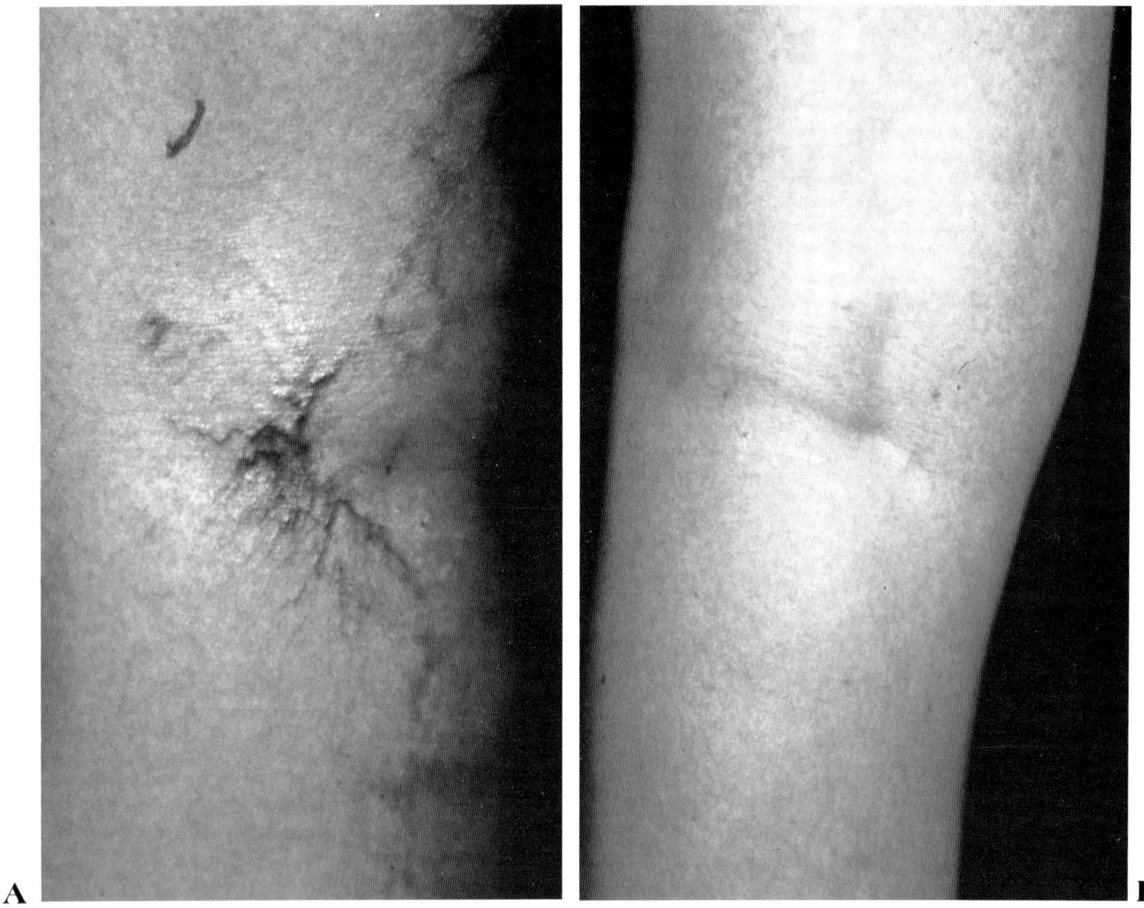

FIG. 14–16. **A.** Complex lesion formed by venules and telangiectasia over the popliteal area. (Courtesy of Dr. D. Duffy.) **B.** Five sessions and 11 months were necessary to eliminate the unsightly lesion. Excellent results can usually be obtained following the principles of sclerotherapy. (Courtesy of Dr. D. Duffy.)

ance levels to the electrical stimuli, we utilize a light epidural anesthesia in patients with extensive telangiectasia on both extremities. In this manner, with the assistance of a second operator in one single session, both extremities can be treated simultaneously. The attractiveness of this modality of treatment is that it saves the patient considerable time, decreases the number of office visits, and, especially, eliminates completely the pain factor.

Lasers were received with great enthusiasm in 1975 and many centers acquired the costly machines which promised to be the solution for the problem of telangiectasia and other skin blemishes. However, the laser's adverse effects, such as cutaneous necrosis, varying degrees of pain similar to electrodesiccation, hypo- or hyperpigmentation, and its relative ineffectiveness compared with other forms of treatment, have been powerful reasons to abandon this method for the management of the blue telangiectasia. Lately, new forms of lasers have been introduced as effective treatment for capillary hemangiomas, such as the portwine stain of some congenital vascular malformations, and in the management of red telangiectasia, postsclerotherapy pigmentation, and other adverse effects of sclerotherapy (17, 18).

DISCLAIMER

These guidelines represent the consensus of a group of physicians with expertise in sclerotherapy. They should not be considered, however, as the only manner in which to practice sclerotherapy. It is recognized that there are alternative techniques that render acceptable results. The statements and recommendations contained in these guidelines are general in nature. Each patient should be considered and treated on an individual basis. The final decision on the procedure of choice rests on the physician after he has analyzed the needs of the patient.

REFERENCES

1. Trendelenburg FV. Über die Unterbindung der Vena Saphena Magna bei Unterschenkelvarizen. Beiträge zur Klinischen Chirurgie 1890;7:195.
2. Keller WL. A new method of extirpating the internal saphenous and similar veins in varicose conditions: a preliminary report. NY Med J 1905;82:385.
3. Mayo CH. The surgical treatment of varicose veins. St. Paul Med J 1904;6:695.
4. Mayo CH. Treatment of varicose veins. Surg Gynecol Obstet 1906;2:385.
5. Babcock WW. A new operation for the extirpation of varicose veins of the leg. NY Med J 1907;86:153.
6. McPheeters HO. Injection treatment of varicose veins by the use of sclerosing solutions. Surg Gynecol Obstet 1927;45:541–547.
7. Dixon FC. The results of injection treatment of varicose veins. Proc Staff Meet Mayo Clin 1930;5:42.
8. McPheeters HO. Injection treatment of varicose veins. Am J Surg 1930;10:19–31.
9. De Takats G. Causes of failure in the treatment of varicose veins. JAMA 1931;96:1111–1114.
10. Smith FL. Varicose veins, complications and results of treatment of 5,000 patients. Military Surg 1939;85:514.
11. Ochsner A, Mahorner HR. The modern treatment of varicose veins. Surgery 1937;2:889.
12. Waugh JM. Ligation and injection of great saphenous veins. Proc Staff Meet Mayo Clin 1941;16:832.
13. Hobbs JT. Surgery and sclerotherapy in the treatment of varicose veins. Arch Surg 1974;109:793–796.
14. Einarsson E, Eklof B, Neglen P. Sclerotherapy or surgery for varicose veins: a prospective, randomized study. Phlebology 1993;8:22–26.
15. Myers TT. Results and technique of a stripping operation for varicose veins. JAMA 1957;163:87.
16. Bishop CCR, Fronek HS, Fronek A, Dile RB, Bernstein EF. Real time color duplex scanning sclerotherapy of the greater saphenous vein. J Vasc Surg 1991;14:505–508.
17. Goldman MP, Fitzpatrick RE. Pulsed dye laser treatment of leg telangiectasiae: with and without simultaneous sclerotherapy. J Dermatol Surg Oncol 1990;16:338–344.
18. Goldman MP. Post-sclerotherapy hyperpigmentation: treatment with a flashlamp excited pulsed dye laser. J Dermatol Surg Oncol 1992;18:417–422.

SUGGESTED READINGS

1. Villavicencio JL, Gomez ER, Coffey JA, Lauer CG, Rich NM. What the vascular surgeon should know about sclerotherapy in the management of varicose veins. In: Veith FJ, ed. Current critical problems in vascular surgery. Vol 3. St. Louis: Quality Medical Publishing Company, 1991:128–134.
2. Bergan JJ, Goldman MP, eds. Varicose and telangiectatic leg veins: diagnosis and treatment. St. Louis: Quality Medical Publishing Company, 1993.
3. Bohler-Sommeregger K, Karnel F, Schuller-Petrovic S, et al. Do telangiectasia communicate with the deep venous system? J Dermatol Surg Oncol 1992;18:403–406.
4. Dodd H, Cockett FB. Pathology and surgery of the veins of the lower limb. 2nd ed. Edinburgh: Churchill Livingstone, 1976:106.
5. Hobbs JT. The management of varicose veins. Surg Ann 1980;12:169.
6. Bodian EL. Techniques of sclerotherapy for sunburst venous blemishes. J Dermatol Surg Oncol 1985;11:696–704.
7. Duffy DM. Small vessel sclerotherapy: an overview. Adv Dermatol 1988;3:221–242.
8. Fegan GW. Treatment of varicose veins by injection compression: a method practiced in Eire. In: Hobbs JT, ed. The treatment of venous disorders. Philadelphia: JB Lippincott, 1977:99–112.
9. Sadick NS. Sclerotherapy of varicose and telangiectatic leg veins: minimal sclerosant concentration of hypertonic saline and its relationship to vessel diameter. J Dermatol Surg Oncol 1991;17:65–70.
10. Weiss RA, Weiss MA. Doppler ultrasound findings in reticular veins of the thigh, subdermic lateral venous system, and implications for sclerotherapy. J Dermatol Surg Oncol 1993;19:947–52.
11. Fegan WG. Continuous compression technique of injecting varicose veins. Lancet 1963;2:109–12.
12. Goldman MP. Sclerotherapy treatment of varicose and telangiectatic leg veins. 2nd ed. St. Louis: Mosby Yearbook, 1995.
13. Carlin MC, Ratz JL. Treatment of telangiectasia: comparison of sclerosing agents. J Dermatol Surg Oncol 1987;13:1181–1184.
14. Browse NL, Burnand KG, Thomas ML. Diseases of the veins: pathology, diagnosis and treatment. Baltimore: Edward Arnold, 1988.
15. Goldman MP, Bennett RG. Treatment of telangiectasia: a review. J Am Acad Dermatol 1987;17:167–182.
16. Imhoff E, Stemmer R. Classification and mechanism of action of sclerosing agents. Phlebologie 1969;22:145–148.
17. Green D. Mechanism of action of sclerotherapy. Semin Dermatol 1993;12:88–97.
18. Bergan JJ, Yao JST. Venous disorders. Philadelphia: WB Saunders, 1991.
19. Goren G. Injection sclerotherapy for varicose veins; history and effectiveness. Phlebology 1991;6:7–11.
20. Neglén P, Einarsson E, Eklof B. High tie with sclerotherapy for saphenous vein insufficiency. Phlebology 1986;1:105–111.
21. Goldman MP, Weiss RA, Bergan JJ. Diagnosis and treatment of varicose veins, a review. J Am Acad Dermatol 1994;31:393–413.

chapter 15

Conservative Management of Chronic Lower Extremity Venous Insufficiency

John C. Mayberry, Gregory L. Moneta, and John M. Porter

Chronic lower extremity venous insufficiency is increasingly recognized as a significant worldwide health problem. Nearly 30% of adults in the United States and up to 55% in Europe exhibit lower extremity venous abnormalities and from one-sixth to one-half of these experience significant clinical manifestations (1–3). An estimated 1.5% of the adult population have or have had venous stasis ulceration (2). Since up to one-third of patients with venous insufficiency have documented limitations in their ability to work outside the home (4, 5), it is not surprising chronic venous insufficiency represents an important cause of time loss from work in Western society (6).

Interestingly, the optimal management of chronic venous insufficiency, including stasis ulceration, remains controversial. Numerous imaginative surgical procedures, bandaging techniques, and wound care protocols have been advocated. Conservative management involves a program of strict adherence to ambulatory compression therapy. A detailed description of this approach to patients with symptomatic venous disease is provided here.

PATHOGENESIS

A familiarity with current theories of the pathogenesis of chronic lower extremity venous insufficiency (CLEVI) is necessary to effectively evaluate appropriate treatment options. Underlying chronic venous insufficiency is the insufficient venous valve (7). Venous valves, which in the normal condition prevent significant distal reflux, exist in both the superficial and deep venous systems of the lower extremity and are believed to be present in the communicating veins of the malleoli and calf. When venous valves are competent, the calf muscle pump augments cephalad ambulatory venous flow, and ambulatory venous pressure

TABLE 15-1

SIGNS AND SYMPTOMS OF CHRONIC LOWER EXTREMITY VENOUS INSUFFICIENCY (CLEVI)

1. Discomfort* (ambulatory or nonambulatory)
2. Edema
3. Lipodermatosclerosis
4. Stasis dermatitis
5. Perimalleolar ulceration

*Including heaviness, fatigue, cramping, burning, itching.

(AVP) at the ankle and foot falls (<30 torr) (8). In patients with deep venous valvular insufficiency the calf muscle pump is disabled and AVP remains high (9–11).

Ambulatory venous hypertension is the presumed basis of the subjective and objective manifestations of chronic venous insufficiency (Table 15.1). Chronically elevated venous pressure is transmitted to the skin and subcutaneous tissues of afflicted patients where it causes dermal capillary proliferation (12), lymphatic destruction (13, 14), excessive colloid filtration (15), and white cell trapping (16). The resultant edema, fibrin deposition, relative hypoxia (17), and inflammation leave the skin discolored, irritated, and prone to ulceration (Fig. 15.1).

In the past, the large majority of lower extremity venous valvular insufficiency was presumed to follow deep venous thrombosis (DVT), hence the term "post-

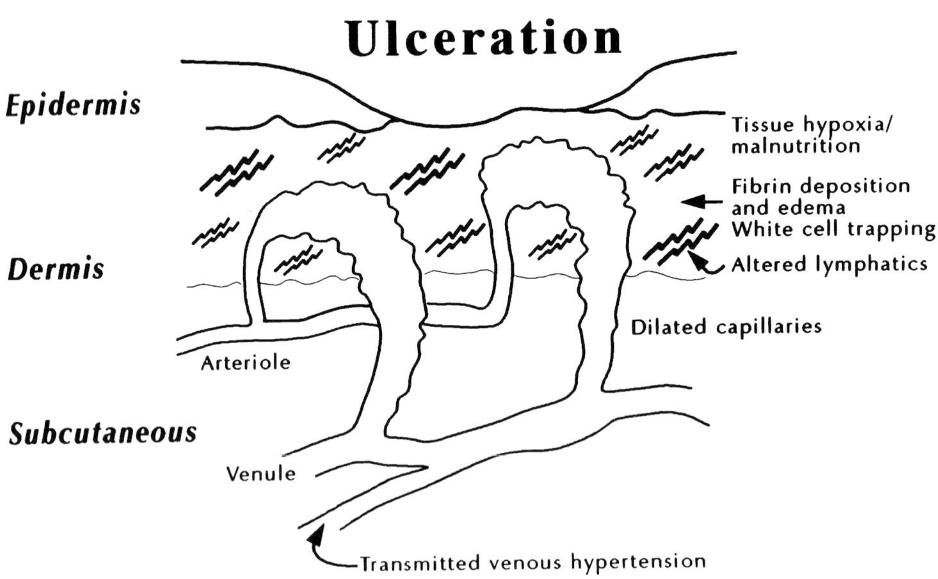

FIG. 15–1. The pathophysiology of venous stasis ulceration. (Adapted and reproduced by permission from Browse NL. The pathogenesis of venous ulceration: a hypothesis. J Vasc Surg 1988;7:470; and Mayberry JC, Moneta GL, Taylor LM, Porter JM. Non-operative treatment of venous stasis ulcers. In: Bergan JJ, Yao JST, eds. Venous disorders. Philadelphia: WB Saunders, 1991:381–395.)

thrombotic syndrome." More recently, however, primary venous valvular insufficiency of unknown, but nonthrombotic, origin has been recognized in an increasing number of patients with venous hypertension (18). In our experience, only 22% of venous stasis ulcer patients have a documented history of lower extremity DVT (19).

Nonthrombotic venous insufficiency may result from genetic defects or developmental anomalies, or may be a consequence of the normal aging process (20). Interestingly, almost two-thirds of venous ulcer patients exhibit venous insufficiency of the contralateral extremity, indicating the largely bilateral nature of this process (19, 21). Patients with insufficiency of one component of the venous system are known to be at increased risk of incompetence throughout the venous system (22–24). Careful vascular laboratory examination of patients believed to have isolated superficial varicosities has revealed a surprising 20% incidence of coexistent deep venous reflux (25).

Superficial venous insufficiency alone, without deep venous involvement, can lead to clinical manifestations of venous insufficiency (26–28), although they are usually mild (29). Discomfort and edema are the most common manifestations and stasis dermatitis and ulceration are rare. In our experience and that of others, isolated superficial venous insufficiency is present in less than 1% of patients with venous ulcers (19, 20).

DIAGNOSIS

Optimal treatment of chronic venous insufficiency is dependent upon the establishment of an accurate diagnosis. There is a myriad of conditions which may mimic the venous insufficiency syndrome (Table 15.2). Confirmatory evidence of venous insufficiency should, therefore, be obtained in the noninvasive vascular laboratory before instituting treatment.

Chronic venous insufficiency is classified according to clinical severity (33). Class 0 identifies those patients who are truly asymptomatic. Class 1 depicts those patients with mild discomfort or edema and minor cutaneous manifestations, while Class 2 includes all patients with hyperpigmentation and brawny edema without ulceration. Class 3 CLEVI describes those with severe discomfort, edema, and ulcerative or preulcerative skin changes.

NONOPERATIVE THERAPY

Nonoperative therapy of chronic venous insufficiency consists of three complementary approaches: the use of ambulatory compression, pharmacologic agents, and selected adjunctive measures.

Ambulatory Compression

The cornerstone of conservative treatment of chronic venous insufficiency is ambulatory limb compression. Preservation of mobility and, ideally, normal ac-

TABLE 15-2

DIFFERENTIAL DIAGNOSIS OF CHRONIC LOWER EXTREMITY VENOUS INSUFFICIENCY (CLEVI)

Arteriopathy	Infection
Scleroderma	Bacterial
Polyarteritis	Tuberculous
Rheumatoid	Tropical
Ischemia	Syphilitic
Lymphedema	Systemic disease
Arteriovenous malformation	Congestive heart failure
Dermopathy	Diabetes mellitus
Allergic	Blood cell dyscrasia
Bullous	Ulcerative colitis
Livido reticularis	Poliomyelitis
Atrophie blanche	Malnutrition
Trauma	Etc.
Pressure ulcer	Neoplasm/Malignancy
Factitious	Orthopedic
Trenchfoot	Osteomyelitic
Insect or animal bite	Paget's disease
	Bony neoplasm
	Paraneoplastic syndrome

tivity is the main advantage of these compression modalities. A number of techniques and devices may achieve this goal.

Elastic Compression Stockings. Although elastic compression stockings have been available since the late 1800s, their efficacy was not widely appreciated prior to the observations and product development of the American engineer Conrad Jobst in the middle of the 20th century (36). Jobst, who himself suffered from recurrent venous ulceration, noted a striking reduction in his lower extremity discomfort and edema during and following ambulation in a swimming pool. The original Jobst stocking was developed to mimic the cutaneous pressure gradient on the lower extremity standing upright submerged in water, i.e., relatively high external compression of the foot and ankle with a gradual decrease toward the knee and thigh. An entire industry is now dedicated to developing the optimum elastic compression stocking. Gradient stockings of varying strengths, lengths, materials, and sizes are readily available (37).

The mechanisms of benefit of elastic compression are unclear (38). While some authors believe elastic compression stockings improve deep venous hemodynamics, others have found no changes or clinically insignificant changes. Studies in our laboratory suggest that while elastic compression augments deep venous blood flow of the lower extremity during ambulation, changes in venous recovery time and ambulatory venous pressure are minimal (38). Even when worn

TABLE 15-3

OREGON PROTOCOL FOR THE TREATMENT OF VENOUS STASIS ULCERATION

1. Initial period of bedrest in hospital or at home.
2. Fitting with pressure gradient elastic compression stockings when edema adequately resolved.
3. Daily ulcer cleansing and dry gauze dressing changes.
4. Corticosteroid ointment to areas of stasis dermatitis surrounding ulcer as needed.
5. Continued use of elastic compression stockings posthealing.

long-term, elastic compression stockings do not appear to prevent the gradual deterioration of deep venous hemodynamics following DVT (39, 40). We believe elastic stockings act primarily by counteracting abnormal Starling forces in the cutaneous microcirculation, thereby preventing or reversing cutaneous damage rather than reversing underlying valvular disease. Cutaneous autoregulation may also be improved. Using the laser-Doppler, Belcaro, et al., demonstrated a near-normalization of the venoarterial reflex and resting skin blood flow after 3 weeks of elastic compression stockings in 80 patients with Class 3 skin changes.

The efficacy of ambulatory compression therapy for chronic venous insufficiency was recently confirmed by our 15-year review of 119 patients with venous stasis ulceration treated solely by elastic compression (19). Our protocol for the conservative treatment of venous ulceration is outlined in Table 15.3. Recognizing the importance of leg elevation in resolving edema and initiating ulcer healing, we recommend an initial period of bedrest, usually 5–7 days, either at home or in the hospital. Patients with large ulcerations, significant edema, cellulitis, or unsatisfactory home situations indicating a low likelihood of compliance with bedrest are recommended for hospital admission. Short-term intravenous or oral antibiotics are utilized if overt infection is present.

Following resolution of edema and initiation of healing, patients are fitted with elastic compression stockings and treated on an ambulatory basis. We begin with 30–40 torr below knee gradient stockings. Only occasional patients require 40–50 torr stockings or above knee stockings. Patients are instructed to wear their stockings at all times during the day and to remove them upon going to bed. Wound care consists of daily soap and water ulcer cleansing and dry gauze dressing changes. All other cleansing agents are avoided because of their potential to harm granulation tissue. A below knee noncompression nylon stocking is placed over the dressing. The compression stocking may then be applied without disrupting the gauze dressing. Saline-soaked or moist dressings are not used, as the resultant skin irritation may exacerbate stasis dermatitis. Stasis dermatitis, when present, is effectively treated with topical corticosteroids. The patients must be cautioned, however, not to place any corticosteroid preparation directly on the ulcer. Other topical preparations such as antiseptics, astringents, or antibiotics are strictly avoided. Patients with unusual ankle anatomy with depressions and crevices not effectively compressed by the stocking may have a sponge-rubber wedge placed locally under the stocking.

Following the resumption of ambulation, periodic elevation of the ulcerated extremity is encouraged. Patients are asked to purchase two pairs of stockings to allow for stocking laundering. Stockings are replaced at least every 6 months, or sooner if the fitting becomes loose. Initially, follow-up is on a weekly basis, then extended monthly until the ulcer heals, and annually or semiannually thereafter. At each visit an ulcer photograph is obtained and the importance of compliance with compression therapy is strongly emphasized. All patients are encouraged to continue wearing gradient elastic compression stockings indefinitely following healing.

Following this protocol we achieved complete healing of venous ulcerations in 105 of 113 (93%) consecutive patients in a mean of 5.3 months (Fig. 15.2) (19). Ninety percent of patients were consistently compliant with elastic stockings while their ulcer healed. Over two-thirds of these patients were healed within 4 months. Following healing, 73 patients were available for long-term follow-up. Of 73 patients, 58 (79%) were compliant with the recommendation for elastic compression stockings posthealing. Nine patients (16%) experienced ulcer recurrence at a mean follow-up of 30 months. Recurrence rate calculated by the life table method was 29% at 5 years (Fig. 15.3). In comparison, all patients who were noncompliant with elastic compression stockings had an ulcer recurrence during the follow-up period (Fig. 15.3).

Thus the routine use of gradient elastic compression stockings can be confidently recommended for all symptomatic patients from the time of diagnosis. We also believe the indication for elastic compression stockings should be extended

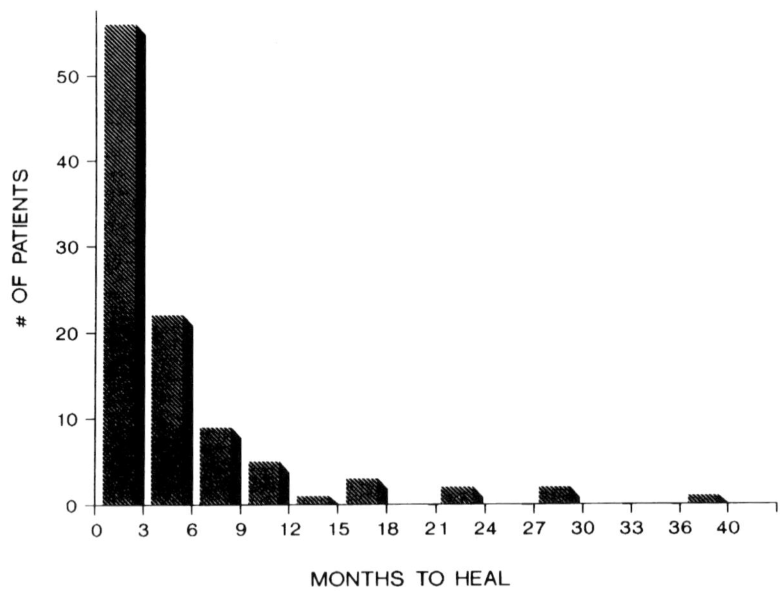

FIG. 15–2. Frequency histogram demonstrating the healing of venous ulcers utilizing the Oregon protocol. The largest group of patients healed in ≤3 months. (Reproduced by permission from Mayberry JC, Moneta GL, Taylor LM, Porter JM. Fifteen year results of ambulatory compression therapy for chronic venous ulcers. Surgery 1991;109:575.)

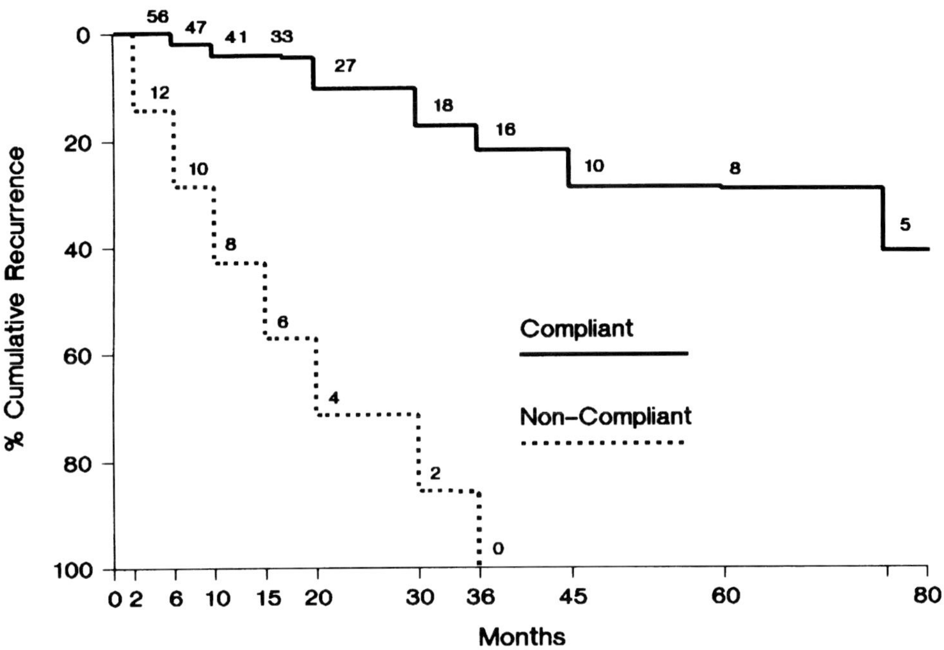

FIG. 15–3. Life table graph demonstrating the recurrence of venous ulceration posthealing comparing those patients compliant with elastic compression stockings and those noncompliant. (Reproduced by permission from Mayberry JC, Moneta GL, Taylor LM, Porter JM. Fifteen year results of ambulatory compression therapy for chronic venous ulcers. Surgery 1991;109:575.)

to asymptomatic patients without varicosities or edema who have vascular laboratory evidence of significant venous insufficiency. The optimal strength and length of stocking to prescribe for a particular patient is unknown and currently is based exclusively on physician preference. In our experience, most patients with severe (Class 3) disease will require at least 30–40 torr gradient stockings. Patients with Class 0, 1, or 2 pathology may find relief and be able to prevent cutaneous deterioration with 20 torr stockings. Unusually configured legs are prescribed stockings by custom fitting (42). For most patients above-knee stockings have no advantage over below-knee stockings (38) and in our practice are rarely prescribed.

Some physicians are reluctant to prescribe elastic stockings because of a perceived high incidence of patient noncompliance. However, in our mixed private/indigent practice, which likely is more representative of venous patients seen in a community vascular practice than many university-based referral centers, we have been able to obtain 79% long-term compliance in patients with Class 3 disease (19). Considerable effort is expended in explaining to our patients the absolute importance of the stocking regimen. We find most patients are quite willing to incorporate elastic stockings into their lifestyle once they understand the basis of their disease. With appropriate persistence, practitioners in the community should expect similar or superior results.

An acknowledged disadvantage of elastic compression stockings is their difficulty in application. This can present an insurmountable hurdle to frail or elderly patients. Several developments in recent years have made a significant impact on this obstacle to treatment. The first is the advent of widespread home nursing care in the United States. Selected patients can be visited daily by nurses and assisted with wound care and stocking placement. We have also begun using stocking placement devices, including the Medi-Butler (Fig. 15.4) and the Sigvaris SOS. These sturdy metal appliances permit the stocking to be loaded by the patient while working on a desktop. By simply stepping into the loaded stocking and lifting the device, the patient is able to apply the tight stocking without significant difficulty. Additionally, the Jobst UlcerCARE system provides a gradient compression stocking with a zipper. Although we have not used this product, satisfactory preliminary results have been reported by others (43).

Unna-style Paste Boots. These time-honored products consist of gauze bandages impregnated with various preparations of glycerin, zinc oxide, and calamine, and are designed to form a firm, yet malleable, compressive shell about the foot and lower leg. Principal advantages are ease of application in an outpatient or home health setting and the option of leaving the boot in place for several days. Although the paste boot is often considered the standard medical treatment for venous ulceration, few long-term studies document its widely perceived efficacy. The limited available data suggest venous ulcer healing rates averaging 30% at 3 months and 70% at 6 months (44, 45). Rubin, et al., obtained 95% ulcer healing at 1 year (46). In the only randomized trial of paste boots versus elastic stockings in the treatment of venous stasis ulcer, no significant difference was found in the resolution of edema, healing percentage, or healing time between the two groups (47).

Disadvantages of paste boot therapy include the development of skin irritation in some patients and the rapid deterioration of compression with time. Blair, et al., found that while initial pressure at the ankle in a series of boot-treated patients averaged 29 torr, after 4 hours ankle pressure averaged only 15 torr and after 24 hours 10 torr ($p < 0.001$) (48). Additionally, since application of the paste boot involves manual wrapping of the impregnated gauze, it is obvious that an optimal declining pressure gradient up the leg will not be reliably obtained. It is, in fact, quite possible to apply the boot erroneously with a reverse gradient tourniquet effect (49).

Ace-type Elastic Bandage. Bandaging ulcerated legs with wraps, elastic or otherwise, dates at least to the time of Hippocrates. In the first half of the 20th century, elastic bandages provided one of the few alternatives to the paste boot. We are aware of only two studies documenting their efficacy in the treatment of venous ulceration. In 1956, Anning, a dermatologist, reported 100% ulcer healing over an unspecified time (50). A similar, more recent study found 65% healing in 12 months but a disappointing 19% 2-month recurrence (51). As might be expected, elastic wraps are also known to rapidly lose their compressive effects with normal activity (52).

Blair, et al., have described the addition of an adhesive, elastic crepe wrap (Coban) to the outer layer of the elastic wrap with the hope that the compressive

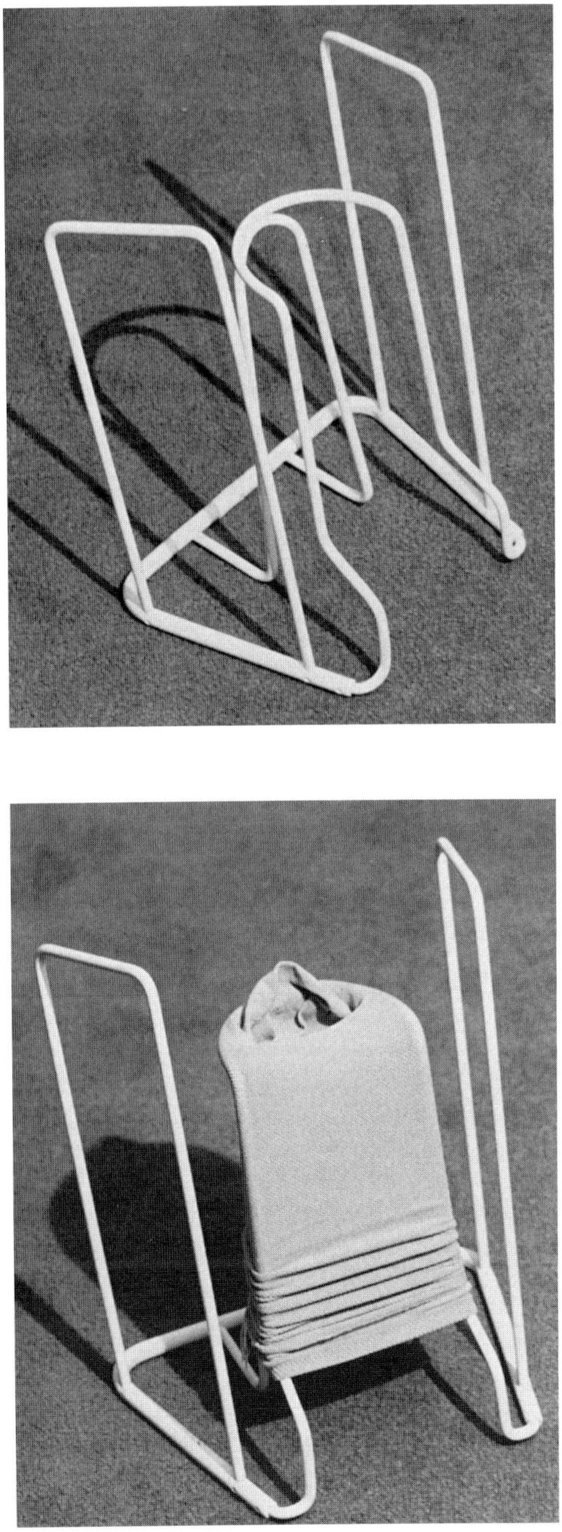

A

B

FIG. 15–4. The Medi-Butler stocking placement device facilitates the application of elastic compression stockings (**A**). **B** through **D** illustrate the stocking being loaded onto the device and sequentially fitted onto the lower leg. (Reproduced by permission from Mayberry JC, Moneta GL, Taylor LM, Porter JM. Non-operative treatment of venous stasis ulcers. In: Bergan JJ, Yao JST, eds. Venous disorders. Philadelphia: WB Saunders 1991:381–395.)

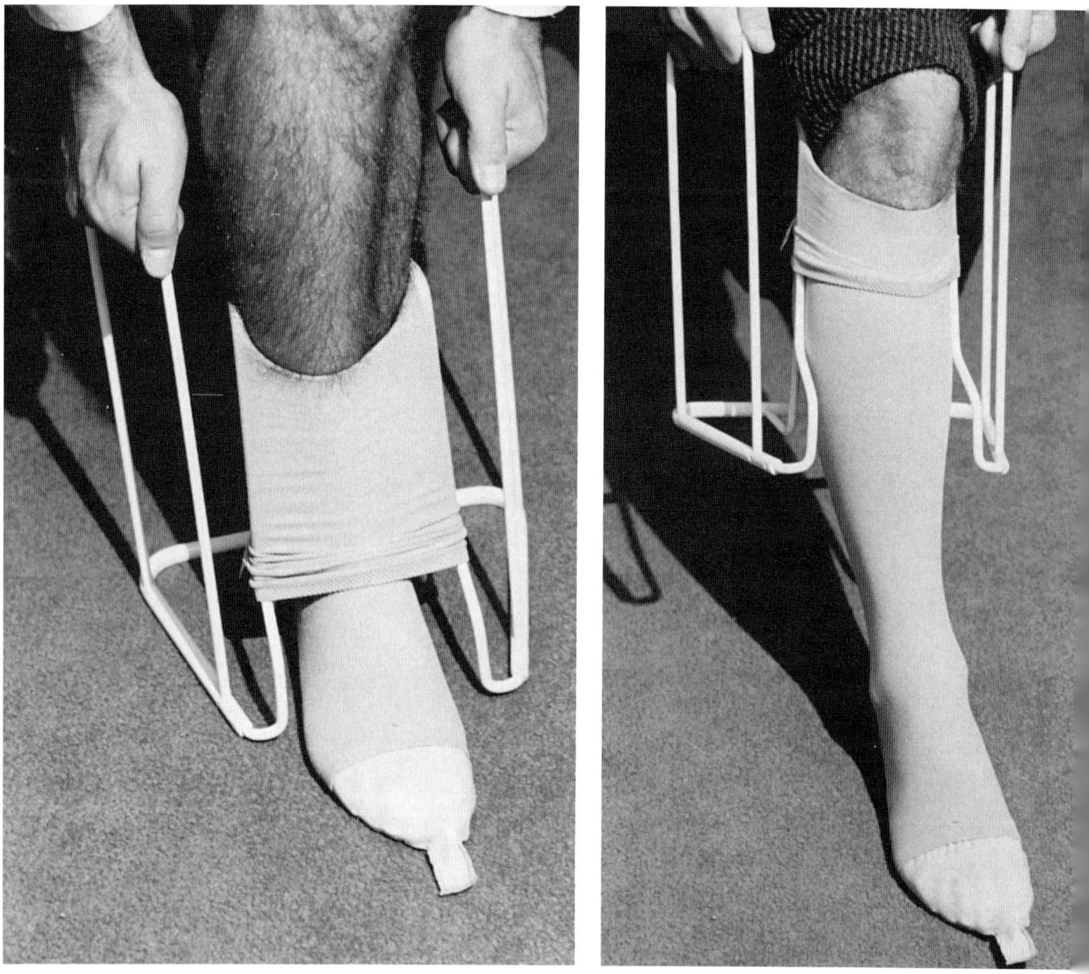

C

FIG. 15–4. Continued.

effect would be more stable (48). Ankle pressure achieved ranged from 33–50 torr initially, and was not significantly changed after 1 week. Seventy-four percent of venous ulcers treated in this fashion healed within 12 weeks.

Circ-Aid Compression Device. The Circ-Aid device is a Velcro-based wrap available in several sizes and designed for simple self-application (53). Although this device is attractive, its usefulness has not been fully evaluated.

Pharmacologic Agents

Pharmacologic treatment of chronic lower extremity venous insufficiency is rapidly evolving. A new class of medications termed "phlebotropic" or "venoactive" have undergone efficacy trials in Europe with preliminary reports of success (Table 15.4) (54). Additionally, several well-known medications used in the treatment of arterial insufficiency, e.g., pentoxifylline and prostaglandin E_1, are being evaluated for use in patients with venous ulceration.

Phlebotropic Medications. The bioflavonoids (a little-known class of vitamins) have long been suspected to produce beneficial microcirculatory effects (55). Their principal action may relate to a decrease in capillary filtration with a resultant decrease in fluid and colloid sequestration in the interstitial space (54). Marketed under several names in Europe, these medications/vitamins contain various combinations of the flavones rutin, oxerutin, diosmin, and hesperidin. None of these is currently approved for prescription use in the United States (56).

Daflon 500 (90% diosmin, 10% hesperidin) is perhaps the most effective and well-studied of the phlebotropic agents. In a double-blind randomized trial conducted at several centers in Europe, Daflon 500 was found more effective than placebo in alleviation of lower extremity discomfort, heaviness, and burning ($p < 0.01$), and in the relief of perimalleolar edema ($p < 0.001$) in patients with CLEVI (54). Improvements in venous capacitance, venous distensibility, and venous outflow time as measured by venous occlusion plethysmography were also found to be statistically significant. These findings are supported by at least three similar trials (57–59).

TABLE 15-4

PHARMACOLOGIC AGENTS USED IN THE TREATMENT OF CHRONIC LOWER EXTREMITY VENOUS INSUFFICIENCY

Class	Drug	Composition	Actions
Phlebotropic	Diosmin/hesperidin (Daflon 500)	Bioflavonoid	? ↓ capillary filtration
	Hydroxyethylrutoside (Paroven, Venoruton)	Bioflavonoid	? ↓ capillary filtration
	Calcium dobesilate (Doxium 500)	Sulfonated benzene	↓ capillary permeability ↑ red cell flexibility ? ↑ lymphatic flow
Hemorrheologic	Pentoxifylline (Trental)	Theobromine derivative	↓ viscosity ↑ fibrinolysis ↓ WBC adhesion
Profibrinolytic	Stanozolol	Anabolic steroid	↑ fibrinolysis
Vasodilatory	Prostaglandin E_1 (Prostavasin)	Prostaglandin	↑ skin blood flow ↑ tc pO_2 ↓ inflammation
Anticoagulant	Heparin	Heparinoid	↑ fibrinolysis
	Low-molecular weight heparin	Heparinoid	↓ viscosity ? ↓ inflammation

Venoruton, a related oxerutin/flavonoid, has been shown in a randomized, controlled trial to improve the response of skin blood flow to heat (the "venoarteriolar response") and increase the transcutaneous PO_2 in patients with chronic venous insufficiency (60). Although ambulatory venous pressure and duplex-determined valvular reflux did not change, total leg volume (i.e., edema) of patients was significantly decreased. However, in a small, double-blind randomized trial of Paroven (virtually equivalent to Venoruton) no significant improvement in venous insufficiency symptomatology or venous ulcer healing was found (61).

Calcium dobesilate (Doxium 500), a sulfonated benzene compound, was previously known in the United States for its antiplatelet effect (62). Recent studies have suggested a prominent edema-reducing effect, possibly due to increased macrophage-mediated proteolysis (63). Increased lymphatic transport and decreased endothelial response to histamine and bradykinin have also been demonstrated (64). In 1982, Hachen and Lorenz performed a double-blind randomized trial of calcium dobesilate in 50 young women with presumed CLEVI and found significant decreases in lower extremity discomfort and edema (65). Patients also demonstrated plethysmographic improvements in maximal venous outflow and capillary filtration. Casley-Smith of Australia recently confirmed these findings in a double-blind placebo-controlled study of 30 Class 3 patients with previous stasis ulceration (66). Clearly these initial studies of the flavonoid compounds and calcium dobesilate are encouraging. These compounds now merit careful review and investigation in the United States.

Pentoxifylline. This well-known hemorrheologic agent, currently approved for use in vasculogenic claudication (67), may be effective in promoting healing of venous ulceration. In a double-blind, randomized, multicenter study, pentoxifylline used in conjunction with compression therapy nearly doubled the 6-month ulcer healing percentage (64% versus 34%) compared to placebo ($p = 0.03$) (68). Angelides has shown that although pentoxifylline does not affect valvular incompetence in patients with postthrombotic venous ulceration, there are statistically significant improvements in skin blood flow at the ulcer perimeter (69). Pentoxifylline's impact on symptomatology and edema of chronic venous insufficiency has, to our knowledge, not been studied.

Stanozolol. The use of the fibrinolytic anabolic steroid stanozolol arose from an attempt to reduce the pericapillary fibrin deposition characteristic of lipodermatosclerosis. Preliminary studies in symptomatic patients were encouraging, with statistically significant reductions in histologic fibrin deposition (70) and total affected skin surface area (71). Stanozolol was not, however, better than placebo in the single randomized trial comparing its effectiveness to placebo in healing of venous ulcers (72).

Prostaglandin E_1. PGE1 has been advocated as an aid to promote the healing of arterial ischemic ulceration (73). It is a potent vasodilator that may also be of benefit in venous ulcer healing. Rudofsky has documented a significant ($p < 0.001$) reduction in venous ulcer surface area with PGE1 over placebo in 6 weeks (74). This study also demonstrated remarkable improvements in CLEVI symptomatology, edema, transcutaneous PO_2, and stasis dermatitis. A significant disadvantage of PGE1, however, is the current necessity for daily intravenous infusion.

Anticoagulants. Both heparin and low-molecular weight heparin have been used in the treatment of chronic venous insufficiency. Sannazzari found significant improvements in lower extremity discomfort, "skin lesions," plethysmographic venous outflow and capacitance, fibrinolytic activity, and plasma viscosity using both agents in patients with Class 1, 2, or 3 disease (75). Low-molecular weight heparin was slightly more effective than heparin and had statistically less hemorrhagic complications ($p = 0.003$). The requirement for parenteral administration and the potential adverse effects associated with prolonged heparin therapy, such as thrombocytopenia and osteoporosis, would appear to limit the utility of heparinoids in the chronic outpatient setting. The usefulness of oral anticoagulants such as warfarin in chronic venous insufficiency is at present unknown.

Antibiotics

The bacteriology of venous stasis ulceration has been well characterized (76, 77). *Streptococcus fecalis, Staphylococcus aureus,* and enteric Gram-negatives including pseudomonas are the most frequent organisms cultured. However, systemic or topical antibiotics do not significantly improve routine venous ulcer healing (78). An exception, of course, is the occasional patient with overt cellulitis or wound drainage (19). These patients are benefitted by an initial several day course of intravenous or oral antibiotics. Lookingbill, et al., performed ulcer biopsies for quantitative bacterial counts and found ulcers containing greater than 10^5 organisms per tissue gram were less likely to heal (76).

ADJUNCTIVE MEASURES

Although any ambulatory treatment protocol for chronic venous insufficiency should include limb compression, several adjunctive measures appear efficacious, particularly in the healing of stasis ulceration. These include the use of certain medical devices usually employed for other indications, compression venous sclerotherapy, and topical preparations.

Medical Devices

Perhaps the most intriguing of these is the sequential gradient intermittent pneumatic compression device (IPC, Fig. 15.5) commonly used in the prevention of postoperative DVT. Two recent studies have documented its additive effectiveness in the healing of venous ulcers. Pekanmaki, et al., studied eight patients with recurrent ulceration demonstrating significantly ($p < 0.05$) decreased healing time with IPC when compared to the patients' own previous venous ulcer healing time without IPC (79). Coleridge-Smith, et al., performed a randomized study in which 21 venous ulcer patients who received daily 4-hour IPC over compression stockings were compared with 24 ulcer patients treated with compression stockings alone (80). All ulcers in 48% of the IPC-treated patients had healed in 3 months versus 11% of the controls ($p = 0.009$). Although the effect of the additional bedrest in the IPC group was not controlled, these results are suggestive of benefit.

Other modalities suggested to aid venous ulcer healing include ulcer ultrasound (44), infrared laser therapy (81), and hyperbaric oxygen (82, 83). We currently feel there are inadequate supporting data to recommend use of these modalities.

Sclerotherapy

The obliteration of superficial varices by compression sclerotherapy is frequently employed in treatment of venous insufficiency for both symptomatic relief and venous ulcer healing (84). Although the improvement in lower extremity discomfort with sclerotherapy is mostly subjective, one study has shown improvements in venous ulcer healing when surrounding varices (if present) are adjunctively sclerosed (85). Queral, et al., randomized 28 patients with perimalleolar ulceration and adjacent varices to Unna paste boot therapy alone or paste boot therapy plus sclerotherapy (85). Ulcers in patients receiving sclerotherapy healed in a mean of 4.3 weeks versus 6.1 weeks for those treated with the paste boot alone ($p < 0.05$). Although the patient groups and the venous ulcers treated in this study were relatively small, these are impressive healing rates.

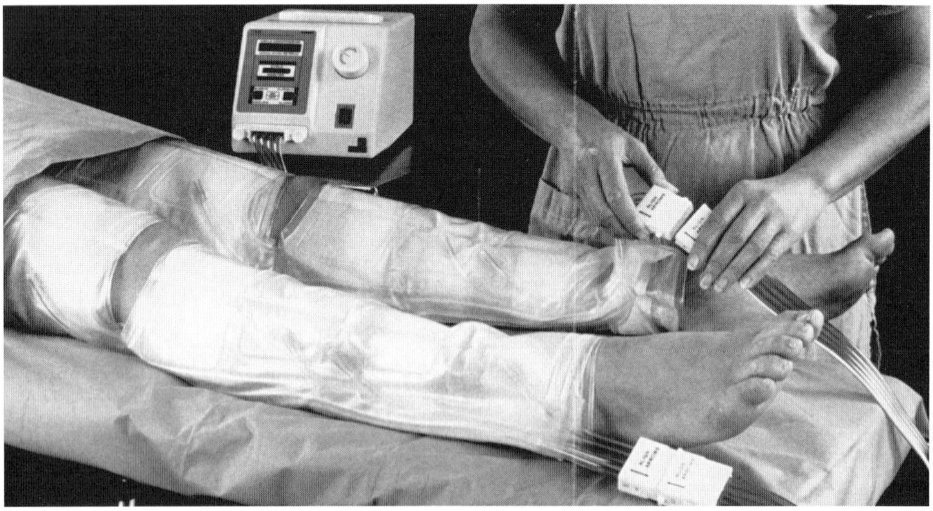

FIG. 15–5. The intermittent pneumatic compression device (IPC) may facilitate venous ulcer healing.

Topical Preparations

Whether a particular dressing or topical agent applied to a venous ulcer can make a significant difference in healing is controversial. Because of the irritable nature of the skin surrounding venous ulcers our preference is to merely cleanse the ulcer daily with a mild soap and water and apply only dry gauze, usually without tape, to the ulcer itself. Topical steroid preparations, although useful in relief of stasis dermatitis, are believed to inhibit wound healing and therefore should not be used on the ulcer itself. Antiseptic solutions such as iodine-containing products and hydrogen peroxide may be more destructive than helpful (86). Clearly, wound sterilization is not necessary for effective healing.

The use of the occlusive, hydrocolloid dressing Duoderm has become popular because of its self-adhesive, semipermeable constitution and creation of a favorable moist healing environment (45). An antipseudomonal effect has also been demonstrated (77). Although the additive effect of a Duoderm dressing beneath elastic stockings has not been studied, Kikta, et al., found 38% venous ulcer healing at 6 months utilizing only Duoderm and intermittent leg elevation (45).

Two topical modalities for wound healing stimulation have shown recent promise. Placental or amniotic growth factors (87, 88) and 2% ketanserin (89), a serotonin antagonist, have been shown in preliminary reports to promote venous ulcer healing. The identification of humoral and local factors instrumental in wound healing appears to be a fertile area of future research in venous disease.

CONCLUSION

Based on our long-term experience, we believe the large majority of chronic venous insufficiency patients, including those with stasis ulceration, can be treated successfully by conservative measures. Ambulatory compression therapy, allowing the continuance of normal daily activity, is the foundation of conservative treatment. We believe the problems of noncompliance and patient dissatisfaction with ambulatory compression have been overemphasized. New pharmacologic agents and nonoperative adjunctive measures show promise for additive, enhanced efficacy of nonoperative therapy, but we remain unconvinced that any combination is superior to elastic compression stockings alone.

REFERENCES

1. Brand FN, Dannenberg AL, Abbott RD, Kannel WB. The epidemiology of varicose veins: the Framingham Study. Am J Prev Med 1988;4:96.
2. Madar G, Widmer LK, Zemp E, Maggs M. Varicose veins and chronic venous insufficiency-disorder or disease? A critical epidemiological review. Vasa 1986;15:126.
3. Widmer LK, ed. Peripheral venous disorders. Bern: Hans Huber, 1978:90.
4. Prevalence of selected chronic conditions, United States 1979–81. Vital and Health Statistics. National Center for Health Statistics. Series 10. No. 155.
5. Gjores JE. The incidence of venous thrombosis and its sequelae in certain districts of Sweden. Acta Chir Scand 1956;206:88.

6. O'Donnell TF, Browse NL, Burnand KG, Thomas ML. The socioeconomic effects of an ileofemoral venous thrombosis. J Surg Res 1977;22:483.
7. Sumner DS. Applied physiology in venous problems. In: Bergan JJ, Yao JST, eds. Surgery of the veins. Orlando: Grune & Stratton, 1985:3–24.
8. Pollack AA, Wood EH. Venous pressure in the saphenous vein at the ankle in man during exercise and changes in posture. J Appl Physiol 1949;1:649.
9. DeCamp PT, Schramel RJ, Ray CJ, et al. Ambulatory venous pressure determinations in post-phlebitic and related syndromes. Surgery 1950;29:365.
10. Sturup H, Hojensgard IC. Venous pressure in the deep veins of the lower extremity of patients with primary and post-thrombotic varicose veins. Acta Chir Scand 1950;99:518.
11. Bjordal RI. Pressure patterns in the saphenous system in patients with venous leg ulcers. Acta Chir Scand 1971;137:495.
12. Burnand KG, Whimster I, Clemenson G, Thomas ML, Browse NL. The relationship between the number of capillaries in the skin of the ulcer-bearing area of the lower leg and the fall in foot vein pressure with exercise. Br J Surg 1981;68:297.
13. Butcher HR, Hoover AL. Abnormalities of human superficial cutaneous lymphatics associated with stasis ulcers, lymphedema, scars and cutaneous autografts. Ann Surg 1955;142:633.
14. Bollinger A, Pfister G, Hoffman U, Franzeck UK. Fluorescence microlymphography in chronic venous incompetence. Int Angiol 1989;8:23.
15. Burnand G, Whimster I, Naidoo A, Browse NL. Pericapillary fibrin in the ulcer-bearing skin of the leg: the cause of lipodermatosclerosis and venous ulceration. Br Med J 1982;285:1071.
16. Coleridge-Smith PD, Scurr JH. Current views on the pathogenesis of venous ulceration. In: Bergan JJ, Yao JST, eds. Venous disorders. Philadelphia: WB Saunders, 1991:36–51.
17. Franzeck UK, Bollinger A, Huch R, Huch A. Transcutaneous oxygen tension, capillary morphology and density in patients with chronic venous incompetence (CVI). Circulation 1984;70:806.
18. Browse NL, Clemenson G, Thomas ML. Is the postphlebitic leg always postphlebitic? Relation between phlebographic appearances of deep-vein thrombosis and late sequelae. Br Med J 1980;281:1167.
19. Mayberry JC, Moneta GL, Taylor LM, Porter JM. Fifteen year results of ambulatory compression therapy for chronic venous ulcers. Surgery 1991;109:575.
20. Raju S. Venous insufficiency of the lower limb and stasis ulceration: changing concepts and management. Ann Surg 1983;197:688.
21. Stacey MC, Burnand KG, Bhogal B, Pattison M. Preclinical changes of lipodermatosclerosis in "normal" limbs [Abstract]. Br J Surg 1988;75:391.
22. Kistner RL. Primary venous valve incompetence of the leg. Am J Surg 1980;140:218.
23. Sumner DS. Site of valve incompetence in chronic venous insufficiency: a possible reason that valve reconstruction may not work. In: Veith FJ, ed. Current critical problems in vascular surgery. St. Louis: Quality Medical Publishing Company, 1989:133–38.
24. Hanrahan LM, Araki CT, Rodriguez AA, et al. Distribution of valvular incompetence in patients with venous stasis ulceration. J Vasc Surg 1991;13:805.
25. Almgren B, Eriksson I. Primary deep venous incompetence in limbs with varicose veins. Acta Chir Scand 1989;155:455.
26. Burnand KG, O'Donnell TF, Thomas ML, Browse NL. The relative importance of incompetent communicating veins in the production of varicose veins and venous ulcers. Surgery 1977;82:9.
27. Sethia KK, Darke SG. Long saphenous incompetence as a cause of venous ulceration. Br J Surg 1984;71:754.

28. Hoare MC, Nicolaides AN, Miles CR, et al. The role of primary varicose veins in venous ulceration. Surgery 1982;92:450.
29. Browse NL, Burnand KG, Thomas ML. Diseases of the veins: pathology, diagnosis, and treatment. London: Edward Arnold, 1988:169–74.
30. Almgren B, Eriksson I. Valvular incompetence in superficial, deep, and perforator veins of limbs with varicose veins. Acta Chir Scand 1990;156:69.
31. Strandness DE, van Bemmelen P. Quantitation of venous reflux using duplex scanning. In: Bergan JJ, Yao JST, eds. Venous disorders. Philadelphia: WB Saunders;1991:137.
32. Abramowitz HB, Queral LA, Flinn WR, et al. The use of photoplethysmography in the assessment of venous insufficiency: a comparison to venous measurements. Surgery 1979;86:434.
33. Porter JM, Rutherford RB, Clagett GP, et al. Reporting standards in venous disease. J Vasc Surg 1988;8:172.
34. Shull KC, Nicolaides AN, Fernandes JF, et al. Significance of popliteal reflux in relation to ambulatory venous pressure and ulceration. Arch Surg 1979;114:1304.
35. O'Donnell TF, McEnroe CS, Heggerick P. Chronic venous insufficiency. Surg Clin N Am 1990;70:159.
36. Bergan JJ. Conrad Jobst and the development of pressure gradient therapy for venous disease. In: Bergan JJ, Yao JST, eds. Surgery of the veins. Orlando: Grune & Stratton, 1985:529–540.
37. Johnson G Jr. The role of elastic support in venous problems. In: Bergan JJ, Yao JST, eds. Surgery of the veins. Orlando: Grune & Stratton, 1985:541–550.
38. Mayberry JC, Moneta GL, De Frang RD, Porter JM. The influence of elastic compression stockings on deep venous hemodynamics. J Vasc Surg 1991;13:91.
39. Lindner DJ, Edwards JM, Phinney ES, Taylor LM, Porter JM. Long-term hemodynamic and clinical sequelae of lower extremity deep venous thrombosis. J Vasc Surg 1986;4:436.
40. Stacey MC, Burnand KG, Layer GT, Pattison M. Calf pump function in patients with healed venous ulcers is not improved by surgery to the communicating veins or by elastic stockings. Br J Surg 1988;75:436.
41. Belcaro G, Grigg M, Vasdekis S, et al. Evaluation of the effects of elastic compression in patients with postphlebitic limbs by laser-Doppler flowmetry. Phlebology 1988;41:797.
42. Horner J, Lowth LC, Nicolaides AN. A pressure profile for elastic stockings. Br Med J 1980;280:818.
43. Young JR, Terwoord BA. Stasis ulcer treatment with compression dressing. Cleveland Clin J Med 1990;57:529–531.
44. Callam MJ, Harper DR, Dale JJ, Ruckley CV, Prescott RJ. A controlled trial of weekly ultrasound therapy in chronic leg ulceration. Lancet 1987;2:204.
45. Kikta MJ, Schuler JJ, Meyer JP, et al. A prospective, randomized trial of Unna's boots versus hydroactive dressing in the treatment of venous stasis ulcers. J Vasc Surg 1988;7:478.
46. Rubin JR, Alexander J, Plecha EJ, Marman C. Unna's boot vs polyethane foam dressings for the treatment of venous ulceration. Arch Surg 1990;125:489.
47. Hendricks WM, Swallow RT. Management of stasis leg ulcers with Unna's boots versus elastic support stockings. J Am Acad Dermatol 1985;12:90.
48. Blair SD, Wright DDI, Backhouse CM, Riddle E, McCollum CN. Sustained compression and healing of chronic venous ulcers. Br Med J 1988;297:1159.
49. Lawrence D, Kakkar VV. Graduated, static, external compression of the lower limb: a physiological assessment. Br J Surg 1980;67:119.
50. Anning ST. Leg ulcers—the results of treatment. Angiology 1956;7:505.

51. Kitahama A, Elliott LF, Kerstein MD, Menendez CV. Leg ulcer: conservative management or surgical treatment? JAMA 1982;247:197.
52. Raj TB, Goddard M, Makin GS. How long do compression bandages maintain their pressure during ambulatory treatment of varicose veins? Br J Surg 1980;67:122.
53. Villavicencio JL, Rich NM, Salander JM, et al. Leg ulcers of venous origin. In: Cameron JL, ed. Current surgical therapy. Toronto: BC Decker Inc., 1989:610–618.
54. Tsouderos Y. Are the phlebotonic properties shown in clinical pharmacology predictive of a therapeutic benefit in chronic venous insufficiency? Int Angiol 1989;8:53.
55. Weininger J, Briggs GM. Bioflavonoids. In: Goodhart RS, Shils ME, eds. Modern nutrition in health and disease. Philadelphia: Lea and Febiger, 1980:279–281.
56. Drug Consultation Service, University Hospital, Portland, OR.
57. Balas P, Pagratis N. Vital capillaroscopy on microcirculation: pharmacologic activity of Daflon 500 mg in venous insufficiency. Int Angiol 1989;8:51.
58. Cospite M, Dominici A. Double blind study of the pharmacologic and clinical activities of 5682 SE in venous insufficiency. Advantages of the new micronized form. Int Angiol 1989;8:61.
59. Guillot B, Guilhou JJ, de Champvallins M, Mallet C, Moccatti D, Pointel JP. A long-term treatment with a venotropic drug: results on efficacy and safety of Daflon 500 mg in chronic venous insufficiency. Int Angiol 1989;8:67.
60. Belcaro G, Rulo A, Candiani C. Evaluation of the microcirculatory effects of Venoruton in patients with chronic venous hypertension by laser-Doppler flowmetry, transcutaneous PO_2 and PCO_2 measurements, leg volumetry and ambulatory venous pressure measurements. Vasa 1989;18:146.
61. Mann RJ. A double blind trial of oral O.B-hydroxyethyl-rutosides for stasis leg ulcers. Br J Clin Pract 1981;35:79–81.
62. Gloviczki P, Fowl RJ, Hollier LH, Dewanjee MK, Plate G, Kaye MP. Prevention of platelet deposition by ibuprofen and calcium dobesilate in expanded polytetrafluoroethylene vascular grafts. Am J Surg 1985;150:589.
63. Casley-Smith JR. The effects of calcium dobesilate on acute lymphoedema (with and without macrophages) and on burn oedema. Lymphology 1985;18:37.
64. Widmer L, Biland L, Barras JP. Doxium 500 in chronic venous insufficiency: a double-blind, placebo-controlled multicentre study. Int Angiol 1990;9:105.
65. Hachen HJ, Lorenz P. Double-blind clinical and plethysmographic study of calcium dobesilate in patients with peripheral microvascular disorders. Angiology 1982;33:480.
66. Casley-Smith JR. A double-blind trial of calcium dobesilate in chronic venous insufficiency. Angiology 1988;39:853.
67. Porter JM, Cutler BS, Lee BY, et al. Pentoxifylline efficacy in the treatment of intermittent claudication. Am Heart J 1982;104:66.
68. Colgan MP, Dormandy JA, Jones PW, Schraibman IG, Shanik DG, Young RAL. Oxpentifylline treatment of venous ulcers of the leg. Br Med J 1990;300:972.
69. Angelides NS, von der Ahe CAW. Effect of oral pentoxifylline therapy on venous lower extremity ulcers due to deep venous incompetence. Angiology 1989;40:752.
70. Browse NL, Jarrett PEM, Morland M, Burnand KG. Treatment of liposclerosis of the leg by fibrinolytic enhancement: a preliminary report. Br Med J 1977;2:434.
71. Burnand K, Clemenson G, Morland M, Jarrett PEM, Browse NL. Venous lipodermatosclerosis: treatment by fibrinolytic enhancement and elastic compression. Br Med J 1980;280:7.
72. Layer GT, Stacey MC, Burnand KG. Stanozolol and the treatment of venous ulceration—an interim report. Phlebology 1986;1:197.
73. Porter JM, Edwards JM, Taylor LM. Drugs in vascular surgery. In: Moore WS, ed. Vascular surgery: a comprehensive review. Orlando: Grune & Stratton, 1986:757–758.

74. Rudofsky G. Intravenous prostaglandin E_1 in the treatment of venous ulcers—a double-blind, placebo-controlled trial. Vasa 1989;28(Suppl):39.
75. Sannazzari P. Low molecular weight heparin in the symptomatic treatment of chronic venous insufficiency. Panminerva Medica 1989;31:127.
76. Lookingbill DP, Miller SH, Knowles RC. Bacteriology of chronic leg ulcers. Arch Dermatol 1978;114:1765.
77. Gilchrist B, Reed C. The bacteriology of chronic venous ulcers treated with occlusive hydrocolloid dressings. Br J Dermatol 1989;121:337.
78. Alinovi A, Bassissi P, Pini M. Systemic administration of antibiotics in the management of venous ulcers. J Am Acad Dermatol 1986;15:186.
79. Pekanmaki K, Kolari PJ, Kiistala U. Intermittent pneumatic compression treatment for post-thrombotic leg ulcers. Clin Exp Dermatol 1987;12:350.
80. Coleridge-Smith P, Sarin S, Hasty J, Scurr JH. Sequential gradient pneumatic compression enhances venous ulcer healing: a randomized trial. Surgery 1990;108:871.
81. Sugrue ME, Carolan J, Leen EJ, et al. The use of infrared laser therapy in the treatment of venous ulceration. Ann Vasc Surg 1990;4:179.
82. Bass BH. The treatment of varicose leg ulcers by hyperbaric oxygen. Postgrad Med J 1970;46:407.
83. Wattel F, Mathieu D, Coget JM, Billard V. Hyperbaric oxygen therapy in chronic vascular wound management. Angiology 1990;41:59.
84. Goldman MP. Compression sclerotherapy and its complications. In: Bergan JJ, Yao JST, eds. Venous disorders. Philadelphia: WB Saunders, 1991:233–249.
85. Queral LA, Criado FJ, Lilly MP, Rudolphi D. The role of sclerotherapy as an adjunct to Unna's boot for treating venous ulcers: a prospective study. J Vasc Surg 1990;11:572.
86. Lineaweaver W, Howard R, Soucy D, et al. Topical antimicrobial toxicity. Arch Surg 1985;120:267.
87. Bennett JP, Matthews R, Faulk WP. Treatment of chronic ulceration of the legs with human amnion. Lancet 1980;1:1154.
88. Burgos H, Herd A, Bennett JP. Placental angiogenic and growth factors in the treatment of chronic varicose ulcers: preliminary communication. J Royal Soc Med 1989;82:598.
89. Roelens P. Double-blind placebo-controlled study with topical 2% ketanserin ointment in the treatment of venous ulcers. Dermatologica 1989;178:98.

chapter 16

Cosmetic Excision and Stripping of Varices

Peter Neglén

Varicose veins are subcutaneous dilated tortuous veins. Due to a primary or secondary incompetence of the valves, reflux is present in the varicosities. This may lead to venous hypertension causing symptoms and skin change. Varicose veins of the lower limbs were observed by Hippocrates as early as 500 BC, and later by Celsius and Galen. However, not until the 19th century did Brodie (1) and Trendelenburg (2) demonstrate retrograde flow from the femoral vein to the saphenous system in patients with varices. Subsequently, directed operative treatment by ligation of the saphenous vein at the saphenofemoral junction was introduced by Homan (3) and Trendelenburg (2), and stripping of the saphenous vein was recommended in the early 20th century (4–6). The present trend is selective stripping of the saphenous veins in combination with stab avulsion of local varicosities.

INDICATIONS

Patients suffering from varicose veins may complain of a variety of symptoms ranging from a few localized varicosities of cosmetic concern to large varicose veins with leg swelling, discoloration, eczema, thrombosis, internal rupture with hematoma, or external rupture with hemorrhage which is sometimes substantial. Rarely, varicosities may be the cause of chronic venous ulceration.

OBJECTIVES

Varicose vein disease is a progressive, incurable entity. Although surgery may have radically removed the identified varicosities, the treatment cannot guarantee a cure. The objectives of surgery are to relieve symptoms, minimize complications, provide a satisfactory cosmetic result, and prevent recurrence by complete removal of diseased incompetent veins and control of the points of reflux. Any mode of treatment should adhere to these objectives.

INVESTIGATIONS

The aim of the examination and investigations is to delineate the distribution of reflux (see Chapter 13). Limbs with varicose veins may have a combination of long saphenous, short saphenous, and calf perforator vein incompetence with varying degrees of varicosities. Thorough examination and simple investigation with a handheld continuous-wave Doppler scanner will delineate the extent of varicosities in many patients. However, the positive predictive value of handheld Doppler to correctly identify long saphenous vein incompetence is 83% and the negative predictive value is only 49% (7). With increased clinical severity, and when a more sophisticated surgical approach is taken, a more accurate mapping of refluxing vein segments is necessary. It is then preferable to use noninvasive duplex Doppler ultrasound scanning. This modality is now standard in most vein surgical clinics in the western hemisphere. Phlebography is usually not indicated, but can be helpful in deciding surgical strategy in the treatment of recurrent veins. The global effect on venous hemodynamics may be determined by measuring the venous refilling time (photoplethysmography) or venous filling index (air plethysmography). These tests will not contribute to the indication or strategy of surgery, but may be used to objectively follow the result of the operation on reflux (8, 9). Before removal of varicose veins it is important to ensure that the veins are not functioning as collaterals in limbs with postthrombotic deep vein obstruction or aplasia of the deep venous system as part of a malformation. If these veins are avulsed, the patient will be in a worse situation than before.

VARICOSE VEIN SURGERY

Following preoperative evaluation of the venous system the most important step is the marking of the refluxing veins. Prior to this, the legs should be shaved and cleaned so the markings are not washed away. With the patient in a standing position an indelible black marker is used to carefully outline all superficial-to-deep incompetence and local varicosities in detail (Fig. 16.1). This is essential, because all veins are collapsed in the supine position at the operating table. With bilateral involvement, both legs may be operated on, although this can be very time-consuming.

Depending on the local tradition, resources, and the patient, surgery can be performed under general, regional (spinal or epidural), or local anesthesia. General or epidural anesthesia, even in day-case on "ambulatory surgical" patients, is preferred for patient comfort, as multiple incisions may be required and the procedure time-consuming. The operating table should be tilted 30° "foot up" to minimize bleeding. The position of the patient depends on the type of operation.

The most common primary surgical interventions are the following:

1. Flush ligation of the saphenofemoral junction;

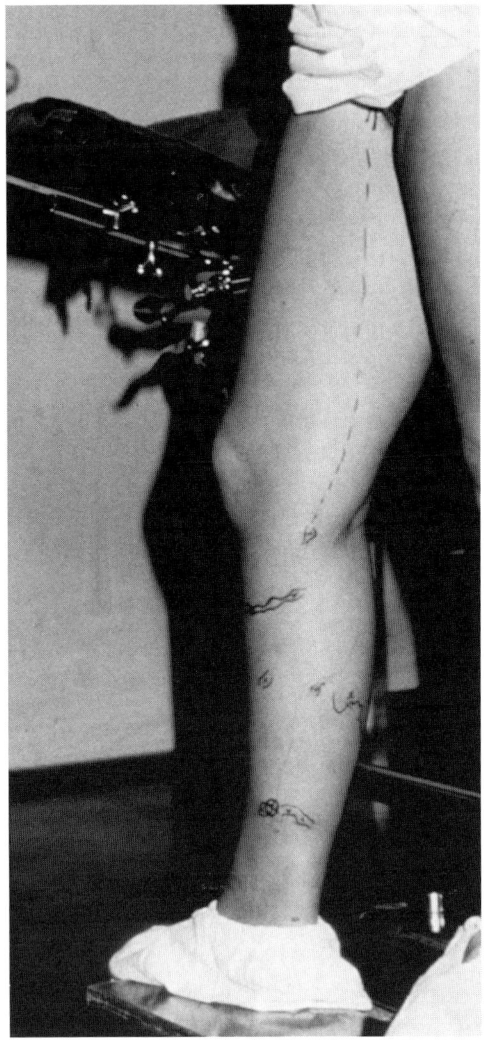

FIG. 16–1. A leg with varicose veins marked-out before surgery. Separate marks (*crosses inside circles*) are used to indicate probable sites of incompetent perforators.

2. Stripping of the long saphenous vein in its entirety or to just below the knee;
3. Local avulsions of isolated varicose vein or branches;
4. Saphenopopliteal ligation and stripping of the short saphenous vein; and
5. Ligation of communicating veins of the medial aspect of the lower leg and elsewhere.

The surgical techniques described in the following sections include steps to prevent as much as possible the recognized causes of recurrence.

Flush "High Ligation" of the Greater Saphenous Vein

Treatment of reflux of the long saphenous vein by ligation near the saphenofemoral junction was introduced at the end of the 1800s. In 1916, Homans pointed out the importance of performing flush ligation of the saphenous vein close to the femoral vein with division of all its tributaries to prevent recurrence (3).

The oblique incision is made just below the crease of the groin over the saphenofemoral confluence. This is the most cosmetic incision because it follows Langer's lines (Fig. 16.2). The length of the incision should be kept as short as possible for cosmetic reasons, but be long enough to assure appropriate visualization of the anatomy of the confluence and subcutaneous veins. By necessity, the incision is longer in obese patients. As the subcutaneous tissue is split and pushed upwards, a large vein is seen, which usually is the main trunk of the saphenous vein. A self-retaining retractor is introduced. The vertically running main trunk is identified and the plane between the subcutaneous fat and the vein's adventitia found. Following this plane proximally, the dissection is simple and bloodless. The branches and saphenofemoral confluence are easily found. The anatomy of the long saphenous vein, its tributaries, and its junction with the femoral vein must be clearly displayed before the main trunk or any large vein is divided. This is the only way to prevent injury or division of the femoral vein or artery with disastrous consequences (10, 11). To use a distally inserted stripper for identification of the long saphenous vein is dangerous, since the stripper may enter the deep system through perforators in a lower position or be pushed too far proximally, leading to dissection and division of the femoral vein (12).

There are six named tributaries joining the long saphenous vein near its termination (Fig. 16.3, *left*). However, there are great variations in number and position. There is not really a "normal" anatomy (13). Therefore, it is necessary to dissect the femoral vein 2 cm above and below the confluence to be sure that no additional branches join the femoral vein directly. The lateral and medial accessory saphenous veins may enter the main trunk anywhere between 0 and 20 cm

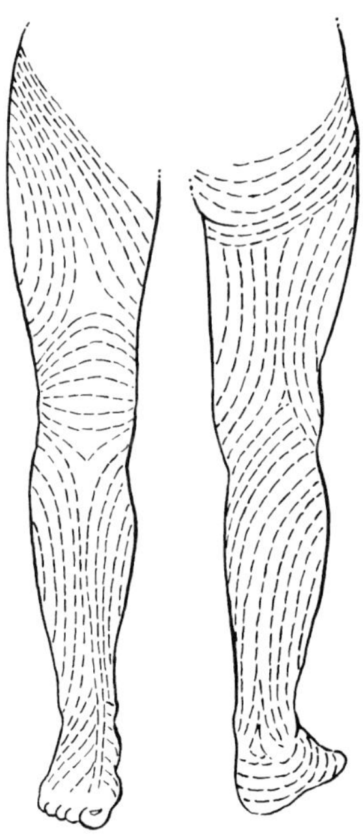

FIG. 16–2. Langer's lines in the lower limb. Skin incisions should be placed along these lines to obtain optimal cosmetic result.

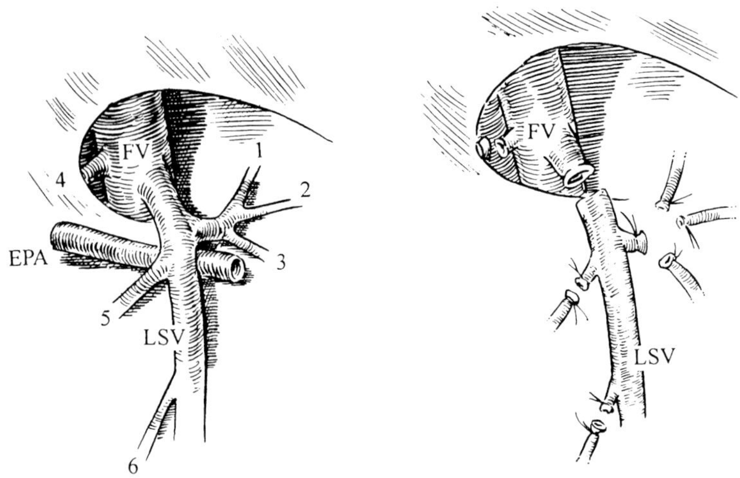

FIG. 16–3. *Left:* This is the most common arrangement of tributary veins at the saphenofemoral junction (38). The external pudendal artery (*EPA*) usually runs between the long saphenous vein (*LSV*) and femoral vein (*FV*), but it may pass above the LSV and is then more liable to be damaged during dissection. *1* = Superficial inferior epigastric vein; *2* = Superficial circumflex iliac vein; *3* = Anterolateral thigh vein (lateral accessory saphenous vein); *4* = Deep external pudendal vein; *5* = Superficial external pudendal vein; *6* = Posteromedial thigh vein (medial accessory saphenous vein). *Right:* All vessels must be individually divided and ligated to prevent recurrence. If no stripping of the LSV is to be performed, the proximal 5–10 cm of the LSV should be resected.

below the confluence. To divide them, it may be necessary to dissect distally for 5–10 cm and retract the skin anteriorly with a right-angled retractor. The external pudendal artery may pass above or below the long saphenous vein. If damaged, it may be ligated and divided with impunity.

The branches are ligated in continuity and divided and tied depending on the exposure. The long saphenous vein is divided and ligated flush to the femoral vein. It is important to avoid narrowing of the femoral vein or placing the tie too far away, creating a stump with risk of thrombus formation. For safety, two ligatures are usually placed on the proximal stump, the second being a transfixion suture. If high ligation of the saphenous vein is the only procedure to be performed, it is important to resect at least 5–10 cm of the saphenous vein (Fig. 16.3, *right*).

The incision is closed by approximation of the subcutaneous tissue using absorbable suture and the skin closed by coapting the edges with fine nonabsorbable or intradermic absorbable suture. The cosmetic result is excellent.

The main intraoperative technical problem is venous injury with copious bleeding. Regardless of the reason, bleeding should be controlled by compression by finger or swab. Under no circumstance should artery forceps be applied blindly or to a side hole in a large vein. More serious venous injuries than the original injury have been made by application of forceps under these circumstances. After a few minutes the compression may be gently removed and the bleeding source located and tied if a branch is bleeding, or directly sutured if a perforation or tear in the vein wall is found.

Stripping of the Greater Saphenous Vein

In the early 1900s, Mayo (4) introduced stripping of the long saphenous vein. The technique was refined by Babcock (5) and later by Myers and Cooley (6). Combined with proper excision of local varicosities with meticulous interruption of all incompetent perforators, this is the "classic" surgery of varicose veins. The recurrence rate is significantly reduced if removal of the vein is performed (13, 14). This is mainly due to interruption of the thigh perforators connecting the deep veins directly with the main saphenous stem. If left in place, they are a source of recurrence. In contrast to these perforators, the calf perforators do not communicate directly with the long saphenous vein, but with the posterior arch vein. Unless the distal saphenous vein is obviously incompetent and varicose, there is no need to remove it. This limited stripping does not endanger the objectives of the operation, leaves a distal vein of potential use for grafting, and avoids injury to the saphenous nerve (Fig. 16.4**A**) (15–17).

With increased demand for autogenous vein graft for reconstructive vascular surgery, saphenous vein-sparing operations have been proposed (18–20). However, it is doubtful that the remaining vein can be used for grafting and the objectives of the varicose vein surgery may be jeopardized with increased recurrence rate (21). For these reasons, most surgeons remove the long saphenous vein at least to just below the knee.

After flush ligation is performed (as described earlier), the divided long saphenous vein is held with an arterial forceps, a transverse venotomy is performed, and a stripper inserted and pushed distally. Either a flexible wire stripper with choice of size of "olives" or a stiffer plastic disposable stripper with reversible heads is used. The passage distally may be facilitated by countertraction of the skin and bending the knee. When the stripper has reached beyond the knee, a small skin incision along Langer's lines is made over the palpable tip. The vein is dissected bluntly, the distal end ligated, and the stripper taken out through a small venotomy. I prefer to strip the vein downwards, since greater lengths of the tributary veins are usually avulsed and the incidence of saphenous nerve injuries is less compared with upward stripping (15).

For cosmetic reasons, the incision below the knee should be kept small. The venous bulk on the stripper may be so large that it needs a large incision to pass through. To avoid this, the vein and stripper can be removed in retrograde direction through the groin incision. The stripper is retrieved by pulling the silk thread attached to the head (22).

If the stripper will not pass distally, the vein must be exposed either medially below the knee or anterior to the medial malleolus. Below the knee the vein is located over the fascia. It is easier to find at the malleolus, but this position should be used only if the intention is to remove the entire vein. It is usually very easy to pass the stripper proximally. If removable heads are used, stripping can still be performed distally after exposing the stripper proximally. After removal, the

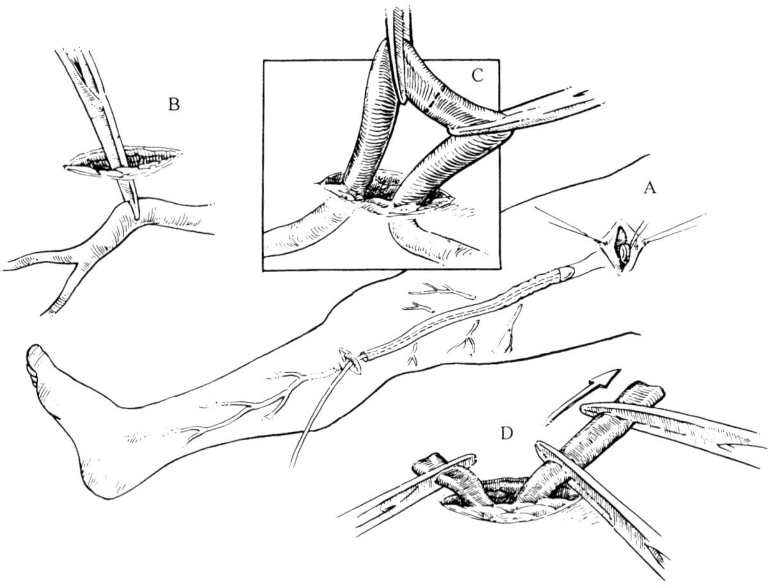

FIG. 16–4. A. Current stripping technique of the long saphenous vein. The removal of the vein is performed in retrograde direction to minimize injury to the nerve and extract longer segments of the torn branches. In most limbs it is sufficient to strip the long saphenous vein to just below the knee, since that interrupts all perforators that connect the superficial femoral vein directly with the proximal long saphenous vein. The calf perforators reach the posterior arch vein, not the distal long saphenous vein. The avulsion of local varicose veins is performed through minimal incisions. The veins are grasped with a fine-tipped artery forceps or vein hook (**B**), pulled out of the wound, divided between forceps (**C**), and carefully avulsed proximally and distally as far as possible (**D**).

vein should be pulled out to assure that it has been totally removed and the site of important tributaries identified. Sometimes a combination of proximal and distal insertion must be used to remove the entire vein. Uncommonly, the stripper will pass in neither direction and the long saphenous vein must be removed piece by piece through several small incisions along Langer's lines.

Bleeding following stripping should be minimized. If blood collects along the stripping channel, the patient may develop a hard, tender cord (pseudothrombophlebitis) in the thigh, which eventually will be absorbed but initially can cause discomfort. To decrease bleeding, the operation table is tilted 30° "foot up" from the start of surgery. Removal of the vein can be performed immediately after insertion of the stripper to allow blood and clots to be expelled by rolling a gauze over the stripping channel. Some surgeons tie a length of roller gauze to the end of the stripper, packing the stripping channel as the vein is removed (22). Others prefer to remove the vein at the end of the operation just before application of compression bandage or after the bandage has been applied. All venous bleeding can be controlled by compression and elevation of the lower limbs. If not, an arterial injury or a bleeding diathesis must be suspected.

Postoperatively, the patient is ambulated as soon as possible. Currently, most varicose vein surgery is performed as day-case surgery with no need for hospitalization. A compression bandage or stocking is worn postoperatively to reduce bruising and edema. Sutures are removed 1 week after surgery.

Excision of Local Varicosities

The flush ligation at the saphenous confluence and stripping of the saphenous veins are most often combined with removal of local varicosities. Traditionally, this was performed through several large incisions, which often left unsightly scars, but the varicose veins were radically removed and recurrence effectively prevented. With increased emphasis on cosmesis, modifications of this technique have been developed. Instead the veins are removed through multiple small (2–5-mm) "stab" incisions (22, 23). Meticulous marking, detailed planning, and great patience are essential. The procedure can be extremely time-consuming with extensive varicose veins. All incisions are small and essentially made along Langer's lines with a fine blade or as a stab incision made with a No. 11 blade. Most incisions are placed longitudinally. In the knee, groin, and ankle region, transverse incisions are preferable. The vein is lifted up with a vein-hook or fine-tipped artery forceps. The vein loop is cleared from fat, double clamped, and divided. Each end of the vein is then gently teased out through the incision and new forceps are placed stepwise until the vein is excised (Figs. 15.4**B**-**D**). Depending on the length of the removed vein, a new incision is made 5–10 cm along the vein and the procedure repeated. A long unsightly varicosity can thus be removed with excellent cosmetic results.

The small skin incisions can be closed by steri-strips or approximated with fine nonabsorbable sutures.

POPLITEAL FOSSA DISSECTION AND SHORT SAPHENOUS VEIN STRIPPING

Some surgeons recommend the entire removal of the short saphenous vein when it is incompetent. Other surgeons only disconnect it from the popliteal vein and resect about 5 cm of its proximal part since it is rarely incompetent throughout its length. It is important to recognize that the position of the saphenopopliteal junction in relation to the knee joint varies greatly (in 57% just above the joint, 33% high above, and 10% below) (Fig. 16.5) (24–26). It is very important to find the level of termination. Clinical examination and continuous-wave Doppler examination are inaccurate. Preoperative duplex ultrasound scan (27) has supplanted varicography (28) and intraoperative phlebography (29) and gives better information.

Preferably, the patient is placed in a prone position to explore the popliteal fossa. When the long saphenous vein is to be stripped during the same procedure, it is advisable to remove the short saphenous first. To avoid turning the pa-

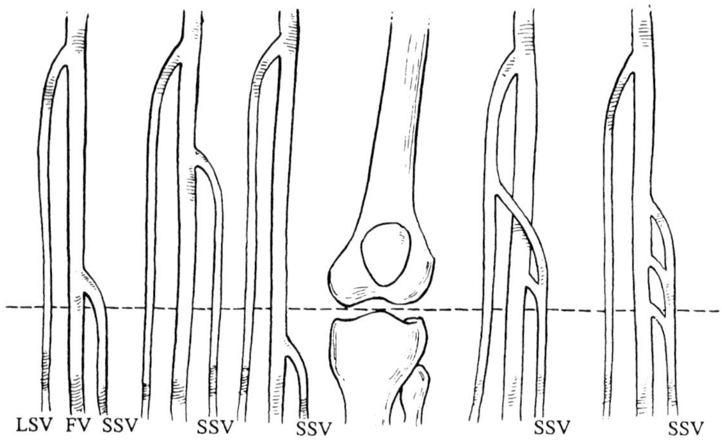

FIG. 16–5. Some types of termination of the saphenous vein in relationship to the knee joint. Giacomini's vein connects the long and short saphenous systems. When multiple connections with the deep system are present, it is difficult to ligate them all.

tient to perform the long saphenous stripping, it is sometimes possible to perform the exploration of the popliteal fossa and the stripping of the short saphenous with the patient positioned on his or her side. After closing the skin, the patient is easily rolled onto the back for the continuation of the operation.

To insert the stripper distally, a short vertical incision is made between the Achilles tendon and the distal fibula. The vein is dissected free from subcutaneous fat and the sural nerve is identified and carefully separated from the vein for several centimeters to avoid injury. The vein is ligated distally, and the stripper is inserted through a transverse venotomy and passed proximally to the popliteal fossa.

A transverse incision is made over the termination of the popliteal vein. The subcutaneous tissue and the fascia are divided, revealing the short saphenous vein as a large vein running vertically in the wound. The stripper can be palpated and used to direct the dissection. Care should be taken to ensure that the stripper has not passed into the popliteal vein, which then may be divided accidentally, with disastrous consequences for the patient. The same rules apply to exploration of the popliteal fossa as to the saphenofemoral confluence, i.e., neither the short saphenous vein nor any large vein should be divided until the confluence is adequately identified.

A large vein often joins the main trunk from above (Giacomini's vein). It must be divided in order to reach the popliteal vein and perform flush ligation (Fig. 16.5). Large veins from the gastrocnemius muscle and other branches may join the short saphenous vein. All tributaries should be ligated. Admittedly, this is sometimes difficult. The dissection may be difficult in a deep and fatty popliteal fossa. After proximal and distal division the short saphenous vein is stripped, preferably in retrograde direction. Great care should be taken to avoid injury of the sural nerve. The skin is closed with attention to cosmesis.

Perforator Ligation

Surgery for perforator incompetence is often required in patients with pigmentation, lipodermatosclerosis, or ulcer. Less commonly, it is done for cosmetic reasons. The site of perforators is difficult to delineate clinically. Pre- or perioperative varicography (30) or preoperative duplex Doppler scanning (31) may be of assistance. The objective is to insure that all perforators are ligated and divided to prevent recurrent varicosities.

If individual perforators can be located, the skin can be incised over the site transversely, following Langer's lines to assure an optimal cosmetic result (32). This is possible only in legs without major skin changes. In other limbs, longitudinal incisions are used. Most commonly, a vertical incision is made 1 inch behind the posterior border of the anteromedial surface of the tibia from the level of the medial malleolus to the midpoint of the calf. The subcutaneous incision is carried straight down without undermining the skin edges. The perforators may be ligated subfascially (Linton's operation) (33) (Fig. 16.6) or extrafascially (Cockett's operation) (34). It appears that the extrafascial procedure is more frequently complicated by necrosis of the skin edges and prolonged healing than the subfascial approach. Dodd, et al., recommend the stocking seam incision posteriorly with the patient in prone position so as to be able to reach medial and lateral perforators through the same incision (35). Others have suggested "blind" subfascial shearing of the perforators through a proximal incision of the leg (36,

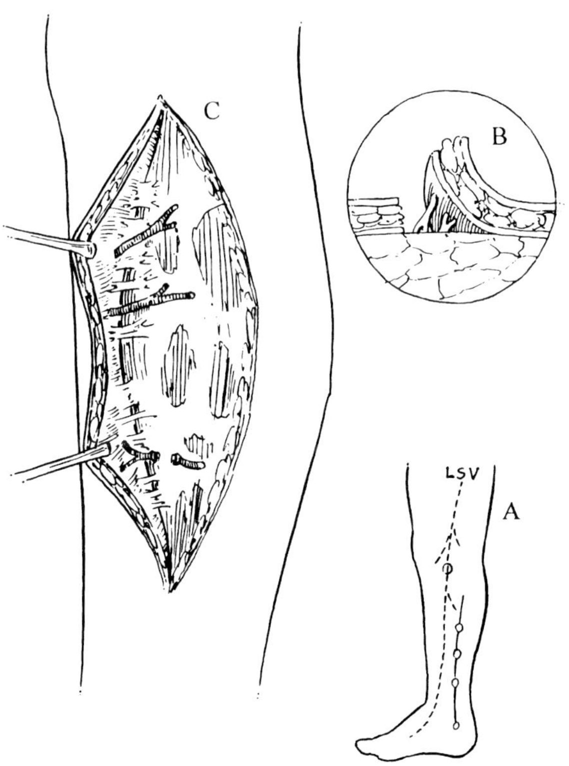

FIG. 16–6. A. The skin is vertically incised along Linton's line over the most common sites of perforators. **B.** The subcutaneous incision is made and the fascia is cut without undermining the skin edges. **C.** The perforators found in the subfascial space are ligated and divided.

37). This is an imprecise method, but one which has been successfully used, especially when the subcutaneous tissue is relatively healthy.

If care is taken to avoid skin necrosis, the cosmetic result is acceptable. It should be remembered that most patients have unsightly pigmentation or venous ulcers and that the cosmetic appearance after surgery is of less importance than the relief of symptoms.

SUMMARY

In varicose vein surgery, it is essential to recognize the expectations of the patient before surgery to correctly inform the patient of the anticipated result. It is also important to warn the patient that varicose vein disease is a progressive disease and that surgery is not a curative but a palliative intervention. The goal of surgery is not only to offer an acceptable cosmetic result, but also to relieve symptoms and prevent recurrences. Therefore, the operation must be directed toward control of the main points of reflux and the permanent removal of varicosities. Using the described techniques insures optimal cosmetic results without compromising functional outcome.

REFERENCES

1. Brodie B. Lectures illustrative of various subjects in pathology and surgery. Vol. III. London: Longmans, Green, and Co., 1846.
2. Trendelenburg F. Über die Unterbindung der Vena Saphena Magna bei Unterschenkelvaricen. Beitr Klin Chir 1890;7:195.
3. Homans J. Operative treatment of varicose veins and ulcers. Surg Gynecol Obstet 1916;22:143.
4. Mayo CH. Treatment of varicose veins. Surg Gynecol Obstet 1906;2:385–388.
5. Babcock WW. A new operation for the extirpation of varicose veins of the leg. NY Med J 1907;86:153.
6. Myers TT, Cooley JC. Varicose vein surgery in the management of the post-phlebitic limb. Surg Gynec Obstet 1954;99:733–744.
7. DePalma RG, Rose SS, Bergan JJ. Treatment of varicosities of saphenous origin: a dialogue. In: Bergan JJ, Goldman MP, eds. Varicose veins and telangiectases: diagnosis and treatment. St. Louis: Quality Medical Publishing Company, 1993:166–188.
8. Christopoulos D, Nicolaides AN, Galloway JMD, Wilkinson A. Objective noninvasive evaluation of venous surgical results. J Vasc Surg 1988;8:683–687.
9. Satin S, Shields DA, Scurr JH, Coleridge Smith PD. Photoplethysmography: a valuable noninvasive tool in the assessment of venous function? J Vasc Surg 1992;16:154–162.
10. Eger M, Goleman L, Torok G, Hirsch M. Inadvertent arterial stripping in the lower limb: problems of management. Surgery 1973;73:23–27.
11. Luke JC, Miller GG. Disasters following the operation of ligation and retrograde injection of varicose veins. Ann Surg 1948;127:426.
12. May R. Varicose veins. In: May R, ed. Surgery of the veins of the leg and pelvis. Stuttgart: Georg Thieme, 1979:82–95.
13. Rivlin S. The surgical cure of primary varicose veins. Br J Surg 1975;62:913–917.
14. Lofgren KA. Management of varicose veins: Mayo Clinic experience. In: Bergan JJ, Yao JST, eds. Venous problems. Chicago: Year Book, 1978:71–83.

15. Jakobsen BH, Wallin L. Proximal or distal extraction of the internal saphenous vein? Vasa 1975;4:240–242.
16. Holme JB, Skajaa K, Holme K. Incidence of lesions of the saphenous nerve after partial or complete stripping of the long saphenous vein. Acta Chir Scand 1990;156:145–148.
17. Negus D. Should the incompetent saphenous vein be stripped to the ankle? Phlebology 1986;1:33–36.
18. Large J. Surgical treatment of saphenous varices, with preservation of the main great saphenous trunk. J Vasc Surg 1985;2:886–891.
19. Hammarsten J, Pederson P, Cederlund CG, Campanello M. Long saphenous vein-saving surgery for varicose veins. A long-term follow-up. Eur J Vasc Surg 1990;4: 361–364.
20. Koyano K, Sakaguchi S. Selective stripping operation based on Doppler ultrasonic findings for primary varicose veins of the lower extremities. Surgery 1988;103:615–619.
21. Neglén P. Treatment of varicosities of saphenous origin: comparison of ligation, selective excision, and sclerotherapy. In: Bergan JJ, Goldman MP, eds. Varicose veins and telangiectases: diagnosis and treatment. St. Louis: Quality Medical Publishing Company, 1993:148–165.
22. Bergan JJ. Surgical procedures for varicose veins: axial stripping and stab avulsion. In: Bergan JJ, Kistner LL. Atlas of venous surgery. Philadelphia: WB Saunders, 1992:61–75.
23. Goren G, Yellin AE. Ambulatory stab avulsion phlebectomy for truncal varicose veins. Am J Surg 1991;162:165–174.
24. Haeger K. The surgical anatomy of the sapheno-femoral and sapheno-popliteal junction. J Cardiovasc Surg 1962;6:420.
25. Kosinski C. The anatomy of the veins of the lower limb. J Anat (Lond) 1926;60:131.
26. Browse NL, Burnand KG, Lea Thomas M. Diseases of the veins: pathology, diagnosis and treatment. 1st ed. London: Edward Arnold, 1988:220.
27. Vasdekis SN, Clarke GH, Hobbs JT, Nicolaides AN. Evaluation of non-invasive and invasive methods in the assessment of short saphenous vein termination. Br J Surg 1989;76:929–932.
28. Lea Thomas M, Bowles JN. Incompetent perforating veins: comparison of varicography and ascending phlebography. Radiology 1985;154:619–623.
29. Hobbs JT. Preoperative venography to ensure accurate sapheno-popliteal ligation. Br Med J 1980;280:1578–1579.
30. Burnand KG. Intéret de la varicographie dans l'appréciation des varices essentielles des membres inférieurs. Phlebologie 1983;1:269–271.
31. Semrow CM, Laborde A, Buchbinder D, et al. Preoperative mapping of varicosities and perforating veins: a preliminary report. J Vasc Tech 1990;14:72–74.
32. DePalma RG. Surgical therapy for venous stasis. Surgery 1974;76:910–917.
33. Linton RR. The communicating veins of the lower leg and the operative technique for their ligation. Ann Surg 1938;107:582.
34. Cockett FB. Diagnosis and surgery of high pressure venous leaks in the leg: a new overall concept of surgery of varicose veins. Br Med J 1956;2:399.
35. Dodd H, Calo AR, Mistry M, Rushford A. Ligation of the ankle communicating veins for the treatment of the venous ulcer syndrome of the leg. Lancet 1957;2:1249.
36. Albanese AR. New instruments of varicose vein surgery. J Cardiovasc Surg 1965;6:65.
37. Edwards JM. Shearing operation for incompetent perforating veins. Br J Surg 1976;63:885–886.
38. Foote RR. Varicose veins: a practical manual. 3rd ed. Bristol: John Wright & Sons Ltd., 1960:55.

chapter 17

Use of Compression and Elastic Devices

George Johnson, Jr.

Compression has been used as therapy for symptoms involving the lower extremity since antiquity (1). Industry's ingenuity in the past 50 years has developed off-the-shelf elastic stockings that will fit more than 80% of patients, yet still deliver a prescribed pressure at the ankle. Durability may vary from company to company and from stocking to stocking. This chapter will help in choosing the correct stocking for a particular problem.

While latex (rubber) was the original stretchable component of elastic stockings, spandex, a synthetic elastic material, is now used almost exclusively. Spandex has been constantly improved so that it will give the same compression over a longer range of stretch. This allows the stocking to render the same compression with variations in size and shape of the leg (sometimes called a low-modulus material). The low-modulus characteristic makes "off-the-shelf" stockings possible; however, most companies still have 6–12 different sizes in addition to custom-made stockings to assure the best fit (1).

The knitting process varies from company to company, but all incorporate some nonelastic material as an inlay. This is usually nylon, but may be cotton or silk.

The Europeans have organized an allegedly independent testing agency, the Hohenstein Institute, that assures the consumer of a certain pressure for a certain fit and also how long the compression will last with usual wear and tear (2). Such information is not available in the United States. A major concern is how long the advertised compression lasts. Some companies assure it will last 6 months under normal wear and tear. Others may not do this, but compensate by a lesser price.

Elastic stockings, to be effective, must have graded compression. If not, the fluid/blood is not pushed caudad, and the funnel-shaped leg causes an increased pressure at the top. This, in effect, is like a constricting band.

Below-the-knee stockings usually give the maximum relief to be expected from elastic compression; however, when the swelling extends above the knee, compression to the thigh is often beneficial. One of the problems with the above-the-knee stocking is that a compression "relief" must be inserted at the knee, causing a relative constriction when the compression resumes.

Although it may be obvious, the stockings must be worn to be effective. The patient should sleep with the foot of the bed elevated and put the stocking on before getting out of bed in the morning. The swelling may occur very rapidly, and thus it is more effective to prevent swelling than to attempt to reduce swelling.

The compression of the stockings is typed by the amount of compression it delivers at the ankle, assuming the proper fit. Different companies use different ranges of compression. This discussion will involve 18 mmHg, 20–30 mmHg, 30–40 mmHg, and 40–50 mmHg, but some companies define the pressure delivered more precisely than this. The higher the compression, the more difficult it is to put the stocking on. For this reason, slippers or devices have been developed to aid the patient, especially with the high compression stocking.

Different problems require different compressions. Support pantyhose, usually worn by women, afford some compression but probably no more than 18 mmHg. The support hose worn by men probably more consistently delivers 8–10 mmHg, although the stocking is not as sheer. This type of stocking does prevent swelling in patients with minimal problems (3). "Antiembolism" stockings usually have this degree of compression, and are not classed as "therapeutic" stockings.

A slightly higher compression (20–30 mmHg) stocking is available for more severe problems such as mild varicose veins or minimal swelling. Although no data are available, they may be more effective than the 18 mmHg compression. They are not frequently prescribed.

Stockings with 30–40 mmHg compression at the ankle are the most frequently prescribed "therapeutic" stockings. They are used for moderate swelling, post-deep vein thrombosis, and after healing of a venous stasis ulcer. They are usually accepted and worn by the patient, although devices to assist in putting them on are helpful.

Stockings with 40–50 mmHg compression are available for lymphedema and difficult-to-control swelling from venous disease. They are difficult to put on, uncomfortable, hot, and not well-accepted by the patient.

There remains little doubt that elastic stockings are effective. We have demonstrated an increase in velocity in the femoral vein in the groin with below the knee 20–30 mmHg stockings, as monitored by Doppler in the supine patient (4). Supphose "off-the-shelf" below-the-knee 18 mmHg compression prevented swelling when compared with a nonstocking leg in a study of medical students and surgeons (3). O'Donnell, et al., demonstrated a decreased systolic venous pressure in patients with venous stasis ulcers when elastic stockings were worn (5). Horner, et al., found a decrease in ambulatory venous pressure when elastic stockings were worn by patients with deep venous insufficiency (6). The greater the compression, the greater the decrease in ambulatory venous pressure. Christopoulos, et al., using the air plethysmograph, found this reduction was due to a reduction in reflux and an improvement in the calf muscle ejection ability during rhythmic exercise (7). Szendro, et al., found these improvements to be related to the severity of the disease, those with milder disease tending to have a more normal pattern with compression (8).

Mayberry, et al., studied venous hemodynamics in patients with and without chronic venous insufficiency, wearing above- and below-the-knee, 30–40 torr and

40–50 torr gradient stockings (9). The authors found no significant improvement in deep venous hemodynamic measurements in patients with deep venous insufficiency.

Intermittent compression pumps for lymphedema or for hard-to-control edema resulting from chronic venous insufficiency have received considerable attention of late. The original device was an inflatable cuff around the extremity that afforded minimal relief in most instances. With the development of a linear pump compression device, results have improved. Although the original pump was bulky, smaller models have been developed that are more acceptable to patients. The pump should be used at least twice a day. Following use of the pump, patients should wear elastic stockings.

Intermittent pneumatic compression boots have been the subject of several prospective randomized trials demonstrating their effectiveness in preventing deep vein thrombosis in high-risk patients (10, 11). Neurovascular compression has been reported to be an unusual complication with these devices (12). CircAid, another innovative compression device, has multiple nonelastic wraparound components held together with Velcro that can be customized to support and compress the lower leg. Although it has been useful in some patients with venous stasis ulcers, it has not been widely evaluated.

Elastic stockings on the lower extremity have been documented by subjective and objective data to be effective for a variety of problems involving the lower extremity. It is the physician's obligation to prescribe the appropriate stocking for the patient and to instruct the patient in the proper use of the stocking.

REFERENCES

1. Johnson G Jr. The role of elastic support in venous problems. In: Bergan JJ, Yao JST, eds. Surgery of the veins. Orlando, FL: Grune & Stratton, 1985:541–550.
2. Johnson G Jr. Role of elastic support in treatment of the chronically swollen limb. In: Bergan JJ, Yao JST, eds. Venous disorders. Philadelphia: WB Saunders, 1991:372–378.
3. Pierson S, Pierson D, Swallow R, Johnson G Jr. Efficacy of graded elastic compression in the lower leg. JAMA 1983;249:242–243.
4. Johnson G Jr, Kupper C, Farrar DJ, Swallow RT. Graded compression stockings. Custom vs noncustom. Arch Surg 1982;117:69–72.
5. O'Donnell TF Jr, Rosenthal DA, Callow AD, Ledig BL. Effect of elastic compression on venous hemodynamics in postphlebitic limbs. JAMA 1979;242:2766–2768.
6. Horner J, Fernandes J, Fernandes E, Nicolaides AN. Value of graduated compression stockings in deep venous insufficiency. Br Med J 1980;280:820–821.
7. Christopoulos DG, Nicolaides AN, Szendro G, Irvine AT. Air-plethysmography and the effect of elastic compression on venous hemodynamics of the leg. J Vasc Surg 1987;5:148–159.
8. Szendro G, Veller M, Fisher C, et al. The effect of elastic compression on the venous tone in patients with varicose veins. Vasa 1992;21:198–202.
9. Mayberry JC, Moneta GL, DeFrang RD, Porter JM. The influence of elastic compression stockings on deep venous hemodynamics. J Vasc Surg 1991;13:91–99.
10. Hull RD, Raskob GE, Gent M, et al. Effectiveness of intermittent pneumatic leg compression for preventing deep vein thrombosis after total hip replacement. JAMA 1990;263:2313–2317.

11. Woolson ST, Watt JM. Intermittent pneumatic compression to prevent proximal deep venous thrombosis during and after total hip replacement: a prospective, randomized study of compression alone, compression and aspirin, and compression and low-dose warfarin. J Bone Joint Surg 1991;73:507–12.
12. Lachmann EA, Rook JL, Tunkel R, Nagler W. Complications associated with intermittent pneumatic compression. Arch Phys Med Rehabil 1992;73:482–485.

chapter 18

Surgery for Perforator Incompetence

Seshadri Raju

Perforator interruption is a controversial surgical procedure. The operation became popular when the theory that perforator incompetence may be a basis for the formation of varicosities came into vogue (1, 2). This "ascending" theory appeared to offer an attractive alternative to the traditional Trendelenburg theory of saphenofemoral incompetence and quickly gained many adherents. This theory appeared to provide an explanation for the persistence and recurrence of varices after saphenofemoral ligation or stripping procedures. Yet, many aspects of the role of perforators in health and disease remain obscure. Functional improvement after interruption, and long-term clinical outcome are controversial. A contributing factor to this state of confusion heretofore has been the absence of an accurate tool to assess perforator function. The advent of duplex scanning has provided a way to assess flow patterns in perforators. The instrument as used at present for perforator assessment provides only qualitative information. Until a more precise method to assess perforator function quantitatively is developed, the surgical approach to perforator incompetence will inevitably remain empirical and clinical.

Traditional teaching has it that the flow in normal perforators is from the superficial to the deep system and the flow reverses only when perforator incompetence develops. Recent duplex studies, however, indicate that flow in the perforators is bidirectional even in normal individuals (3). In a large number of patients referred to our center for treatment of refractory stasis ulceration, a 70% incidence of perforator incompetence was found (4); in 92% of such patients perforator incompetence was "secondary," associated with underlying deep venous valve incompetence. Published reports with but one exception (5) indicate that there is little change in ambulatory venous pressure after perforator interruption (6–8). This does not necessarily invalidate clinical use of the procedure for treatment of stasis ulceration. A number of other conservative and surgical measures, such as compression therapy, saphenous vein stripping, and deep valve reconstruction, are known to result in healing of stasis ulceration even when they result in little or no change in ambulatory venous pressure (8). A significant improvement in Valsalva foot venous pressure after perforator interruption can, however, be demonstrated (6). The reduction of venous pressure with ambulation is generally ascribed to column segmentation and reduction of hydrostatic pressure from valve closure, but this fundamental explanation may be incorrect (see Chapter 23). A better understanding based on the nonlinear volume pressure relationship that exists in collapsible tubes such as the calf venous pump provides the foundation for unraveling the role of perforators in normal and disease states.

Reported clinical results after perforator interruption have been inconsistent. Both excellent results with lower recurrence (9–12) and poor results with higher recurrence (6, 7, 13) can be found in the literature.

TECHNIQUE

Perforator ligation by the traditional approach through a long medial incision results in a high incidence of wound complications. These complications can be minimized by blunt disruption of the perforators in the subfascial plane (14–16), utilizing a 2-inch long transverse or oblique incision in the upper calf (Figs. 18.1 and 18.2). If the stasis ulcer is medial in distribution, the procedure may be limited to disruption of medial perforators only. In some patients, the ulcer is circumferential or atypically located on the lateral aspect of the leg. In such instances, perforators may be circumferentially disrupted or limited only to the lateral perforators, respectively. Figure 18.1 illustrates the steps in the technique, in which a malleable retractor is used, riding on the posterior edge of tibia for about a centimeter and proceeding distally to the medial malleolus.

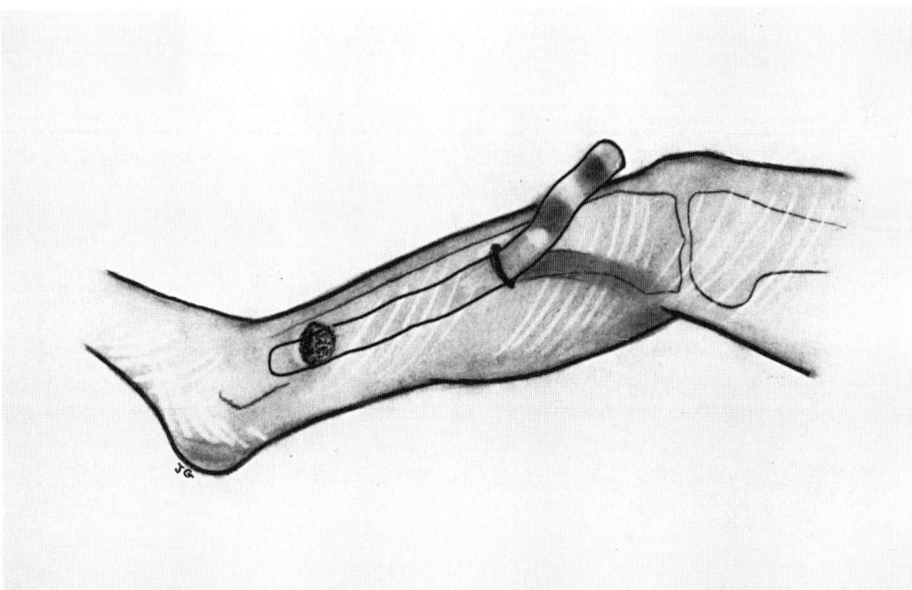

FIG. 18–1. Blunt subfascial interruption of perforators through a limited upper calf incision.

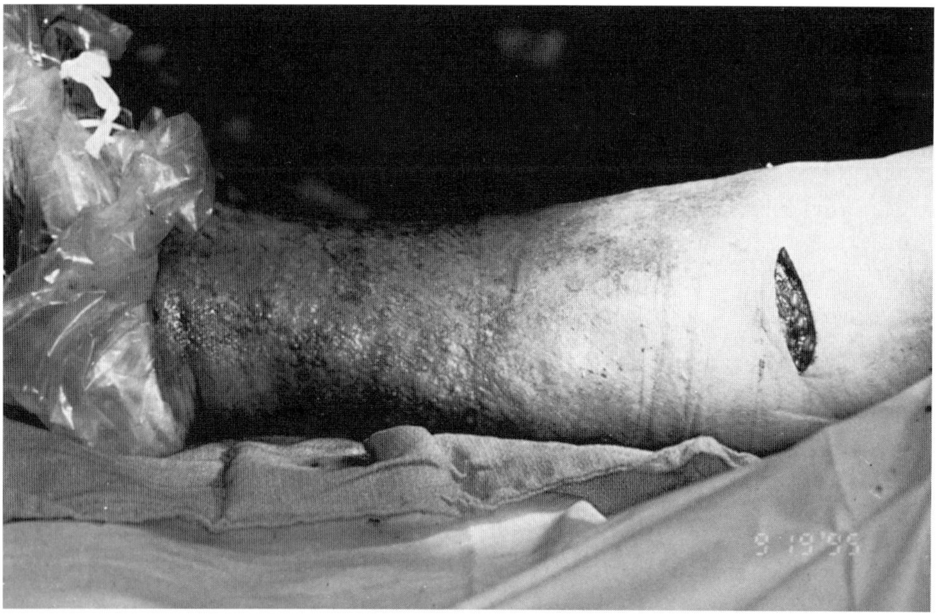

FIG. 18–2. Modified Linton technique is patent with extensive dermatitis and induration of the lower leg. The incision has been placed in the upper calf away from the skin changes.

With the advent of endoscopic surgery, perforator interruption is being performed under endoscopic visualization (17–19). More precise division of perforators and hemostatic control superior to that of the blunt disruption technique are obvious advantages with the newer method. Although satisfactory as an independent procedure, the endoscopic technique probably is not a suitable method as an adjunctive measure concurrent with valve reconstruction because of time considerations.

RESULTS

Results of perforator interruption performed in patients with stasis ulceration due to reflux are shown in Figure 18.3. The procedure can also be safely employed for treatment of ulcer in the presence of significant venous obstruction. Because perforators may function as collaterals in the presence of deep venous obstruction, there was initial concern that the procedure might exacerbate hemodynamic obstruction. These fears, however, were not realized as the level of obstruction did not worsen (6). Approximately one-half the patients appeared to have benefitted from the procedure with the healing of stasis ulceration. The incidence of recurrence after perforator interruption appears to be higher than that after venous valve reconstruction.

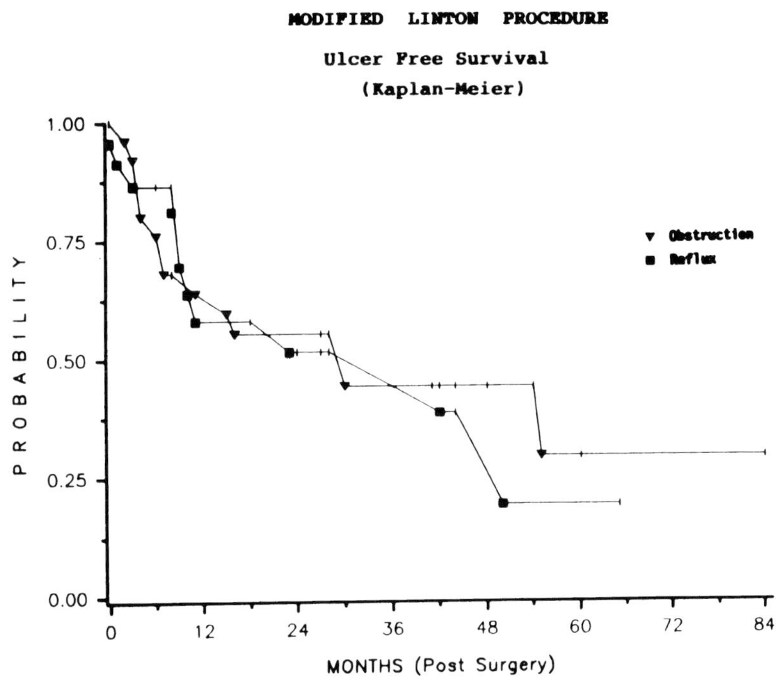

FIG. 18–3. Ulcer healing after modified Linton procedure in patients with reflux (Kaplan-Meier) or obstruction, respectively.

REFERENCES

1. Cockett FB. The pathology and treatment of venous ulcers of the leg. Br J Surg 1955;43:260–278.
2. Linton RR. The communicating veins of the lower leg and the operative technique for their ligation. Ann Surg 1938;107:582.
3. Sarin S, Scurr JH, Coleridge-Smith PD. Medial calf perforators in venous disease: the significance of outward flow. J Vasc Surg 1992;16:40–46.
4. Raju S, Fredericks R. Valve reconstruction procedures for nonobstructive venous insufficiency. J Vasc Surg 1988;7:301–310.
5. Almgren B. Nonthrombotic deep venous incompetence with special reference to anatomic, hemodynamic and therapeutic aspects. Acta Universitatis Upsaliensis 1990;256:IV-1–IV-14.
6. Raju S, Fredericks R. Venous obstruction: an analysis of one hundred thirty-seven cases with hemodynamic, venographic, and clinical correlations. J Vasc Surg 1991;14:305–313.
7. Burnand KG, O'Donnell TF, Thomas ML, Browse NL. The relative importance of incompetent communicating veins in the production of varicose veins and venous ulcers. Surgery 1977;82:9–14.
8. Raju S, Fredericks R. Hemodynamic basis of stasis ulceration—a hypothesis. J Vasc Surg 1991;13:491–495.
9. DePalma RG. Surgical therapy for venous stasis: results of a modified Linton operation. Am J Surg 1979;137:810–813.

10. Hyde GL, Hull DA. Long-term results of subfascial vein ligation for venous stasis disease. Surg Gynec Obstet 1981;153:683–686.
11. Johnson WC, O'Hara ET, Corey C, Widrich WC, Nabseth DC. Venous stasis ulceration; effectiveness of subfascial ligation. Arch Surg 1985;120:797–800.
12. Wilkinson GE, Maclaren JF. Long-term review of procedures for venous perforator insufficiency. Surg Gynec Obstet 1986;163:117–120.
13. Nash TP. Venous ulceration: factors influencing recurrence after standard surgical procedures. Med J Aust 1991;154:48–50.
14. Lacour RA, Cigorraga JR, Haedo MS, Cigorraga JA. Perforating vein insufficiency: long term results in 4494 cases with different surgical techniques. Phlebology 1995;(Suppl) 1:959–961.
15. DePalma RG. Surgical therapy for venous stasis. Surgery 1974;76:910.
16. Edwards JM. Shearing operation for incompetent perforating veins. Br J Surg 1976;63:885–886.
17. Fischer R. Surgical treatment of varicose veins; endoscopic treatment of incompetent Cockett veins. Phlebologie 1989;1040–1041.
18. Gloviczki P, Cambria RA, Rhee RY, Canton LG, McKusick MA. Surgical technique and preliminary results of endoscopic subfascial division of perforating veins. J Vasc Surg 1996;23:517–523.
19. Hauer G. The endoscopic subfascial division of the perforating veins—preliminary report (in German). Vasa 1985;14:59–61.

chapter 19

Present Status of Surgical Intervention for Chronic Venous Insufficiency

Robert L. Kistner

The person who has well-established chronic venous insufficiency (CVI) sufficient to limit activity at work or in the conduct of life has traditionally been destined to remain that way permanently. Typically, recurrent episodes of ulceration or lipodermatosclerosis are expected and require more restrictions with rest, elevation, doctor visits, and occasional hospitalization. The physician's role has been to train the individual in the use of well-fitted support and to suit the patient's way of life to the limitations imposed by the CVI state.

The purpose of treatment in CVI should be to restore the individual to a normal way of life free of ulceration, pain, and swelling. When this can be done with the use of elastic stockings, no further treatment is required.

During the past 40 years, progress has been made in the surgical treatment of many of these far-advanced, lifestyle-limiting problems. We have learned to differentiate obstructive venous problems from reflux-dominated problems, and to bypass the former and repair valves in the latter. We have learned that obstruction is the cause of problems at the common femoral vein (CFV), iliac, and inferior vena cava (IVC) levels, while reflux is the dominant problem below the CFV. For about 30% of the reflux group, surgery will be sufficient and elastic stockings will be discarded when total repair of axial reflux is performed, including saphenous, deep, and perforator veins.

To be successful with surgery in CVI, thorough diagnosis of the venous abnormality is necessary. The surgeon must determine whether the dominant problem is one of reflux or obstruction, or a combination of these. The sites of involvement above or below the inguinal ligament, and the exact venous segments involved must be identified. The position of valves in the patent veins and their functional state must be known. When this information is coupled with the clinical symptoms and confirmed by physiologic tests, an accurate plan of surgery can be developed for most patients with CVI.

The surgical plan in CVI should aim at correction of as much reflux as possible below the common femoral vein, and bypass of as much obstruction as is needed in the common femoral, iliac, and IVC vessels. All reflux is important, and clinical improvement occurs progressively as this is treated in the saphenous, perforator and deep veins of the thigh and leg. In advanced cases, it is not possible to restore the veins to a normal state, but improvement of part of the reflux and obstruction leads to a state of clinical compensation in the face of retained disease.

The published results of success in surgery for reflux disease are very good. Conventional ligation and stripping of the saphenous system is clearly successful. Interruption of large incompetent calf perforator veins is also successful. Direct valvuloplasty for primary valve reflux of the deep veins is successful for over 10 years in 73% of cases. Transplantation of valved vein segments is successful in 50% or more of appropriate candidates up to 4 years and perhaps indefinitely.

Surgery for obstructive disease of the iliac vein is also successful in appropriate cases. The femoral-femoral or femoral-iliac bypass for iliac vein obstruction has been widely reported to have 70% good results. Prosthetic bypass of the IVC and high iliac vein is much less frequent and clear statements about its long-term success await further analysis. Bypass for obstruction below the common femoral vein is rarely indicated.

With the published reports of improvement in the clinical condition that results from an aggressive surgical approach to the CVI state, it is time to establish controlled randomized interinstitutional study of surgical versus nonsurgical treatment. The potential economic and social benefits of improvement in this area are great. Unfortunately, such a study could not be performed today because we lack consensus agreement about the classification and distribution of venous insufficiency states and the diagnostic criteria that are needed to support a given diagnosis.

The clarion call at this time should be to develop a universally agreed upon classification of chronic venous insufficiency with diagnostic criteria for each diagnosis. With this basis, randomized studies of various combinations of venous reflux and obstruction can be done to define morbidity with each problem and to test treatment alternatives. Only then will we be able to communicate clearly about the optimal method of management of advanced chronic venous insufficiency states.

chapter 20

Bypass Procedures for Venous Obstruction: Palma and May-Husni Bypasses, Raju Perforator Bypass, Prosthetic Bypasses, and Primary and Adjunctive Arteriovenous Fistulae

J.D. Gruss and W. Hiemer

Chronic venous insufficiency is due either to obstruction, or reflux, or a combination of the two. In all cases of severe chronic venous insufficiency with trophic changes to the skin, chronic swelling and ulceration, an accurate diagnostic evaluation must be carried out before any reconstructive surgery is planned. A bypass procedure is indicated only when venous obstruction can be unequivocally documented to have a hemodynamic effect. Photoplethysmography can be employed at best only as a screening procedure in the presence of short filling time. While ascending phlebography is capable of providing accurate morphologic information, it provides no information about the functional effect of an obstruction. Both Doppler ultrasound and descending phlebography are able to demonstrate reflux, but are unable to validate its pathophysiologic significance. Even the technique of venous occlusion plethysmography, or venous pressure measurement at rest, is not enough to diagnose chronic venous obstruction. Even with extensive obstructions, irrespective of their localization, venous capacity and maximum outflow may lie within normal limits. In the presence of adequate collateralization, the resting pressure may be normal. The hemodynamic effect of a venous obstruction often manifests under conditions of stress. Suitable test procedures in this context have proved to be venous pressure measurement under standardized exercise or after hyperemia and plethysmographic volumetry performed while the patient performs heel-raising exercises.

PREOPERATIVE INVESTIGATION

The methods of ascending phlebography and duplex scanning provide information about the pathologic anatomy, i.e., about the site of obstruction, and thus permit determination of operability purely from the technical point of view. The functional indication for surgery is provided by pressure measurements. Irrespective of the site of the obstruction, venous pressure can be measured after puncturing a vein on the dorsum of the foot with the patient standing, at rest, and under conditions of exercise. Resting pressure should be clearly higher on the affected side than on the healthy limb. In response to exercise (10 tiptoe movements), the pressure on the affected side should decrease by not more than one-third of the pressure decrease on the unaffected side. A lesser decrease in pressure—or even an increase—improves the surgical indication and the postoperative chances of success (gradient increases).

In the event of a unilateral iliac vein obstruction, the planning of a Palma procedure is preceded by pressure measurements in the recumbent patient, involving puncture of the common femoral vein in the groin. In a healthy limb, the pressure at this site is 4 mmHg. A pelvic vein obstruction with functional relevance produces an increase in resting pressure to 6 mmHg or more. On activating the calf muscle pump by having the patient flex and extend the ankle joint in rhythm with a metronome, the venous pressure in the groin should increase to at least twice the resting pressure in the presence of significant obstruction. Again, higher values mean a better surgical indication.

Venous pressure measurements following reactive hyperemia also provide a very good functional indication for operation. The measurement is performed in the recumbent patient, and involves puncture of the vein on the dorsum of the foot. In the horizontal position, the venous pressure corresponds to the pressure in the femoral vein (about 4 mmHg). In the event of a functional obstruction, the resting pressure is higher. A cuff applied to the thigh is inflated to a pressure of more than 300 mmHg for 2 minutes. Five seconds after deflating the cuff, the pressure measurement is repeated. The increase in pressure to values of up to 30 mmHg reflects the functional severity of the venous obstruction. In the most severe cases of postthrombotic syndrome (stages V–VI), the increase in pressure either does not take place, or is only very small, which is puzzling. Raju uses the term paradoxical reaction. The reason for this paradoxical reaction is that the expected reactive hyperemia does not take place or is delayed. The lack of reactive hyperemia can be documented by venous occlusion plethysmography. The reasons for this phenomenon are not clear, although it is suggested that venous hypertension produces a backup via the venous capillaries, extending into the arterial capillary limb; and that maximum filling of the peripheral circulation prevents any further filling, thus abolishing the reactive hyperemia response.

The same examination design also permits a quantification of the venous reflux. While Doppler techniques and descending phlebography merely document the presence of a reflux, the increase in peripheral pressure represents a parameter that reflects the pathophysiologic effect of the reflux. Again, the pressure is measured with the patient recumbent via a needle inserted into a vein of the dorsum of the foot. The patient is requested to perform a Valsalva maneuver and maintain it for 5 seconds. An increase in pressure exceeding 4 mmHg—in severe cases up to more than 10 mmHg—reflects the magnitude of the reflux (see Chapter 12).

From the morphologic perspective, there are three operable venous conditions in the lower extremity. Reconstructive procedures on the inferior vena cava will not be discussed. The three operable conditions are the following: (a) unilateral pelvic venous obstruction with the patent contralateral side, (b) obstruction of the superficial femoral vein, and (c) obstruction of the bifurcation of the popliteal vein associated with varying degree of perforating vein insufficiency of the calf. Isolated unilateral iliac vein obstruction is corrected using the Palma bypass (Fig. 20.1) operation (1, 2); circumscribed superficial femoral vein obstruction is treated by the May-Husni operation (3–6); and obstruction of the popliteal bifurcation by the Raju perforator bypass (7–9). Some authors (see Chapter 32) have advocated construction of a bypass early after the onset of obstruction to prevent the development of valve reflux from obstructive venous hypertension. In our opinion, however, none of these procedures should be carried out without a delay of at least 1 year after the onset of the acute thrombotic event for these reasons: (a) the possible spontaneous recanalization and collateralization, and (b) the fact that the construction of an adjuvant AV fistula with the bypass at an early stage may re-

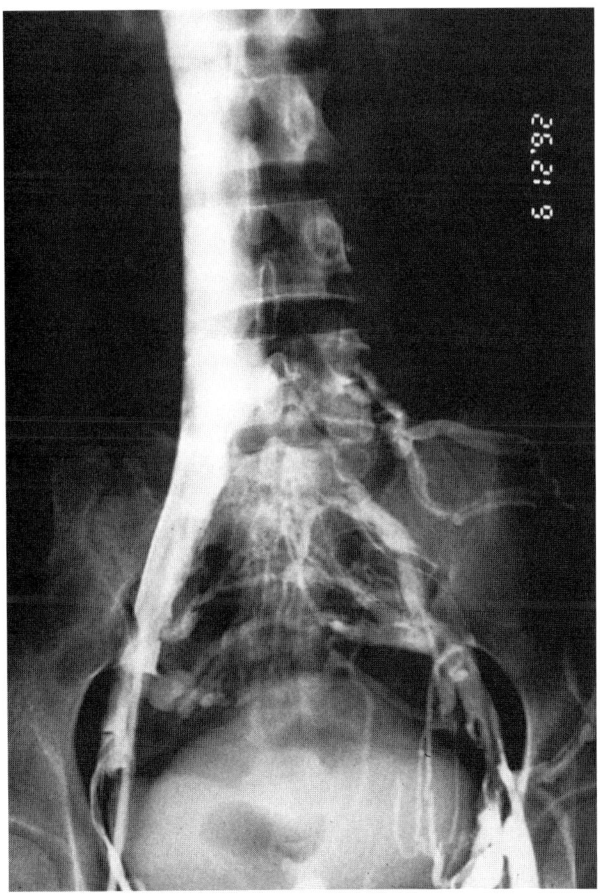

FIG. 20–1. Preoperative venographic appearance of unilateral iliac vein occlusion in a patient who underwent a Palma operation.

sult in recanalization of the iliac vein and thus a failure of the bypass. It goes without saying that surgery is indicated only in the presence of severe clinical symptomatology, with chronic swelling, pain, or venous claudication. Development of stasis ulceration occurs late after the onset of acute obstruction and is thought to be the result of postphlebitic reflux rather than to the hemodynamic obstruction per se (see Chapter 23).

PALMA PROCEDURE

The first attempts at venous reconstruction were undertaken by Carrel and Guthrie (10, 11) in 1906 and 1910, and by Jeger (12) in 1913. In 1955, Wanke (13) made an unsuccessful attempt to perform a direct reconstruction of a chronic iliac vein obstruction. In 1953, Kunlin (14) attempted to interpose the long saphenous vein to treat obstruction of an external iliac vein. In 1959, Eduardo Palma (1), the South American urologist, treated a 35-year-old woman with intractable ulcus cruris by performing a femoro-femoral crossover bypass with the saphenous vein. In 1960, Palma and Esperon (2) published a report on seven more patients operated on using the same technique. In 1967, the same authors reported on 14 cases, seven of whom were still patent (2). In 1963 and subsequently, Dale and Scott (16–18) presented supporting experimental work on "venous grafting." In 1968, Dumanian et al. (15) recommended the construction of a temporary adjunctive AV fistula as a protective measure (20, 21) to maintain patency of the venous bypass. In 1979, Gruss published the first report using externally supported PTFE prostheses as a conduit in Palma procedures (20).

On account of the extensive nature of the operation and the poor results obtained, direct procedures on the iliac vein itself failed to prevail over the elegant principle of the Palma operation.

"Classic" Palma Operation Using the Contralateral Long Saphenous Vein

The long saphenous vein of the unaffected side is dissected and mobilized to about the level of the knee. All the tributaries must be divided. Only its junction with the temporal vein on the healthy side is left intact. The graft is passed through a subcutaneous tunnel to the affected side, avoiding kinking. The vein is anastomosed end-to-end or end-to-side with the common femoral vein. The anastomosis is constructed with monofilament suture material (5–0/6–0), with precautions similar to the handling of autologous material. That is, only the adventitia of the vein is grasped during handling, carefully avoiding damage to the intima with the forceps. The donor side, as far as possible, must remain integrated within the tissues and is not dissected circumferentially (Fig. 20.2). In all cases we construct a "bucket handle" arteriovenous fistula, using either a large lateral tributary of the long saphenous vein or the long saphenous vein of the affected side. The anastomosis between the vein and the adjoining superficial femoral artery is constructed transversely end-to-side, employing a continuous 7–0 or 8–0 PTFE suture. The AV fistula is tagged with a wire loop which is embedded within the

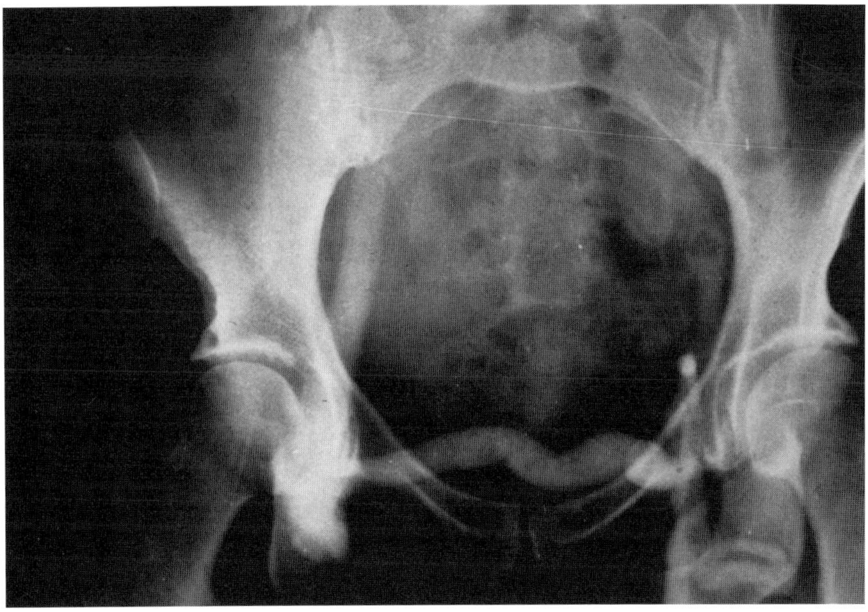

FIG. 20–2. The classic saphenous vein Palma bypass at 10 years after operation.

subcutaneous tissue. This facilitates surgical closure of the fistula 3 months later. Raju has suggested that the AV fistula may be retained longer to enlarge the size of the saphenous conduit (7). AV fistulae that are retained beyond 3 months carry the risk of bacterial infection of the fistula, distal venous hypertension (7) and possibly acceleration of distal valvular incompetence. The placement of a 4-mm prosthetic sleeve around the venous limb of the fistula may help to limit fistula flow avoiding venous hypertension therefrom. With the sleeve in place, percutaneous closure of the fistula may be achieved by embolization of occluding coils larger than the sleeve size.

It is not absolutely necessary to select the common femoral vein of the affected side as the site of the anastomosis. In the interest of a kink-free bypass, the superficial femoral vein, or even the profunda femoris, can be employed for the anastomosis. It makes no sense to construct the anastomosis at a site where substantial mural changes are present. In exceptional cases, an anastomosis with the long saphenous vein can be performed when the vessel has taken a collateral function. Palma, himself, occasionally chose the distal femoral vein for the construction of the anastomosis. We have little experience with this site. Our main objective is to keep the graft as short as possible.

Modified Palma Procedure Using Spirally Reinforced PTFE Prostheses

In 1979, Gruss proposed the use of plastic material, namely, PTFE, for Palma grafts. Initially, spirally reinforced PTFE "ring" prostheses (IMPRA) of

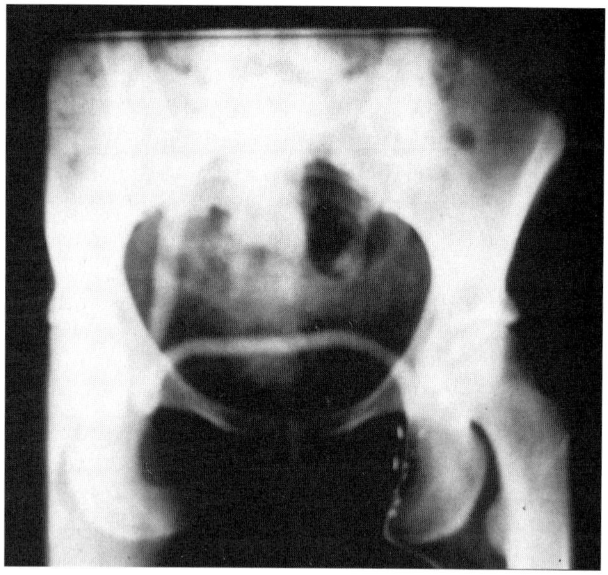

FIG. 20–3. An early PTFE Palma bypass performed in the classic way (femoro-femoral).

10–12-mm diameter were employed for crossover femoro-femoral bypass (Fig. 20.3). Later, we moved the recipient site to the external iliac vein and positioned the graft behind the abdominal muscles in front of the bladder, passing it to the opposite side through the Retzius' space. This surgical strategy has three advantages: (a) avoids a groin incision, (b) protects the graft by the abdominal muscles, and (c) improves the hemodynamics of the graft (24, 25) (Fig. 20.4).

In 1980, Hutschenreiter and Vollmar (26) modified the procedure as an ilio-iliac, so-called high Palma procedure. In this technique, the prosthesis has a diameter of 10–12 mm (Fig. 20.4). The same principles are also applied as in the case of the original Palma procedure. Handling of the vein and prosthesis must be as atraumatic as possible. Dissection of the vein from its tissue bed should be kept to a minimum and circumferential dissection should always be avoided. The anastomosis should be constructed in an area free of thrombotic damage to the wall of the vein. Depending upon phlebographic criteria, end-to-end and end-to-side anastomosis are equally possible. Fine 5–0 or 6–0 suture material, preferentially PTFE sutures, is employed. Both experimental investigations and our own experience have shown that, in particular, the prosthetic grafts used in venous surgery can benefit from the protection of an arteriovenous fistula. The increased flow in the area of the anastomosis and the graft itself provides protection against graft thrombosis. This is of particular importance in the initial postoperative phase, during sleep, when the calf muscle pump is inactive. The arteriovenous fistula is fashioned as in the original Palma procedure, either by employing a large tributary or the long saphenous vein of the diseased side. In this case, the superficial femoral artery of the affected side should be used as the arterial donor. As in the original Palma procedure, the fistula is marked with a wire loop that should be palpable through the skin, or with commercially available vessel loops. A particular property of the loops is that they do not incorporate into the tissues, facilitating subsequent closure of the fistula. The follow-up treatment is similar to that of the original Palma procedure. Before concluding the operation we introduce, via a branch of the superficial femoral vein or the profunda femoris, or even a tributary of the AV-fistula itself, a thin venous catheter, the end of which is placed exactly opposite the Palma anastomosis. Through this fine catheter, we initiate heparin irrigation of the anastomosis and the graft during the intraoperative phase. This catheter may also be used for intraoperative phlebography. During the first postoperative days, the dose of heparin is increased from 400 u/hr to 1500 u/hr by the fifth postoperative day. If wound healing proceeds normally, the patient is changed over to oral anticoagulation. When a prothrombin Quick test value of 25% is achieved, the venous catheter is removed after performing followup angiography. This examination is supplemented by an ascending phlebographic study of the diseased leg, preferentially using the digital subtraction technique, to document the patency of the graft. As a result of the increased flow produced by the AV fistula, in rare cases a descending thrombosis may develop in the superficial femoral vein. Such an occurrence should be detected at an early stage and treated accordingly. In some cases, the arteriovenous fistula is the cause of persistent or even progressive swelling of the diseased leg. This swelling disappears when the arteriovenous fistula is closed. The venographic examinations carried out in the immediate postoperative phase (on duplex scanning) are repeated shortly before the AV fistula is closed. After closure, anticoagulation treatment and the use of compression stockings are continued for at least 6 more months. Further treatment is decided on the basis of the clinical and hemodynamic findings. The final objective is to discontinue anticoagulation treatment, although further monitoring must be continued.

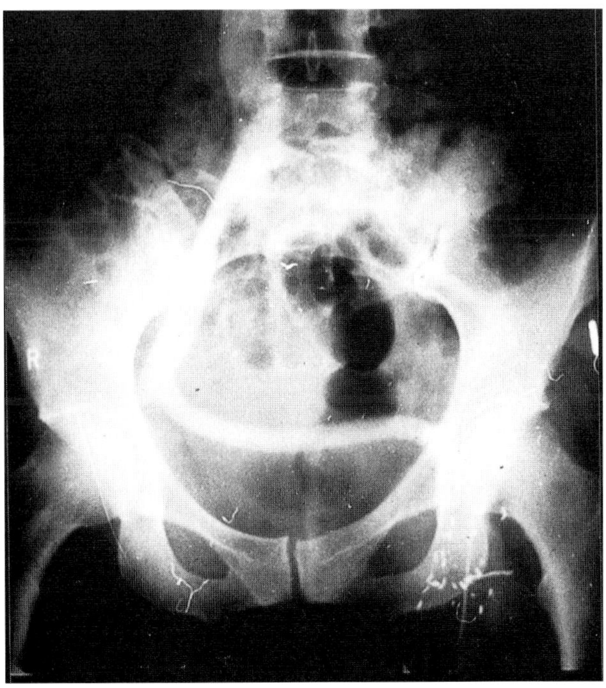

FIG. 20–4. The modified PTFE Palma bypass (retropubic ilio-iliac) immediately postoperation.

Results

The long-term patency rates of venous reconstructions tend to be empirical observations, since large groups studied prospectively are lacking. Good retrospective studies on functional duration have been published by Halliday, et al. (27), in the United States and Gruss (24, 25) in Europe. Both authors have performed original Palma grafts using vein as well as PTFE prostheses, and have reported durable results (Fig. 20.5). The results reported by these authors have been quite similar. The patency rate after 5 years based on the life table method is about 70%, both for the vein and the synthetic grafts (Table 20.1). Clinically, most patients with a patent graft appear to have benefitted from the operation (Fig. 20.6). Bypass obstruction correlates quite well with the return of symptoms. Addi-tionally, Halliday reports that the nature of the venous inflow has an obvious effect on the patency rate. Thus, occlusion of the superficial femoral vein on the inflow side (that is, a two-level occlusion) clearly impairs the prognosis with respect to patency, at least in the initial phase. After 5 years, this difference becomes blurred. It must be said, however, that the group is too small to permit any final statement on this point. In only 4 of 50 patients, Halliday (27) carried out an AV fistula following the Krug modification (28). We share May's (29) view that the Krug modification, where the venous Palma transplant is anastomosed side-to-side to the common femoral vein and end-to-side with the common femoral artery, has more hemodynamic disadvantage than the AV fistula with a high branch of the saphenous vein. The results are comparable with the 1972 results of Robert May (15, 29, 30), who reported a long-term patency in 16 of 22 cases. After perfecting his

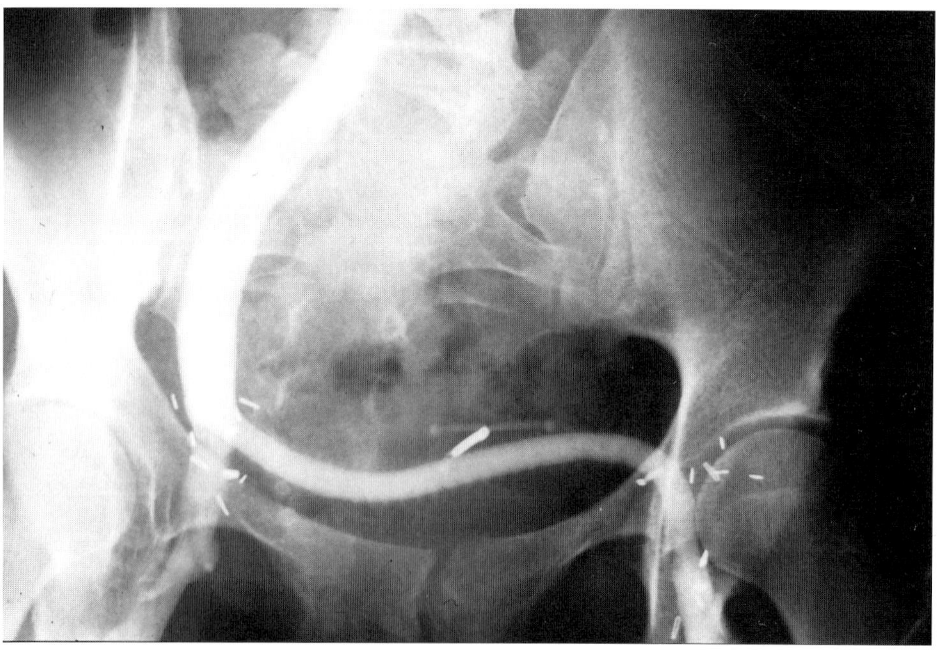

FIG. 20–5. A modified PTFE Palma bypass at 7 years postoperatively.

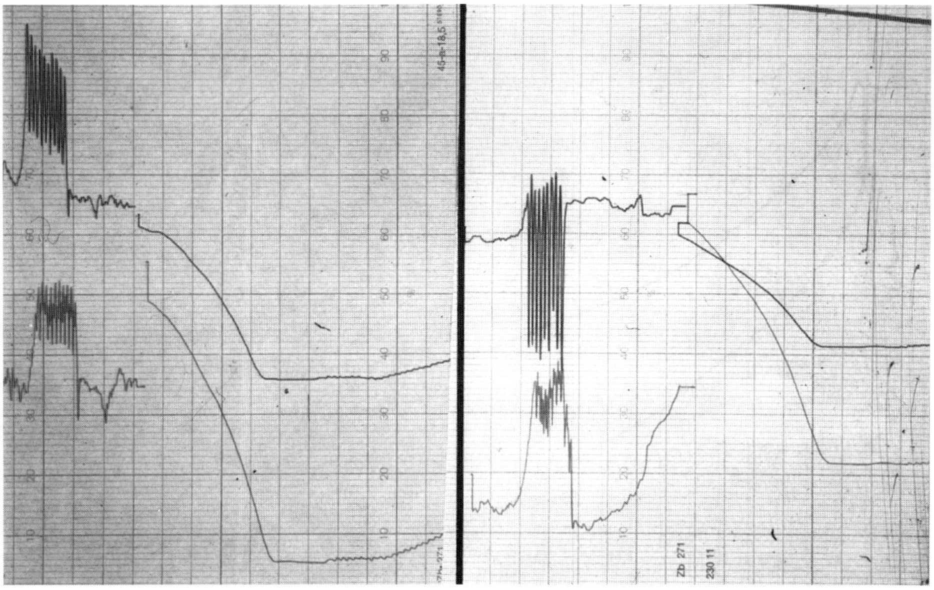

FIG. 20–6. Strain-gauge plethysmography (*left panel*) 7 years after Palma bypass. *Top curve* represents obstructed left leg and the *bottom curve* the normal right leg. Note obstructive pattern preoperation which normalized after surgery.

technique, in 1980 May reported a long-term patency of 13 grafts in 14 operations. As Table 20.1 also shows, our own experience since 1978 demonstrates that the autologous graft is not superior to the synthetic one. On the basis of this observation, we now employ PTFE prostheses strengthened with a PTFE "ring" coil, which saves the long saphenous vein for other possible uses (Tables 20.2, 20.3, and 20.4).

TABLE 20-1

FIVE-YEAR FOLLOW-UP OF THE PALMA OPERATION

Author	Material	No.	5-Year Patency Rate %	% Patients with AV-Fistula
May 1971	Vein	22	73	No AVF
May 1980	Vein	14	92	No AVF
Hutschenreiter, et al. 1982	PTFE	9	78	100%
Ijima, et al. 1985 (31)	PTFE	26	84	With AVF
	PTFE	26	75	No AVF
Halliday 1985	Vein	34	75	20%
Gruss, et al. 1988	PTFE	27	77	100%
Gruss 1993	Vein	20	71	100%

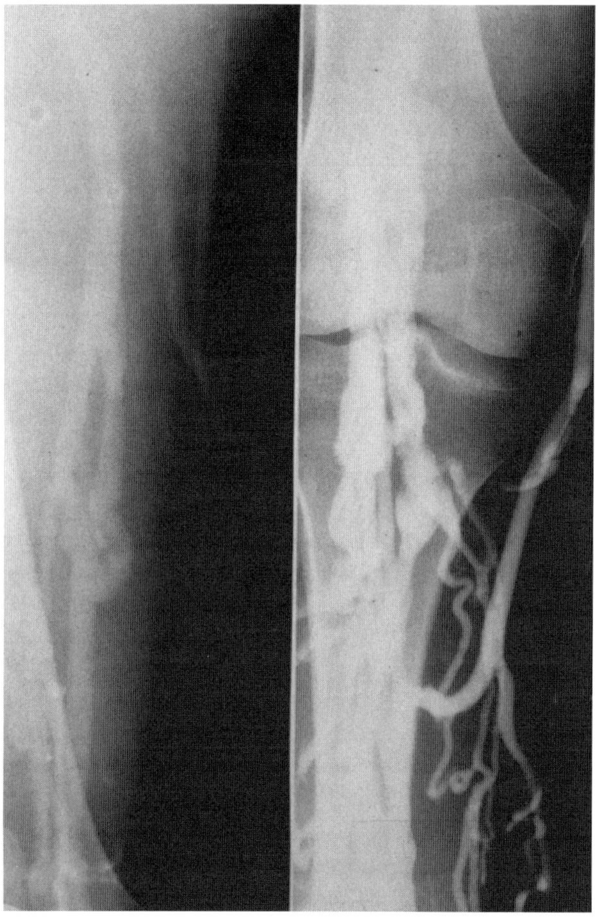

FIG. 20–7. May-Husni Bypass for femoral venous obstruction at mid thigh level (not shown).

MAY-HUSNI PROCEDURE

As early as 1954, Warren and Thayer (32) reported on the possibility of reconstructing circumscribed superficial femoral vein obstructions by anastomosing the ipsilateral long saphenous vein to the patent popliteal vein. This first report was completely forgotten, and the femoral bypass was not rediscovered

TABLE 20-2

LONG-TERM FOLLOW-UP (<5 YEARS) OF THE PALMA OPERATION (PROF. J.D. GRUSS SERIES)

Material	No. Patients	No. Operations
Vein	19	20
PTFE	32	33

TABLE 20-3

LONG-TERM FOLLOW-UP (<5 YEARS) OF THE VEIN GRAFTS IN THE PALMA OPERATION (PROF. J.D. GRUSS SERIES)

	No. Patients	No. Operations	No. Follow-up	No. Patent	No. Lost
Vein PALMA	19	20	14	10	5

until the 1970s, independently by Husni (1970) (5) in the United States, Frileux (1972) (33) in France, and by May (1972) (3, 4) in Austria. In 1975, we modified the procedure by constructing an AV fistula at the level of the ankle (34).

The procedure (Fig. 20.7) is performed under general endotracheal anesthesia. The patient is placed in the supine position, the affected leg is flexed at the hip and knee joints, and the operating table is slightly tilted toward the affected side. A longitudinal skin incision is made on the medial side of the proximal calf, about 1 cm behind the edge of the tibia. Preoperative duplex examination assures an accurate placement of the incision over the saphena vein. The long saphenous vein is carefully dissected and a moistened rubber sling applied; the branches are divided between metal clips. The fascia is then split and the medial tendons (pes anserinus) are divided. The popliteal vein is also dissected and a sling applied. In the case of a duplicated popliteal vein, the larger one is selected; in the presence of postthrombotic changes, the least affected one is used. Following systemic heparinization (5000 units), the blood flow is interrupted by digital compression or with the aid of a rubber sling. The anastomosis of the long saphenous vein is performed end-to-side or, obliquely, end-to-end, depending upon the anatomic situation present and the diameter of the vessels. In the case of a deep-lying popliteal vein and a well-developed long saphenous vein, the end-to-end anastomosis is preferred, since acute angulation of the saphenous vein can be avoided. The anastomosis is created with a continuous 6–0 or 7–0 PTFE suture.

After reestablishing blood flow, the distal long saphenous vein is exposed and mobilized at the ankle through an S-shaped incision. Through the same incision, the posterior tibial artery can be exposed. After applying atraumatic clamps, the artery is carefully opened by a longitudinal arteriotomy. The transversely divided long saphenous vein is then anastomosed, end-to-side, to the posterior tibial artery using a continuous 8–0 PTFE suture. The posterior suture line of the anastomo-

TABLE 20-4

LONG-TERM FOLLOW-UP OF 33 PALMA OPERATIONS USING PTFE GRAFTS (<5 YEARS) (PROF. J. D. GRUSS SERIES)

	No. Patients	No. Operations	No. Follow-up	No. Patent	No. Lost
PTFE PALMA	32	33	26	22	6

sis is applied from the luminal side. The AV fistula results in an increased blood flow in the saphenous vein and, via the perforating veins, in the deep veins of the calf. The increased flow is propagated to the saphenopopliteal anastomosis and ensures its patency, even when the calf muscle pump is inactive during sleep and in particular during the first few postoperative days.

When closing the fascia of the tibial region, care must be taken to leave a large gap, to prevent compression of the venous graft. For the same reasons, the tendons of the pes anserinus are not reconstructed.

The patient receives anticoagulation treatment from day one, initially with heparin in increasing doses, and after the sixth postoperative day, with coumarin. The patient is mobilized from the fourth postoperative day. Patients with a peripheral AV fistula must not be given an elastic bandage or compression stocking.

In one-half of the cases, the AV fistula closes spontaneously within the first 3 postoperative months. In 14 May-Husni procedures, we constructed an AV fistula in 10. Among the five patients in whom spontaneous fistula closure did not occur, we initially attempted to promote closure by the application of a firm elastic compression bandage with a pad applied locally to the medial side of the ankle joint (medial malleolus). In two cases, this proved successful, while in three patients operative closure of the fistula was necessary.

Results and Assessment

Among 14 May-Husni procedures, early thrombotic occlusion with persistent severe postthrombotic syndrome occurred in three cases. In four cases, varicose changes and loss of function occurred after some time in the vein graft (Fig. 20.8). In these four cases, a severe postthrombotic syndrome recurred. Varicose degeneration developed about 6–7 years after the operation. In seven patients, the bypass remains patent, as demonstrated by a substantial improvement in the vein pressure curves, although four of these grafts already show signs of varicose changes. In five cases, we combined the May-Husni operation with a Palma procedure (Fig. 20.9). Of these, only two have remained patent over the long term, that is, up until the present (19 and 14 years after surgery). Because of a noticeable difference between the fistula and nonfistula group and the small number of cases, it cannot be ascertained whether the construction of a peripheral AV fistula brings about an improvement in long-term patency or not. Because of the poor late results, the combined Palma/May-Husni approach probably should not be employed. While in the Palma procedure the varicose dilatation with loss of venous-valvular function has no functional effect, varicose degeneration of the May-Husni bypass is accompanied by a loss of function. This fits in well with normal physiology; the iliac veins in most cases are without valves. This also fits in well with the observation that primary valveless synthetic grafts employed for venous crossover bypasses provide very favorable results. In view of the stated long-term results, the decision to use the May-Husni procedure should be carefully considered (35, 36).

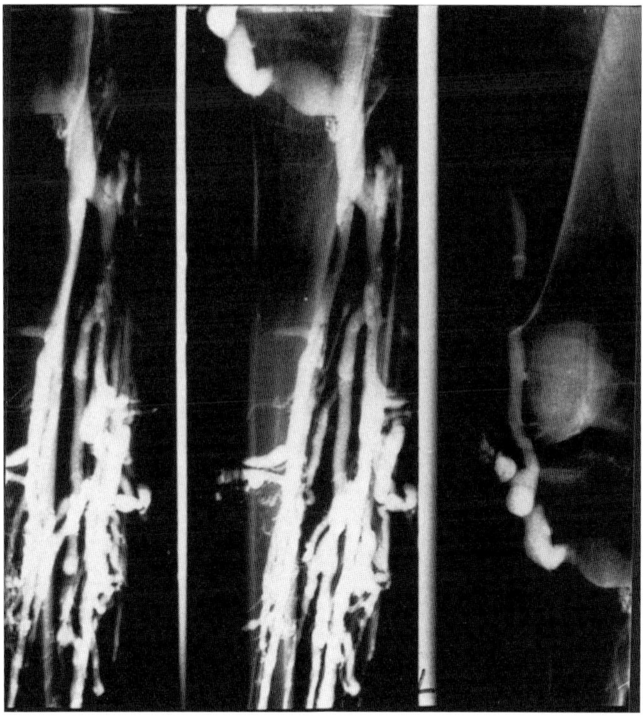

FIG. 20–8. A May-Husni bypass at 7 years. Note early varicose changes.

RAJU PERFORATOR BYPASS

The indication for the Raju perforator bypass is a severe postthrombotic syndrome with obstruction in the region of the bifurcation of the popliteal vein, and occlusion of the popliteal vein that extends into the proximal parts of the veins of the calf. The rationale of this procedure is that, in severe cases, although multiple perforating veins drain the blood from the deep veins toward the long and short saphenous veins, the capacity of these radiologically documented perforating vessels is insufficient. The phlebographic demonstration of perforating veins tells us nothing about their functional capacity, as the frequently tortuous connecting veins may be kinked, or stenotic, or have valves that hinder the blood flow from the deep to the superficial system. The valves are oriented to conduct flow from the superficial to the deep system in the normal individual. The inadequate collateral function of the perforating veins in this syndrome is again documented by venous pressure measurement. High pressure values of at least 6 mmHg measured after reactive hyperemia are considered a functional indication for the Raju perforator bypass. The operation was described by Raju (7) in 1986, who reported on the six patients treated successfully (Fig. 20.10). The procedure involves the mobilization of the peripheral long saphenous vein in the calf. Via the same incision, the posterior tibial vein is dissected distal to the occluded segment and below the incompetent perforating veins. The peripherally divided long

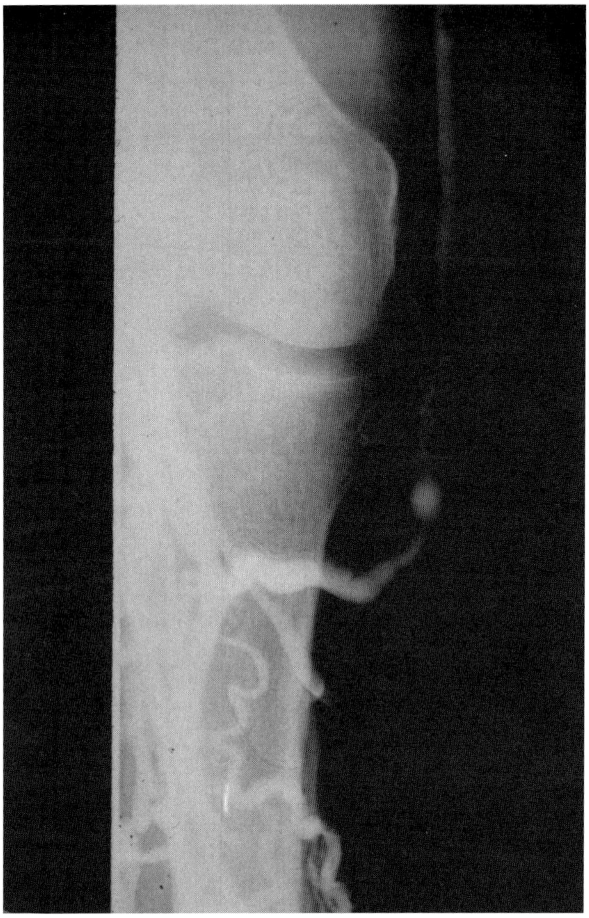

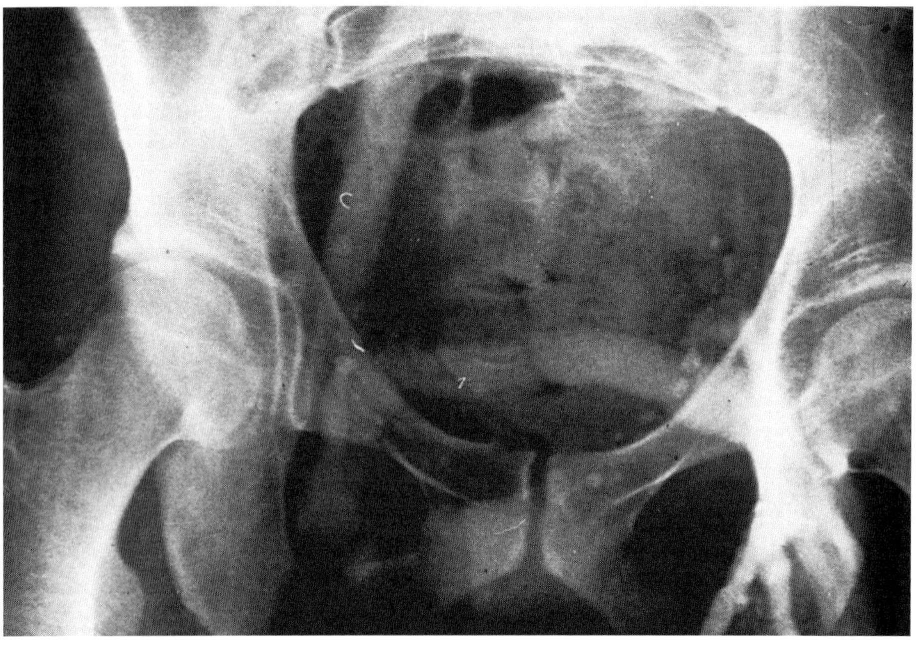

FIG. 20–9. A combined May-Husni and Palma transplant at 11 years.

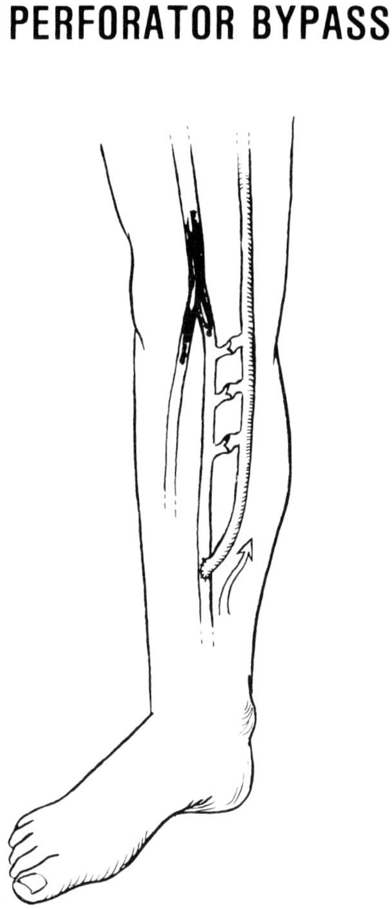

A

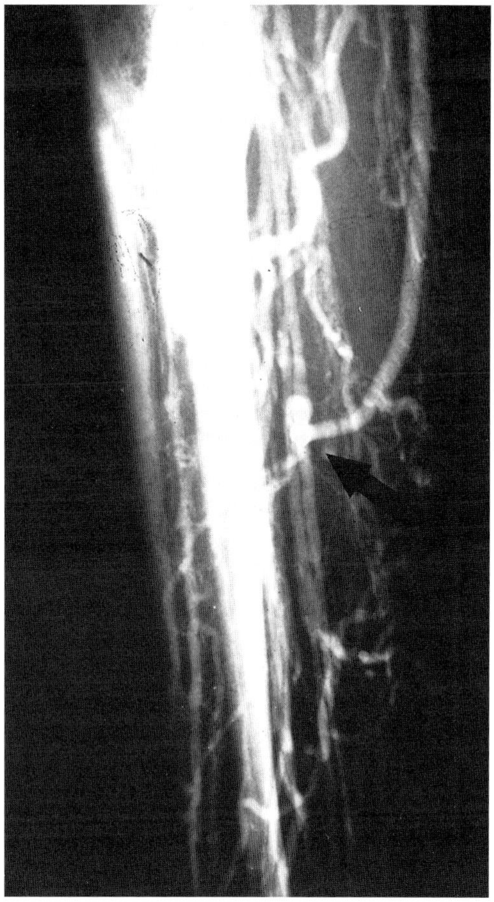

B

FIG. 20–10. Raju Perforator Bypass. A: Perforator collaterals may be poorly functional due to valve orientation. B: Patent bypass one year after surgery. (By permission from Raju S. Venous reconstruction. In Current Surgical Therapy, Fourth Edition. ed. Cameron JL. Mosby. St. Louis. 1992:780–784.)

saphenous vein is anastomosed end-to-side to the posterior tibial vein. A running suture with 8–0 monofilament suture material is employed. By grafting the long saphenous vein to the peripheral posterior tibial vein, the functionally insufficient perforating veins and the proximal venous obstruction are bypassed. Later, Raju combined his procedure with a peripheral AV fistula between the peripheral long saphenous vein or posterior tibial vein and the posterior tibial artery. On account of the high rate of spontaneous fistula closure, however, this adjunctive procedure was later abandoned. In a series of six cases, Raju reports a 100% long-term patency (7, 9, 37) even though many of the grafts thrombosed in the immediate postoperative period only to recanalize later. This striking observation may be related to the high rate of spontaneous thrombolysis known to occur in the calf.

Since the number of patients in this series is small and long-term results are not available, this procedure—as in the case of the May-Husni operation—should be employed only after careful consideration.

Primary Arteriovenous Fistula

A primary AV fistula to enlarge existing collaterals and relieve symptoms of venous obstruction has been proposed (7, 38). This procedure should be considered only when other bypass options are unavailable or have failed, as a high rate of spontaneous fistula closure has been observed and the long-term functional improvement is inferior to a well-performed bypass procedure (9).

REFERENCES

1. Palma EC, Esperon R. Tratamiento del sindrome postthrombo-flebitico mediante transplante de safena interna. Angiologie 1959;11:87.
2. Palma EC, Esperon R. Vein transplants and grafts in surgical treatment of the postphlebitic syndrome. J Cardiovasc Surg 1960;1:94–107.
3. May R. Der Femoralisbypass beim postthrombotischen Zustandsbild. Vasa 1972;1:267.
4. May R. Venentransplantation beim postthrombotischen Zustandsbild. Aktuelle Chir 1972;7:1.
5. Husni EA. In situ saphenopopliteal bypass graft for incompetence of the femoral and popliteal veins. Surg Gynec Obstet 1970;130:297.
6. Husni EA. Clinical experience with femoralpopliteal venous reconstruction. In: Bergan JJ, Yao JST, eds. Venous problems. Chicago: Year Book Medical Publishers, 1978:485.
7. Raju S. New approaches to the diagnosis and treatment of venous obstruction. J Vasc Surg 1986;4:42–54.
8. Raju S. A pressure-based technique for the detection of acute and chronic venous obstruction. Phlebology 1988;3:207–216.
9. Raju S. Experience with venous reconstruction in patients with chronic venous insufficiency. In: Bergan JJ, Yao JST, eds. Venous disorders. Philadelphia: WB Saunders, 1991:296–305.
10. Carrel A, Guthrie CC. Uniterminal and biterminal venous transplantations. Surg Gynec Obstet 1906;2:266.
11. Carrel A. Graft of the vena cava on the abdominal aorta. Ann Surg 1910;52:462.
12. Jeger E. Die Chirurgie der Blutgefässe und des Herzens. Berlin: Hirschwald, 1913:112, 138, 323–324.
13. Wanke R. Die operative Therapie der chronischen Beckenvenensperre. Chirurg 1955;26:161.
14. Kunlin J. The reestablishment of venous circulation with grafts in cases of obliteration from trauma or thrombophlebitis. Mem Acad Clin 1953;79:109.
15. May R. Venenplastiken bei postthrombotischen Zuständen. Acta Chir Austriaca 1972;(Suppl):4.
16. Dale WA, Scott HW. Grafts of the venous system. Surgery 1963;53:52–84.
17. Dale WA. Reconstructive venous surgery. In: Veith FJ, ed. Critical problems in vascular surgery. New York: Appleton-Century-Crofts, 1982:199–213.
18. Dale WA. Crossover vein grafts for relief of iliofemoral venous block. Surgery 1965;57:608–612.
19. Dumanian AV, Santschi DR, Park U, et al. Cross-over saphenous vein graft combined with a temporary femoral arteriovenous fistula. Vasc Surg 1968;2:116.
20. Gruss JD, Bartels D, Kawai S, Karadedos C, Tsafandakis E. Anwendung von Kunststoff bei der Palma-Operation. Angio 1979;1:51–57.
21. Gruss JD, Vargas-Montano H, Bartels D, Hanschke D, Fietze-Fischer B. Direct reconstructive venous surgery. Int Angio 1985;4:441.

22. Gruss JD, Laubach K. Modifikation der Operationstechnik bei tiefer Becken- und Oberschenkelvenenthrombose. Thoraxchirurgie 1971;19:508.
23. Gruss JD, Bartels D, Tsafandakis E, et al. The AV fistula operation technique. In: May R, Weber J, eds. Pelvic and abdominal veins. Amsterdam: Excerpta Medica, 1981:215.
24. Gruss JD. Venous bypass for chronic venous insufficiency. In: Bergan JJ, Yao JST, eds. Venous disorders. Philadelphia: WB Saunders, 1991:316–330.
25. Gruss JD. Pontage pre-pubien croisé (Operation de Palma). In: Branchereau A, Jausseran JM, eds. Chirurgie des veines profondes. Marseille: Edition Chirurgie Vasculaire Nouvelle, 1993:123–128.
26. Vollmar JF, Hutschenreiter S. Der quere Beckenvenenbypass ("hoher Palma"). Vasa 1980;9:62.
27. Halliday P, Harris J, May J. Femoro-femoral crossover grafts (Palma operation): a long term follow-up study. In: Bergan JJ, Yao JST, eds. Surgery of the veins. Orlando, FL: Grune & Stratton, 1985:241–254.
28. Krug A, Lehmann U, Zaborsky F. Modifizierte temporäre A.V. Fistel beim venösen suprapubischen cross-over-shunt wegen einseitiger Beckenvenensperre. Chirurg 1974;45:389.
29. May R. Chirurgie der Bein- und Beckenvenen. Stuttgart: Georg Thieme Verlag, 1974:178–185.
30. May R, Weber J, eds. Pelvic and abdominal veins: progress in diagnostics and therapy. International Congress Series 550. Amsterdam: Excerpta Medica, 1981:192–197.
31. Ijima H, Kodana M, Hori M. Temporary arteriovenous fistula for venous reconstruction using synthetic graft: a clinical and experimental investigation. J Cardiovasc Surg 1989;26:131–136.
32. Warren R, Thayer T. Transplantation of the saphenous vein for postphlebitic stasis. Surgery 1954;35:867.
33. Frileux C, Pillot-Bienaymé P, Gillot C. Bypass of segmental obliterations of ilio-femoral venous axis by transposition of saphenous vein. J Cardiovasc Surg 1972;13:409.
34. Gruss JD. Zur Modifikation des Femoralisbypass nach May. Vasa 1975;4:59.
35. May R. Spätergebnisse nach venösem Femoralisbypass. Vasa 1979;8:67.
36. Gruss JD. The saphenopopliteal bypass for chronic venous insufficiency (May-Husni operation). In: Bergan JJ, Yao JST, eds. Surgery of the veins. Orlando, FL: Grune & Stratton, 1985:255–265.
37. Raju S, Fredericks R. Venous obstruction: diagnosis and treatment. In: Veith FJ, ed. Current critical problems and new horizons in vascular surgery–III. St. Louis: Quality Medical Publishing Company, 1991:151–155.
38. Edwards WS. Femoral arteriovenous fistula as a complementary or primary procedure for iliac venous occlusion. In: Bergan JJ, Yao JST, eds. Surgery of the veins. New York: Grune & Stratton, 1985:267–274.

chapter 21

Venous Valve Surgery—An Overview

Robert L. Kistner

Direct repair of the incompetent valve in lower extremity veins has been practiced since the first repair in 1968 (1). The procedure is performed on a highly selective basis to correct reflux in patients with advanced symptoms due to primary valve incompetence (PVI), but is not useful in the destroyed valves of the postthrombotic veins. Several surgical methods have been developed to achieve competence in these primary incompetent valves, and there are various valve locations where the procedure can be done, including the superficial femoral vein (SFV), deep (profunda) femoral vein (PFV), popliteal vein (PV), posterior tibial vein (PTV), and the common femoral vein (CFV).

BACKGROUND

The concept of repairing incompetence in the lower extremity veins has its origins in the works of John Homans and Robert Linton in the United States and Gunnar Bauer in Sweden. Homans' observations in 1916 (2) provided the basis for understanding that ulcers follow thrombophlebitis and perforator vein incompetence. In the 1940s, Bauer (3) described severe valve leakage in both the postthrombotic state and in an idiopathic nonthrombotic state. He introduced the concept of descending phlebography by placing contrast in the femoral vein of the semierect individual. He observed that the symptoms were the same in both the idiopathic and the postthrombotic reflux cases. Bauer found that the severe symptoms of deep vein reflux were controlled by interruption of the popliteal vein. His concept that proximal valve incompetence is important in chronic venous insufficiency was examined and discarded in England in favor of attention to superficial saphenous incompetence and distal perforator vein incompetence (4).

Linton (5), in the United States, in the 1950s became convinced of the importance of proximal deep vein reflux and advocated ligation of the SFV as part of the treatment for postthrombotic recanalized veins in patients with advanced ulcer disease. He recommended treatment of superficial, perforator and deep veins in these patients by stripping of the incompetent greater saphenous vein, radical interruption of the communicating veins and ligation of the SFV. These SFV ligations were done because he thought all cases of SFV thrombophlebitis resulted in recanalization of the SFV, which left a valveless vein with reflux into the calf. He theorized that this reflux gave rise to severe chronic venous insufficiency and ulceration. His experience with SFV ligation, combined with treatment of the saphenous and perforator veins, yielded superior results.

Linton's experience was not studied with phlebography to prove its indications or its results. His use of SFV ligation and Bauer's use of popliteal vein ligation have both been criticized by later analyses of their patients. In Lindhagen and Hallbook's analysis (6) of a small sample of Bauer's cases 20 years later, it was found that reflux by way of deep collaterals had overcome the popliteal ligation in all but one of the 38 patients. It is important to note that during the period when the ligation was dominant over reflux, the clinical results apparently were very good.

These studies were the background from which experience with deep venous valve repair evolved. The controversies over the validity of interruption of major venous channels ultimately led to the restoration of valve competence and preservation of the venous drainage by direct valve repair when this became feasible.

RATIONALE OF DEEP VEIN VALVE SURGERY

In the patient with chronic venous insufficiency (CVI) and venous ulceration, the dominant finding is axial valve incompetence in most cases. When the incompetence is limited to the saphenous vein, stripping of the vein provides relief. If the perforator veins are large and incompetent, they are interrupted and the patient improves. In the deep veins, Bauer (3) and Linton (5) tried interruption with good results in the early course even though this was followed by late recurrence in some cases.

The rationale for valve repair is to eliminate as much of the incompetence in the proximal veins as possible without introducing obstruction. In addition to the deep vein valve repair, it is still necessary to treat the diseased saphenous and perforator veins according to conventional methods because these veins are diseased and their persistence will lead to poor results after valve surgery. The importance of perforator repair was noted in the analysis of our cases in 1982 (7), and was demonstrated by the experience at Northwestern University (8) where large incompetent perforator veins were purposely left untreated in a series of transposition operations, and early recurrence of symptoms was found in a majority of patients.

In an erect individual, the venous pressure in the resting foot is equal to a fluid column from the heart to the foot. It has been reasoned that a single valve placed in the femoral vein divides this column approximately in half and is an appropriate place to insert a competent valve. The choice of the upper end of the SFV for valve repair is based partly on the presence of a valve at this point that is frequently repairable. More importantly, a competent valve in the SFV prevents reflux from the CFV, and thereby avoids the possibility of a circus flow of blood up the profunda vein into the CFV and then down the SFV.

Although the functional disadvantage of deep valve incompetence seems obvious, there is no test that accurately quantitates its physiologic severity. The importance of unidirectional flow in the venous system is clinically apparent in the lower extremity of the erect human where the need to have a mechanically efficient mechanism of venous return flow is so important. In the erect individual with incompetent valves, to-and-fro flow is easily monitored by Doppler and duplex scan in incompetent veins. Even a single competent valve at the superficial femoral or the popliteal level does much to interrupt the to-and-fro flow pattern in the lower extremity veins, and thereby works to improve the mechanical efficiency of venous return.

PRIMARY VERSUS SECONDARY VALVE INCOMPETENCE

Direct surgery on the venous valve can be done only when the valve cusps are intact and repairable. In secondary valve incompetence, the phlebitic process will have scarred and deformed the valve to such an extent that repair is seldom possible. The finding that there is a significant population with primary valve incompetence of the deep veins was noted first in Bauer's cases (3) and later in our early series (9), and is now corroborated in multiple other series in the world (10–13). In these cases, the valve is thin, pliable and normal in structure but its cusps are stretched and it is incompetent; this is the valve that can be repaired to a full competent state by direct surgery on the valve.

In addition to pure primary and secondary valve incompetence, there is a significant population of patients who have proximal primary valve incompetence in the upper femoral veins associated with distal secondary valve incompetence due to postthrombotic disease (deep vein thrombosis [DVT]) of the tibial, popliteal and even the distal superficial femoral veins. This is a category where proximal valve repair can be done even though the distal veins are deformed by phlebitis. In our population of patients with chronic venous insufficiency due to reflux disease, about one-third are primary, one-third are secondary, and the other one-third are combined primary/secondary deep vein disease.

The valve of primary valve incompetence (PVI) is thin, pliable, and normally formed. Its defect is that the cusps have been stretched and their leading edges are elongated, and these long edges prolapse under pressure, resulting in loss of effective valve function. This valve is entirely different from the scarred, contracted valve of the postphlebitic state from a morphologic standpoint, but it is functionally the same (Figs. 21.1, 21.2, and 21.3). Since the function of the two valves is the same, the late clinical sequelae are also similar and the condition of chronic venous insufficiency with pain, swelling, induration, and ulcer may be due to either cause.

The occurrence of PVI is diagnosed by descending phlebography, which is about 90% accurate in its ability to distinguish the PVI valve from the post-thrombotic syndrome's (PTS) scarred valve. When the valves identified by descending phlebography are exposed at surgery, those with PVI are found to have a normal valve architecture with elongated stretched cusps. Additionally, some

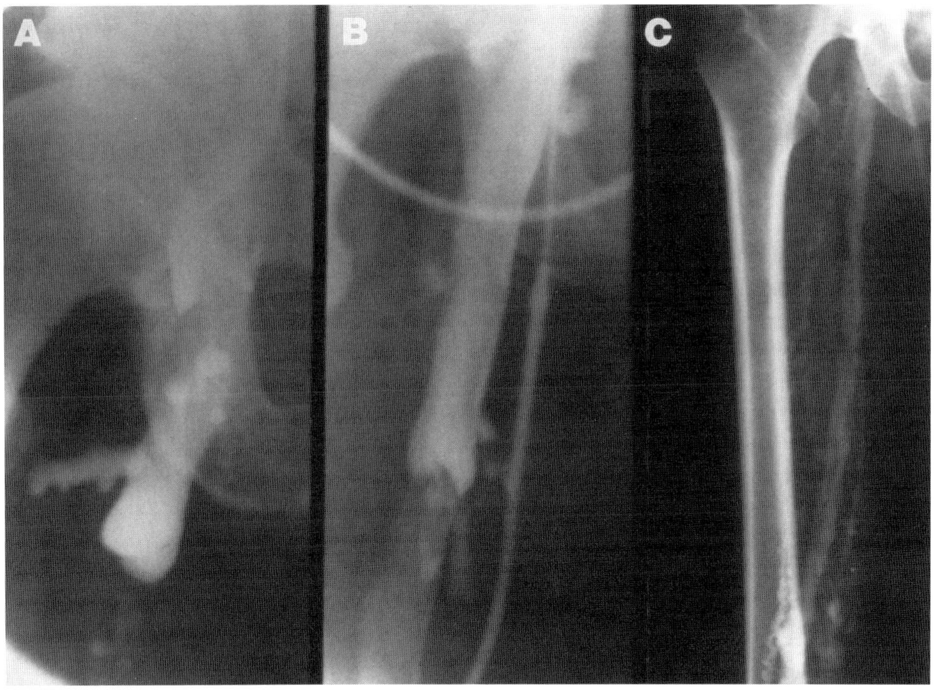

FIG. 21–1. A. Competent valve of superficial femoral vein (SFV). **B.** Refluxing occurring through a repairable valve. **C.** Postthrombotic appearance of SFV with secondary incompetence. (Reproduced by permission from Kistner RL. Descending phlebography: the Straub technique. In: Bergan JJ, Kistner RL, eds. Atlas of venous surgery. Philadelphia: WB Saunders, 1992:107–108.)

of these veins exhibit a thin dilated vein wall that is stretched below the cusp, resulting in separation of the cusps with widening and flattening of the normal angle at the valve commissure. In contrast, the postthrombotic veins show scarred, thickened walls and deformed or destroyed valve cusps.

DIAGNOSIS OF PRIMARY VALVE INCOMPETENCE

Proper selection of patients for valve surgery requires a thorough evaluation of the lower extremity veins. An organized approach begins with a detailed history and physical examination with special reference to previous venous disease and coagulation abnormalities. The extent of swelling, pain, stasis changes, and ulceration should be determined. Previous varicose vein disease and operations are important. Possible episodes of previous DVT, including the extent of the problem and whether definitive diagnosis had been made, may help in the interpretation of later tests. A thorough Doppler interrogation of the veins should be part of the physical examination to give the physician a working impression of the location and degree of both occlusion and reflux in the saphenous, perforator, and axial deep veins.

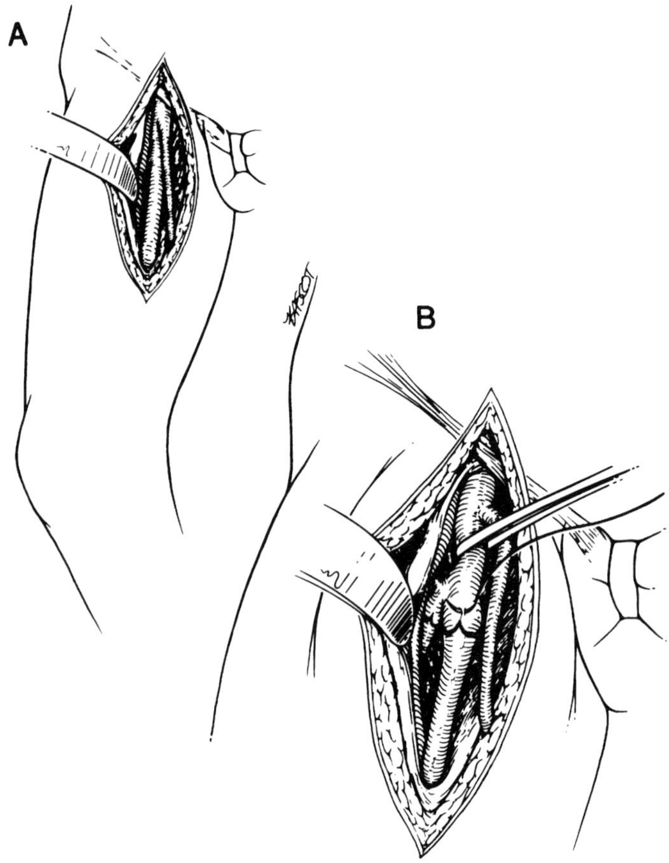

FIG. 21–2. Transvalvular method of Kistner for internal valve repair. **A.** Vertical incision in thigh for valve repair. **B.** Marking suture placed at valve commissure. **C.** Venotomy begins below commissure. **D.** Advance the venotomy carefully. **E.** Venotomy completed, floppy valve cusps exposed. **F.** First suture. Needle passes from outside vein to inside at apex of medial commissure. **G.** Inside vein; needle engages edge of cusp 2 mm away from commissure. **H.** Needle passes through valve cusp and through vein wall at apex of commissure. **I.** First suture tied on outside of vein. Valve cusp shortened by 2 mm. **J.** Suture being placed in lateral commissure. **K.** Two sutures placed and tied down to shorten lateral commissure. **L.** Suture being placed in cusp on posterior wall of vein. Posterior suture engages both cusps with a single suture. **M.** Completed repair with multiple sutures at commissures. Shortened cusp restores cup-like effect to valve. **N.** First suture being placed in closure to reconstitute the valve commissure. **O.** Venotomy being closed in cephalad direction with running suture. **P.** Caudad part of venotomy being closed. **Q.** Competent valve postrepair as proven by strip test. (Reproduced by permission from Kistner RL. Valve reconstruction for primary valve insufficiency. In: Bergan JJ, Kistner RL, eds. Atlas of venous surgery. Philadelphia: WB Saunders, 1992:127–129.)

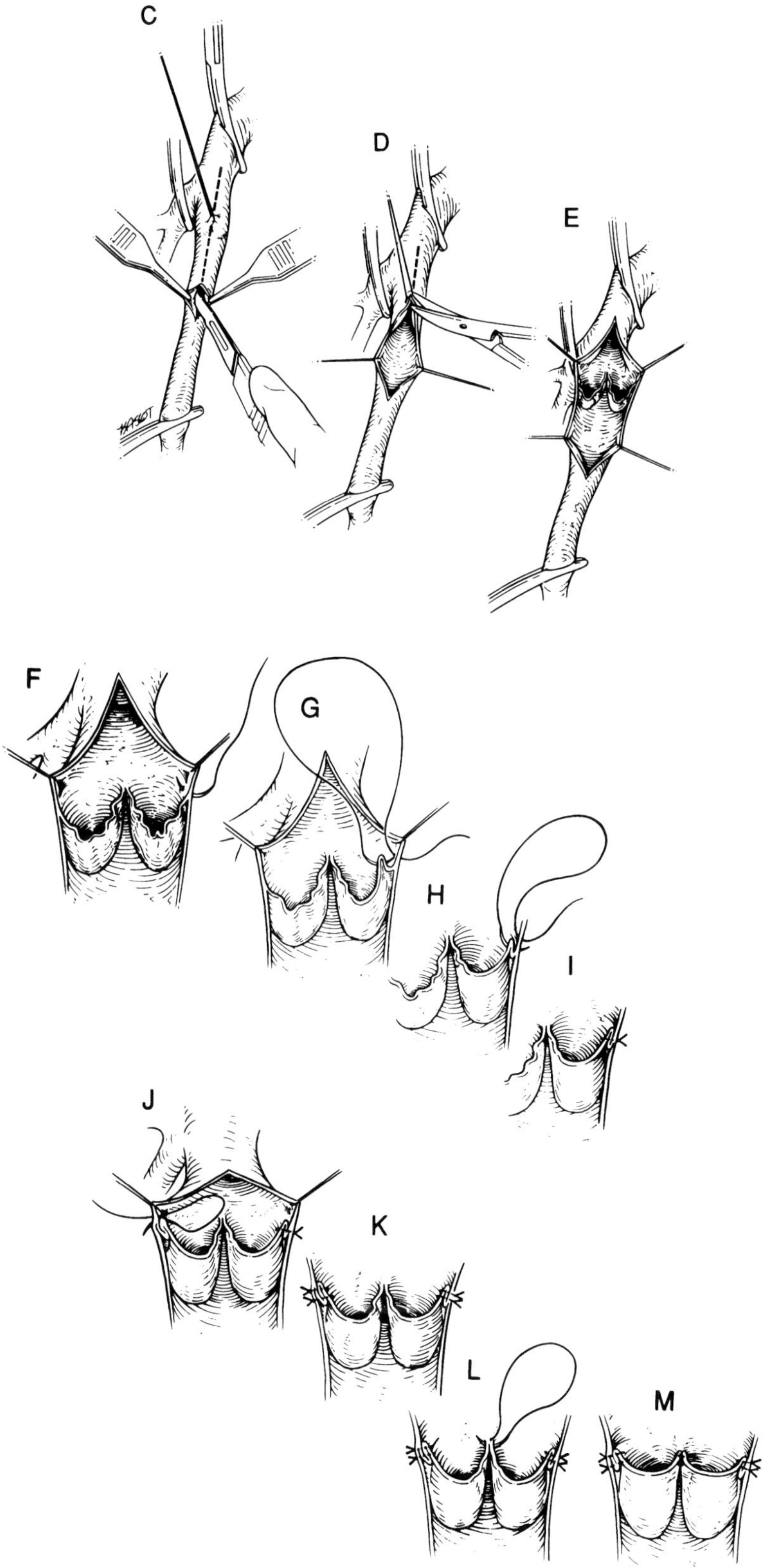

FIG. 21–2. Continued

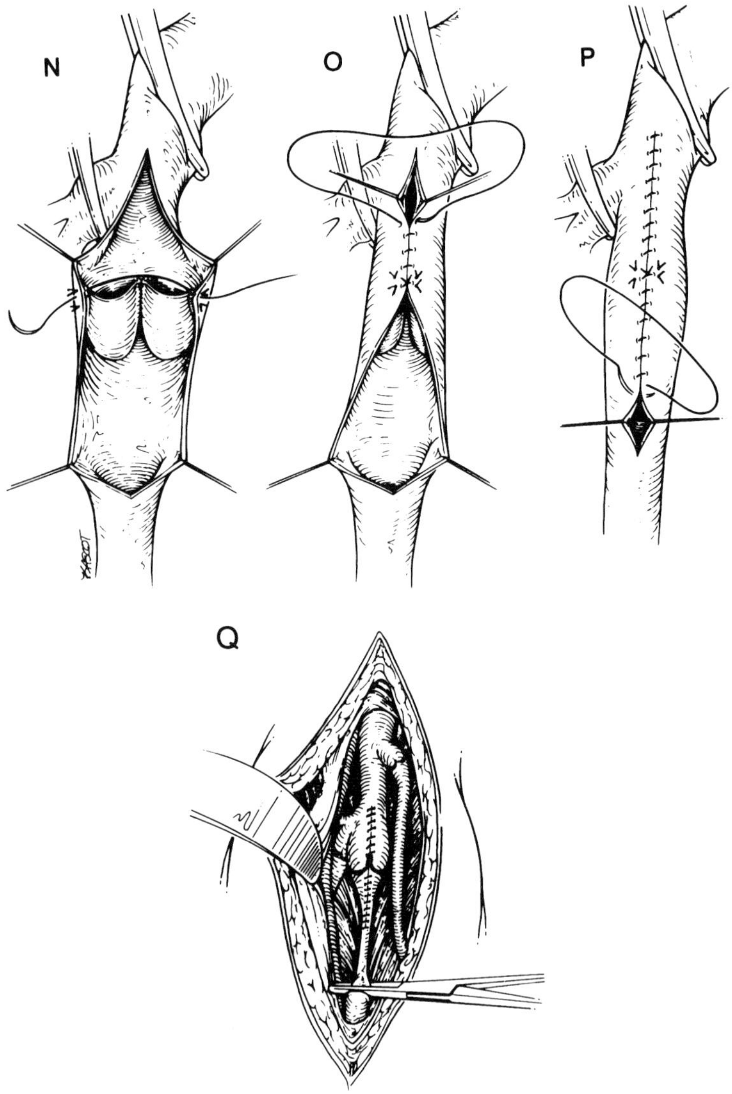

FIG. 21–2. Continued

The vascular laboratory is used to confirm physiologic abnormalities of the venous system by pressure and plethysmographic techniques and to image the veins for patency and reflux by duplex scan. The role of these techniques is still evolving. Venous pressure studies identify the patient with abnormal veins and can be of use in differentiating reflux from obstruction, but are not able to discriminate causes or sites of reflux disease or degrees of reflux disease. Photoplethysmography has similar limitations. The air plethysmography does provide discrimination between reflux and obstruction in the venous system and will probably prove to be very useful in the workup of the CVI patient. The well-equipped laboratory will provide most, if not all, of these modalities.

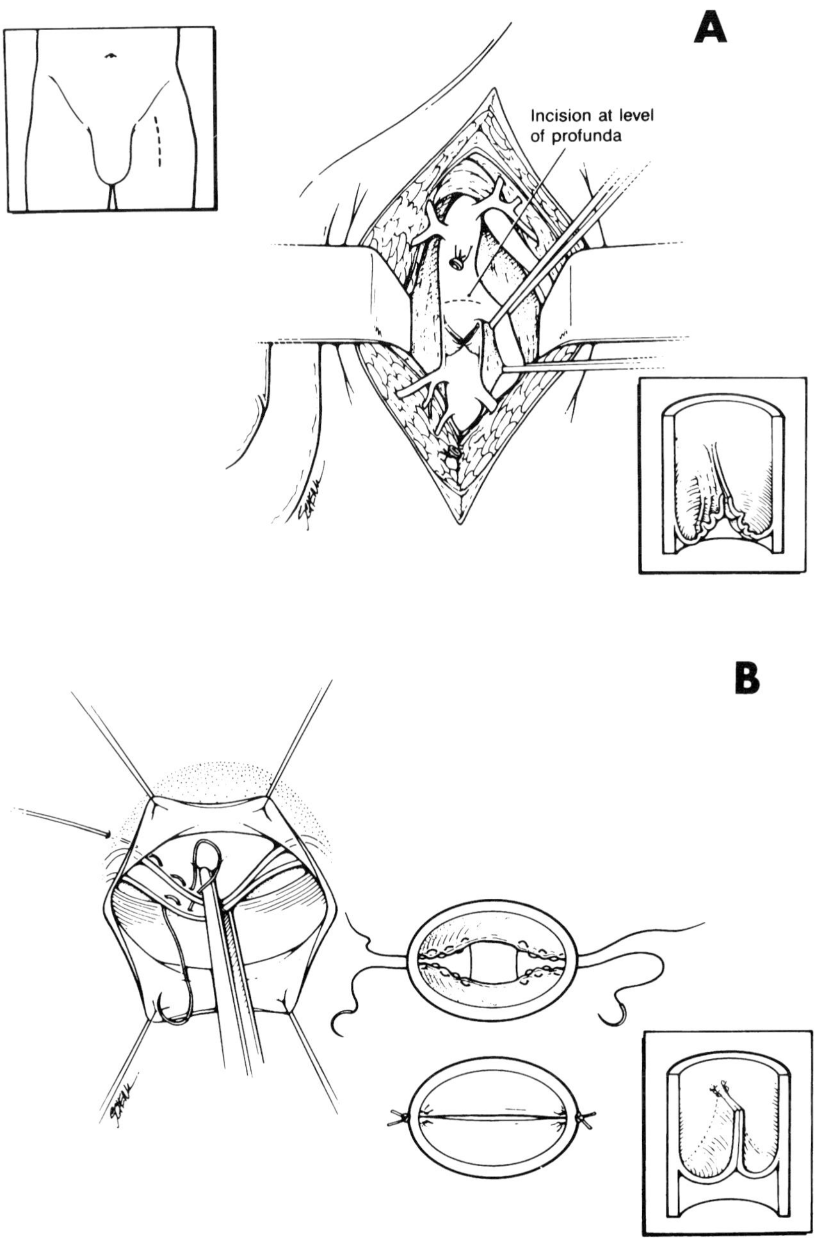

FIG. 21–3. Raju method of supravalvular internal valve repair. **A.** Femoral vein exposure is through a longitudinal incision. The vein is incised transversely above the cusp. Redundant valves are clearly seen (*inset*). **B.** Continuous suture using double needles allows shortening of valve leaflets and subsequent knot placement externally. Alternatively, single sutures may be taken (*inset*). (Reproduced by permission from Kistner RL. Supravalvular incision for valve repair in primary valvular insufficiency. In: Bergan JJ, Kistner RL, eds. Atlas of venous surgery. Philadelphia: WB Saunders, 1992:136.)

Imaging with the duplex scanner is an important part of the workup. This allows identification of occlusion and reflux in every segment of the deep and superficial venous systems. It is the single best test in the vascular laboratory due to its ability to discriminate reflux from obstruction, segment by segment, in the lower extremity veins. In time, it may become a quantitative as well as a qualitative test. Color Doppler adds a major dimension to this test by making it quicker and easier.

A complete imaging study will visualize the saphenous, perforator, tibial, popliteal, SFV, PFV, and CFV veins, and assess each segment for reflux and patency.

Phlebography remains a necessary part of the CVI evaluation for the potential surgical candidate. Ascending phlebograms demonstrate patency of the axial veins and competence of the perforator veins. These should be done with fluoroscopy to demonstrate perforator vein flow from deep to superficial to locate incompetent perforator veins. One can utilize a semierect position of the patient, contrast injection by way of a dorsal foot vein, an ankle tourniquet to prevent filling of superficial veins, and fluoroscopy of the calf to study the perforators. Under these conditions, contrast in the deep system should not pass through the deep fascia into surface veins unless the perforator veins are incompetent. Using fluoroscopy, the exact sites and sizes of incompetent perforators are discovered. Perforators can be studied further and corroborated with the duplex scanner. The ascending venograms will usually identify those cases with postthrombotic changes in the tibial-popliteal-SFV segments. The presence and extent of postthrombotic disease and perforator incompetence on this study will weigh heavily in the decisions for various types of surgical treatment.

Descending phlebography is the hallmark for identifying primary valve incompetence in a given valve. This study pinpoints the site of the various valves in the saphenous and femoral veins. It is done with the patient semierect. Contrast is placed in the common femoral vein and the patient is taught to do a standardized Valsalva maneuver. Under fluoroscopy, one can see the stress placed on proximal competent valves with the Valsalva maneuver. When the proximal valve is competent (Fig. 21.1**A**) in the saphenous, SFV, or PFV veins, this study will not identify more distal problems in these segments because the contrast does not reflux down the vein. When the proximal valve is incompetent (Fig. 21.1**B**), contrast flows through these valves and down the vein until a competent valve is encountered or until the contrast is diluted out in the calf veins. The study is accurate only when done under fluoroscopy as a dynamic study. Under these conditions one can usually see the valve cusps actively leaking in patients with PVI and this finding is diagnostic for the presence of PVI. In the patient with postthrombotic scarring or destruction of the valves, the picture is very different and readily discriminated from PVI because cusp leaflets are not seen, and longitudinal septa are often visible in a recanalized vessel (Fig. 21.1**C**).

With this complete evaluation of the patient from clinical, physiologic, and imaging perspectives, the surgeon can identify which segments are patent and normal, which are patent and incompetent, which have primary valve incompetence as compared to postthrombotic incompetence, and which are obstructed. These data are compared to the physiologic information and placed in the perspective of the clinical setting. From these considerations, recommendations for surgery can be made on a selective and reasonable basis.

INDICATIONS FOR DEEP VEIN SURGERY

The basic indication for repair of the deep venous valve is the patient whose occupation or normal way of life is impaired by venous disease, and in whom repairable defects are found. The intent of surgery is to restore the patient to full activity free of aching, swelling, and ulceration and, in the ideal case, to relieve the patient of the need to wear elastic support.

The clinical evaluation identifies those patients whose venous disease limits their activity, whether the limitation is due to aching, swelling, or ulceration, alone or in combination. The physiologic tests confirm the presence of disease in the venous system, and the imaging studies identify the details of primary versus secondary incompetence, and the sites of obstruction, segment by segment.

In planning surgery, all segments of the venous system are taken into account. In the majority of CVI cases, surgical treatment of the saphenous or perforator veins, or both, will control the problem and restore function, and deep valve repair is not needed. Overall, it is estimated that fewer than 10% of CVI patients will need valve surgery. In those patients who have a severe CVI problem and are most limited by their disease, however, the conversion of an incompetent deep proximal system to a competent state by valve repair can be dramatic in helping to restore the individual to a full functional condition.

When planning valve surgery, the surgeon is best advised to identify all incompetent segments and try to control them all. The saphenous and perforator veins are treated with interruption techniques. The SFV is controlled by valve repair of any single valve in the segment from CFV to popliteal vein. The most frequent repairable valve is in the proximal SFV, but it is not unusual to find another repairable valve in the mid-SFV or at the adductor canal level. While some surgeons prefer to repair more than one valve, the necessity to do this awaits further study. When the PFV has significant reflux, it should be repaired at the same time as the SFV repair. This can often be done by an external repair technique. An alternative method to control PFV reflux is to interrupt the large collaterals between the PFV and the upper popliteal vein at the adductor canal level when they are present. A third approach to combined PFV and SFV reflux is to perform repair in the popliteal veins when a satisfactory valve can be found there, or to transplant a valve-containing segment from the arm to the popliteal vein.

The concept of multiple valve repair is being explored by several investigators (14, 15) and may be shown to give an improvement in long-term results.

METHODS OF PRIMARY VALVE REPAIR

The original method of valve repair was an internal (16) repair with the vein being opened by a transvalvular incision (Fig. 21.2; Table 21.1). This method remains the author's current choice of definitive repair because it is a precise anatomic repair with known long-term results.

TABLE 21-1

REPAIR OF VALVE INCOMPETENCE

Methods
Valvuloplasty
Internal
Transvalvular (Kistner)
Supravalvular (Raju)
Supravalvular with T-extension (Sottiurai)
External
Suture Technique (Kistner)
External Cuff (Lane) Dacron Sleeve (Raju)
Angioscopic Repair (Gloviczki)
Transposition (Kistner)
Transplantation
Axillary Vein Transfer (Taheri), (Raju)

Raju modified the transvalvular approach to a supravalvular incision (17) in which access to the valve is gained from a position on top of the valve (Fig. 21.3). Sottiurai modified both of these methods by a supravalvular incision (Fig. 21.4) with a vertical limb down into a valve cusp (18).

These methods have been reported by various surgeons (7, 10, 11, 19, 20) and the long-term results at 4 years are similar, with good results in 70% of primary valve patients. Lane (21), in Australia, developed an external silastic wrap, called a venocuff, to provide valve competence without the need for opening the vein. This work was supported by extensive animal research and is presently in clinical trials. Raju (10) described a much simpler external wrap technique with readily available prosthetic grafts such as dacron or PTFE. The technique was more selectively used than the venocuff and was restricted to valves that become competent with venoconstriction induced by surgical manipulation. The advantage of these external techniques is that the valvuloplasty procedure is simplified and anticoagulants are not needed. The disadvantage is that it is not an anatomic repair and it places a foreign body around the vein. The long-term effects will determine the usefulness of this procedure.

In 1987, an external suture technique was devised (22) where a series of sutures are placed along the diverging cusp margins on both sides of the bicuspid valve (Fig. 21.5). This procedure results in a competent valve and avoids the need for opening the vein, but it is not an anatomic repair of the defect; its long-term effects remain to be proven.

A more recent report (23) describes a technique to achieve anatomic repair by external suture technique guided from within the vein by an angioscope. This procedure combines the benefits of external suture with precise anatomic repair.

In addition to these methods of direct valve repair, the operation of transposition (24) allows the surgeon to transfer an incompetent SFV or PFV vein to an adjacent saphenous or femoral vein which has competent valves and thereby provide proximal competence to the incompetent segment.

Transplantation of vein segments that contain a valve can also be done (12, 25, 26), but is not the procedure of choice in primary valve incompetence. It has been the consensus experience that valve repair is preferable to valve transplant in PVI when a repairable valve is available because the long-term results have been more durable (10, 12, 19, 20).

RESULTS

Similar results 2–4 years after direct internal valve repair have been reported by five authors constituting more than 170 collective cases with the finding of 70–90% good results (Table 21.2) (7, 10, 11, 19, 27). In most cases, the deep vein repairs have been accompanied by control of reflux in saphenous and large incompetent perforator veins, and the good results are attributable to the total

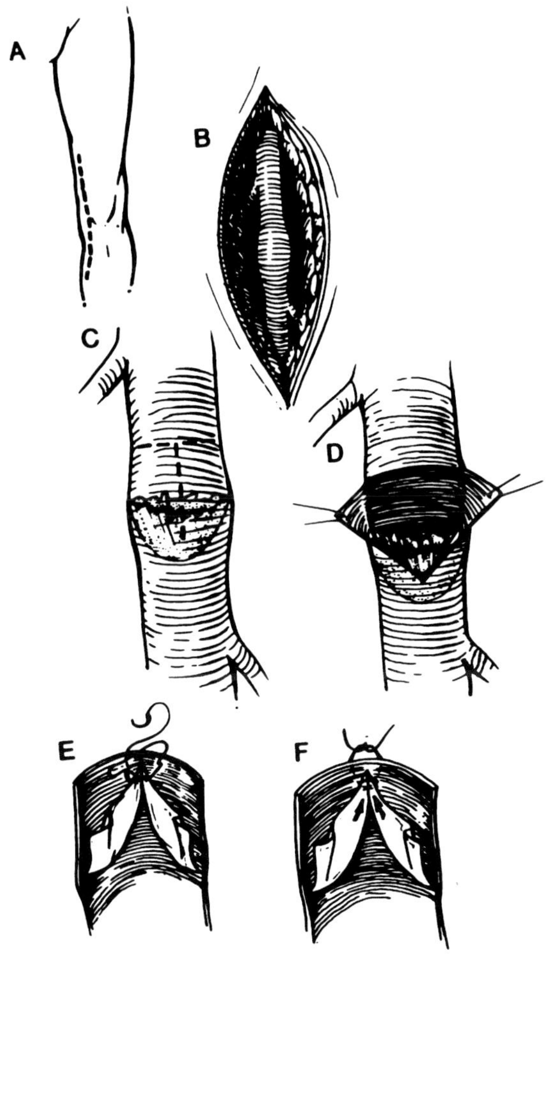

FIG. 21–4. Sottiurai supravalvular method of internal valve repair. **A.** Vertical skin incision placed at medial aspect of distal thigh. **B.** Femoral vein exposed through a vertical incision. **C.** Transverse and vertical venotomies as indicated by broken lines. **D.** Vein flaps retracted laterally with suture to display the valve cusps. **E.** Double-ended suture used to suspend valve cusps at the commissure. **F.** Ties placed at outside of vein to tack valve cusps to the venous wall. (Reproduced by permission from Kistner RL. Supravalvular incision for valve repair in primary valvular insufficiency. In: Bergan JJ, Kistner RL, eds. Atlas of venous surgery. Philadelphia: WB Saunders, 1992:139.)

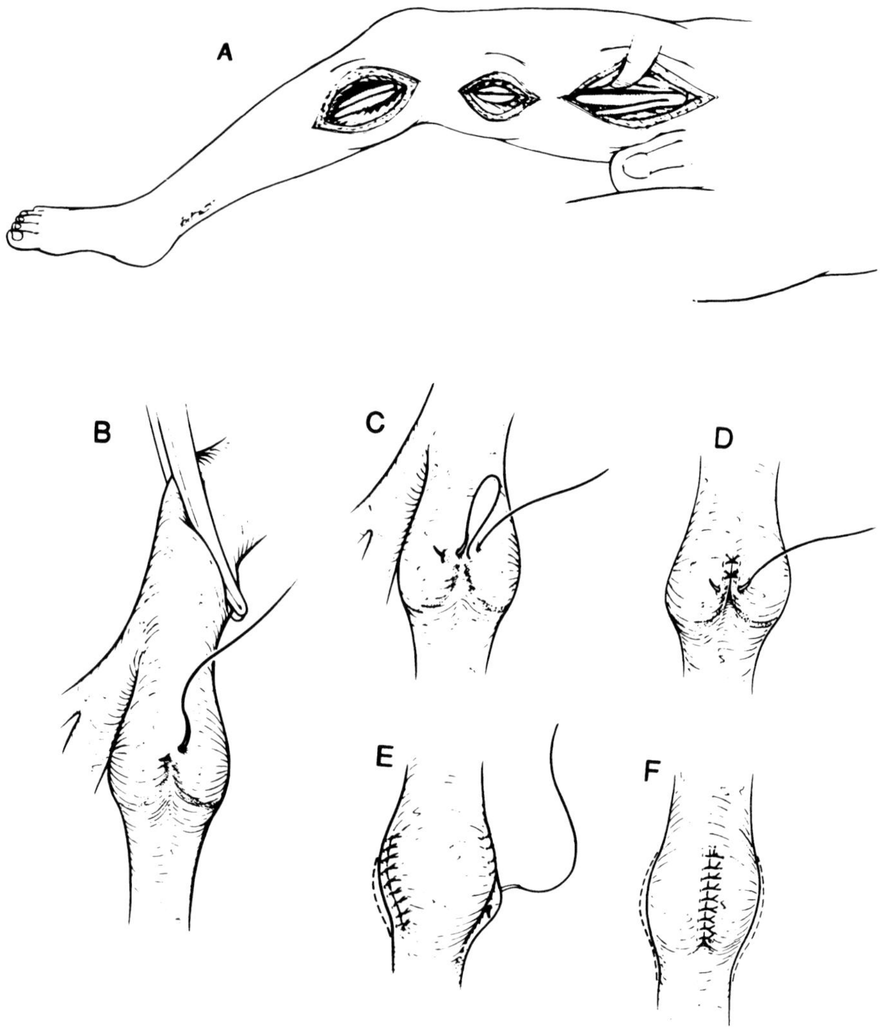

FIG. 21–5. Suture method of external valve repair. **A.** Incisions for repair of valves at various levels. **B.** First suture engages cusp margin. **C.** First suture engages both cusp margins. **D.** First suture tied outside vein. Multiple sutures coapting cusp margins. Intervening tissue is imbricated. **E.** Sutures placed in both commissures. **F.** Completed repair. Vein narrowed slightly. (Reproduced by permission from Kistner RL. Valve reconstruction for primary valve insufficiency. In: Bergan JJ, Kistner RL, eds. Atlas of venous surgery. Philadelphia: WB Saunders, 1992:132.)

control of reflux in the extremity. The deep vein repairs were performed for PVI of the thigh veins in all cases. In all cases, the popliteal and tibial veins were also incompetent; in some cases, this distal incompetence was due to PVI, and in others it was due to postthrombotic disease of the more distal segments. Since these results reflect similar long-term efficacy of the internal repair of the incompetent valve by the different techniques of Raju, Sottiurai, and Kistner, it appears that the choice of technique does not alter the ultimate result.

TABLE 21-2

LATE RESULTS OF VALVULOPLASTY 2–4-YEAR FOLLOW-UP GOOD RESULTS (CLASS 0–1)

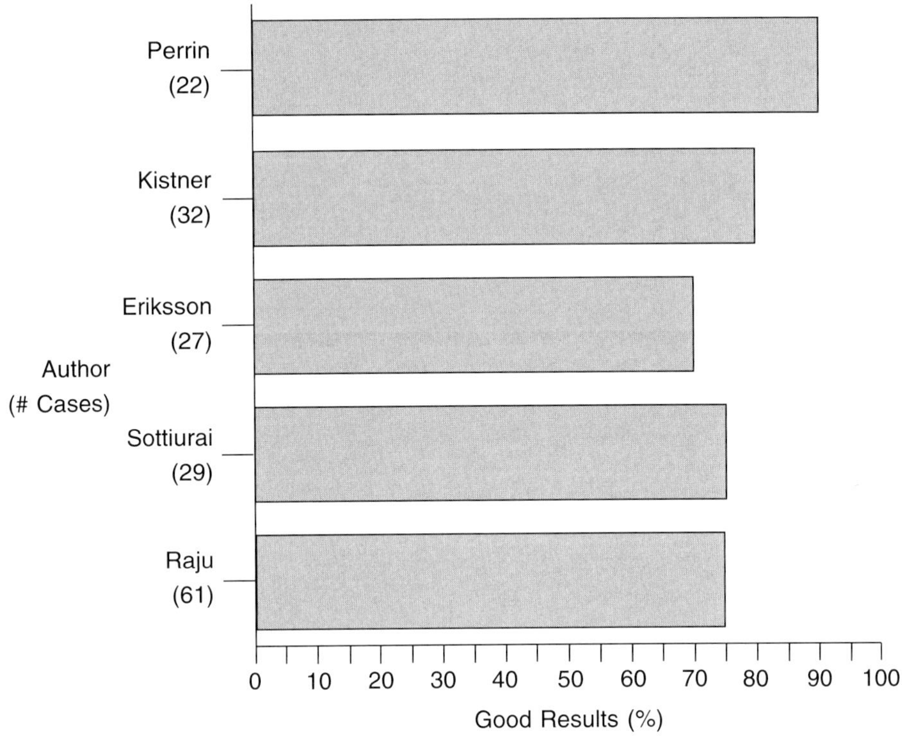

The long-term results of external repair are yet to be reported. The external suture technique was first done in 1987 (22) and its 4-year results will be forthcoming in the near future. The external cuff repair remains under clinical trial in Australia and the United States. Angioscopic repair was described in the literature in 1991 (23) and will require additional time for analysis of results.

The results of transposition and transplantation surgery are not applicable to patients with PVI since they are used in the main for postthrombotic incompetence. The 4-year results with these procedures for postthrombotic disease have been less encouraging than direct valve repair for PVI disease. From analysis of six series of transplantation (Table 21.3) (10–12, 27–29) and seven reports of transposition (Table 21.4) (8, 10, 11, 19, 27, 30, 31), it appears that long-term good results have been achieved in about 50% of these cases rather than the demonstrated 75% good results for PVI. This suggests that extensive postthrombotic disease represents a more severe insult to the deep veins than does pure PVI disease.

There are questions about deep valve repair in PVI that remain to be answered. Those who have repaired multiple valves rather than a single valve point out the possibility of improved results with this approach. Lane (14) has suggested that three competent repaired valves give better results than a single valve. Raju (15) has found repair of the SFV, PFV, and posterior tibial vein simultaneously gives better correction of the venous pressure test in the postoperative period when compared to single valve repair.

The choice of correcting a valve in the SFV versus one in the CFV or in the popliteal vein has not been tested in PVI. Restoring competence in the popliteal vein is indicated when both the SFV and PFV are incompetent, or when large collaterals between the popliteal and incompetent PFV exist. When the PFV is competent, there is not likely to be any difference between restoring competence in the SFV versus the popliteal vein since there are no major branches between these two sites that would lead to significant reflux. The advantage of providing the competent valve in the upper SFV is to prevent circus movement of blood that flows through the PFV into the CFV and then down the SFV. This type of circus

TABLE 21-3

LATE RESULTS OF VALVE TRANSPLANT 2–4-YEAR FOLLOW-UP GOOD RESULTS (CLASS 0–1)

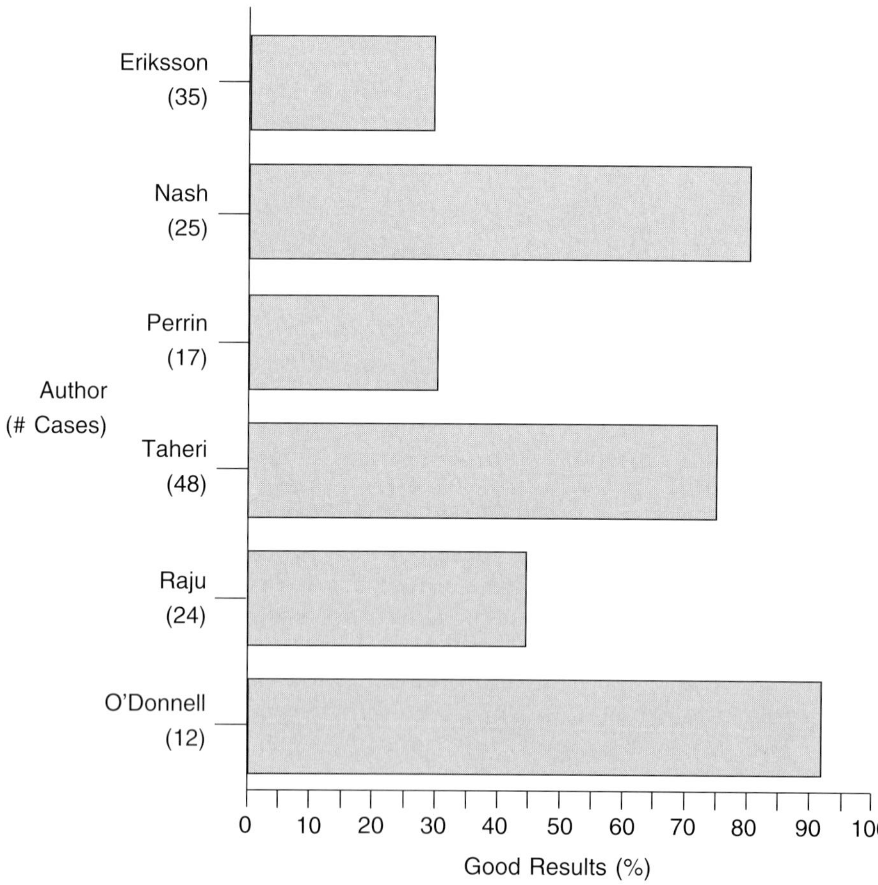

TABLE 21-4

LATE RESULTS OF VENOUS VALVE TRANSPOSITION 2–4-YEAR FOLLOW-UP GOOD RESULTS (CLASS 0–1)

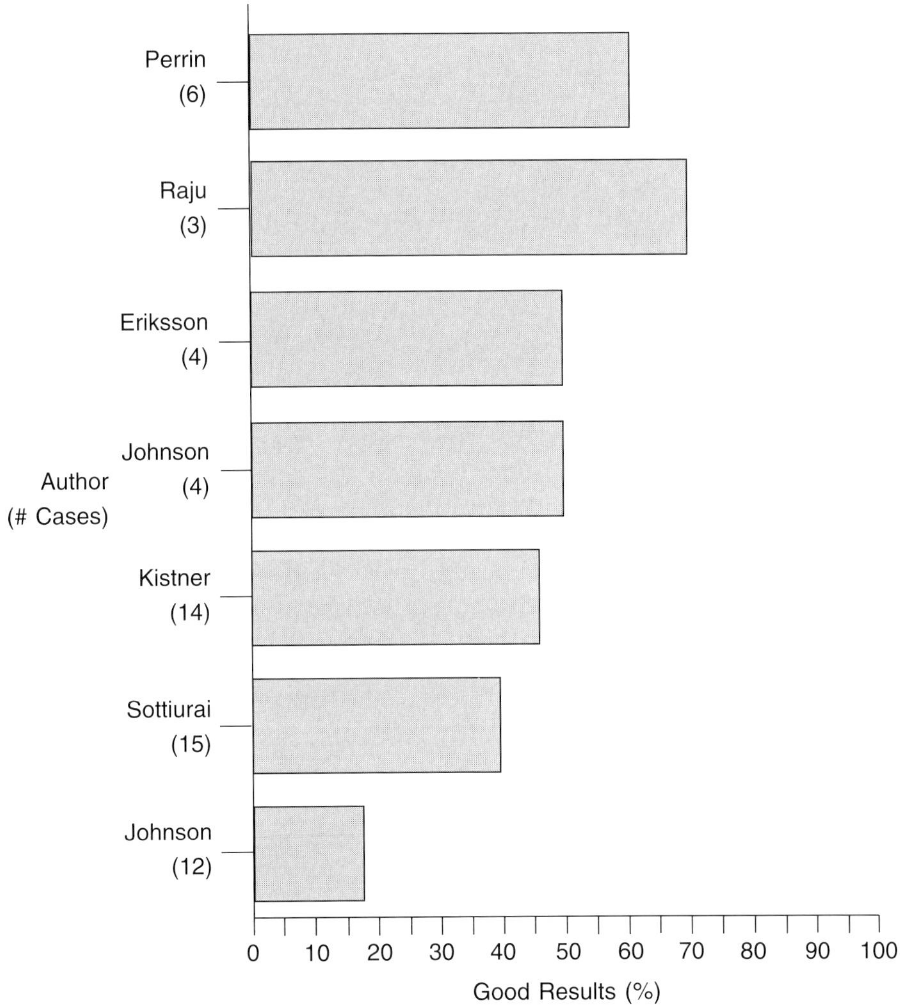

flow has been shown to occur in the incompetent saphenous system (32) and may also occur in the deep system.

In our recent analysis of very long-term (4–21 year) results of valve repair for PVI, there were 51 extremities in 48 patients followed for a median of 12 years and a range of 4–20 years (30). The important findings were that 60% of the extremities maintained good results free of recurrent pain, swelling, and ulcerations, and half of these did not even use elastic support postoperatively. Of those that did develop recurrent ulcer, two-thirds of the cases had only a single ulcer recurrence over the duration of the followup; this single ulcer recurrence did not necessarily indicate a long-term poor clinical result in these patients even though they do constitute a poor statistical result. Some of the single recurrent ulcers were seen at the 1-year or 2-year followup and never recurred again over many years of subsequent follow-up. Of the entire group, there were 17% with two or more recurrences, and it was this group who had inadequate response to the surgical approach of valve repair.

When imaging results were compared to the clinical results, we found those whose valve repairs remained competent by late imaging studies enjoyed the best long-term results. In the 35% of patients with excellent results who did not require elastic stockings in late follow-up, there were competent or near competent valves by late postoperative imaging study in all cases. The physiologic improvement as reflected in the late postoperative venous pressure studies did not correlate as well with clinical improvement. Some improvement of the ambulatory venous pressure was seen in 75% of the cases. Although there was a strong tendency for those with significantly improved venous pressure tests after surgery to show good clinical results, there were enough patients with good clinical results who showed no improvement in venous pressure to reduce the statistical evaluation to nonsignificant levels. We interpret the lack of clear correlation with physiologic tests to demonstrate that residual abnormalities are still present in these extremities even though they may not present as clinical problems, and these abnormalities produce abnormal venous pressure. The results of pre- and postoperative evaluation with the air plethysmograph may shed some light on the results of valve surgery, but this will have to await an adequate series of cases.

SUMMARY

The experience of the past 24 years with deep vein valve repair combined with control of saphenous and perforator vein incompetence in advanced clinical insufficiency due to PVI is that the majority of these cases can be returned to a healthy state of full activity. One-third will be able to discard elastic support. One-third of ulcer cases will have a single recurrent ulcer, or mild-to-moderate symptoms, and will require elastic support to maintain a really good result. In the one-third with continuing symptoms, half of these will have multiple recurrent ulcerations. Although these are not ideal results, they do represent a significant improvement for many venous cases who previously lived with severe lifestyle impairment due to their venous disease.

REFERENCES

1. Kistner RL. Surgical repair of a venous valve. Straub Clin Proc 1968;34:41–43.
2. Homans J. Operative treatment of varicose veins and ulcers. Surg Gynecol Obstet 1916;22:143–158.
3. Bauer G. The etiology of leg ulcers and their treatment by resection of the popliteal vein. J Int Chir 1948;8:937–967.
4. Cockett FA. The pathology and treatment of venous ulcers of the leg. Br J Surg 1955;43:260–278.

5. Linton RR. The post-thrombotic ulceration of the lower extremity: its etiology and surgical treatment. Ann Surg 1953;138:415–430.
6. Lindhagen A, Hallbook T. Venous function in the leg 20 years after ligation and partial resection of the popliteal vein. Acta Chir Scand 1982;148:131–134.
7. Ferris EB, Kistner RL. Femoral vein reconstruction in the management of chronic venous insufficiency: a 14-year experience. Arch Surg 1982;117:1571–1579.
8. Johnson ND, Queral LA, Flinn WR, et al. Late objective assessment of venous valve surgery. Arch Surg 1981;116:1461–1466.
9. Kistner RL. Primary venous valve incompetence of the leg. Am J Surg 1980;140:218–224.
10. Raju S, Fredericks R. Valve reconstruction procedures for nonobstructive venous insufficiency: rationale, technique, and results in 107 procedures with two- to eight-year follow-up. J Vasc Surg 1988;7:301–310.
11. Eriksson I. Reconstructive surgery for deep vein valve incompetence in the lower limb. Eur J Vasc Surg 1990;4:211–218.
12. O'Donnell TF. Popliteal vein valve transplantation for deep venous valvular reflux: rationale, method and long-term clinical, hemodynamic and anatomic results. In: Bergan JJ, Yao JST, eds. Venous disorders. Philadelphia: WB Saunders, 1991:273–295.
13. Perrin M, Bayou JM, Castells-Fender P, Hiltbrand B. Resultats de la chinangie veinease restaura trice daws les reflux veineus profonds. Proc XI World Congress, Union Internationale de Phlebologie. Montreal: John Libbey, 1992:1212–1213.
14. Lane RJ. Presentation. Australian and New Zealand Society of Phlebology. Sydney, Australia, May 4, 1991.
15. Raju S. Experience with venous reconstruction in patients with chronic venous insufficiency. In: Bergan JJ, Yao JST, eds. Venous disorders. Philadelphia: WB Saunders, 1991:296–305.
16. Kistner RL. Valve reconstruction for primary valve insufficiency. In: Bergan JJ, Kistner RL, eds. Atlas of venous surgery. Philadelphia: WB Saunders, 1992:125–130.
17. Raju S. Supravalvular incision for valve repair in primary valvular insufficiency: method of Raju. In: Bergan JJ, Kistner RL, eds. Atlas of venous surgery. Philadelphia: WB Saunders, 1992:135–137.
18. Sottiurai VS. Supravalvular incision for valve repair in primary valvular insufficiency: method of Sottiurai. In: Bergan JJ, Kistner RL, eds. Atlas of venous surgery. Philadelphia: WB Saunders, 1992:137–144.
19. Sottiurai VS. Comparison of surgical modalities in the treatment of recurrent venous ulcer. Int Angiol 1990;9:231–235.
20. Perrin M, Hiltbrand B, Bolor JE, et al. Resultats de la chirurgie veineuse restauratrice dans les reflux de lu voie veinende profonde au niveau des membres inferieurs. Proc 10 EME Congress Mondial Union Internationale de Phlebologie. Strasbourg: John Libbey, 1989:1085–1086.
21. Jessup G, Lane RJ. Repair of incompetent venous valves: a new technique. J Vasc Surg 1988;8:569–575.
22. Kistner RL. Surgical technique of external venous valve repair. Straub Found Proc 1990;55:15–16.
23. Gloviczki P, Merrell SW, Bower TC. Femoral vein valve repair under direct vision without venotomy: a modified technique with angioscopy. J Vasc Surg 1991;14:645–648.
24. Kistner RL. Transposition techniques. In: Bergan JJ, Kistner RL, eds. Atlas of venous surgery. Philadelphia: WB Saunders, 1992:153–156.
25. Raju S. Axillary vein transfer for postphlebitic syndrome. In: Bergan JJ, Kistner RL, eds. Atlas of venous surgery. Philadelphia: WB Saunders, 1992:147–152.
26. Taheri SA, Pendergast DR, Lazar E, et al. Vein valve transplantation. Am J Surg 1985;150:210–202.

27. Perrin M, Hiltbrand B, Bayou JM. La reparation valvulaire au niveau du reseau vein eux profond sous-inguinal Ganget technique on intervention efficace. Phlebologie 1991;44:649–660.
28. Nash T. Long-term results of vein valve transplants placed in the popliteal vein for intractable post-phlebitic venous ulcers and pre-ulcer skin changes. J Cardiovasc Surg 1988;29:712–716.
29. Taheri SA, Elias SM, Yacobucci GN, et al. Indications and results of vein valve transplant. J Cardiovasc Surg 1986;27:163–168.
30. Masuda E, Kistner RL. Long-term results of venous valve reconstruction: a 4 to 21 year follow-up. Presented at the Society of Vascular Surgery. Chicago, June 1992.
31. Johnson WC, Nabseth DS, Bush HL, Widdick WC. Direct venous surgery for venous valvular insufficiency of the lower extremity and updated experience. Contemp Surg 1985;26:35–43.
32. Bjordal RI. Blood circulation in varicose veins of the lower extremities. Angiology 1972;23:163–173.

chapter 22

Angioscopic Valvuloplasty

Agustin A. Rodriguez and Thomas F. O'Donnell

Interest in deep venous reconstructive surgery has heightened over the last 5 years. Several large reviews of the etiology of deep venous involvement show that valvular incompetence is the cause of deep venous insufficiency in more than 70–80% of patients (1–3). While valvular incompetence had been related to postthrombotic valvular damage alone in earlier reports (4, 5), increasing evidence from several authors demonstrates that primary valvular incompetence is the cause of valvular reflux in 30–60% of patients with chronic venous insufficiency (6–8). Primary valvular incompetence (PVI) appears to be due to a fibroelastic tissue defect rather than thrombotic injury (8). PVI differs from postthrombotic valvular destruction not only in the technique required for repair, but also in long-term results. Kistner (9) was the first to describe a direct approach to rendering a valve competent rather than replacing the incompetent segment with a competent valve "borrowed" from either a local or distant venous segment. His initial report in 1975 stimulated interest in the surgical repair of primary valvular incompetence.

PATHOLOGY OF VALVULAR INCOMPETENCE

Although deep venous reflux is assumed to be related to recanalization and subsequent valve destruction which occur as sequelae to a previous episode of deep venous thrombosis, Bauer (4) reported in 1948 that valvular reflux could arise from a primary degeneration of the valve. Using high quality descending phlebograms Kistner (9) observed that approximately 40–50% of limbs with deep venous reflux had an entity he described as primary valvular incompetence (PVI).

Our general knowledge of vein valve function has been expanded greatly by the popularity of the in situ femoral-popliteal vein bypass, which has restimulated research on venous valves. In the deep venous system, the vein valves are usually bicuspid. The semilunar-shaped cusps may either bob in the moving venous blood stream or retract back against the vein wall. The convex margin of the vein is directed cephalad and the straight free margin caudad. When a Valsalva maneuver is performed and blood flow is directed caudad, supravalvular pressure increases so that the valve cusp fills with blood. The valve closes as it is pushed toward the midline to meet the opposite valve cusp. Reflux of blood down the vein is prevented (Fig. 22.1).

On gross examination, primary valve incompetence presents with a normal appearing vein from the exterior. None of the adhesive attachments to the surrounding tissue characteristic of previous thrombosis are observed. The vein wall on the exterior is normal although somewhat dilated. The valve commissure has been described by several authors to have a widened angle (8). The valve area bulges, par-

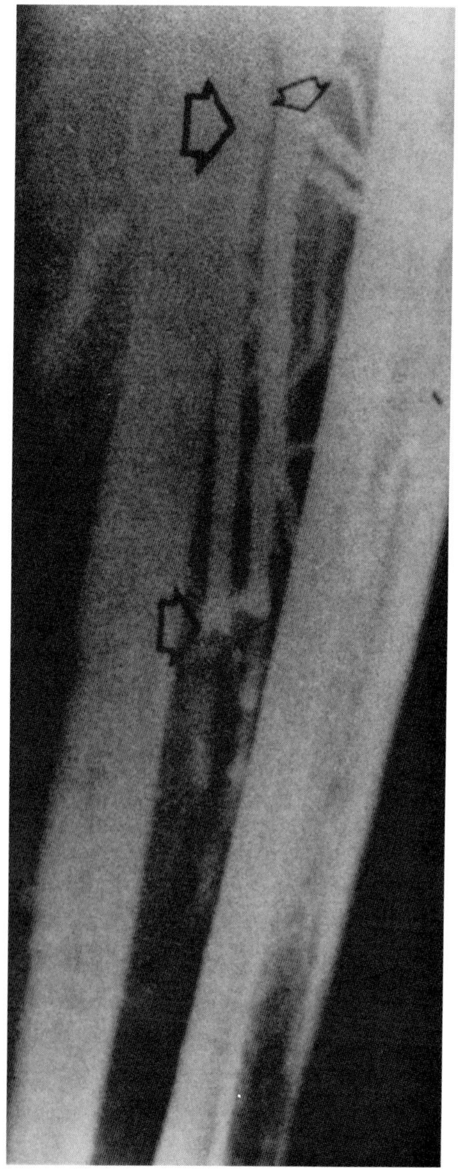

FIG. 22–1. Ascending phlebogram of a patient with competent venous valves. *Lower arrow* points to valve of deep calf vein arresting dye column. Both semilunar cusps coapt so that no dye appears below on proximal compression. (Reproduced by permission from O'Donnell TF Jr, Shepard AD. Chronic venous insufficiency. In: Jarrett F, Hirsch SA, eds. Vascular surgery of the lower extremity. St Louis: CV Mosby, 1985:206–238.)

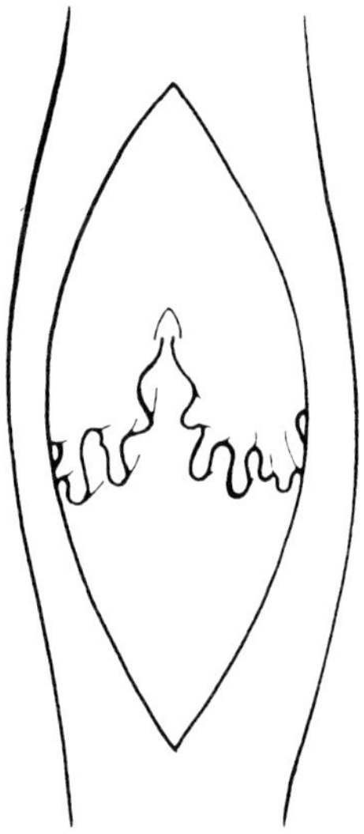

FIG. 22–2. Congenital valvular incompetence. The redundant valve edge resembles a cauliflower, as visualized through a longitudinal venotomy. (Reproduced by permission from O'Donnell TF Jr, Shepard AD. Chronic venous insufficiency. In: Jarrett F, Hirsch SA, eds. Vascular surgery of the lower extremity. St. Louis: CV Mosby, 1985:229.)

ticularly with Valsalva. The internal aspect of the vein when examined through venotomy shows floppy redundant valves. The valves have no evidence of an inflammatory response and resemble gossamer wings. The valve margin is redundant, much like a cabbage leaf (7) (Fig. 22.2). Kistner (9) has theorized that primary valve incompetence is an abnormality of fibroelastic tissue. This defect produces redundancy so that normal coaptation of the valve cusp is prevented. Supportive evidence for the developmental nature of this process is that patients with Klippel-Trenaunay syndrome quite commonly have primary valve incompetence.

In contrast to the sequelae of acute thrombophlebitis, in which the valve may be either totally destroyed by recanalization changes or thickened and frozen so that it ineffectually collapses with a Valsalva maneuver, the patient with "primary" valvular insufficiency has a redundant valve edge that resembles a lettuce leaf (7). In this condition, the valves are unable to close properly and become incompetent. Kistner (9) and Raju (7) have observed that the valves of the superficial femoral veins are involved most frequently. With increased back pressure, both the veins and valves distal to the incompetent proximal superficial femoral vein valve progressively dilate, so that insufficiency of the distal venous system eventually results. A global valvular defect has been postulated since concomitant axillary valvular incompetence may be present (7). Descending phlebography has demonstrated morphologically normal but incompetent venous valves in contrast to the scarred valveless segments or frozen valves seen in the postthrombotic limb.

PRIMARY VALVULAR INCOMPETENCE

Pathophysiologic Sequelae

The primary circulatory abnormality in patients with primary valvular incompetence is the transmission of the high pressures generated during ambulation from the deep system to the superficial system. Valvular reflux increases ambulatory venous pressure. Incompetence of the communicating or perforating veins is usually necessary to develop the well-recognized pathophysiologic sequelae of primary valvular incompetence. During the systolic phase of the calf muscle pump cycle, abnormal transmission of pressure and flow occurs from the deep to the superficial venous system via incompetent perforating veins (10). Such abnormal circulatory hemodynamics result in sustained venous hypertension in the subcutaneous and cutaneous tissues. There is debate as to how these large vessel circulatory abnormalities relate to the ultimate microcirculatory changes. Burnand, et al. (11), have theorized that this pressure leads to development of a capillary block due to defective fibrinolysis with subsequent pericapillary fibrin deposits. Altered delivery of oxygen and nutrients to the subcutaneous tissue and skin ensues, leading to cell death. Alternatively, Wilkinson, et al. (12), have shown that white blood cells are trapped within the microcirculation, releasing cytotoxic agents and producing cell damage.

Evaluation Methods

Clinical Examination. Characteristically patients with valvular reflux in the deep venous system have recognizable features. Pain is described as a heaviness rather than the intense bursting pain experienced by the patient with deep venous obstruction. The patient may develop the sensation of heaviness upon arising from bed. After prolonged standing the pain may develop into a severe form of heaviness localized to the calf, which can be quite incapacitating. The calf heaviness occurs irrespective of whether the patient is ambulating, which is in distinct contrast to the situation with obstructive venous disease and venous claudication. Edema is a frequent finding in patients with deep venous reflux and is of the mild-to-moderate degree. The edema is predominantly distributed in the perimalleolar area. Cutaneous sequelae occur frequently in patients with incompetent perforating veins. Skin pigmentary changes secondary to hemosiderin deposits are the first sign. As the condition advances, eczematous dermatitis ensues and, finally, loss of epithelial integrity (venous ulcer) appears.

Diagnostic Noninvasive and Phlebographic Evaluation. In our experience, deep venous valvular reconstruction is indicated in patients with stage 3 disease (venous ulcer), while a smaller segment of patients with advanced stage 2 disease are candidates. We are more aggressive in offering valve reconstruction to patients with stage 2 disease who have "primary" valve insufficiency, than to patients with postthrombotic valvular damage. Duplex ultrasound and air plethysmography are used to evaluate reflux. Venous reflux can be tested most physiologically in the upright rather than the supine position. Tests that quantify the degree of reflux are best performed with the patient standing.

Duplex Assessment of Venous Reflux. Duplex scanning answers several questions: (a) what pathologic process is the cause of deep venous involvement; (b) what are the levels involved; and (c) who are candidates based on the degree of reflux? The advantage of this technique is related to its speed and the fact that it is patient independent; disadvantages include the initial capital cost, as well as operator and interpreter dependency.

Quantitative evaluation of venous valvular reflux is performed as described by van Bemmelen, et al. (13). Patients are examined in the standing position with their weight supported by the contralateral leg. An ATL Ultramark 9 high-definition imaging color duplex scanner (Advanced Technology Laboratories, Bothell, WA) is used to scan the superficial femoral vein and popliteal veins. Venous flow is recorded proximal to the area of rapid pneumatic cuff deflation. For evaluation of the superficial femoral vein, a thigh cuff is inflated to 80 mmHg and then rapidly deflated. When evaluating the popliteal vein, a cuff is applied to the calf, inflated to 100 mmHg, and rapidly deflated. Both color Doppler and spectral analysis are recorded and used to quantify the amount of reflux.

Van Bemmelen assessed 30 clinically normal limbs and found that the usual reflux time was less than 0.5 second. The tourniquet compression tests of van Bemmelen have become the "gold standard" for evaluating reflux by duplex scan. Masuda and Kistner (14) recently examined 133 venous segments in 18 patients and compared duplex scanning by duration and velocity of reflux to descending phlebography. They found that competence of the valve segment correlated best with a reflux duration of less than 1 second. By contrast, phlebographic incompetence was associated with reflux duration of greater than or equal to 2 seconds or a reflux velocity ≥30 cm/sec.

Air Plethysmography. Air plethysmography is performed with an ACI Medical APG model CR101 (ACI Medical, Inc., Sun Valley, CA), and patients are examined by the standard technique in an upright position. The venous filling index (VFI; in ml/sec), ejection fraction, and residual volume fraction are calculated. The VFI relates directly to the degree of venous reflux and is independent of the venous volume reservoir. Christopoulos, et al. (15), demonstrated that the normal VFI was usually <2 ml/sec, while VFI in patients with popliteal vein reflux ranged from 7–28 ml/sec. Additionally, air plethysmography provides information about the calf muscle pump function by measurement of the ejection fraction.

We feel that these noninvasive studies should be carried out not only prior to valve reconstruction as a method of selection for subsequent phlebography and hemodynamic characterization, but also afterwards to assess postoperative results. We carried out a prospective trial comparing air plethysmography and quantitative duplex scanning to the gold standard of descending phlebography in a group of normal limbs and in limbs of patients with severe chronic venous insufficiency. The latter patients were stratified according to the degree of reflux on phlebography into mild and severe reflux. VFI accurately distinguished between normal limbs and those with reflux, but could not differentiate between mild and severe reflux. By contrast the combination of the valve closure time at the superficial femoral vein and popliteal vein levels—the total valve closure time—had an excellent discriminant value. The total valve closure time as assessed by receiver operator characteristic curves had a sensitivity of 90% and specificity of 94% for distinguishing mild from severe reflux. All patients with advanced stage 2 and stage 3 disease who are candidates for surgery should undergo phlebographic studies.

Phlebography. Ascending phlebography is performed with multiple tourniquets to maximize visualization of the deep system. The superficial system is occluded at the ankle and below the knee with tourniquets, and contrast material is injected by hand into a foot vein. Visualization of contrast material in the superficial system usually indicates incompetent perforating veins. Additionally, valve sites may be seen in the superficial femoral vein. If no deep venous obstruction or obvious recanalization is identified, descending phlebography is performed.

Descending phlebography is performed under fluoroscopy with the patient on a 75° tilt table. The contralateral femoral vein is punctured and the catheter is directed into the common femoral vein on the affected leg. Contrast material is hand-injected while the patient performs a Valsalva maneuver. The reflux of contrast material is followed by fluoroscopy and cut films are taken. The use of multiple tourniquets maximizes visualization of the deep venous system and is carried out first during descending phlebography.

NEW ENGLAND MEDICAL CENTER SERIES

Open Surgical Technique

The common femoral, superficial femoral, profunda femoris, and greater saphenous veins (if present) are approached through a longitudinal incision placed over the common femoral vein (15). We prefer to perform the dissection with a scalpel rather than with scissors in order to avoid venospasm (16). As opposed to veins that have been involved by a previous episode of thrombophlebitis, the veins of a patient with "primary" valve incompetence usually do not have the intense perivenous scarring unique to postthrombotic veins. The various branches of the major veins are ligated so that approximately 4 cm of superficial femoral vein is isolated. The proximal valve is identified by its characteristic bulge in the upper superficial femoral vein. The vein is then stripped of blood to test its competence. An incompetent valve will permit blood flow down to the clamp distal to the valve. Following heparinization, soft, noncrushing vascular clamps are placed on the common femoral, profunda femoris, and superficial femoral veins below the valve.

A transverse venotomy according to the method of Raju and Fredericks (16) is placed proximal to the valve structure, usually at the level of the orifice of the profunda femoris and the common femoral veins. Care should be taken to avoid damage to the valve commissure. In primary valve incompetence, a wispy gossamer-like valve with marked redundance of its free edge is encountered. We prefer to place 7–0 monofilament sutures through the vein wall for retraction in order to visualize the valve structures. The redundant valve cusp is then "reefed" to the valve commissure by placing a 7–0 monofilament mattress suture at each commissure (Fig. 22.3). Rather than passing the same suture through the valve structure to shorten it, we prefer interrupted mattress sutures. Raju recommends shortening the valve cusp length by about 20% at each commissure. This suture advances the valve cusp in a cephalad direction, shortening the valve cusp. The double-needled stay sutures that were placed previously in the vein wall are then

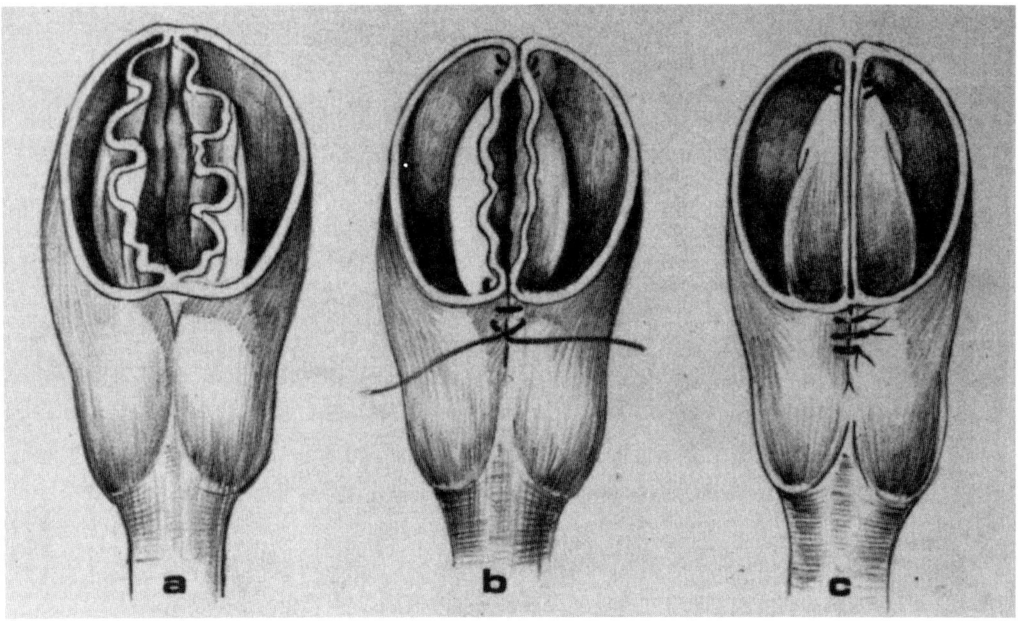

FIG. 22–3. Valvuloplasty by the open technique. A venotomy has been made above the valve, the valve is seen to be incompetent and floppy (A); one suture has been placed at either side (B); the valve cusps have been reefed with three interrupted 7-0 nonabsorbable (Prolene) sutures and competency has been achieved (C). (Reproduced by permission from Rodriguez AA, O'Donnell TF Jr. Advances in the noninvasive diagnosis and surgical management of chronic venous insufficiency. In: Whittemore AD, ed. Advances in vascular surgery. Vol. 2. St. Louis: Mosby Yearbook, 1994.)

used to repair the venotomy in an interrupted manner. The repair is performed under adequate heparin anticoagulation (5000 unit bolus) with a transverse venotomy just above the valve leaflets (15). Valve competence is then tested by the strip test.

Angioscopic Valve Repair

The scope is inserted through a large tributary of the proximal greater saphenous vein, which is invariably absent, or via a branch of the femoral vein down into the superficial femoral vein (Fig. 22.4). Saline solution is infused through the angioscope and the valve leaflets are observed for incompetence, which, when present, is both obvious and dramatic. Failure of valve coaptation with saline reflux into the infravalvular segment is easily observed. After the diagnosis is confirmed, valve repair is performed. Monofilament sutures are placed across the commissure of the valve leaflets from the outside, while the angioscope is used within the lumen to observe and guide the suture placement (17, 18). A suture needle that enters the lumen from outside at the commissure is allowed to take bites of the free edge of both valve cusps under angioscopic visualization be-

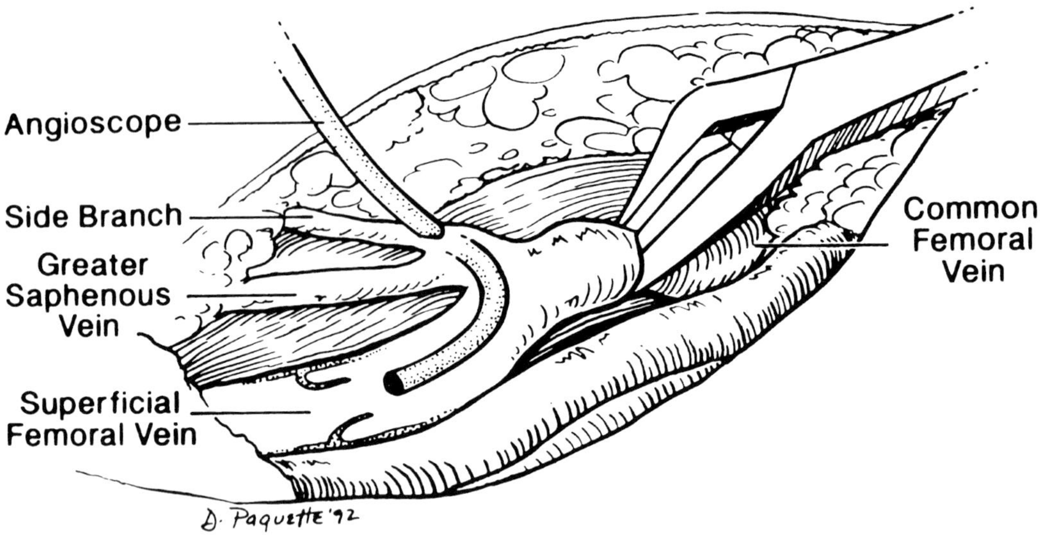

FIG. 22–4. Technique of angioscopic valvuloplasty. The angioscope is inserted through the tributary or stump of the previously ligated greater saphenous vein into the superficial femoral vein. Diagnosis of valvular incompetency is made, the valve is repaired, and competency of repair is assessed uder direct visualization with the angioscope. (Reproduced by permission from Welch HJ, McLaughlin RL, O'Donnell TF Jr. Femoral vein valvuloplasty: Intraoperative angioscopic evaluation and hemodynamic improvement. J Vasc Surg 1992;16:694–700.)

fore exiting to the outside, close to the entry point, to be tied. After placing two or three sutures on each side of the valve, repair is tested for competence by infusing saline solution through the scope.

Angioscopic Evaluation

Eight of our patients have undergone angioscopic evaluation of the valve before and after valve repair. The first three patients underwent an open valvuloplasty through a transverse venotomy with angioscopic examination pre- and postrepair. After repair of the valve and closure of the venotomy, the angioscope was reinserted to directly observe the valve repair, under saline infusion, to test the competence of the valvuloplasty. In two of these patients, an additional suture was needed to render the valve totally competent. In the last five patients, angioscopic repair technique was used. Common to the patients who have undergone angioscopy is the use of the angioscope rather than the strip test to judge the competence of the repair.

Postoperative Care. All but the initial two patients were treated with heparin and pneumatic compression boots in the immediate postoperative period, with a subsequent conversion to warfarin therapy for 6 months. Elastic compression stockings were worn for at least 6 months after surgery, although none of the eight patients have worn them continuously since surgery.

Valvuloplasty: A Review of Worldwide Experience

There are seven recent series that attempt to define the indication, role, efficacy, and long-term outcome of direct valvular reconstruction for valvular incompetence.

The first series, and that with the longest follow-up, is that of Kistner and his group (14), who pioneered the development of valvular reconstruction. This series looked at clinical, physiologic, and imaging results following venous valve reconstruction in 51 limbs (48 patients). Indications for surgery were ulceration or severe stasis in 57% of cases, and severe pain and edema in 43% of cases. These patients were characterized anatomically into three groups: primary venous insufficiency (PVI) (47%), postthrombotic syndrome (PTS) (29%), and mixed (PVI/PTS) (24%).

All these patients had clinically class 2 or 3 disease as defined by SVS/ISCVS criteria, and all had grade 3 or 4 venous reflux on descending phlebography. Twenty-two had preoperative air plethysmography (APG), and all were severely abnormal. All limbs had direct valvular repair by the open technique, many with ligation of perforating veins. Outcome was graded 0–3 based on clinical observation.

0 (Excellent result): Asymptomatic extremity without need for elastic support.
1 (Good result): Mild symptoms of swelling, pain, or indurative change.
2 (Fair result): Moderate symptoms of swelling, pain, or skin changes, but no ulcerative change.
3 (Poor result): Any ulceration and/or severe disabling edema or pain.

Fifty-nine percent went from class 3 or 2 to class 1 or 0, with 33% of patients restored to full activity without elastic support. The 10-year cumulative success rate by life table analysis was 60%. Ambulatory venous pressure (AVP) normalized in 67% of PVI patients versus 29% of PTS patients, although no significant correlation was found between AVP results and clinical outcome.

Duplex scan and/or descending phlebography documented competent valves (or mild reflux) in 86% of class 0 or 1 patients versus 47% of class 2 or 3 patients ($p = 0.0011$), suggesting that recurrence of symptoms and/or ulcers is highly dependent on achieving structural competence of the valve at the time of surgery. In patients with preoperative ulcers, the ulcer recurrence rate seemed to be lower for cases in which no incompetent perforators could be demonstrated or in which they had been interrupted (36%) versus those with untreated incompetent perforators (69%), but this difference did not attain statistical significance. Kistner observed that failure of reconstruction occurred within 4 years in the majority of cases (12/15), and 18 postoperative ulcers (15 recurrent, 3 new) developed, which necessitated five redo procedures.

The largest reported series is that of Raju (16), who studied 107 venous valve reconstructions, followed over a period of 2–8 years. The most common cause of venous insufficiency in this series was PVI. Arm/foot venous pressure differences and reactive hyperemia foot venous pressure were used to both rule out and to grade degree of obstruction. Valsalva foot venous pressure and ambulatory venous pressures were employed as indices of reflux. Patients with obstructive venous insufficiency were not considered candidates for valvuloplasty, and stasis ulceration was the primary indication for surgery in 73 limbs (71%). Patients underwent direct valvular repair through a transverse venotomy, as well as ligation of the saphenofemoral junction. If the previously incompetent vein was found to gain competence following venospasm from handling, the repair was not attempted, and a dacron "jacket" was placed around the vein to maintain the competent luminal dimension. Sixty-nine percent of patients in this series had clinical healing of the ulcer or marked symptomatic improvement. There was no mortality, while morbidity consisted of a 7% incidence of DVT with loss of valve repair in two of eight limbs. Eleven patients (10%) underwent a secondary procedure for recurrent ulcer or symptoms. Interestingly, two recurrences were due to recanalization of the saphenous vein, and saphenofemoral disconnection resulted in long-term healing. Raju points out that the presence of abnormal lymphangiographic findings did not jeopardize the results of valvular reconstruction for relief of edema. The most consistent test to judge reflux in this series was the Valsalva foot venous pressure measurement, not ambulatory venous pressure.

Perrin (19) and colleagues from France studied 52 limbs in 42 patients who underwent superficial femoral venous valvuloplasty for recurrent venous ulceration or severe stasis. Forty-four of these limbs had adjunctive surgery to the superficial or perforating veins. Twenty-one limbs had intractable venous ulceration, while 31 limbs had pain, swelling, and lipodermatosclerosis. All had grade 3 or 4 reflux on descending venography. Patients were excluded if they proved to be hypercoagulable. All patients had direct valvuloplasty using Sottiurai's technique (18), and 14% had simultaneous interruption of the perforating veins. All patients underwent phlebography on postoperative day one to rule out thrombosis (four valves thrombosed in the first 24 hours). Patients were followed up with duplex scanning and photoplethysmography. At 1-year follow-up, 85% were free of reflux on duplex scanning and 68% had normalization of their venous recovery time. At more than 1-year follow-up, one patient (9%) from the ulcer group had recurrent ulceration. In patients without ulceration, the procedure has been successful in alleviating the symptoms of venous insufficiency.

Eriksson and his group (20) from Sweden have summarized their experience with valvuloplasty in 20 patients (22 limbs) with severe deep venous insufficiency (class 2 or 3) and multiple previous procedures on their superficial system. All patients with superficial venous insufficiency (SVI) had undergone perforator ligation prior to valve reconstruction. The group was studied with ambulatory venous pressure and ascending and descending phlebography prior to surgery (grade 3 or 4 reflux), and only patients with primary valve incompetence were operated upon. The valve most commonly repaired was the most proximal superficial femoral vein according to the technique of Kistner. All patients were heparinized, and received dextran daily for 3 days. Patients were followed with clinical and Doppler examinations, reserving phlebography for those suspected of having thrombosis or reflux. Their results were good after follow-up, which ranged from 6–84 months. Nearly two-thirds (64%) of limbs showed marked improvement at 6 months, while 53% of limbs maintained improvement at 84 months. Doppler examination showed competent valves in all repairs at 6 months. Seven clinical failures were observed and all of these patients had documented incompetence of the repaired valve by phlebography. These investigators were the first to call attention to the role of profunda femoris vein competence.

Persistent incompetence of the profunda femoris vein, despite competent repair of the superficial femoral vein valve, resulted in no improvement in postoperative physiologic measurements (AVP, VRT), whereas those limbs with competent profunda femoral valve showed a marked improvement in these parameters ($p < 0.01$). There was no mortality and only minor morbidity.

Sottiurai (18) described a combined transverse and vertical venotomy to attain better exposure for direct valvuloplasty and reported on his experience with 20 patients. All patients had recurrent ulcers (class 3), and had a mean follow-up of 37 months (range of 10–73 months). Eighty percent healed their ulcers, with 7 of 20 having good results and 9 of 20 having fair results. There was no mortality and only minor morbidity.

Simkin (21) and his group from Argentina have reported their experience with seven patients, three of whom underwent Kistner valvuloplasty, and four of whom underwent intraluminal femoral and popliteal valvuloplasty. This latter technique, described by the author, diminishes the caliber of the vein through its length by placing multiple U-shaped polypropylene sutures. Fifty percent of the patients were ulcer-free at long-term follow-up (unspecified), the other 50% having return of edema after 6 months.

Our group (15) recently reported results for superficial vein valvuloplasty in six patients (nine limbs), all of whom were clinically stage 3 with severe venous stasis and skin changes with ulceration. Preoperative descending phlebography documented grade 4 reflux in six limbs, grade 3 reflux in one limb, and grade 2 reflux in two limbs. In addition to valvuloplasty, five limbs also underwent subfascial ligation of perforators, three limbs underwent ligation and stripping of superficial varicosities, and two valves had external PTFE "wraps" (16). The last five valvuloplasties had angioscopic evaluation of the repair, and the last two in the series had closed, angioscopically-guided repair. Mean follow-up was 20.3 months (range of 2–51 months). All patients healed their ulcer without recurrence. There was no mortality. Morbidity consisted of perioperative DVT in the two patients who had the PTFE "wrap" and no anticoagulation. Follow-up evaluation included duplex scan (all repairs patent by duplex), as well as venous recovery time by light-reflected rheography, which did not improve postoperatively, and venous filling index (by APG), which improved to near normal following angioscopically-guided valvuloplasty. Duplex quantitation of venous reflux was also normalized in the angioscopically-evaluated group. It is interesting to note that in this group, two patients required an additional suture to render the valve totally competent, which may not have been appreciated without the benefit of angioscopy. The angioscopically-evaluated valvuloplasties also had much shorter valve closure times for both the superficial femoral and popliteal valves.

Summary of Experience. Over 170 patients in this review underwent open valvuloplasty for recurrent venous stasis ulcer. All had grade 3 or 4 reflux on descending phlebography. Most underwent an adjunctive procedure (e.g., ligation of incompetent perforators or the saphenofemoral junction). Ulcer healing rates varied from 50–100% (mean 72%), with no mortality and minimal morbidity. These results show that venous valvuloplasty for reflux of a deep venous segment in patients with stage 3 disease is associated with healing of ulcers, as well as hemodynamic improvement in patients who have a competent profunda femoris vein. Furthermore, angioscopic evaluation of vein valve repair appears to improve hemodynamic and functional results.

Role of Perforating Veins

We believe, like Kistner, that perforating veins should be ligated when shown to be incompetent. It is extremely unusual to encounter patients with advanced stage 2 or stage 3 disease without incompetent perforating veins. Whether these should be ligated prior to deep venous reconstruction is immaterial, but correction of superficial system incompetence optimizes outcome.

The data presented thus far suggest that the ideal candidate for valvuloplasty is someone with primary valvular insufficiency, who has grade 3 or 4 reflux and clinical stage 2 or 3 disease. The use of angioscopy and judicious anticoagulation, as well as adjunctive procedures as needed (i.e., ligation of incompetent perforators in patients with recalcitrant ulcers), will also lead to improved results.

Although significant advances have been made in arterial reconstruction over the last two decades, advances in venous reconstruction have been slow. The reasons for this phenomenon are many. The results of venous surgery are not as dramatic or immediate as for arterial surgery. Venous problems are not seen as limb- or life-threatening. Venous reconstruction suffered from lack of a thorough understanding of venous insufficiency, and the variable underlying pathology was hitherto unknown. No vascular surgeon would think of attempting a difficult vascular reconstruction without a road map, and venous surgery should be afforded the same. Improvement in our imaging ability, refinement of duplex scanning technology, and development of new techniques to evaluate venous physiology (APG, VRT), as well as application of new technology such as angioscopy, should allow the surgeon to define the site and extent of the problem so that appropriate therapy can be instituted. Venous surgery is technically demanding and as unforgiving as arterial surgery, perhaps even more so. The accurate preoperative evaluation and careful selection of patients (e.g., PVI or PVI/PTS), followed by meticulous surgery by an operator experienced in the technique, and guided by angioscopy to eliminate the need for venotomy will all result in improved outcome.

REFERENCES

1. McEnroe CS, O'Donnell TF, Mackey WC. Correlation of clinical findings with venous hemodynamics in 386 patients with chronic venous insufficiency. Am J Surg 1988;156:148–152.
2. Ferris EB, Kistner R. Femoral vein reconstruction in the management of chronic venous insufficiency. Arch Surg 1982;117:1571–1579.
3. O'Donnell TF, Mackey WC, Shepard AD, Callow AD. Clinical, hemodynamic, and anatomic follow-up of direct venous reconstruction. Arch Surg 1987;122:474–482.
4. Bauer G. The etiology of leg ulcers and their treatment by resection of the popliteal vein. J Int Chir 1948;8:937–967.
5. Kistner R. Surgical repair of a venous valve. Straub Clin Proc 1968;34:41–43.
6. Darke SG. Reconstructive surgery for chronic venous insufficiency in the lower limbs. In: Greehalgh RA, Jamieson CW, Nicolaides AN, eds. Vascular surgery issues in current practice. London: Grune & Stratton, 1986.

7. Raju S. Venous insufficiency of the lower limb and stasis ulceration. Changing concepts and management. Ann Surg 1983;197:688–697.
8. Leather RP, Powers SR, Karmody AM. A reappraisal of the "in situ" saphenous vein arterial bypass: its use in limb salvage. Surgery 1979;86:453.
9. Kistner R. Surgical repair of the incompetent femoral vein valve. Arch Surg 1975;110:1336–1342.
10. Raju S, Fredericks R. Hemodynamic basis of stasis ulceration—a hypothesis. J Vasc Surg 1991;13:491–495.
11. Burnand KG, Whimster IW, Clemenson G, et al. The relationship between the number of capillaries in the skin of the venous ulcer bearing area of the lower leg and the fall in foot vein pressure during exercise. Br J Surg 1981;68:297–300.
12. Wilkinson LS, Bunker C, Edwards, JCW, Seurr, JH, Smith, C. Leukocytes: their role in the etiopathogenesis of skin damage in venous disease. J Vasc Surg 1993;17:669–675.
13. van Bemmelen PS, Bedford G, Beach K, Strandness DE. Quantitative segmental evaluation of venous valvular reflux with duplex ultrasound scanning. J Vasc Surg 1989;10:425–431.
14. Masuda EM, Kistner R. Long-term results of venous valve reconstruction: a 4 to 21 year follow-up. Presented at the 46th annual meeting of the Society for Vascular Surgery. Chicago, June 8–9, 1992.
15. Christopoulos D, Nicolaides AN, Galloway JMD, Wilkinson A. Objective noninvasive evaluation of venous surgical results. J Vasc Surg 1988;8:683–687.
16. Raju S, Fredericks R. Valve reconstruction procedures for nonobstructive venous insufficiency: rationale, techniques, and results in 107 procedures with two- to eight-year follow-up. J Vasc Surg 1988;7:301–310.
17. Gloviczki P, Merrell SW, Bower TC. Femoral vein valve repair under direct vision without venotomy: a modified technique with use of angioscopy. J Vasc Surg 1991;14:645–648.
18. Sottiurai VS. Technique in direct venous valvuloplasty. J Vasc Surg 1988;8:646–648.
19. Cheatle TR, Perrin M. Venous valve repair: a report of 52 cases. Personal communication.
20. Eriksson I. Vein valve surgery for deep valvular incompetence. In: Eklöf B, Gjöres JE, Thulesius O, Berquist D, eds. Controversies in the management of venous disorders. London: Butterworths, 1989:267–279.
21. Simkin R, Esteban JC, Bulloj R. By-pass veno-venosos y valvuloplastas en el tratamiento quirurgico del sindrome post-trombotico. Angiologia 1988;1:30–34.

chapter 23

Venous Valve Reconstruction

Seshadri Raju

RATIONALE AND CONTROVERSIES

In 1968, Robert Kistner reported the first successful repair of a deep femoral vein valve (1). A subsequent report comprising 17 such repairs was presented before the Joint Meeting of Vascular Societies in June 1975, inaugurating a new era in reconstructive venous surgery (2). Until that time, deep venous surgery had been considered inadvisable, beset by fears of thrombosis and embolism. This pioneering report, along with the Vietnam registry experience reported by Dr. Norman Rich (3), allayed fears on this score. Controversies and questions, however, have continued to swirl around valve reconstruction for venous stasis. The value of proximal valve reconstruction has been questioned because distal valvular reflux is statistically more frequently associated with venous stasis than is proximal reflux (4). Most patients with venous stasis disease suffer from multilevel, multisystem reflux (5). Clinical experience indicates that elimination of the proximal component results in resolution of stasis ulceration and dermatitis. Since perforator ligation and/or saphenous stripping was often combined with femoral valve reconstruction (2), the question of specific therapeutic benefit from the valvuloplasty has been raised. Long-term follow-up after valve reconstruction (6–9) indicates that the results are durable, more so than could be expected from the ancillary procedures by themselves. Postexercise pressure did not always improve (6, 7, 10) after valve reconstruction despite resolution of stasis ulceration. Without uniform improvement in this important physiologic measure, some have suggested that healing of stasis skin changes could be due to enhanced aftercare and stocking use bestowed on the operated limb rather than the valve reconstruction per se. Lack of improvement with elimination of reflux in ambulatory venous hypertension, despite obvious clinical improvement after valve reconstruction, is probably due to the nonlinear volume pressure relationship in collapsible leg veins that govern the regulation of ambulatory venous pressure. Stocking use clearly declines after valve reconstruction surgery (6, 7). We cannot ascribe clinical improvement to continued stocking use. Patients presenting with bilateral leg ulcers experience healing of stasis ulcers only on the operated side despite use of compression therapy and medical attention meted out in similar measure to both limbs after surgery. Because of these fundamental controversies, several centers eschew a surgical approach, preferring traditional compression therapy instead (11). It is well-recognized, however, that compression therapy is not uniformly successful and recurrences are common. Some of these patients require hospitalization, sometimes repeatedly, to control exacerbation of pain, swelling, or infection associated with the ulcers that have recurred or failed to heal despite compression therapy. Many such patients become dependent on pain medication on a chronic basis. The direct and indirect cost of compression therapy, including the cost of chronic disability and man hours lost in the work force, is probably substantial. When rigidly enforced, a regimen of conservative measures incorporating compression stockings yields results with about 60% healing in the short run (11). However, data regarding the long term are as yet unavailable despite such conservative measures having been in vogue for several decades longer than valve reconstruction. Ironically, such long-term data for valve reconstruction are now available from varied sources (6, 9).

A major difficulty in assessing the outcome of conservative therapy is the lack of a reliable technique to monitor patient compliance in an outpatient setting. Failure of the conservative regimen indicates that it did not work or that the patient would not or could not comply with the rigid regimen for some reason. Some patients, especially the younger ones, may not comply because of cosmetic considerations. An active lifestyle, warm weather, poor fit, or other forms of real or perceived physical discomfort associated with compression stockings may result in noncompliance. Elderly patients may be unable to use them because of physical frailty, arthritis, or other ailments that prevent application of stockings without help. Lesser surgical procedures, such as saphenous vein stripping (12, 13) and perforator ligation (14), may yield good results, at least in the short term, raising questions about the need for a more complex valve reconstruction procedure. Despite these many controversies, valve reconstruction as a therapeutic approach to stasis ulceration has survived as direct correction of reflux pathology is appealing and supportive data from multiple centers have accumulated, validating excellent clinical results and durability. From these data it appears that valve reconstructions yield higher success rates that are sustained much longer than published results for conservative therapy or other surgical measures for severe venous stasis. Because of the lack of standardization in assessing severity of reflux and clinical grades, a double-blind trial involving valve reconstruction and several alternative methods, both conservative and surgical, is yet to be undertaken.

INDICATIONS FOR SURGERY AND SELECTION OF PATIENTS

Patients who fail conservative therapy should be considered for deep valve reconstruction. In the younger patient, rapid healing of a stasis ulcer by surgery offers the potential for speedy return to the work force. A decision for surgery should be quickly made in this group of patients when conservative therapy is slow to heal the ulcer or it results in frequent absences from the workplace for bed rest, leg elevation, and treatment of stasis-related complications. Surgery should also be considered in the elderly patient who may be unable to comply with compression regimens due to infirmity or other ailments such as arthritis. In the absence of institutional care or adequate family support, such patients pose a severe nursing problem and may be considered for surgery if overall general health permits. Patients who suffer frequent complications during conservative therapy regardless of age and other socioeconomic considerations are also candidates for deep venous surgery. Such complications include recurrent or chronic cellulitis, ascending lymphangitis, recurrent phlebitis (superficial or deep), intractable pain requiring chronic pain medication, and nonthrombotic recurrent attacks of pain and swelling. All of these complications can occur in patients with severe venous stasis, even in the absence of overt skin ulceration. Curiously, some patients present with episodic sudden leg swelling and pain suggestive of deep venous thrombosis, but duplex examination and ascending venography show a normal venous tree without thrombosis. Some of these patients perhaps harbor calf vein thrombi not detected by these techniques. In others, it appears probable that the sudden onset of edema and pain is due to episodic decompensation and disequilibrium in Starling forces that govern microcirculation. The mechanism is unknown. Correction of reflux by valve reconstruction provides relief.

Deep venous reconstruction should be approached with some caution in very obese patients because the results seem inferior, presumably due to compression of the vena cava by adiposity. Poor results can be expected in elderly patients who are not ambulatory, but spend a considerable part of the day sitting in a chair with legs dependent and with little calf muscle activity. Correction of reflux alone is unlikely to relieve dependent venous hypertension in such patients. Long-term physical therapy directed toward calf muscle exercise and strengthening with ambulatory training should be an integral part of care after surgery in these patients.

Caution is required in choosing patients for surgery when the presenting symptom is dependent pain without overt stasis skin changes. Many patients in this group have a low pain threshold due to chronicity and have become addicted to pain medication. Some are malingerers who are seeking disability qualification and others who are vying for an excuse to receive pain medication. Surgery is contraindicated unless duplex and descending venography can document severe reflux and significant ambulatory venous hypertension is present. When patients are properly selected in this fashion, successful pain relief can be achieved. Patients with painless swelling are not candidates for surgery. Swelling often becomes worse immediately after surgery and gradually improves over succeeding months. When surgery is offered for painful swelling and pain relief is achieved with surgery, patients appear to tolerate well the temporary postoperative exacerbation of swelling. Multilevel, multisystem reflux is typically present in patients with severe venous stasis (15). Patients with a large saphenous reflux component benefit from an initial saphenectomy procedure without concurrent valve reconstruction for deep reflux when the latter abnormality is mild (16). Removal of the saphenous component may allow the patient to compensate for and to tolerate the residual deep reflux (17). Currently available techniques for differential quantitative assessment of reflux in various venous segments are not reliable. In the absence of an objective method for reliable assessment, we tend to choose younger patients for initial saphenectomy procedure, with the clear warning that they may require an additional deep venous reconstruction as a second stage procedure if they do not obtain adequate resolution of their symptoms after the initial operation. Older patients who are unable to tolerate multiple hospitalizations and surgeries probably should undergo the combined single stage procedure.

It is not uncommon to encounter venous stasis ulcers in elderly patients with significant arterial insufficiency. A suitable arterial bypass procedure is the initial procedure of choice in this select group of patients. It has been our experience that venous ulcers often heal with rearterialization without the need for a subsequent venous procedure. If venous surgery is undertaken before revascularization, poor healing of distal incisions (e.g., Linton procedure incision) may ensue.

Valve reflux may be due to congenital, "primary," or postthrombotic causes. In congenital reflux, refluxive conduit duplication is more common than dysplastic valve abnormalities (Fig. 23.1). Simple ligation of the refluxive conduit produces relief provided the remaining conduit is large enough to supply adequate outflow. Valve reconstruction was initially employed in "primary" reflux. Clearly, equally good results can be obtained in postthrombotic patients as well (9, 18). Valve reconstruction techniques have evolved since the original description of internal valvuloplasty. We can now employ a technique optimally suited to address any of the above reflux pathologies and tailored to the particular patient (19). Currently, all patients who have deep reflux and meet the stated indications are considered for surgery without exclusion, regardless of the venographic appearance or expected pathology. With an occasional exception, we can successfully reconstruct most patients employing one or the other of the many techniques currently available.

WORKUP

Color duplex examination is the initial screening technique of choice and the definitive tool as well, in most centers addressing venous reconstructive

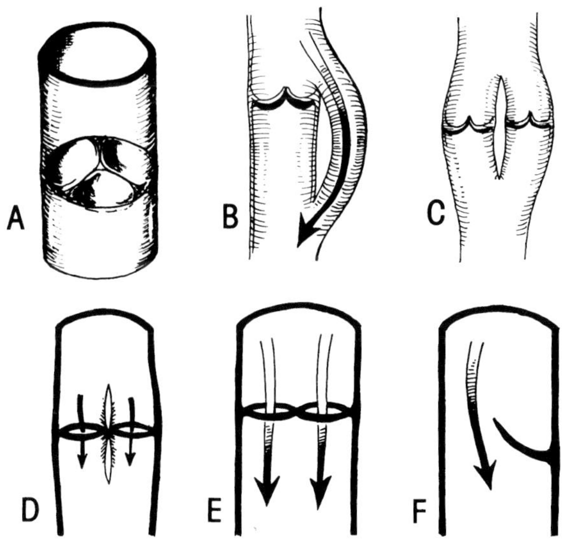

FIG. 23–1. Congenital anomalies of the venous conduit and the valve structure. These are frequently associated with venous reflux. **A.** Tricuspid valve. **B.** Avalvular duplication conduit. **C.** Duplication conduit with refluxive valves. **D.** Duplication of the valve with an intervening septum. **E.** Duplication of the valve without a septum. **F.** Refluxive monocuspid valve. Refluxive duplication conduits account for 80% of congenital anomalies; valvular dysplasias are present in 20%.

surgery. Ascending and descending venography are obtained before surgery because they provide a composite detail of venous and valve station anatomy that is essential for the surgical approach. Nucleotide lymphangiography reveals reduced or absent nodal activity in about 20% of patients with chronic venous stasis (7). This may be congenital or acquired due to repetitive indolent infections in the affected extremity. No untoward sequelae have been noted in patients with reduced lymphatic activity after correction of associated deep venous reflux. Provided strong indications for venous reconstruction are present, we do not consider reduced lymphatic activity a contraindication for surgery.

SURGICAL TECHNIQUE

The original technique of valve reconstruction is internal valvuloplasty as described by Kistner in 1968. Modifications of the original technique (20) and other techniques as well (7, 19, 21) have since been described. The internal valvuloplasty technique (Fig. 23.2) is well-established with a proven track record and as such remains the "gold standard." It is durable and arguably provides the best chance of cure for stasis ulceration compared with other surgical approaches. However, it is time-consuming and, therefore, not well-suited for multiple valve reconstructions when required; it cannot be performed in small caliber veins or in situations in which exposure and mobilization of the valve station are limited.

A prosthetic sleeve applied to the valve station to restore competency was experimentally proposed by Hallberg (22) in 1972. Professor Roger Lane of Australia has developed a prosthetic device based on the same principle (23). This technique evokes some reticence because of the fear of substituting an obstruction for reflux at the valve station. We have used the method selectively, restricting it to those cases in which surgically induced venospasm restores competency to the previously refluxive valve (7). In these cases the commissural valve angle is 11° or less (24), no different from "normal" competent valves in healthy individuals. Valve stations with commissural valve angles of greater than 11° remain overtly

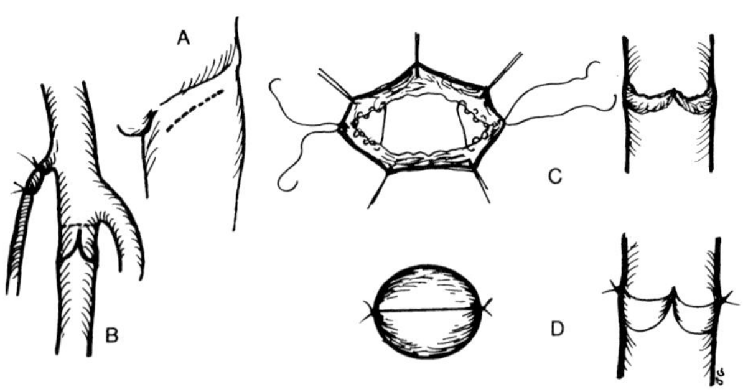

FIG. 23–2. Technique of internal valvuloplasty. **A.** An oblique groin incision provides access to the superficial and deep femoral veins and the saphenofemoral junction as well. **B.** The transverse venotomy is placed just above the commissural apex. **C.** Placement of valvuloplasty sutures. **D.** Appearance of valve cusp after the valvuloplasty sutures are tied. By permission: Raju S. Local management and surgical treatment of superficial and deep chronic venous insufficiency of the leg. In: Nyhus LM, Baker RJ and Fischer JE, ed. Mastery of Surgery. Little, Brown and Company. Boston 1996:2133–2139.

refluxive despite surgically-induced venoconstriction. The phenomenon occurs in about 15% of superficial femoral valves and progressively more often as the caliber of the vein decreases (19). It is seen in about 50% of cases of posterior tibial reflux. We apply a prosthetic sleeve of either Dacron or ringed PTFE around the valve segment to maintain its competency in the slightly constricted position (Fig. 23.3). When utilized in this fashion, long-term clinical results and Doppler competence of valves repaired by the prosthetic sleeve technique appear comparable to those repaired by internal valvuloplasty without producing hemodynamic stenosis at the valve site. This technique is fast and can be used in small caliber veins where internal valvuloplasty is often not feasible. A technique of angioscopic valvuloplasty (21) has been recently described (see Chapter 22). The valve cusps are tightened and the valve attachment lines are brought together with closure of the commissural angle by interrupted through-and-through sutures placed under angioscopic visualization (Fig. 23.4). The technique is a modification of external valvuloplasty (Fig. 23.5) that closes the commissural angle by externally placed transmural sutures. In the angioscopic technique, sutures are placed transluminally under guidance. This allows tightening of the valve cusps in addition to coaptation of valve attachment lines and closure of commissural angle. The angioscope is introduced through the saphenous vein stump or more conveniently through a 3-mm venotomy controlled by a transmural pursestring suture of 5–0 Prolene. The latter technique allows an optimal introduction site for the angioscope and is less restrictive than the saphenous entry site; mobilization of the adjoining venous segments for vascular control is also considerably lessened. We have found that this type of "transcommissural repair" with transluminal sutures can be performed "blindly" without angioscopy (Fig. 23.4). This is useful when angioscopy may be difficult or impossible, such as in small caliber veins, and in instances in which adequate exposure and mobilization of the valve station cannot be easily achieved. Angioscopy, when feasible, adds a useful dimension to the technique: valve and luminal pathology can be observed, correct placement

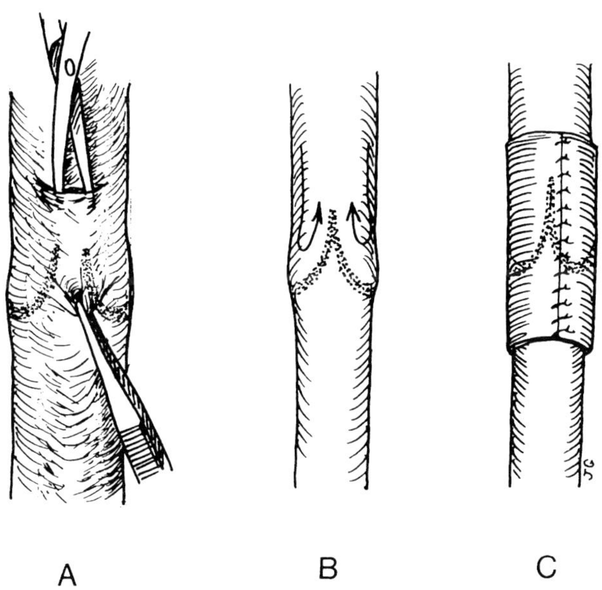

FIG. 23–3. Prosthetic sleeve in situ. **A.** Dissection around the refluxive valve leading to **B.** venoconstriction and restoration of valve compliance. **C.** Application of prosthetic sleeve to maintain valve competence in the slightly contracted position of the valve station. By permission: Raju S. Local management and surgical treatment of superficial and deep chronic venous insufficiency of the leg. In: Nyhus LM, Baker RJ and Fischer JE, ed. Mastery of Surgery. Little, Brown and Company. Boston 1996:2133–2139.

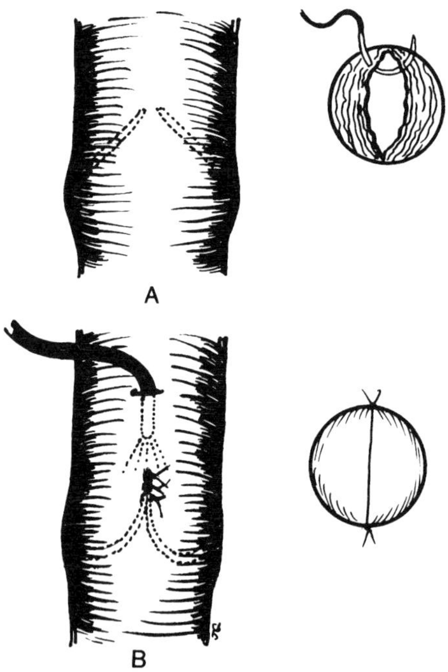

FIG. 23–4. Transcommissural valvuloplasty. A. Initial appearance of valve attachment lines and placement of transcommissural transluminal sutures that traverse the valve cusps near their attachment to the vein wall. B. Appearance after repair. The use of angioscope is optional. By permission: Raju S. Local management and surgical treatment of superficial and deep chronic venous insufficiency of the leg. In: Nyhus LM, Baker RJ and Fischer JE, ed. Mastery of Surgery. Little, Brown and Company. Boston 1996:2133–2139.

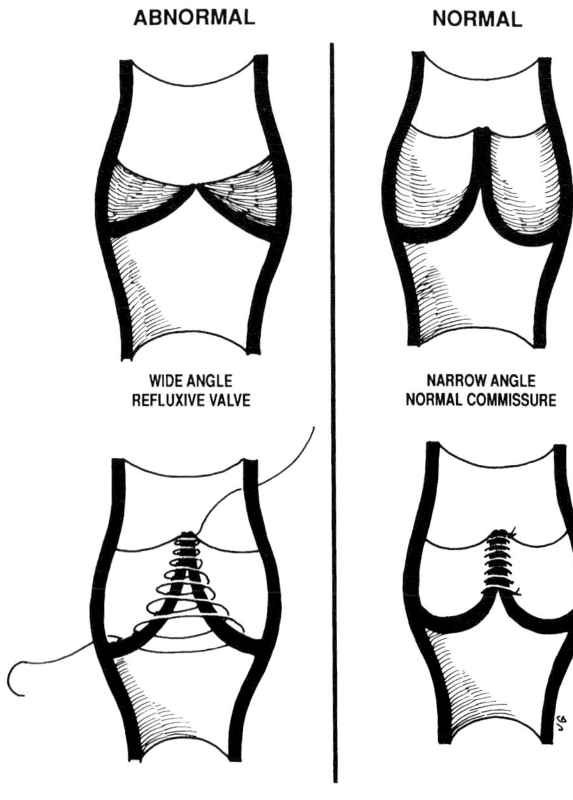

FIG. 23–5. External valvuloplasty. The commissural angle is normally acute. It becomes widened in cryptogenic reflux. The *lower panel* depicts the technique of external valvuloplasty. The valve attachments are brought together by running suture applied to the external vein wall. The space between the valve attachments is thus obliterated at both commissures. Transmural sutures are used in this repair, which differs from the transcommissural repair technique in which transluminal sutures are used. By permission: Raju S. Venous reconstruction. In: Cameron JL. ed. Current Surgical Therapy. Fourth Edition. B.C. Decker/ Mosby. St. Louis 1992:780–784.

of sutures can be assured, and the degree of valve tightening required for restoration of competency can be progressively monitored with angioscopic irrigation. It is our practice to use angioscopy during the actual repair wherever feasible or at least before and after the repair if continuous angioscopic observation and guidance during the actual placement of valvuloplasty sutures are difficult or impossible due to technical reasons.

These techniques were primarily devised for the repair of "primary" valve reflux. We have employed the same techniques in postthrombotic cases as well, where valve structure anatomy is preserved (25).

Regardless of existing valve pathology or the particular repair technique to be employed, the first step in valve reconstruction is to gain adequate exposure of the valve station and to mobilize the segment, with division of small branches and vascular control of larger ones. Our preference is an oblique incision in the groin along skin lines through which valve stations in the common, superficial, and profunda femoral veins can be exposed. The saphenofemoral junction can be dealt with through the same incision. The uppermost valve in the superficial femoral vein is nearly constant in position below the profunda takeoff. A characteristic bulge, when present, is a pointer to the location of the valve station. Valve station bulge is often obscured or absent when postthrombotic wall thickening is present. Valve station wall changes impose additional technical difficulties in the procedure and may offer etiologic clues to the reflux pathology. Despite considerable wall thickening, an intact valve apparatus may be present and amenable to direct valvuloplasty (25). In extreme cases of postthrombotic syndrome, especially when there has been prior surgical intervention, the affected venous segment may have completely dissolved, leaving no more than a fibrous cord as a remnant. Valve station fibrosis may result in "secondary" valve redundancy (Fig. 23.6) due to wall restriction, a phenomenon that may explain the onset of reflux in venous segments not directly affected by prior thrombosis.

When wall thickening is not present, the valve attachment lines can be clearly visualized through the glistening adventitia. When wall thickening is present, the thick adventitia surrounding the valve station must be peeled or excised with a number 15 blade or Potts scissors before valve attachment lines can be visualized (Fig. 23.7). Identification of valve attachment lines sets the stage for optimal placement of transverse venotomy for internal valvuloplasty and the definition of necessary valve station anatomy for carrying out transcommissural, angioscopic, or external valvuloplasty repairs. Absence of valve attachment lines despite adequate adventitial dissection denotes postthrombotic dissolution of valve cusps. Further

'SECONDARY' VALVE REFLUX

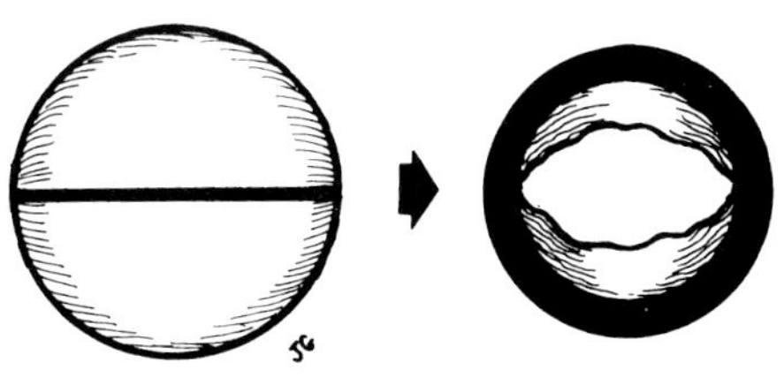

FIG. 23–6. "Secondary" valve reflux. May be produced by restrictive postthrombotic wall thickening and contraction at the valve station. By permission: Quality Medical Publishing Company. St. Louis (25).

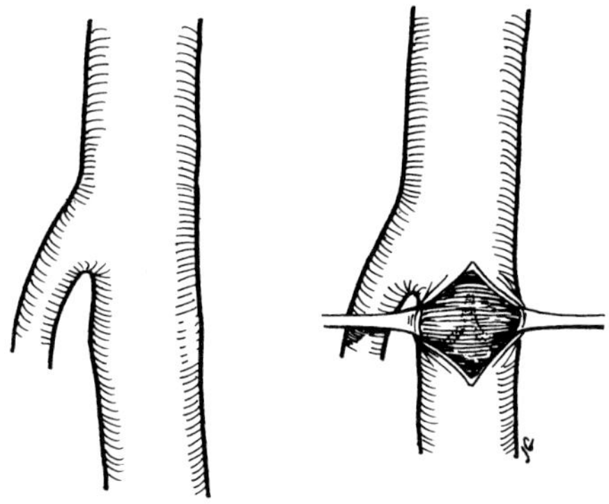

FIG. 23–7. Definition of valve attachment lines is a necessary preliminary step in most valve reconstruction techniques. Wall thickening at the valve station can obscure the lines (*left*) requiring adventitial dissection to expose the attachment lines (*right*).

time should not be wasted by carrying out a venotomy to look for nonexistent valve cusps in such instances. When valve cusps are absent, axillary vein transfer offers the hope of restoring competency to the refluxive venous segment. One axilla is always kept prepared for use in such an eventuality. The axillary vein is exposed through a transverse incision along the skin lines high in the axilla. The axillary vein carries one or more valves close to the first rib which are usually an adequate size match for the superficial femoral vein. Axillary venospasm is common with surgical manipulation and may be relieved by irrigating the segment with a dilute solution of nitroglycerine. In exposing the axillary vein, considerable care should be exercised to avoid disturbing the adjoining brachial plexus and branches to preclude irksome postsurgical neuropathy. Thirty to 40% of exposed axillary vein valves, however, will be found refluxive (7). This may be related to the shallow cusp architecture of the axillary vein valve. Refluxive axillary vein valves can, however, be successfully repaired by the transcommissural technique before transfer. "Bench" repair of the axillary valve by the external valvuloplasty technique has been less successful. Restoring continuity to the axillary vein after excision of the valve segment is not necessary. In our experience of more than 100 axillary vein valve transfers, there have been no instances of arm swelling or hemodynamically significant axillary vein obstruction. The rich collaterals with which the axillary vein segment is endowed appear adequate to compensate well for the loss of the excised venous segment.

The excised axillary valve segment is transposed to the superficial vein in the groin or other chosen site in proper orientation. The technique of axillary vein transfer may appear deceptively simple, but requires exacting technique for insertion of the valve segment under optimal tension without axial distortion (Fig. 23.8). Owing to the shallow nature of the axillary vein valve cusps, even minor technical infractions can result in incompetence of the valve in the transferred position. Since some venospasm of the donor and/or recipient venous segments is usually present, interrupted sutures are mandatory. Suture line stenosis may result after the spasm is relieved if a continuous suture technique is used. Late dilatation and failure of the transferred axillary valve segment is a well-recognized complication (26). This apparently results from a compliance mismatch between donor-recipient venous segments. We recommend placement of a restrictive prosthetic sleeve around the transferred valve (26), especially when a severe compliance mismatch is present, such as when an axillary vein segment is transferred to a rigid, postthrombotic venous segment. Axillary vein transfer to a location other than the proximal superficial femoral vein may sometimes be required. When the superficial femoral vein is severely compromised in postthrombotic syndrome, the profunda femoral vein frequently enlarges, assuming a size as large as or larger than the postthrombotic superficial femoral vein (axial transformation) (19). In such instances, a large collateral connection exists between the profunda and popliteal veins. The rapid appearance of this tributary connection when the superficial femoral vein occludes suggests an embryologic basis for the collateral connection (Fig. 23.9) (27). This tributary collateral is a direct line for outflow and reflux as well. A profunda reconstruction is required in such cases, in addition to dealing with any existing postthrombotic reflux in the superficial femoral vein. A proximal valve in the profunda femoral vein amenable to repair can usually be found in such cases. The precise location of this valve in relationship to the profunda-femoral junction, however, is quite variable ranging 1–10 cm distally. Repair of refluxive valves in distal locations is technically quite difficult because of exposure requirements, especially in obese patients. In about 5% of patients, a common femoral valve is present. Repair of this valve is technically simpler than and offers a functional equal of a profunda repair.

In some patients with postthrombotic syndrome, a repairable valve may not be present and an axillary vein valve may be absent or unusable (e.g., a previous mastectomy, Erb's palsy, small caliber, etc.). In such patients, a de novo valve reconstruction (19) may be considered (Fig. 23.10).

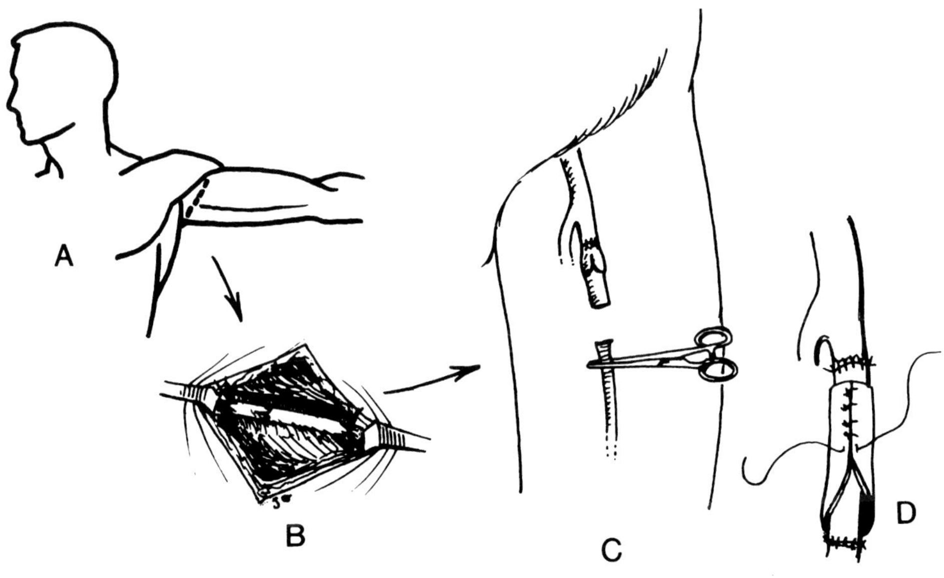

FIG. 23–8. Axillary vein transfer. **A.** Axillary vein near the axilla is exposed through an incision along skin lines. **B.** Isolation of the valve-bearing segment. Reconstitution of the axillary vein after harvest of the segment is not required. **C.** The segment is transplanted to the superficial femoral vein without axial rotation and under proper tension. **D.** Prosthetic sleeve to prevent dilatation of the transplanted venous segment from compliance mismatch. By permission: Raju S. Local management and surgical treatment of superficial and deep chronic venous insufficiency of the leg. In: Nyhus LM, Baker RJ and Fischer JE, ed. Mastery of Surgery. Little, Brown and Company. Boston 1996:2133–2139

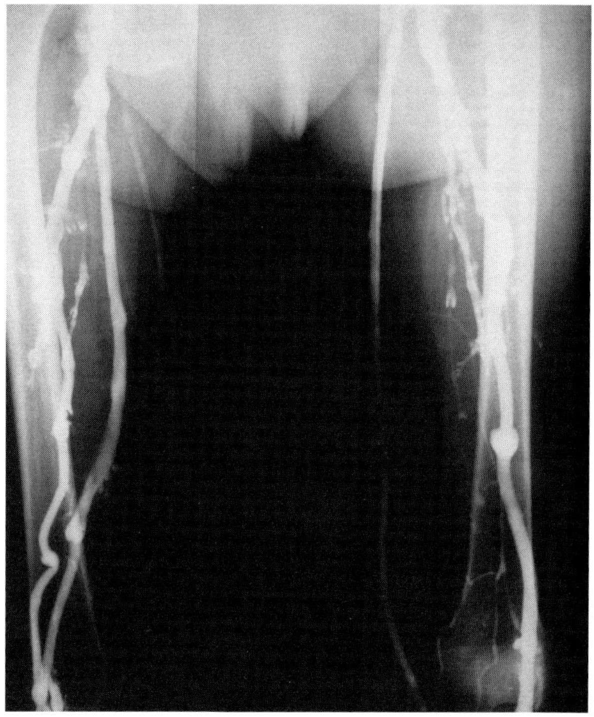

FIG. 23–9. Axial transformation of the profunda femoral vein. In a patient with bilateral postthrombotic changes, the profunda femoral vein has markedly enlarged and has become the axial vein (*right*). The superficial femoral vein is totally occluded on the right and is present as a recanalized vessel on the left. The profunda femoral vein communicates with the popliteal vein on the left through a large collateral.

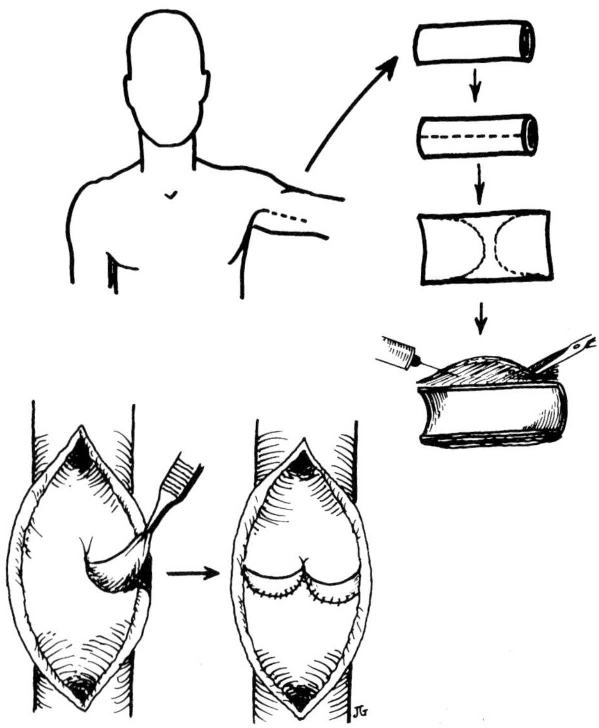

FIG. 23–10. De novo valve reconstruction. New valve cusps are fashioned out of a harvested segment of donor vein, preferably axillary vein. Transmural saline injection is used to thin out the donor vein in preparation for use as valve cusps.

SPECIAL CONSIDERATIONS IN POSTTHROMBOTIC SYNDROME

Collateral reflux is a prominent feature of postthrombotic syndrome. Collaterals may be axioaxial or tributary-axial. Axial transformation of the profunda vein may be present. Additionally, significant reflux may be present in the recanalized superficial femoral vein. Postthrombotic changes in the calf venous pump compound these multiple reflux pathologies (Fig. 23.11). Organized thrombus or fibrotic contraction of the venous lumen may reduce venous capacitance in the calf. Postthrombotic compliance changes may impair venous pump function and contribute to ambulatory venous hypertension. Ligation of a refluxive collateral in an attempt to abolish reflux may result in outflow obstruction. Direct valve reconstruction procedures in refluxive collaterals is seldom technically feasible. A strategy for controlling collateral reflux is to perform multiple valve reconstructions at sequential sites in the venous tree to control both the entry and exit points of reflux collaterals. In a postthrombotic patient with a large refluxive profunda-popliteal collateral with reflux in the recanalized superficial femoral vein as well, a multiple reconstruction procedure with repair of the superficial femoral, profunda, and posterior tibial veins would be ideal (Fig. 23.12). This can be approached through an oblique groin incision and a small tibial incision. A proximal saphenectomy and a modified Linton procedure can be accomplished at the same time when indicated through the same incisions and within reasonable operative times (Fig. 23.12). The prevailing view that a thrombus in a valve station inevitably results in valve destruction appears incorrect. Valve structure has been adequately preserved for performing a direct valvuloplasty technique in several postthrombotic cases, even when some trabeculae are present in the lumen (25). The preservation of valve cusp anatomy within the lumen of a thickened postthrombotic venous segment raises important pathologic questions. Preservation of the valve apparatus in such a setting implies rapid resolution of the thrombus from anticoagulant therapy without residual damage to the cusp

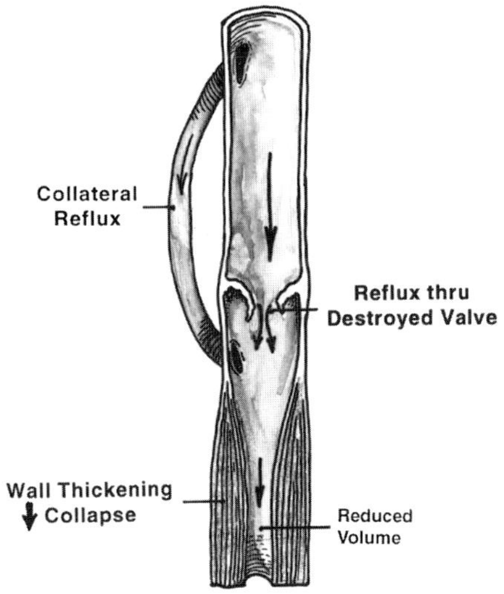

FIG. 23–11. Pathophysiology of postphlebitic syndrome. Reflux through the postphlebitic valve and through collaterals is compounded by postphlebitic abnormalities of the calf venous pump. Reduced venous capacitance and postthrombotic compliance changes decrease the efficiency of the calf venous pump and produce ambulatory venous hypertension.

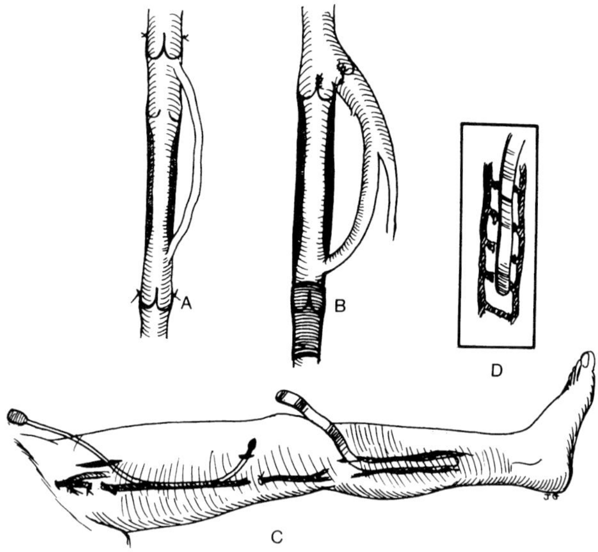

FIG. 23–12. Multiple valvuloplasty to control collateral reflux in postthrombotic syndrome. **A.** Axioaxial collaterals. **B.** Profunda and femoral repairs to control tributary-axial collateral reflux. Different valve repair techniques may be combined in such multiple valve reconstructions. **C.** Saphenectomy and perforator interruption can be added to the procedure through the groin and crural incisions used for valve reconstruction. **D.** Detail of modified perforator interruption technique utilizing a malleable blade inserted through a limited upper calf incision. By permission: Raju S. Local management and surgical treatment of superficial and deep chronic venous insufficiency of the leg. In: Nyhus LM, Baker RJ and Fischer JE, ed. Mastery of Surgery. Little, Brown and Company. Boston 1996:2133–2139.

anatomy. This is contrary to the current concept that thrombosis in a valve station invariably leads to valve destruction. Alternatively, the noted wall changes may extend more proximally than the level of a luminal thrombus to induce secondary valve redundancy and reflux from restriction (Fig. 23.7). This would explain the presence of intact valve cusps in a thickened venous segment. The noted wall changes may also be due to phlebosclerosis of "primary" reflux rather than postthrombotic thickening (28). The nature of wall thickening frequently encountered during valve reconstruction remains an enigma and merits further study.

Significant reflux may be present below an obstructed iliac vein segment resulting in reflux venous stasis changes in the skin. Valve reconstructions carried out at the femoral level, below an obstructed iliac vein, surprisingly remain patent and functional with relief of stasis symptoms (19).

Combined Superficial, Perforator and Deep Reflux

When reflux is generally present in multiple superficial and deep venous segments, correction of all points of reflux is required for complete relief of symptoms and durable healing of stasis ulceration. In a selected group, saphenectomy without concurrent valve reconstruction may provide substantial if not complete relief. Saphenectomy, when performed, is currently limited to the thigh segment. This is easily combined with the deep valve reconstruction when indicated. In those requiring valve repair at more than one level, different reconstruction techniques can be combined according to the optimal choice for a given location and valve pathology. Perforator incompetence is often secondary to deep valve reflux (7). When large medial perforators are present, these can be interrupted subfascially, using a malleable retractor for this purpose, through the calf incision, and little time is added to the overall operative procedure. Multiple valve reconstructions with correction of saphenous and perforator reflux can be performed through the same thigh and tibial incisions used for valve reconstruction with an acceptable operative time.

REDO VALVE CONSTRUCTION

Valvuloplasty is a durable antireflux procedure (6, 9). Clinical recurrences appear to be low even when deterioration of Doppler competence occurs with the passage of time. Recurrences are often transient and easily manageable after valve reconstruction in the few patients who have recurrences (28). Patients with recurrences should be fully investigated with ascending and descending venography after initial duplex examination. Often reflux in a venous segment not previously addressed because it is new or was missed during previous surgery is found and easily corrected (e.g., saphenous, perforator). Sometimes the original valve repair has simply failed (Fig. 23.13) with the passage of time and a "redo"

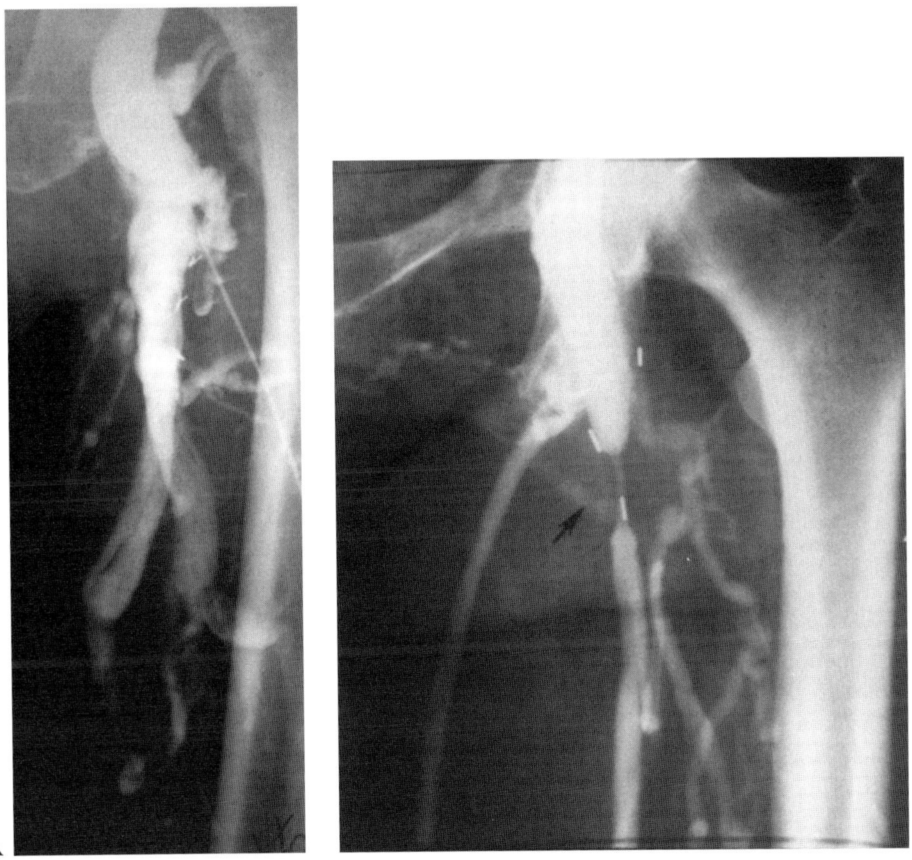

A B

FIG. 23–13. Failure of axillary valve transplant after several years of satisfactory function. **A.** Late dilatation and recurrent reflux. **B.** Late stenosis.

valve reconstruction may be required. This was necessary in 4% of valve reconstructions in our experience.

It is seldom technically possible to perform a "redo" repair at a valve station that has been previously reconstructed. Cicatrix formation may render dissection difficult and dangerous. It is preferable in such instances to approach an adjoining venous segment unmolested by previous surgery. The second superficial femoral vein valve found 1–2 inches below the first valve is a good candidate for "redo" surgery. This valve can be approached by extending the original groin incision in a caudate direction. A valve is frequently present in the superficial femoral vein at the adductor hiatus. This location is also a good choice for "redo" valve repairs.

MANAGEMENT OF VENOUS ULCER AFTER VALVE RECONSTRUCTION

Even very large venous ulcers rapidly heal after valve reconstruction. It appears that islands of follicular epithelium surviving in the midst of venous stasis ulceration proliferate rapidly to epithelialize the surface. Misguided attempts to "debride" superficial ulcers that are relatively clean and free of slough before valve reconstruction may slow the process. When reepithelization is slow, it may be preferable to speed the process by application of split thickness skin graft after valve reconstruction surgery.

POSTOPERATIVE MANAGEMENT

Patients undergoing venous valve reconstruction, especially those with a history of venous thrombosis, receive low molecular weight heparin (Lovenox) 15 mg BID subcutaneously before surgery. This regimen may be continued postoperatively for several days, or, alternatively, patients may be placed on a low dose intravenous heparin (400–700 u/hr). Oral anticoagulation with warfarin sodium at low dosage (2.5 mg daily) is started the day after the surgical procedure. Long-term low-dose Coumadin has been shown to be effective in a variety of situations that predispose to deep venous thrombosis (29). Protime is seldom prolonged at this dosage and routine Protime determinations at frequent intervals are not necessary. While effective as a prophylaxis for recurrent deep venous thrombosis, this low-dose warfarin regimen appears to be associated with a significantly reduced risk of bleeding complications. No serious bleeding complications have developed in 400 reconstruction procedures in which this regimen was employed. Pneumatic compression devices are routinely employed in the postoperative period as an antiembolism measure and to control postoperative limb edema. Activity and ambulation are resumed as soon as possible after surgery, usually the next day. Patients are discharged with a semirigid leg support (Circaid) for control of temporary exacerbation of limb edema that often follows valve reconstruction surgery. A month or two after surgery most patients discard leg support devices with resolution of symptoms.

MORBIDITY AND MORTALITY

The incidence of complications after valve reconstruction surgery is low. Even elderly patients tolerate the surgery well. There have been no operative deaths after valve reconstructions in our institution. In a total experience of 379 patients undergoing valve reconstructions, two patients, both with hypertension on medication, died suddenly 2 months after recovering from surgery, but pulmonary embolic cause could not be ruled out. The incidence of deep venous thrombosis was 4.5%. In four patients (<1%), the repaired valve was involved in the thrombosis. Others were silent and were detected during routine duplex and venous pressure testing at follow-up. There was one known case of pulmonary embolism that resolved without sequelae. Fifty-six percent of reconstructed valves were considered postthrombotic. The incidence of these thromboembolic complications is particularly noteworthy because this group is prone to recurring thrombosis, yet the incidence does not appear to be different from unoperated patients with the disease or other types of surgery at high risk for thromboembolic complications. Technical failures, complications, and mortality after the procedure are quite low (Table 23.1). The incidence of deep wound infections (<2%) is comparable to the reported incidence in "clean" nonvenous surgery, even though 30% of patients undergoing valve reconstruction had active stasis ulcers at the time of surgery and in 41% a recently healed ulcer with persistent skin changes or dermatitis was present. Only two prosthetic sleeves had to be removed for infection among 210 sleeve implantations.

Improvement in venous function studies after valve reconstruction is shown in Table 23.2. While there is no postexercise pressure, recovery time (VFT) is signif-

TABLE 23-1

TECHNICAL DATA AND COMPLICATIONS IN 582 VALVE RECONSTRUCTIONS IN 379 LIMBS*

Operative mortality	0%
Intraoperative technical failure	4%
Repaired valve totally refluxive	
Repair valve slightly refluxive after repair	10%
Less refluxive than before	
Competent repair	86%
Hemodynamically significant suture line stenosis	4%
Early postoperative thrombosis of repaired valve	1%
Postoperative DVT not involving repair	3.5%
Hematoma/seroma requiring drainage or aspiration	5%
Wound infection	2%
Infection involving prosthetic sleeve requiring removal	1%

*30% had active ulcers at time of surgery and another 41% had stasis dermatitis or recently healed ulcers at time of surgery.

TABLE 23-2

VENOUS FUNCTION AFTER VALVE RECONSTRUCTION

Type of Valve Repair	Number	Test	Pre-operation	Post-operation	P Significance
Single	61	Ambulatory venous pressure (mmHg)	64 ± 15	61 ± 16	Not significant
Multiple	57	Ambulatory venous pressure (mmHg)	57 ± 17	54 ± 16	Not significant
Single	61	Median recovery time (seconds) (VFT)	10 ± 08	13 ± 07	<.02
Multiple	57	Median recovery time (seconds) (VFT)	14 ± 12	21 ± 18	<.005
Single	81	Valsalva foot venous pressure (mmHg)	6.4 ± 5.5	3.7 ± 4.0	<.005
Multiple	60	Valsalva foot venous pressure (mmHg)	5.1 ± 4.6	3.6 ± 2.7	<.02

icantly prolonged after reconstructive surgery. This dichotomy is thought to be due to the nonlinear volume pressure relationship that exists in collapsible venous tubes of the calf venous pump. Postoperative improvement in VFT was more impressive after multiple valve reconstructions. Improvement in VFT was durable, extending up to and beyond 5 years. Valsalva foot venous pressure elevation also improved significantly. There was little change in plethysmographic parameters. Since VFI90 measures passive reflux in the absence of Valsalva, no improvement after repair could be expected in this parameter. Valve reflux is a postejection event. Therefore, ejection related parameters (ejection fraction, residual volume fraction) measured with air plethysmography are not to be expected to show an improvement after correction of reflux.

CLINICAL RESULTS

Excellent results with healing of stasis ulcer that is sustained over time are achieved with venous valve reconstruction (Fig. 23.14). Similar excellent results for relief of pain and swelling are obtained (6, 7). There was no difference between postthrombotic and "primary" reflux in actuarial ulcer healing rates (9). A variety of different techniques yielded equally good results. Use of stockings declines after successful valve repair (6, 7).

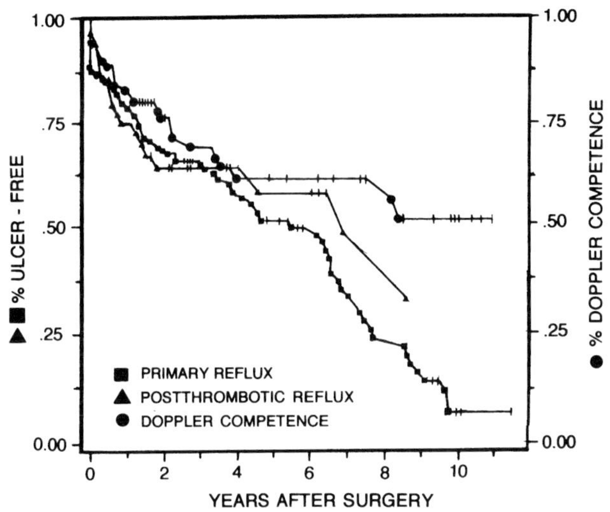

FIG. 23–14. Ulcer-free survival curves (Kaplan-Meir) after valve reconstruction in "primary" and postthrombotic reflux. There is a time lag between recurrence of ulcer and Doppler competence after valve repair.

There is a slow deterioration, spanning over years, in competence of repaired valves when monitored by serial duplex examination. A deterioration of repair, however, does not invariably lead to ulcer recurrence in that there is a lag between Doppler failure and clinical ulcer recurrence (14). In Doppler competence, postthrombotic repairs appear to be less durable than "primary" reflux cases. Some differences among the various techniques are also seen. The techniques could be ranked as follows in decreasing order of Doppler durability: (a) internal valvuloplasty, (b) prosthetic sleeve in situ, (c) external valvuloplasty, and (d) axillary vein transfer. The experience with angioscopic repair is too recent for adequate evaluation.

REFERENCES

1. Kistner RL. Surgical repair of a venous valve. Straub Clin Proc 1968;34:41–43.
2. Kistner RL. Surgical repair of the incompetent femoral vein valve. Arch Surg 1975;110:1336–1342.
3. Rich NM, Spencer FC. Vascular trauma. Philadelphia: WB Saunders, 1978.
4. Gooley NA, Sumner DS. Relationship of venous reflux to the size of venous valvular incompetence: Implications for venous reconstructive surgery. J Vasc Surg 1988;7:50–59.
5. Raju S, Fredericks R. Hemodynamic basis of stasis ulceration—a hypothesis. J Vasc Surg 1992;15:938.
6. Masuda EM, Kistner RL. Long-term results of venous valve reconstruction: a four- to twenty-one-year follow-up. J Vasc Surg 1994;19:391–403.
7. Raju S, Fredericks R. Valve reconstruction procedures for non-obstructive venous insufficiency: rationale, techniques, and results in 107 procedures with 2–8 year follow-up. J Vasc Surg 1988;7:301–310.
8. Bry JDL, Muto PA, O'Donnell TF, Isaacson LA. The clinical and hemodynamic results after axillary-to-popliteal vein valve transplantation. J Vasc Surg 1995;21:110–119.

9. Raju S, Fredericks RK, Neglén PN, Bass JD. Durability of venous valve reconstruction techniques for "primary" and postthrombotic reflux. J Vasc Surg 1996;23:357–367.
10. Bergan JJ, Yao JST. Perforating vein interruption in the postphlebitic syndrome. In: Bergan JJ, Yao JST, eds. Surgery of the veins. New York: Grune & Stratton, 1985:194–196.
11. Mayberry JC, Moneta GL, DeFrang RD, Porter JM. The influence of elastic compression stockings on deep venous hemodynamics. J Vasc Surg 1991;13:91–100.
12. Hobbs JT. A random trial of the treatment of varicose veins by surgery and sclerotherapy. In: Hobbs JT, ed. The treatment of venous disorders. Philadelphia: JB Lippincott, 1977:195–207.
13. Sethia KK, Darke SG. Long saphenous incompetence as a cause of venous ulceration. Br J Surg 1984;71:754–755.
14. DePalma RG. Surgical therapy for venous stasis: results of a modified Linton operation. Am J Surg 1979;137:810–813.
15. Raju S. Valve reconstruction procedures for chronic venous insufficiency. Semin Vasc Surg 1988;1:101–106.
16. Darke SG, Penfold C. Venous ulceration and saphenous ligation. Eur J Vasc Surg 1991;6:4–9.
17. Walsh TC, Bergan JJ, Beewan S, Moulton SL. Proximal venous reflux adversely affects distal venous function. Surgery 1995;8:566.
18. Raju S. Surgical management of postphlebitic syndrome. In: Veith FJ, ed. Current critical problems in vascular surgery. Vol. 6. St Louis: Quality Medical Publishing Company, 1994:108–112.
19. Raju S. Technical options in venous valve reconstruction. Am J Surg (in press).
20. Raju S. Axillary vein transfer for postphlebitic syndrome. In: Bergan JJ, Kistner RL, eds. Atlas of venous surgery. Philadelphia: WB Saunders, 1992:147–152.
21. Gloviczki P, Merrell SW, Bower TC. Femoral vein valve repair under direct vision without venotomy: a modified technique with use of angioscopy. J Vasc Surg 1991;14:645–648.
22. Hallberg D. A method for repairing incompetent valves in deep veins. Acta Chir Scand 1972;138:143–145.
23. Lane RJ, McMahon C, Cuzilla M. The treatment of varicose veins using the venous valve cuff. Phlebology 1994;9:136–145.
24. Raju S. Multiple-valve reconstruction for venous insufficiency: indications, optimal technique, and results. In: Veith FJ, ed. Current critical problems in vascular surgery. Vol. 4. St. Louis: Quality Medical Publishing Company, 1992:122–126.
25. Raju S. Optimal technique for venous valve repair: Which patients should have the procedure? In: Veith FJ, ed. Current critical problems in vascular surgery. Vol. 7. St. Louis: Quality Medical Publishing Company, 1996:502–506.
26. Raju S. Venous insufficiency of the lower limb and stasis ulceration: changing concepts and management. Ann Surg 1983;197:688–697.
27. Raju S, Fredericks R. Venous obstruction: an analysis of one hundred thirty-seven cases with hemodynamic, venographic, and clinical correlations. J Vasc Surg 1991;14:305–313.
28. Kistner RL. Personal communication. September, 1994.
29. Bern MM, Lokich JJ, Wallach SR, et al. Very low doses of warfarin can prevent thrombosis in central venous catheters. Ann Int Med 1990;112:423–428.

chapter 24

Modern Interventional Techniques: Endoscopy, Balloon Dilatation and Stents

S. Raju and J.L. Villavicencio

Major advances in percutaneous interventional radiologic techniques have contributed to the successful treatment of vascular lesions that traditionally would have required a traumatic open surgical approach (1). The experience with endoscopic vascular techniques has been primarily concentrated in the treatment of arterial disease. These techniques include: balloon angioplasty for arterial stenosis or occlusion (2–4), atherectomy of occluded arterial segments (5,6), application of stents after failed or complicated balloon angioplasty (7–9), endovascular repair of false aneurysms, traumatic arteriovenous fistulas and aortic aneurysms (10–13), and catheter-directed intra-arterial thrombolysis. The latter has been of great value in cleaning debris after difficult vascular procedures and in the management of acute or sub-acute graft thrombosis (14,15). The excellent results obtained in the arterial system have prompted vascular surgeons and interventional radiologists to develop endovascular techniques to address the challenging pathology of the venous system. The latter, with its low pressure, low velocity flow presents special problems for the investigator. Nonetheless, the early results of this emerging technology in the management of some venous problems are encouraging. An outline of the techniques used in the venous system and the results obtained will give us a good perspective of the advances in this new field and the exciting opportunities for future research.

To a great extent, the development and success of the new endovascular technology are closely related to the dramatic progress in imaging techniques of the vascular system. One must have a clear picture of the anatomy of the lesion to be treated. The introduction of real time color Doppler sonography with its capability to determine direction and velocity of blood flow has been of pivotal importance for a better understanding of the pathophysiology and hemodynamics of the arterial and venous circulation and to monitor some endovascular procedures (16).

Computerized three-dimensional spiral computed tomography (CT) has greatly improved our ability to evaluate the arterial, venous and lymphatic systems (17). High-speed computerized tomography developed in the 1970s has increased the scope and usefulness of conventional CT by providing information on the size, extent and character of the endovascular lesions (18). Magnetic resonance imaging (MRI) with the use of contrast material has been of great value in the diagnosis and assessment of the distribution and magnitude of the lesions of congenital vascular malformations. In some centers, it has been the only preoperative imaging technique in peripheral vascular surgery (19).

The capability of imaging the vessel wall and its lumen with intraluminal ultrasonography (IU) has increased the potential for exploration and assessment of the nature and extent of the vascular lesions. IU is a valuable tool in monitoring the actual endovascular procedure and its outcome (20,21). Vascular angioscopy has been used extensively in Europe to monitor the results of venous thrombectomy (Fig. 24.1). After completion of the surgical procedure, Fogarty balloons are used to achieve a bloodless field. The thrombectomized segment is examined angioscopically. Adherent residual thrombus can then be removed under direct vi-

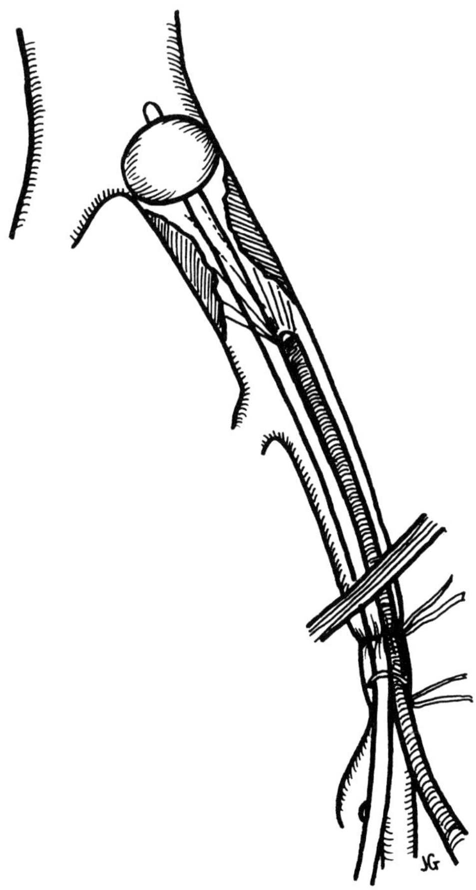

FIG. 24–1. Completion angioscopy after iliofemoral thrombectomy. Vascular control is achieved by proximal balloon occlusion and distal clamp. Residual thrombus can be removed with angioscopic visualization.

sualization with an alligator forceps or with a Fogarty adherent thrombectomy catheter as illustrated in Figure 24.1. The angioscope has been employed in the procedure of valve reconstruction for primary valvular insufficiency. Previous to valve repair, angioscopic examination and irrigation of the vein provide valuable information on the pathology, valve configuration, and the presence and magnitude of reflux. Under angioscopic guidance, the placement of the valvuloplasty sutures can be done with accuracy. After valve repair, confirmation of the precise placement of the sutures can be observed. With irrigation, restoration of valve competence can be observed, and the desired degree of valve tightening can be precisely controlled by progressive observation of the valve structure as the valvuloplasty sutures are sequentially placed (22).

Success in this procedure depends to a great extent on the ability of the surgeon to judge the competency of the valve repair. The advantage of this method is the avoidance of venotomy and the possibility to operate on more than one valve, if considered necessary. The long-term results of valvuloplasty, through a venotomy, are excellent in published retrospective series. Preliminary results with the angioscopic technique are encouraging (23). Long term results are not available.

Angioscopy, as an adjunctive technique, has been successfully used to evaluate valve disruption during in-situ saphenous vein bypass (24,25). One wonders in these cases how much damage is produced to the venous endothelium by the angioscopic manipulations! Despite this concern, the role of angioscopy has been investigated in several centers in the endoscopic intra- and extraluminal ligation of saphenous tributaries for infrainguinal in-situ bypass. One of the feared postoperative complications of in-situ bypass techniques has been skin necrosis and wound infection secondary to extensive dissection and flap undermining. This is particularly severe in the case of diabetic patients. With minimal skin disruption, as practiced with the endoscopic techniques, this complication may be largely eliminated. The endoscopic extraluminal ligation of saphenous tributaries with laparoscopic technique and CO_2 insufflation was investigated in cadavers and in the swine model by our group (JLV) in late 1993 and 1994 (26). Recently, this technique was used successfully by Rosenthal in a patient with severe limb ischemia (27). Other angioscopically guided methods to eliminate the saphenous tributaries in preparation for in-situ bypass include coil embolization of tributaries. Coil "recoil" has occurred in some cases requiring endovenous retrieval or flushing of the free coils (28).

The beneficial impact of the interventional radiologic advances has extended to the field of pelvic venous disorders. Patients with the pelvic venous congestion syndrome and pelvic varices secondary to massive gonadal and hypogastric tributaries reflux, who in the past have been treated by extraperitoneal resection of the ovarian vein and intrapelvic ligation of incompetent internal iliac vein tributaries (29,30), can benefit by less aggressive nonsurgical methods. These include coil and/or balloon embolization of the ovarian vein and the incompetent hypogastric vein tributaries. These methods have been also successfully used in the treatment of male varicocele (31,32).

The division of incompetent leg perforators in the management of primary and post-thrombotic chronic venous insufficiency has been practiced ever since Linton described a technique for subfascial ligation of the perforators in 1938 (33). It is recognized that incompetent perforators larger than 3 to 4 mm in diameter should be interrupted either as a single procedure, or as a part of the treatment of chronic venous insufficiency. Traditionally, all the operations designed for the subfascial ligation of perforators required wide dissection and elevation of skin flaps that often resulted in skin necrosis and painful postoperative recovery. In 1985, Hauer described an endoscopic technique using a specially designed mediastinoscope without the use of CO_2 insufflation (34). Saetler and Fischer presented a video describing the endoscopic division of perforators during the Vth European American Symposium on Venous Diseases that took place in Vienna, Austria, in November 1990. Saetler's technique included the use of a special thigh pneumatic tourniquet that allowed operation in a bloodless field. Division of perforators was accomplished with diathermia and without the use of CO_2 insufflation. Partial fasciotomy was performed at the end of the procedure. Other techniques have incorporated the use of laparoscopic instruments and infusion of saline solution under the fascia to expand the subfascial space (35). Most European investigators do not use CO_2 insufflation (36). However, in the United States and Australia (37,38), the procedure is performed using CO_2 insufflation and a pneumatic tourniquet to achieve a bloodless field, as described by Saetler. It is clear that this endoscopic technique has the appeal of being less traumatic and less incapacitating than the traditional subfascial open procedures. However, there are many patients with severe chronic venous insufficiency and leg ulceration in whom it is impossible to safely introduce the endoscopic instruments under lipodermatosclerotic tissues, which have practically fused the fascia with the periosteum.

In these cases, the involved area must be resected enbloc to be grafted in a subsequent operation. It is clear that a well-designed prospective study comparing long-term endoscopic ligation of perforators to a group of patients managed by conservative measures and to a third group treated by small incisions placed directly over areas of Duplex localized incompetent perforators is needed. This type of study should be performed in a population of patients with chronic venous insufficiency who share similar hemodynamic venous parameters. Some of these studies are currently in progress.

The Use of Stents, Balloon Dilatation, and Other Techniques on the Venous System

The success obtained with endovascular procedures in the arterial system has been difficult to reproduce in the venous system due to the special characteristics of the venous wall and the venous circulation. Expandable metallic stents (EMS) have been used experimentally and clinically in the coronary and peripheral arterial system, vena cava, portal vein, bile duct, trachea and bronchial tree, gastrointestinal system and urethra (39–46). Percutaneous endovascular stent insertion in the management of superior vena cava obstruction has been attempted by several investigators. In a recent study (47), stent insertion was attempted in 13 patients. Twelve patients had known malignant disease. In two patients, it was not possible to cross the lesion with a guide wire and this prevented stent insertion. Primary success was achieved in 11 patients with associated symptomatic relief. There was some recurrence of symptoms in 5 of the 11 patients (45.5%) after a time interval from 14 to 183 days. Patency was re-established in all cases with symptomatic recurrence with the use of thrombolysis and/or further stent insertion. This study reveals that percutaneous management of complete superior vena cava obstruction with a combination of thrombolysis followed by stent insertion is effective and produces sustained symptomatic relief.

Self-expandable endovascular stents have been used in the treatment of patients with venous stenosis secondary to chronic hemodialysis. Quinn placed 25 modified self-expandable endovascular stents in 20 hemodialysis access sites to treat 21 stenoses and 4 occlusions in 19 patients. All stenoses were initially dilated with a high-pressure balloon. The initial success rate was 90% (18 of 20 access sites). The long-term success was as follows: primary (25%), secondary (34%) and tertiary (42%). The best results occurred in patients in whom the stenosis or occlusion affected a large vein that had no acute angle and was away from venous confluences, such as the femoral and iliac region (48).

Numerous and different stents are now in use: self-expanding, balloon expandable, stainless steel, tantalum, flexible and articulated stents, and, more recently, heparin-coated stents. All stents are foreign bodies and may induce spasm and thrombosis. Careful drug treatment may help to reduce the side-effects of the stent. New designs with improved fluid dynamics and optimal conformability are now being successfully tested. Optimal implantation strategy aiming at an absolutely perfect primary result with no residual narrowing, absence of dissections and complete stent expansion, has reduced dramatically the complication rate after stenting as well as reduced the need for heavy anticoagulation. Stents hold great promise as local drug delivery devices and have opened a new field in endovascular management of arterial and venous lesions (49).

An interesting variation of the utilization of stents is the use of temporary stenting (50). This modality appears to be an attractive potential therapy that combines some of the benefits of permanent stenting without the need for permanent endovascular prosthesis and oral anticoagulation. The devices used for temporary stenting are still evolving. The Flow Support Catheter (50) was promising during the early clinical trials. However, the device was associated with a high rate of thrombosis and suboptimal overall success rate. The experience with In-Stent has been limited and its safety and reliability still needs to be proved. The HARTS™ device is currently in the preclinical phase, but available data from animal studies show it to be a feasible device for coronary use. Its potential applications include its use as a permanent or temporary stent, a repositionable stent, a primary lesion-dilating device or a local drug delivery vehicle. Clinical trials are likely to begin in the foreseeable future for one or more of these applications.

Venous stenosis and occlusions of benign etiology have been treated successfully with endovascular stents of the Wallstent type. The use of percutaneous transluminal angioplasty (PTA) in the venous system in combination with implantation of self-expanding vascular endoprosthesis offered a new therapeutic modality to massage venous stenosis or occlusion of benign etiology without surgical intervention. Eight patients (7 female and 1 male) suffering from stenosis or occlusion of the pelvic or superficial femoral veins after surgical or percutaneous interventions were treated successfully with endovascular stents. Phlebographic control showed patency of all stented lesions at follow-up times between 3 and 82 months (average 27 months) (51).

The advent of better techniques and improved stent materials have opened new avenues in the management of portal hypertension secondary to cirrhosis or congenital malformations. The Budd-Chiari syndrome, whose surgical management required a formidable operation, has been managed successfully by inferior vena cava dilatation and the placement of an expandable metal stent (52). The transjugular intrahepatic portosystemic shunt has revolutionized the management of acute esophageal varices bleeding in patients with advanced stages of portal hypertension (53). Other areas of the venous system where stents have been used successfully have been the points of compression of arteries on the veins. These "dangerous crossings" may be the cause of symptoms and venous thrombosis. The iliac compression syndrome produced at the crossing of the right common iliac artery over the left common iliac vein may produce edema and incapacitating symptoms in some patients. There are reports on the successful management of this syndrome with expandable stents (54).

A new, exciting field of stent utilization, still in the experimental stages, is the endovascular valve transplantation of either autogenous or prosthetic valves carried in a stent. The search for an ideal substitute for segments of the venous system has led to numerous experimental and clinical studies using a variety of materials and techniques. Interventional radiology and new endovascular techniques may offer new alternatives of management to the challenging disorders of the venous system. The following cases illustrate the indications and the potential for these emerging technologies.

THROMBOLYSIS

Therapeutic anticoagulation with heparin followed by warfarin remains the current method of treatment for deep venous thrombosis (DVT). While this regimen undoubtedly decreases mortality and morbidity from progression of thromboses and embolism, incidents of post-thrombotic syndrome with this regimen is probably substantial. Short-term studies indicate that one-third of patients with DVT develop severe symptoms and another third develop moderate symptoms of post-thrombotic syndrome within a few years after the onset of thrombosis (55). Because recurrent thrombosis years or decades after the initial attack is quite common, long-term incidence may be worse than that indicated by these preliminary data. Meta-analysis of several series using systemic Streptokinase or Urokinase appear to be associated with lesser incidence of post-thrombotic syndrome. Careful follow-up studies after surgical thrombectomy and temporary arterial venous fistula also indicate a superior clinical outcome to systemic anticoagulant or thrombolytic therapy. Restoration of luminal patency and flow by rapid lysis of thrombus or surgical removal appears to be the key to lessening the incidence of post-thrombotic syndrome. The widespread use of Urokinase therapy and attendant success in treating arterial thrombosis is encouraging application of this technique in venous thrombosis.

CATHETER-DIRECTED THROMBOLYSIS

Case

A 55-year-old salesman developed extensive ilio-femoral thrombosis in the contralateral unoperated limb 2 weeks after undergoing a valve reconstruction procedure for stasis ulceration. Venous profile scans strongly suggested pulmonary embolus, but the patient was clinically stable. He underwent catheter-directed thrombolysis of the occluded iliac vein by infusion of Urokinase through a side-hole catheter directly placed into the clot. Thrombolysis with restoration of flow was achieved within 48 hours with resolution of pain and swelling in the affected limb (Fig 24.2). The repeat venogram 10 days later showed a small residual nonocclusive thrombus that resolved completely with a short duration catheter-directed thrombolytic therapy. At 6-month follow-up, the patient's limb continued to be asymptomatic with normal function.

BALLOON DILATATION AND STENTING

Case 1

A 27-year-old grocery store manager sustained severe ilio-femoral thrombosis following appendectomy for acute appendicitis. He was initially treated with heparin/Coumadin anticoagulation therapy at another institution. When he was referred 2 months after the event, massive painful swelling of the affected left lower extremity was present with severe dependent pain. The patient was unable to stand for more than a few minutes at a time, even with support stockings. A side-hole catheter over a guide wire was successfully manipulated into the occluded iliac vein segment by the transfemoral approach. After 72 hours of Urokinase therapy, a small channel was opened through the previously occluded iliac vein segment (Fig 24.3). This channel was enlarged by a balloon angioplasty, but several areas of residual stenosis persisted. He was maintained on oral anticoagulant therapy and was brought back after 3 weeks at which time the iliac vein segment was dilated and a stent placed (Fig 24.3B and C). The procedure resulted in an excellent clinical result with resolution of pain and swelling. A repeat venogram 4 months later confirmed patent stent without rethrombosis and normal flow. The patient has resumed full-time work with support stockings prescribed as a precaution.

Case 2

A 42-year-old active housewife sustained massive iliac vein thrombosis 2 weeks after having been treated for bladder infection. She received standard heparin/Coumadin anticoagulation therapy and was referred 4 months later for persistent limb swelling and pain. Pain was particularly severe when the limb was in the dependent position. She was unable to stay on her feet for more than 10 to 15 minutes at a time. Even with support stockings, she had to sit down to prop her feet. She was using pain medication at frequent intervals to carry her through required household activities. An initial attempt at cannulation of the occluded iliac vein

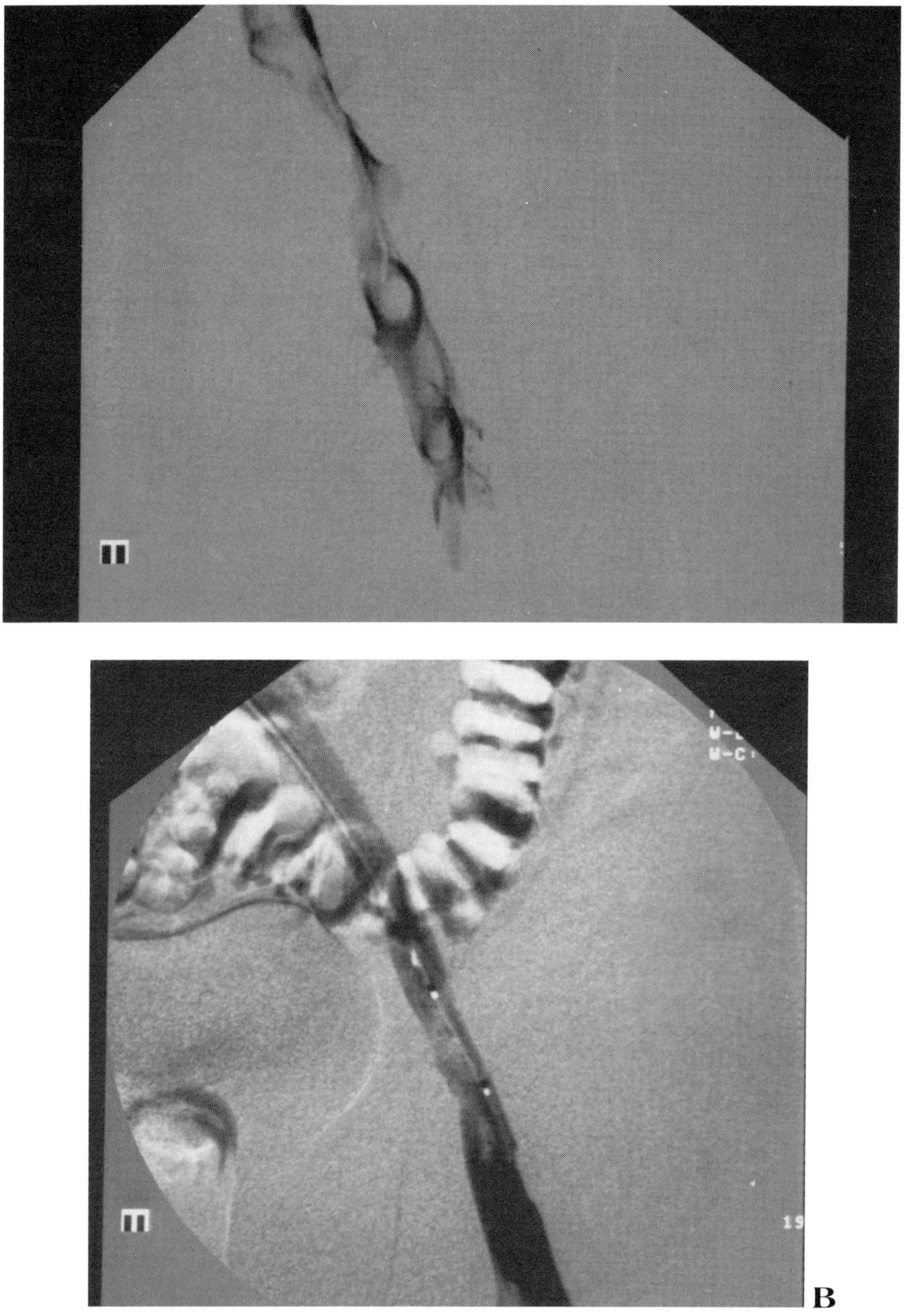

A

B

FIG. 24–2. **A.** Patient with iliofemoral thrombosis; initiation of catheter directed through thrombolysis. **B.** Completion venogram after successful thrombolysis.

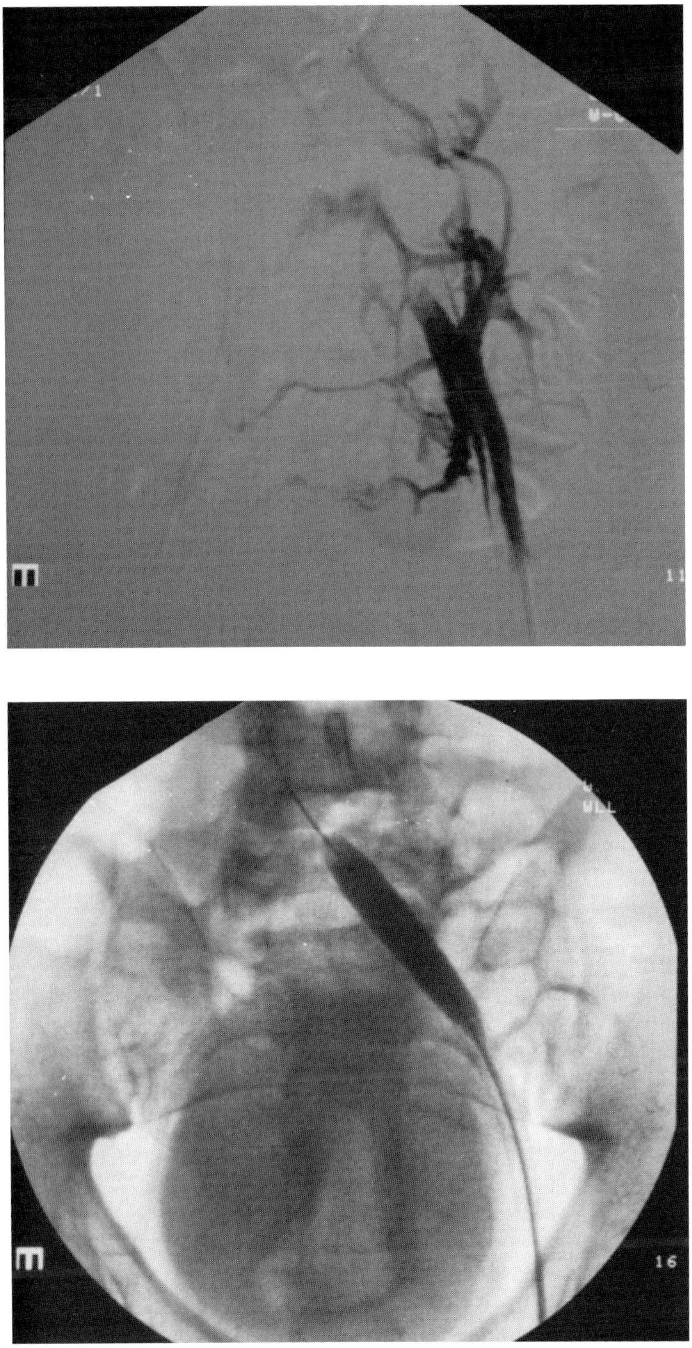

A

B

FIG. 24–3. Case 2: Stenotic iliac venous segment with collaterals after catheter-directed thrombolysis of a 2-month-old thrombosis **(A).** Balloon dilatation followed by stenting **(B and C)** reestablished luminal patency and flow. Note disappearance of collaterals.

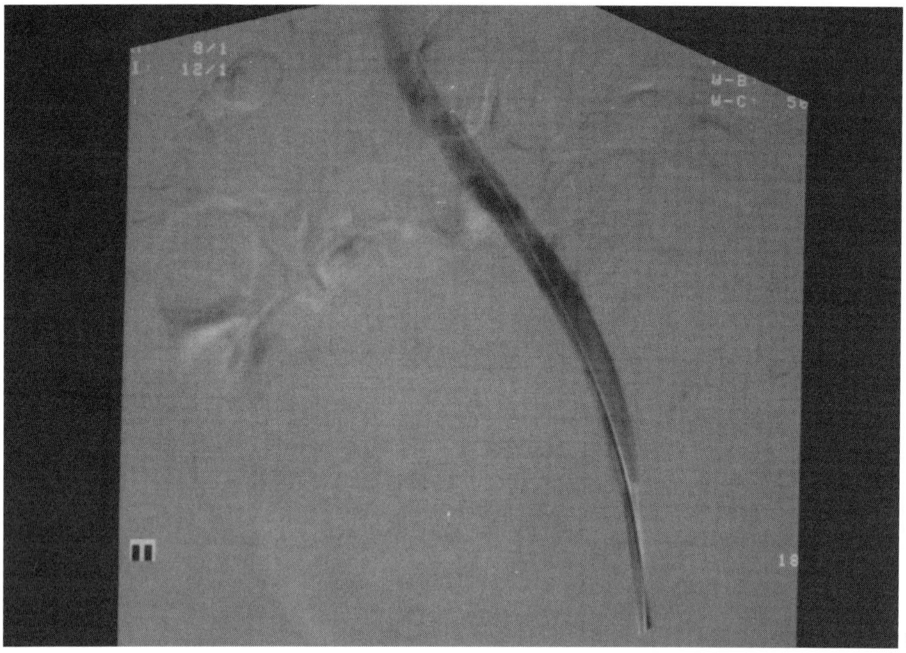

C

FIG. 24–3. Continued

through a transfemoral approach from the opposite side was unsuccessful. Ipsilateral femoral flow cannulation also failed, as femoral flow was absent. She was admitted 3 weeks later and was infused with Urokinase through a peripheral foot vein for 48 hours. With this treatment, femoral venous flow at the groin level reappeared, allowing successful cannulation of the occluded vein segment. Balloon dilatation of this segment was successful and a Wallstent was placed to maintain patency of the dilated venous segment. The patient has been maintained on oral anticoagulation. Pain relief was immediate, and the regression of swelling was apparent to the patient at discharge, 72 hours after the procedure. She has resumed her normal activities, once again with compressive leg support. She has not required pain medication after placement of the stent.

Comments

These cases represent preliminary and encouraging results. They indicate the luminal patency and flow can be re-established several months after onset of thrombosis. Long-term outcome and complications remain to be determined. Clinical experience with traditional therapeutic approaches in the group of patients typified by the examples cited had been disappointing. By and large, these classes of patients have remained semi-invalid, disabled to greater or lesser extent by severe post-thrombotic sequelae. Aggressive, early intervention that can achieve thrombolysis and maintain venous patency may forestall the development and/or sequelae of this debilitating syndrome.

REFERENCES

1. Moore WS. Endovascular surgery: state of the art. Introduction. World J Surg 1996;20:621.
2. Kalman PG, Johnston KW, Sniderman KW. Indications and results of balloon angioplasty for arterial occlusive lesions. World J Surg 1996;20:630–634.
3. Johnston KW. Iliac arteries: reanalysis of results of balloon angioplasty. Radiology 1993;186:207.
4. Wilson SE, Wolf GL, Cross AP. Percutaneous transluminal angioplasty versus operation for peripheral arteriosclerosis. J Vasc Surg 1989;9:1.
5. Ahn SS, Concepcion B. Current status of atherectomy for peripheral arterial occlusive disease. World J Surg 1996;20:635–643.
6. Sapoval MR, Gaux JC, Bruneval P, Peronneau P. Animal Evaluation of the prototype OmniCath atherectomy catheter. Cardiovasc Intervent Radiol 1994;17:226.
7. Palmaz JC, Laborde JC, Rivera FJ, Encarnacion CE, Lutz JD, Moss JG. Stenting of the iliac arteries with the Palmaz stent: experience from a multicenter trial. Cardiovasc Intervent Radiol 1992;15:291.
8. Robinson KA, Roubin G, King S et al. Correlated microscopic observations of arterial responses to intravascular stenting. Scanning Microsc 1989;3:665.
9. Ahn SS, Concepcion B. Indications and results of arterial stents for occlusive disease. World J Surg 1996;20:644–648.
10. Parodi JC, Palmaz JC, Barone HD. Transfemoral intraluminal graft implantation for abdominal aortic aneurysms. Ann Vasc Surg 1991;5:491.
11. Chuter T. Bifurcated endovascular graft insertion for abdominal aortic aneurysms. In: Greenhalgh RM, ed.Vascular and endovascular surgical techniques. Philadelphia: WB Saunders, 1994:92.
12. Marin ML, Veith FJ, Sanchez LA, et al. Endovascular aortoiliac grafts in combination with standard infrainguinal arterial bypasses in the management of limb-threatening ischemia: preliminary report. J Vasc Surg 1995;22:316.
13. Colburn MD, Moore WS. Endovascular repair of abdominal aortic aneurysms using the EGS tube and bifurcated graft systems. World J Surg 1996;20:664–672.
14. Quinones-Baldrich WJ, Zierler RE, Hiatt JC. Intraoperative fibrinolytic therapy: an adjunct to catheter thromboembolectomy. J Vasc Surg 1985;2:319.
15. Nilsson L, Albrechtsson U, Jonung T, et al. Surgical treatment versus thrombolysis in acute arterial occlusions: a randomized controlled study. Eur J Vasc Surg 1992;6:189.
16. Cluley SR, Brener BJ, Hollier L, et al. Transcutaneous ultrasonography can be used to guide and monitor balloon angioplasty. J Vasc Surg 1993;17:23.
17. Rubin GD, Walker PJ, Dake MD, et al. Three-dimensional helical CT angiography. Radiographics 1994;14:905.
18. Agatston AS, Janowitz WR, Hildner FJ, Zusmer NR, et al. Quantification of coronary artery calcium using ultrafast computed tomography. J Am Coll Cardiol 1990;15:827.
19. Carpenter JP, Baum RA, Holland GA, Barker CF, et al. Peripheral vascular surgery with magnetic resonance angiography as the sole preoperative imaging modality. J Vasc Surg 1994;20:861.
20. Gussenhoven WJ, Essed CF, Frietman P, et al. Intravascular echographic assessment of vessel wall characteristics: a correlation with histology. Int J Cardiol Imaging 1989;4:105.

21. Fitzgerald PJ, Yock PG. Mechanisms and outcomes of angioplasty and atherectomy assessed by intravascular ultrasound imaging. J Clin Ultrasound 1993;21:570.
22. Gloviczki P, Merrell SW, Bower TC. Femoral vein valve repair under direct vision without venotomy: a modified technique with use of angioscopy. J Vasc Surg 1991;14:645–648.
23. Welch HJ, McLaughlin RL, O'Donnell TF Jr. Femoral vein valvuloplasty: intraoperative angioscopic evaluation and hemodynamic improvement. J Vasc Surg 1992;16:694–700.
24. Parent FN III, Gandhi RH, Wheeler JR, Gregory RT, et al. Angioscopic evaluation of valvular disruption during in situ saphenous vein bypass. Ann Vasc Surg 1994;8:24–30.
25. Clair DG, Golden MA, Mannick JA, et al. Randomized prospective study of angioscopically assisted in situ saphenous vein grafting. J Vasc Surg 1994;19:992–1000.
26. Villavicencio JL, Wherry D, Sidawy A, Neville R, Martin J, Rob CN. Endoscopic extraluminal ligation of saphenous tributaries for in situ bypass in the lower extremities. Experimental study. Discussion of Rosenthal D. video presentation: Improved endovascular techniques for in situ vein bypass. Annual Montefiore meeting: Current Critical Problems in Vascular Surgery, New York NY, November 1993.
27. Rosenthal D, Tucker JG, Atkins CP, Walters AS, et al. Extraluminal endoscopic-assisted ligation of venous tributaries for infrainguinal in situ saphenous vein bypass: a preliminary report. Cardiovasc Surg 1996;4:512–514.
28. Rosenthal D, Dickson C, Rodriguez FJ, et al. Infrainguinal endovascular in-situ saphenous vein bypass: ongoing results. J Vasc Surg 1994;20:389–95.
29. Lechter A. Pelvic and vulval varices: pelvic congestion syndrome. In: Bergan JJ, Goldman MP, eds. Varicose veins and telangiectasias. St Louis MO. Quality Med Publ 1993:353–369.
30. Gomez ER, Villavicencio JL, Coffey JA, Rich NM. Pathogenesis and surgical management of varicose veins of the vulva and upper thigh: the internal iliac venous insufficiency syndrome. In: Veith FJ, ed. Current Problems in Vascular Surgery. St Louis MO Quality Med Publ 1990:141–142.
31. Edwards RD, Robertson IR, MacLean AB, Hemmingway AP. Case report: Pelvic pain syndrome. Successful treatment of a case by ovarian vein embolization. Clin Radiol 1993;47:429–431.
32. White RI, Kaufman SL, Barth KH, Kadir S, et al. Occlusion of varicoceles with detachable balloons. Radiology 1981;139:327–334.
33. Linton RR. The communicating veins of the lower leg and the operative technique for their ligation. Ann Surg 1938;107:582–593.
34. Hauer G. The endoscopic subfascial division of the perforating veins—preliminary report. VASA 1985;14:59–61.
35. O'Donnell TF. Surgical treatment of incompetent communicating veins. In: Bergan JJ, Kistner RL, eds. Atlas of Venous Surgery. Philadelphia: W.B. Saunders, 1992;111–124.
36. Pierik EGJM, Wittens CHA, van Urk H. Subfascial endoscopic ligation in the treatment of incompetent perforating veins. Eur J Vasc Endovasc Surg 1995;9:38–41.
37. Gloviczki P, Cambria RA, Rhee RY, Canton LG, McKusick MA. Surgical technique and preliminary results of endoscopic subfascial division of perforating veins. J Vasc Surg 1996;23:517–523.
38. Conrad P. Endoscopic exploration of the subfascial space of the lower leg with perforator vein interruption using laparoscopic equipment: a preliminary report. Phlebology 1994;9:154–157.
39. Sawada S, Fujiwara Y, Koyama T, Kobayashi M, et al. Application of expandable metallic stents to the venous system. Acta Radiologica 1992;33:156–159.
40. Yoshioka T, Sakaguchi H, Yoshimura H, Tamada T. et al. Expandable metallic biliary endoprostheses: preliminary clinical evaluation. Radiology 1990;177:253–257.

41. Carrasco CH, Nesbitt JC, Charnsangavej C, Ryan MB, et al. Management of tracheal and bronchial stenosis with the Gianturco stent. Ann Thorac Surg. 1994;58:1012–1017.
42. Watkinson AF, Ellul J, Entwisle K, Mason RC et al. Esophageal carcinoma: initial results of palliative treatment with covered self-expanding endoprostheses. Radiology 1995;195:821–827.
43. Song HY, Cho KS, Sung KB, Han YM, et al. Self-expandable metallic stents in high risk patients with benign prostatic hyperplasia: long-term followup. Radiology 1995;195:655–660.
44. Mathias K, Bolder U, Liehlein D, Jager H. Percutaneous transhepatic angioplasty and stent implantation for prehepatic portal vein obstruction. Cardiovasc Intervent Radiol 1993;16:313–315.
45. Nishibe T, Katoh H, Satoh K, Hirano S, Tanaka E, et al. Expandable metallic stent for portal stenosis and biliary obstruction caused by gallbladder carcinoma (Japanese with English abstract). J Jpn Soc Clin Surg 1994;55:3157–3160.
46. Chan O, Marchbank AJ, Bhagat K, Wood AJ. Pulmonary arterial obstruction caused by recurrent tumour treated with endovascular stenting. Clin Radiol 1996;51:228–229.
47. Crowe MT, Davies CH, Gaines PA. Percutaneous management of superior vena cava occlusions. Cardiovasc Intervent Radiol 1995;18:367–372.
48. Quinn SF, Schuman ES, Hall L, Gross GF, et al. Venous stenosis in patients who undergo hemodyalisis: treatment with self-expandable endovascular stents. Radiology 1992;183:199–504.
49. Sigwart U. Coronary stents. Z Kardiol 1995;84 suppl 2:65–77.
50. Dev V, Eigler N, Litvack F. Current status and prospects for the use of temporary stents. Coron Artery Dis 1994;5:597–604.
51. Janssen HJ, Antonucci F, Stuckman G, Tatalovic S, et al. (Treatment of venous stenoses and occlusions of benign etiology with vascular endoprostheses: a new, non-operative therapeutic concept.) Behandlung von Venenstenosen und verschlussen benigner Atiologie mit vaskularen Endoprothesen: Ein neues nichtoperatives Therapiekonzept. VASA 1994;23:66–73.
52. Gillams A, Platts DR, Irving D, Hobbs K. Dilatation of the inferior vena cava using an expandable metal stent in Budd-Chiari syndrome. J Hepatol 1991;13:149–151.
53. Laberge JM, Ring ET, Gordon RL, et al. Creation of transjugular intrahepatic portosystemic shunts with Wallstent endoprosthesis. Results in 100 patients. Radiology 1993;187:413–420.
54. Berger A, Jaffe JW, York TN. Iliac compression syndrome treated with stent placement. J Vasc Surg 1995;21:510–514.
55. Strandness DE Jr., Langlois Y, Cramer M, Randlett A, Thiele BL. Long term sequelae of acute venous thrombosis. JAMA 1983;250:1289–1292.

section IV

Clinical Features: Pathology and Management

chapter 25

Superficial Varicose Veins: Therapeutic Options

J. Leonel Villavicencio, David Gillespie, Emmanouil Pikoulis, and Norman M. Rich

Varicose veins may appear in any area affected by venous hypertension. Most epidemiologic studies dealing with the prevalence of varicose veins in the general population point out the large number of patients afflicted with venous disorders. Widmer, et al. (1) , reported that 22% of apparently healthy working individuals from the Basel Chemical Industry had signs and symptoms of chronic venous insufficiency. In a health survey in the United States, venous disease was one of the 10 most frequently diagnosed ailments in a group of 28 chronic diseases (2). Wright, et al. (3), reported that in a community sample of 2103 individuals from West London who completed a self-administered questionnaire, 31% reported having some form of venous disease. Among them, 25% had important varicose veins. The questionnaire was validated by selected clinical examination studies. In another study in the United States (4), the prevalence of venous insufficiency grade I was 12.9% in males and 25.9% in females. There was a 7.4% incidence of males and 16.7% of females suffering from grade II–III venous insufficiency. This important epidemiologic study was carried out in three phases. Phase I involved 8641 individuals, Phase II involved 9236, and Phase III, 6021 individuals. In a disease so prevalent, it is not strange that throughout the history of medicine a wide variety of methods and techniques have been tried to treat these disorders. Varicose veins constitute a progressive disease that becomes steadily worse. There is never remission of the disease except after pregnancy and delivery, when many of the dilated varicosities may disappear. During its course, the disease produces complications which usually induce the patient to seek medical care. The most frequent complications are superficial thrombophlebitis; acute bleeding originating in one of the thin dilated varices; eczema; and, finally, skin ulceration. Depending on age, general health condition, and symptomatology, patients with varicose veins may be offered one of the following alternatives of management: no treatment, conservative management, or surgical treatment.

No treatment is selected in patients with minimal, asymptomatic varicosities; athletes with dilated, prominent, cylindrical venous trunks; and patients over 65 years of age with asymptomatic, moderate varicosities that are a cosmetic nuisance.

Conservative treatment is recommended in these conditions: pregnancy; obesity greater than 20% of the ideal body weight; febrile illnesses representing either an acute or chronic disease; hemorrhagic diatheses; and poor general health. These patients receive the same general measures recommended to all patients with varicose veins. The extremities should be washed daily with a neutral soap and the skin should be lubricated with any preparation containing lanolin. The extremities should be elevated whenever possible; at night, the bed should be elevated, placing a 6-inch block between the floor and the foot of the bed. A good elastic compression should be an essential part of the treatment.

External elastic support is the single most important therapeutic measure in the management of venous disorders of the extremities (5). It has been demonstrated by several authors that ambulatory pressures of 100 mmHg are developed in areas of incompetent ankle perforators (6, 7). Hargens (8) has established that the normal pressure in the interstitial tissue is about 30 mmHg. With the use of a slit catheter, Taheri, et al. (9), found that 83% of patients with venous insufficiency have elevated deep compartment pressures (a mean of 55.8 mmHg). In their series, normal individuals had pressures in the range of 28–42 mmHg. Using foot volumetry and ^{24}Na, Jones, et al., reported that hosiery that exerted a pressure of 22 mmHg at the ankle was less effective than that exerting pressures of 30–50 mmHg in both primary and secondary varicose veins (10).

In patients with severe postphlebitic syndrome or primary varicose veins with advanced skin lesions, the use of a heavy rubberized elastic bandage wrapped from the base of the toes to just below the knee, or a good elastic stocking with pressures between 30 and 40 mmHg, is recommended (11). Elastic bandages or stockings should be applied before the patient gets up from bed and must be worn the entire day. If possible, there should be two periods of rest of at least 30 minutes each. These periods of rest contribute to eliminate the edema accumulated from morning to the time that the patient lies down. Elastic stockings should be fitted to the individual leg. They are usually easy to apply and more comfortable than the elastic bandages. They are highly recommended for most patients with uncomplicated varicose veins and for those with varicose veins during pregnancy and in the late postoperative period. For patients whose work requires long periods of standing, elastic stockings are often a necessity. At present, there are available very satisfactory light and heavy elastic stockings that are both effective and attractive.

Nonelastic compression systems are available in the form of low stretch elastic bandages, Unna boot and CircAid. The best indication for a Unna boot is the patient who has a physical impairment that prevents him/her from bandaging the limb, such as individuals with rheumatoid arthritis, senility, obesity, etc. Unna boots should never be applied in patients with borderline arterial circulation. CircAid consists of a series of custom-made Velcro bands that have a minimum life of 18 months and produce an unyielding compression that has the advantage of being adjustable to the volume changes of the patient's extremity and can also be removed at any time to monitor the course of the condition.

SCLEROTHERAPY

Sclerotherapy is a nonsurgical method of treating varicose veins that has definite indications. The use of sclerotherapy has been the center of controversy from two groups of advocates. On one side are physicians who use the method as a sole form of treatment of varicose veins of all sizes and etiology. In regard to this group, Dodd states "the worst aspects of injection therapy are seen when 'varicose vein cases' are herded into 'injection clinics,' often seen by junior or even temporary staff or by part-time practitioners; injections are given to all who attend, and there is little attempt at real diagnosis and minimal follow-up, and the science of management of venous disorders falls to a low ebb in such circumstances" (12). In an effort to elucidate the real place of sclerotherapy and surgery in the management of venous insufficiency, Hobbs carried out a random trial of treatment of varicose veins by surgery and sclerotherapy at St. Mary's Hospital in London (13). He treated 404 legs by injections and 275 legs by surgery. The patients had follow-up studies during a 6-year period. At the end of the sixth year, fewer than 10% of the injected legs were cured; of the patients treated by surgery, 84% had been without recurrences. Fegan in Ireland (14) and Sigg in Switzerland (15) have been the strongest advocates of total sclerotherapy. Sigg used this method exclusively in the treatment of all kinds and sizes of varicose veins in more than 500,000 instances. The indications, contraindications, techniques, and types of sclerosing agents have been thoroughly described in Chapter 14. Intermittent sequential pneumatic compression has been utilized in certain cases of severe chronic venous insufficiency with skin changes or accompanied by an important lymphatic component. There are reports of enhancement of ulcer healing and, in our experience, this form of therapy has been effective in controlling the lymphatic component of chronic venous insufficiency (16, 17).

OPERATIVE MANAGEMENT

Keller in 1905 (18) removed the internal saphenous vein by passing a wire loop through the vein and attaching a ligature to the end. Mayo in 1906 (19) and Babcock (20) used vein strippers to excise the varicose saphenous vein. Because of the considerable postoperative morbidity and mortality rates from sepsis and thromboembolism, this form of treatment was abandoned 20 years later and replaced by sclerotherapy. It soon became apparent, however, that this form of therapy was accompanied by a high incidence of recurrence. Sclerotherapy was then combined with high ligation of the saphenofemoral junction and retrograde injection of a sclerosing agent at the time of surgery (21–23).

Sclerotherapy as a single form of treatment, or in combination with high ligation of the saphenofemoral junction, was not the answer to the problem. There was a high incidence of recurrences (24). With the introduction of antibiotics and improved surgical instrumentation, saphenous vein stripping regained popularity in the 1950s. An extensive operation, involving long and short saphenous stripping and complete excision of all varicose vein clusters, was popularized by T.T. Myers and the Lofgren brothers from the Mayo Clinic (25). The Mayo Clinic procedure became the standard method of treatment for most forms of varicose veins of the extremities and has been performed in many thousands of patients during the last four decades. During the last two decades, there has been a steady and significant increase in our knowledge of venous diseases. A great deal of the progress has been the result of a technological revolution that has allowed us to examine and understand the venous system and its pathophysiology in a much better way than previously. To a great extent, these advances have been responsible for the renewed interest in venous diseases. The introduction of air plethysmography, bidirectional Doppler ultrasound, and real-time, B-ultrasound imaging system with pulsed Doppler detector provided us, for the first time, with the necessary tools to study the physiology and anatomy of the venous system in the living patient. We are now able to observe the fascinating movements of a venous valve and its relationship with the respiratory cycle. The use of the noninvasive diagnostic methods to study the vascular system has provided us with reliable means of assessing reflux or obstruction of the deep and superficial venous systems. The judicious use of varicography, ascending and descending phlebography under direct fluoroscopic control, and often by video angioscopy has given us the ability to establish a precise diagnosis of the site of incompetence in the venous system and plan a rational surgical approach. We have learned that it is possible to preserve valuable venous segments which in the past were routinely excised.

Success in the management of patients with chronic venous insufficiency and varicose veins depends on establishing with accuracy the etiology of the varicose veins. We have recognized the following types of varicose veins: (a) primary or familial; (b) secondary or postphlebitic; (c) varicosities associated with congenital venous malformations without detectable arteriovenous fistulas; and (d) varicose veins associated with arteriovenous fistulas, either traumatic or congenital. Telangiectases, or spider veins, are cutaneous blemishes with a striking familial tendency that usually do not require surgical treatment.

Primary, familial, and essential are all terms used to describe a form of varicosities that appear early in life, sometimes during childhood and more often during pregnancy, and that usually involves one or more members of a family (Fig. 25.1). Secondary, postthrombotic or acquired varicose veins are the late sequelae of an episode of deep venous thrombosis. The clinical manifestations of the syndrome depend on the extent and location of the original thrombus and the damage to the valvular mechanism of the venous system. The Klippel-Trenaunay syndrome is a congenital malformation with large varicose veins, hypertrophy of the limb, and a portwine malformation usually located over the lateral aspect of the extremity. There are no detectable arteriovenous fistulas, and for this reason this type of patient should not be confused with the Parkes-Weber syndrome in which congenital arteriovenous communications are present.

Acquired, traumatic, or iatrogenic arteriovenous (AV) fistulas are the source of large venous dilatations in the vicinity of the arteriovenous communication. The hemodynamic effects on the circulatory system depend to a great extent on the location, size, and duration of the AV fistula.

Venous spiders, venous stars, and telangiectasia are skin blemishes that appear mostly in women and were described by Osler as "a collection of small veins converging upon a central bright nodule projecting a little beyond the skin." They appear especially on the medial, posterior, and lateral aspects of the thigh, and

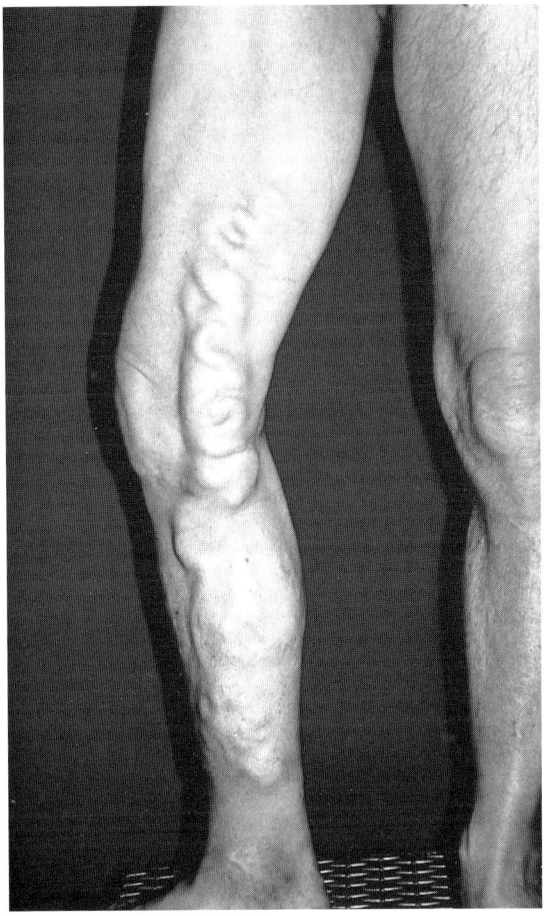

FIG. 25–1. Typical patient with primary, familial, or essential varicose veins. Large venous dilatations are observed along the territory of the greater saphenous vein. In this patient, there was overt insufficiency of the main trunk of the saphenous vein, incompetent Hunterian perforator, and striking absence of skin changes.

less often in the lower leg and calf (Fig. 25.2). Bean described the morphologic aspect of these lesions as "the star shape is over idealized, since linear, angular and polymorphous ones or those arranged like a cascade, flare, rocket or a tangle, may embellish an otherwise undecorated leg."

Each of the clinical types of varicose veins described has a different origin and a specific type of treatment. It stands to reason that many failures of surgical management result from performing the wrong type of surgical procedure for the particular etiology of the varicosities.

IMPORTANCE OF A THOROUGH ANATOMIC KNOWLEDGE

One of the most important causes of failure in the management of varicose veins is the lack of knowledge of the anatomy and pathophysiology of the venous system. We have been impressed by the lack of interest and understanding of the venous pathology that exists in our vascular fellowships and general surgery training programs. The new generations of vascular surgeons are being

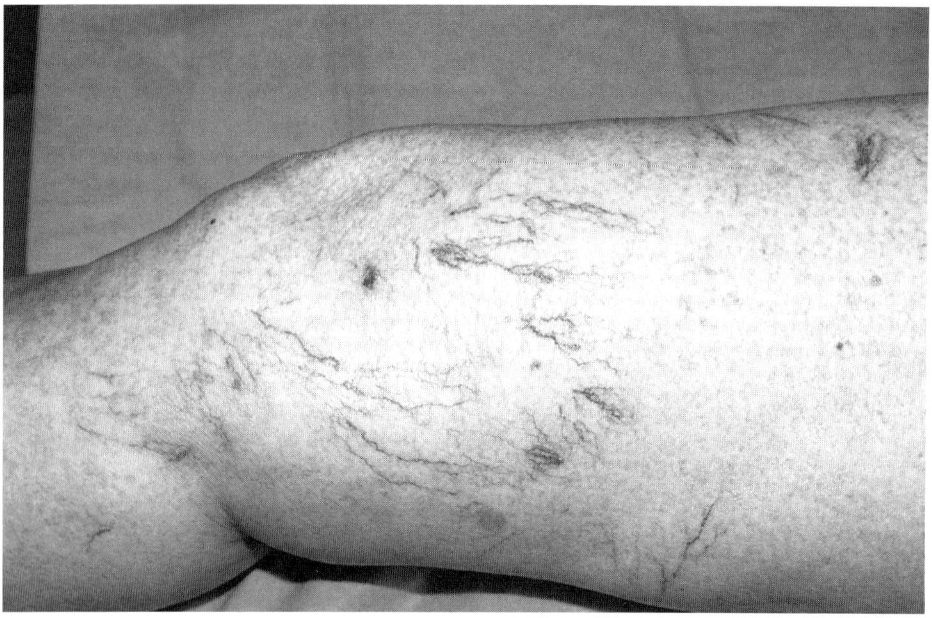

FIG. 25–2. "Venous spiders," venous stars, or telangiectasia are skin blemishes that appear mostly in women and have a striking familial tendency. Sclerotherapy is particularly effective in the treatment of this type of varicosity.

trained essentially as "arterial surgeons." The consequence is a benign neglect of the venous and lymphatic pathology, which comprises diseases that are difficult to understand and whose surgical management is often belittled because it is not as profitable or glamorous as an arterial operation. As a result, we are graduating vascular surgeons who have a gap in their training program representing as much as two-thirds of the vascular pathology. In an effort to expand the knowledge of our surgical trainees in the field of venous diseases, venous and lymphatic teaching clinics have been established at two of the major teaching hospitals of our medical school (Walter Reed Army Medical Center and National Naval Medical Center).

In the human cadaver studies performed at the Anatomy Department of the Uniformed Services University of the Health Sciences, we have recognized the three classic groups of veins of the lower extremity, and have added a fourth group which includes the gonadal and iliac venous systems. The three classic groups are: (a) the superficial system, which comprises the long and short saphenous veins and their tributaries; (b) the deep venous system, which consists of veins that lie under the muscular fascia; and (c) the communicating system, which connects the superficial and deep systems. The anatomy and pathology of the "perforating system," as it is known, have received a great deal of attention as a result of the anatomic studies of Cockett (26) and May (27). The system of the iliac pelvic veins, either alone or in combination with gonadal insufficiency, produces vulvar and gluteal varices that extend to the posteromedial aspect of the thigh and may be responsible for a distinct type of nonsaphenous varicosities that may reach a large size (Fig. 25.3). This system is responsible for the pelvic congestion syndrome which is associated with vulvar varices in some women. The clinical and phlebographic observations on a patient with vulvar varices led us to study the valvular system of the iliac venous system in 72 human cadaver specimens. The presence of valves was demonstrated in the main trunk of the internal iliac vein in 10% of the cases and in 9.8% of the tributaries dissected. The investigations of Eger and Casper (28) on the valves of the iliofemoral segment showed that nearly 40% of the world population have the potential to develop varicose veins in the area of the long saphenous vein. They examined the valves of the external iliac and common femoral veins in 38 cadavers. No vein contained more than one valve. This means that only one valve typically protects the saphenous vein against the high intra-abdominal pressure developed during the many phases of our daily activities. The valve was absent bilaterally in nearly 8% of the cases and unilaterally in about 29%. Since the inferior vena cava and common iliac vein rarely have valves, individuals with this variation are exposed to the high intra-abdominal pressures exerted directly on the saphenofemoral junction. Patients with a family history of varicose veins and weakness of the vein walls have a high possibility of developing varicose veins.

The following anatomic information is relevant in the surgical management of varicose veins: (a) the greater saphenous vein in the thigh is duplicated in 35% of the cases (29). This important information became evident during the phlebographic studies carried out by Leather's group in Albany, New York, to investigate the saphenous vein as an arterial substitute for in situ bypass. (b) During a study performed by our group on human cadavers at the Uniformed Services

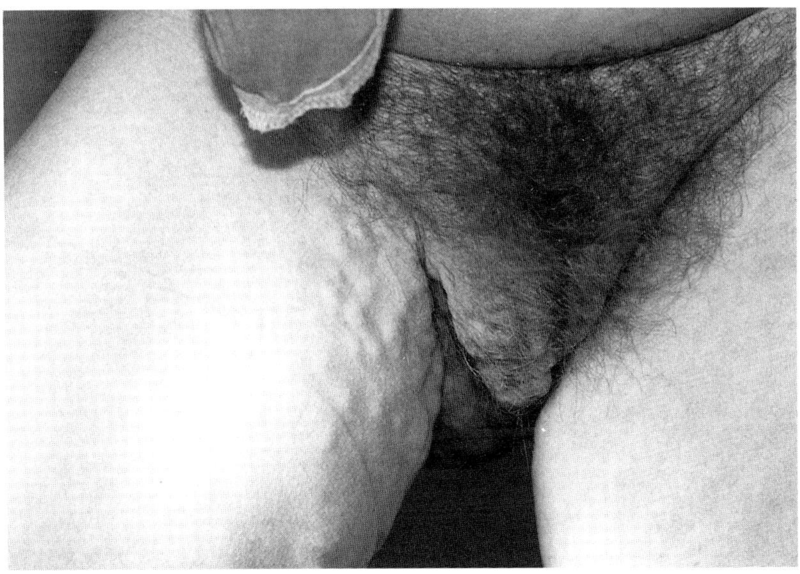

FIG. 25–3. Grotesque varicosities of the labia majora and medial aspect of the thigh. There was massive pelvic reflux secondary to gonadal and internal iliac venous insufficiency by duplex scanning. The saphenous trunk was competent.

University of the Health Sciences, we found a duplicated femoral system in 20% of the specimens. The duplicated segment often was valved. The duplicated femoral vein may be used as an arterial or venous substitute. (c) The lower limb has 150 perforators of different sizes (27), the majority of which are in the calf. Only a few are of clinical significance and they do not connect with the main trunk of the saphenous vein, but with the posterior arch veins (Fig. 25.4). The existence

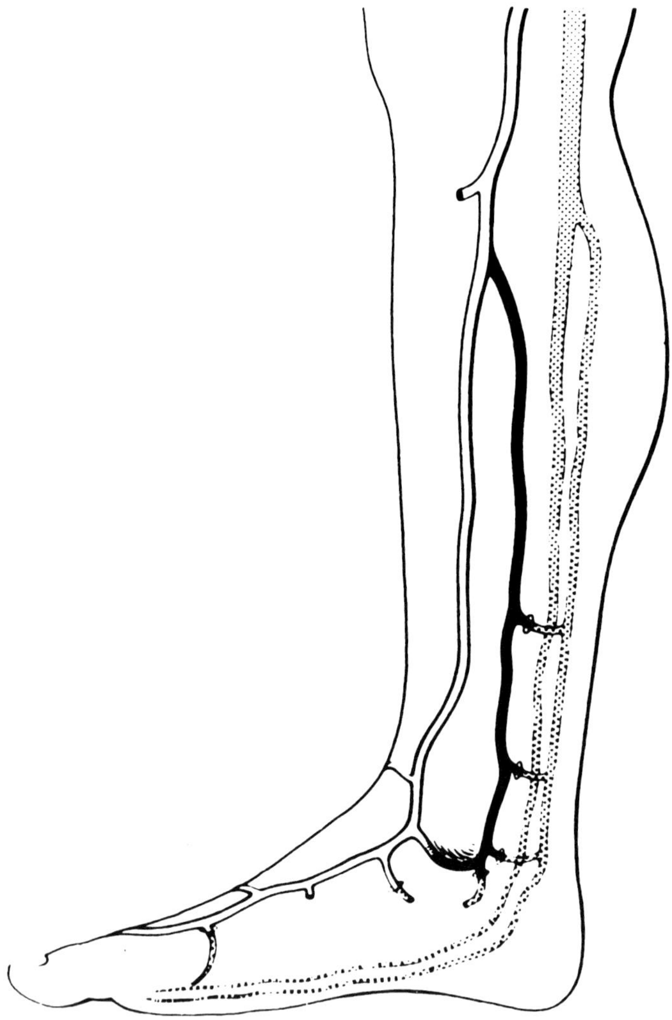

FIG. 25–4. Perforators of the distal third of the leg communicate the deep system with the posterior arch tributary of the greater saphenous vein. Stripping of the saphenous trunk at this level is of little benefit in the treatment of perforator incompetence. This is one of the reasons why modern stripping techniques recommend stripping from groin to just below the knee. Sparing injury to the saphenous nerve is another good reason to use this technique. (Reproduced by permission from May R, Partsch H, Staubesan D. Perforating veins. Baltimore: Urban & Schwarzenburg, 1981:9.)

of a large number of perforators may explain the recurrence of varicose veins and/or venous ulcers after an apparently successful perforator ligation. If the deep system is incompetent, it is a matter of time until a recurrence appears. This anatomic information reveals the importance of performing a complete duplex examination of both venous systems in all patients with chronic venous insufficiency. The anatomic localization of the leg perforators has become essential in the developing field of endoscopic perforator ligation.

NEW TRENDS AND OPERATIVE TECHNIQUES IN THE MANAGEMENT OF VARICOSE VEINS

Save the Saphenous vs. Stripping to Below Knee vs. Selective Stripping

The advances in noninvasive diagnostic vascular technology have allowed us to study with accuracy the anatomy and pathophysiology of the venous system. With the use of the bidirectional Doppler, color-flow duplex scanner, and air plethysmography, we can investigate the venous pathology in a very precise manner and plan the appropriate treatment. As a result of these technological advances, we have learned that the main trunk of the saphenous vein may be quite healthy despite the presence of large clusters of varicose veins in one or more of its tributaries. Sparing a healthy saphenous trunk has become of importance for two main reasons: the first reason is that it makes no sense to excise a healthy organ that is performing its assigned function in a satisfactory manner (30). The second reason is that the saphenous vein is the most important autogenous conduit utilized as bypass, patch, or substitute in the arterial system.

Despite these reasons, surgery for primary varicose veins with preservation of the saphenous trunk is controversial. There are several published reports that support sparing the saphenous vein. Large (30) studied 202 patients in whom he performed stab avulsion and proximal ligation only in cases of saphenofemoral incompetence (51.5%). There was a 10.5% recurrence rate at 3 years. Hanrahan, et al. (31), performed duplex examination of 54 lower extremities with varicose veins. Seventy-two percent of these patients manifested branch incompetence alone. The relationship of incompetence of the saphenofemoral junction to the presence of superficial varices was inconsistent. Deep venous incompetence was present in 41% of the extremities. These data support the position that the preoperative assessment of reflux in vein segments is more appropriate than routine stripping of the main trunk or ligation of the saphenofemoral junction. Koyano and Sakaguchi (32) studied 337 legs of 208 patients using Doppler and calf compression-release. They found that 66% of these patients had incompetence of the long saphenous vein. They were able to demonstrate reflux in segments of the saphenous vein. Based on Doppler findings, they performed selective stripping in 80 limbs in which only the segments with venous reverse flow were selectively removed. Their follow-up studies showed that selective stripping operations were as satisfactory as those in which the standard stripping operation was carried out (189 limbs). Additionally, the incidence of saphenous neuritis was 4.8% in patients with selective stripping versus 27% in patients submitted to full stripping.

Other studies have challenged the preservation of the saphenous vein. Munn, et al. (33), reported that routine greater saphenous vein stripping had a lower incidence of recurrent varicosities (18%) than was seen in patients in whom the saphenous vein was preserved (29% recurrence). Of interest, however, was the finding that the patients were more satisfied with the results of the leg that was not stripped. This was the result of a high incidence of nerve injuries in the legs which had full stripping.

Sutton and Darke (34) performed perioperative retrograde saphenography to study 80 incompetent long saphenous veins in 60 patients with primary varicose veins. They found that there were varicose changes in 65% of the greater saphenous veins and stated that the incompetent vein did not appear to be a suitable arterial replacement. They concluded that insufficiency of the saphenous valves may contribute to the development of venous ulceration. In these studies, Hunterian perforators of variable size were seen on 70 saphenograms (87%) and these investigators concluded that stripping of the incompetent greater saphenous vein would certainly disconnect such perforators and reduce the incidence of both recurrent varicose veins and persistent ulceration. The diagnosis of saphenous incompetence was performed with Doppler and Valsalva maneuver and confirmed by intraoperative phlebography.

MacFarlane, et al. (35), performed phlebography in 35 extremities that were going to be operated on for varicose veins. They demonstrated that the segment of saphenous vein below the knee does not undergo varicose dilatation. In 7 of 9 patients examined postoperatively, the segment remained patent after the vein above had been stripped. Additionally, 75% of the greater saphenous veins above the knee were not dilated or tortuous. These authors concluded that varicose veins resulting from saphenofemoral incompetence can be treated surgically by stripping the long saphenous vein only to the knee and yet still leave a nonvaricose segment for possible future utilization. In 75% of their cases, the greater saphenous vein above the knee was incompetent, but not grossly dilated or tortuous. In the remaining 25%, the above knee portion was severely diseased and would have been unsuitable for any form of bypass grafting.

McMullin, et al. (36), studied 54 limbs with duplex scanning before high ligation and multiple avulsion of primary varicose veins. Duplex scanning confirmed saphenofemoral incompetence and excluded short saphenous incompetence. Of interest is that in 24 of the 52 limbs in which the junction had been ligated, there was persistent reflux down the long saphenous vein. In only two limbs was this reflux attributable to mid-thigh perforating veins. Photoplethysmography was performed before and after surgery and the venous refilling time measured. Using this method to evaluate results, the authors concluded that high ligation without stripping fails to control significant reflux within the long saphenous vein in a high proportion of cases. However, van Bemmelen and Strandness (37, 38), by applying graded pressure in a cuff placed proximal to the valve segment investigated, have shown that a velocity exceeding 30 cm/sec is necessary to prompt the normal valve to close. With velocities lower than this, the valves will not regularly close and reflux can persist, giving a false impression of the status of the valves in question. After ligation of the saphenofemoral junction, there is not enough pressure or sufficient blood velocity to close the valves below the junction. For this reason, trunk reflux may be detected by color duplex scanning after compression-release at the calf.

At our institution, patients who are going to be submitted to varicose vein surgery for primary venous insufficiency have examination of their saphenous system by duplex scanning in the upright position before surgery. The saphenous diameter is measured at the femoral junction, and upper, middle, and distal thirds of the thigh. Depending on the height and weight of the individual, saphenous veins which are found dilated, tortuous, and irregular, and which demonstrate reflux, are routinely stripped from groin to just below the knee (Fig. 25.1). However, a saphenous vein trunk of normal size, which tapers down uniformly without tortuosity or aneurysmal dilatations, is preserved.

Even though there is evidence in the literature and in our clinical experience that the saphenous vein can be spared in those cases of patients with varicose veins in whom the saphenous trunk is found to be healthy, the definitive answer to the controversy of stripping the saphenous trunk or preserving it in a selective manner must await prospective randomized studies using duplex scanning and air plethysmography to evaluate long-term results. The diameter of the vein at different levels and the soundness of the trunk are considered in the randomization to strip or to preserve.

Another method of achieving competence of the saphenofemoral junction in patients with varicose veins has been the application of venous cuffs at the first centimeter of the saphenofemoral junction. The cuff is tightened until competence is achieved. The cuffs are made of dacron or other prosthetic materials. Again, long-term results in a sizable sample of patients with hemodynamic information are lacking. Besides, the insertion of prosthetic material in young individuals, which form the majority of patients with primary varicose veins, is costly and, in our opinion, not justifiable.

Varicose Vein Surgery in a Bloodless Field

During the last three decades, we have learned to appreciate the benefits of a bloodless field as practiced by the orthopaedic and plastic surgeons. In vascular surgery, the pneumatic tourniquet has been utilized to avoid clamping calcified vessels during the performance of distal anastomosis in bypass surgery. We have used the pneumatic tourniquet extensively during the resection of hemangiomas and other vascular malformations in patients with congenital vascular anomalies. More recently, the pneumatic tourniquet has been utilized to render a bloodless field during the endoscopic subfascial ligation of perforators. At our institution, we have used the pneumatic tourniquet in patients with extensive and grossly dilated varicose veins. In the past, patients with extensive varicose veins occupied several hours of our operating time. The introduction of the tourniquet has dramatically reduced the operating time and has allowed us to perform a complete removal of all varicosities without blood loss. The technique consists of exposure of the saphenofemoral junction before applying the tourniquet. After division of the saphenous vein, in those cases in which stripping is to be performed, a flexible stripper is introduced through a small incision below the knee and retrieved at the groin. The vein is prepared for invaginated stripping, the wound is closed in layers and a pneumatic tourniquet is applied at the upper thigh after wrapping the leg with an Esmarch rubber bandage (Fig. 25.5). The tourniquet is inflated at 300 mmHg and the operation can then be performed in

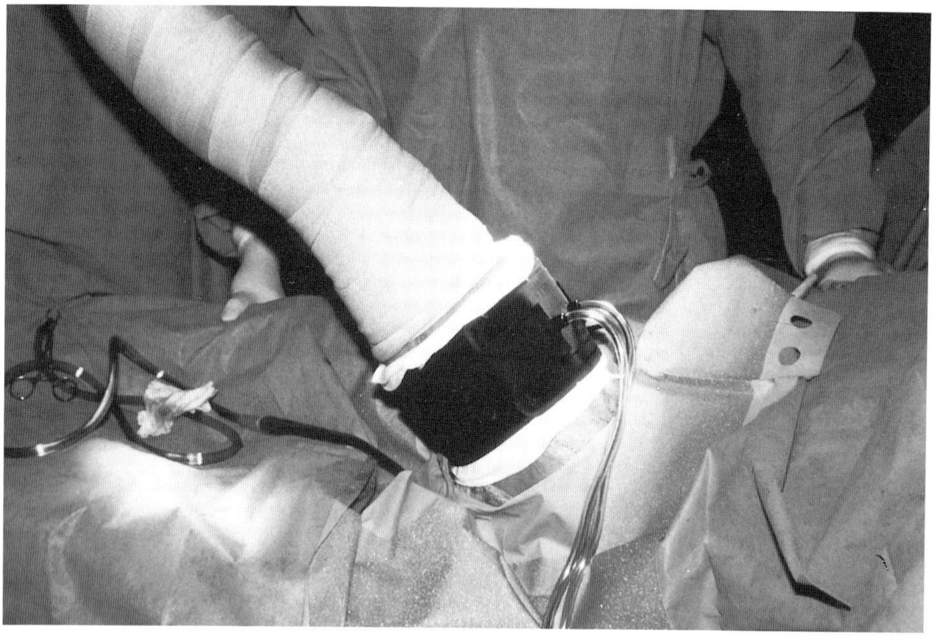

FIG. 25–5. Surgery of extensive varicose vein disease can be performed safely and expeditiously with the use of a pneumatic tourniquet. An Esmarch rubberized bandage is applied from toes to groin and a pneumatic tourniquet inflated at the pressure of 300 mmHg. The average operating time is 55 minutes (range: 45–80 minutes). When stripping is indicated, the procedure is carried out with the tourniquet inflated. The stripper slides easily under the tourniquet. These procedures are now performed on an outpatient basis.

a bloodless field. In 55 patients with extensive varicose veins, the average operating time has been 55 minutes (range: 45–80 minutes). When necessary, stripping is performed with the tourniquet inflated. The vein stripper slides easily under the tourniquet (Fig. 25.6). The wounds are usually closed with steri strips, the extremity is carefully padded and a compression bandage applied. The patient remains in the hospital for a few hours and goes home during the late afternoon.

Ambulatory Venous Surgery

Ambulatory venous surgery has been practiced for many years. In 1930, De Takats (21) published his experiences with this technique. Nabatoff (39), in 1972, described his method of complete stripping of the varicose veins as an outpatient procedure. The competition for hospital beds, the long waiting lists for varicose vein surgery and financial considerations have stimulated surgeons to seek options to operate as many cases as possible without compromising the hospital capacity. There are numerous reports in the literature dealing with this subject (40–44). In a recent publication, Baccaglini, et al. (45), conducted a multicenter trial in 2568 extremities with varicose veins. Different anesthesia techniques were utilized (local, spinal, general, and local plus sedation). Postoperative hospitalization was required in only two cases. Postoperative complications included headache after spinal anesthesia and residual paraesthesia after femoral nerve block. The consensus of surgeons participating in this protocol confirms that surgery of varicose veins can be carried out on an outpatient basis with similar complications as observed in hospitalized patients. The authors conclude that outpatient surgery is cost-effective and diminishes the demand for hospital beds, while assuring that the quality of patient care is maintained.

Crochet-hook Vein Excision

In 1957, Thomas T. Myers, of the Mayo Clinic, reported that extensive removal of all varicosities, followed by ligation and stripping of the greater and lesser saphenous veins, was accompanied by 85% good-to-excellent results at 10 years. Since then, many thousands of patients throughout the world have been submitted to this procedure. The extensive scarring of the operation and the length and tediousness of the procedure have prompted the surgical community to seek new avenues of treatment for varicose veins. In 1975, Rivlin (46) reported the use of mini-incisions and fine pointed forceps for the extraction of the varicose tributaries of the saphenous vein. Since then, the method of stab avulsion through

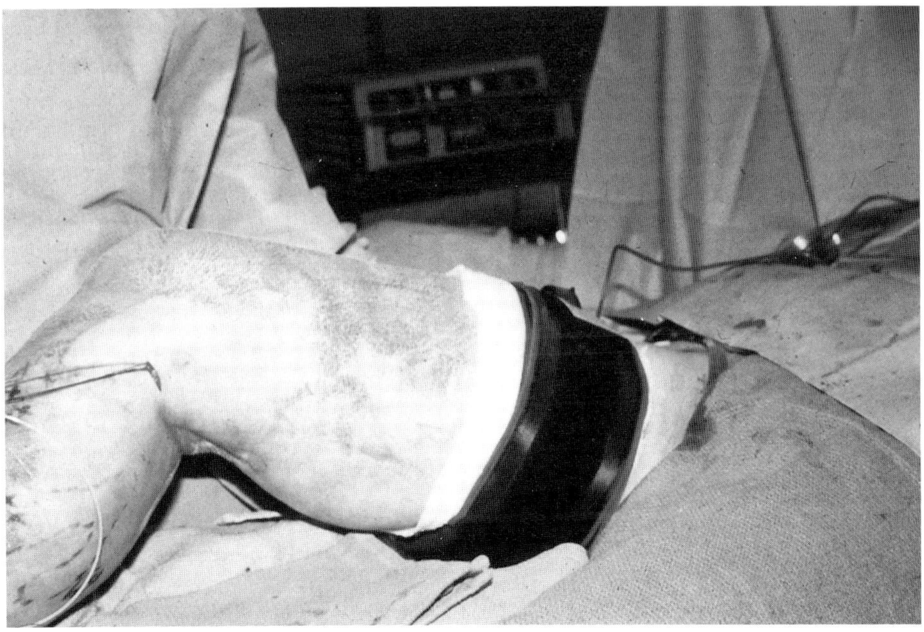

FIG. 25–6. Stripping from groin to just below the knee in a bloodless field. In this patient, the saphenofemoral junction has been dissected, the saphenous trunk and its tributaries have been divided, and the stripper passed through a small incision just below the knee to the groin. The stripping procedure, when necessary, is carried out at the end of the operation.

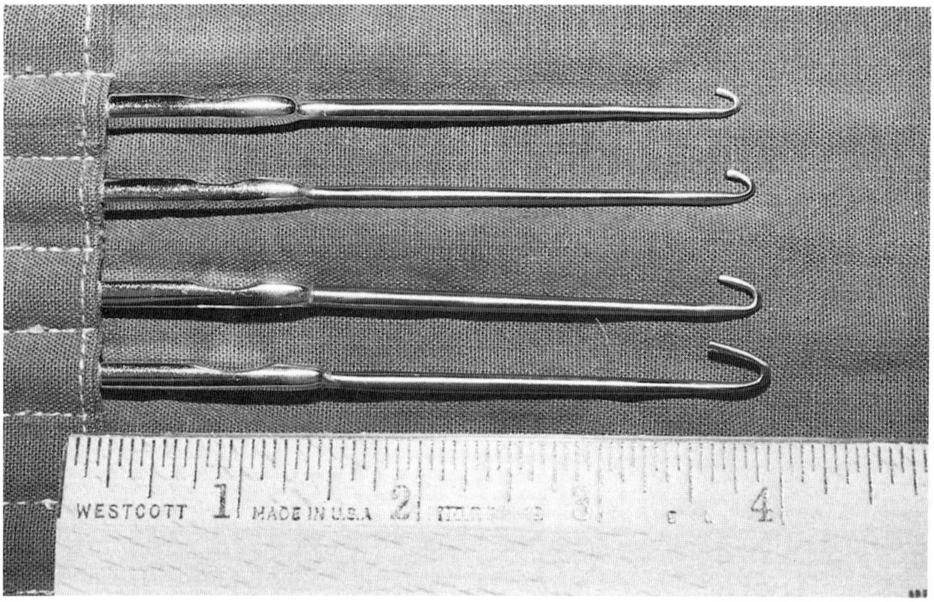

FIG. 25–7. Set of vein hooks designed by Dr. Villavicencio. Through a 2–3-mm stab incision with a number 11 blade, the vein hook is introduced under the vein and, with a pull-back maneuver, the varicosity is pulled out through the skin incision. Large segments of varicose veins can be removed through multiple mini-incisions which heal extremely well.

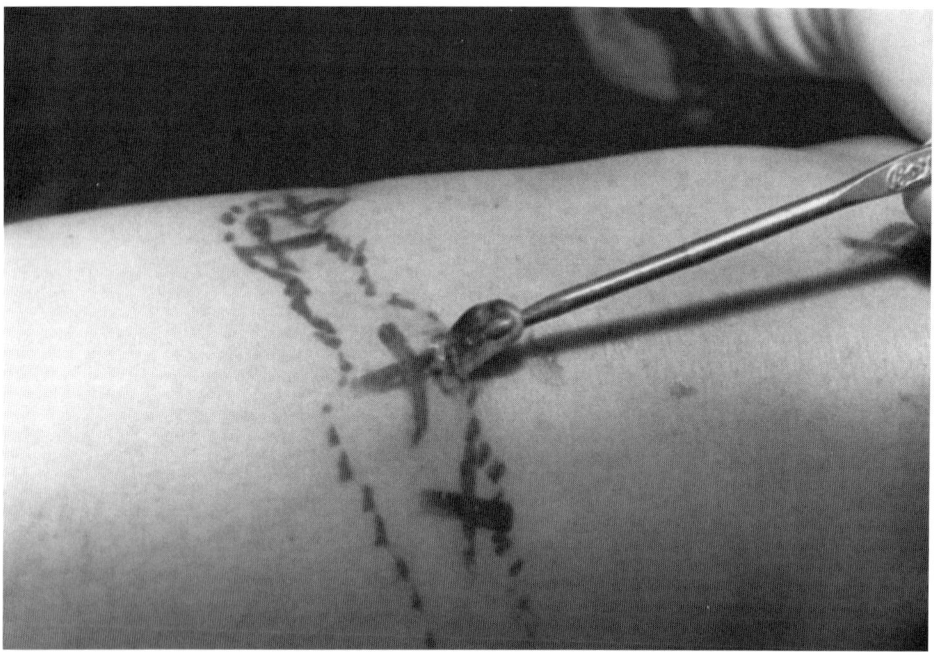

FIG. 25–8. A small 2–3-mm incision has been made parallel to a previously marked vein. The vein hook has successfully captured the vein loop which is pulled out gently through the skin. A mosquito forceps is applied at each limb of the loop which is divided. The operation is repeated at intervals of 1–2 inches until the entire varicose segment has been excised.

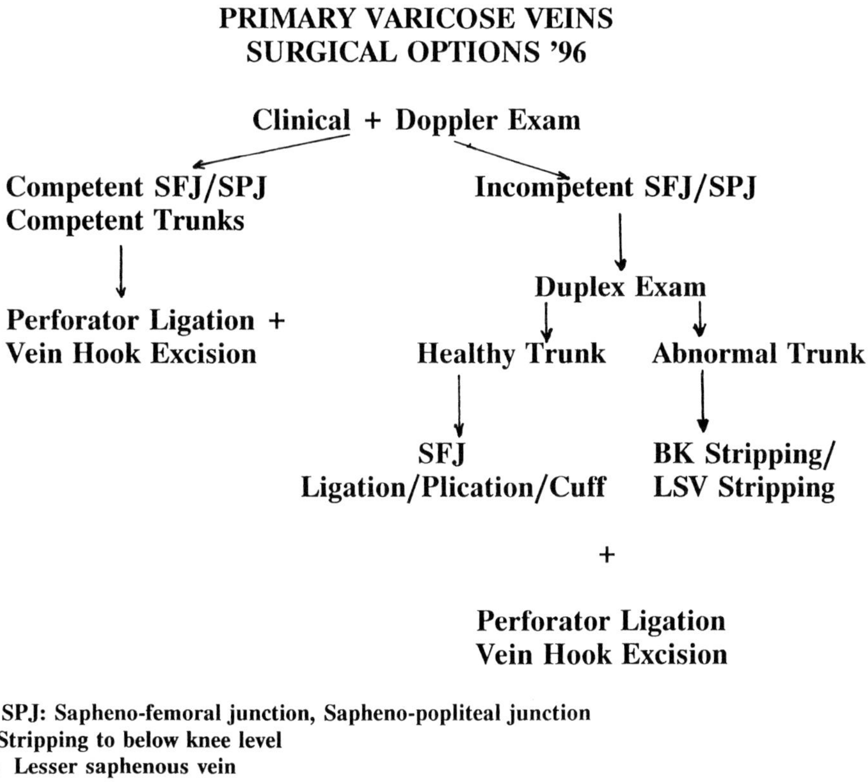

FIG. 25–9. Algorithm depicting the modern policy for the management of primary varicose veins based on the principle of selective venous surgery. The saphenous vein is examined with duplex color-flow, its diameter measured at different levels of the thigh, and its anatomic configuration recorded. Healthy saphenous trunks are preserved. Abnormal, varicose, dilated saphenous trunks are stripped from groin to just below the knee. Other alternatives of management are analyzed in the algorithm.

mini-incisions has been extensively practiced throughout the world. Special hooks have been developed by Müller (40, 41), Oesch (42), Varady (47), and Villavicencio (48). The technique of stab avulsion phlebectomy has been used extensively over the last 20 years by Villavicencio. A set of specially designed hooks has been routinely utilized in every case of varicose vein surgery during the last 13 years.

Technique. With the patient in the upright position and the extremity shaved, the varicose veins are marked with indelible ink. The operating surgeon should mark the patient. The extremity is placed in the Trendelenburg position, and the crochet hook phlebectomy is performed through 2–3 mm incisions done with a number 11 scalpel blade. Incisions must be made parallel to the axis of the vein to prevent piercing it. The hook is introduced with its flat side under the vein. Once the tip of the hook has passed on the other side of the vein, it is rotated so its tip is pointing toward the skin. At this point, it is pulled back, lifting the hooked vein while counterpressure is applied over the skin. The loop of vein is exteriorized by pulling gently (Fig. 25.7). The maneuver is repeated through several incisions placed along the course of the vein until the complete venous segment has been excised. Incisions are placed approximately 1–2 inches apart, and at the end of the procedure are closed with steri-strips. Compression pads are placed over the wound and the extremity is wrapped with a thick roll of gauze and a firm elastic bandage. The small incisions heal uneventfully and are practically invisible after several months (Fig. 25.8).

In summary, great advances have occurred in the management of venous disorders. The surgical management of varicose veins is more objective and based on sound hemodynamic and anatomic principles. However, the most important aspect of this progress is its continuous evolution. Research protocols are in progress to solve some of the most important problems in the management of these diseases. This is an exciting time in which technological advances have provided the necessary tools for sound investigation. In the algorithm illustrated in Figure 25.9, are represented the modern surgical options for the management of primary varicose veins. The surgical procedures should be planned depending on the findings of the clinical and noninvasive vascular diagnostic tests. The algorithm represents the principle of selective venous surgery and the policy for the management of varicose veins currently in use at our institutions.

REFERENCES

1. Widmer LK, Mall TH, Martin H. Epidemiology and social medical importance of peripheral venous disease. In: Hobbs JP, ed. The treatment of venous disorders. Philadelphia: JB Lippincott, 1977:33.
2. Borschburg E. The prevalence of varicose veins in the lower extremities. Basel: Karger, 1967:22.
3. Wright FPJ, Moffat CJ, Stirling J, et al. Prevalence of venous disease: a community study in West London. Eur J Surg 1992:158:143–147.
4. Coon WW, Park W, Kellerer JR. Venous thromboembolism and other venous disease in the Tecumseh community health study. Circulation 1973;48:839–846.
5. Beninson J, Jobst CB. The support of the venous circulation. Angiology 1982;33:442.
6. Filatov VN, Bogachev VN. Methods of determining pressure on tissues from elastic stockings used for the prevention and treatment of chronic venous diseases of the lower limbs. Polim Med 1981;11:95.
7. Bjordal RI. Circulation patterns in incompetent perforating veins of the calf in venous dysfunction. In: May R, Partsch H, Staubesan D, eds. Perforating veins. Munich: Urban & Schwarzenberg, 1981:71–88.
8. Hargens AR. Interstitial fluid pressure in muscle and compartment syndromes in man. Microvasc Res 1976;14:1.
9. Taheri SA, Yacobucci GN, Williams J, Elias S. Deep posterior compartment pressure in the evaluation of venous insufficiency of the lower extremity: a preliminary report. Angiology 1984:35;173.
10. Jones NAG, Webb PJ, Rees RI, cited in Negus D. Claims about compression treatment of venous disease [Letter]. Br Med J (Clin Res) 1982;285:439.
11. Stemmer R. The choice of compressive stockings. Phlebology 1982;35:107.
12. Dodd H, Cockett FB. Pathology and surgery of the veins of the lower limb. 2d ed. Edinburgh: Churchill Livingston, 1976:106.
13. Hobbs JT. The management of varicose veins. Surg Ann 1980;12:169.

14. Fegan WG. Treatment of varicose veins by injection compression: a method practiced in Eire. In: Hobbs JT, ed. The treatment of venous disorders. Philadelphia: JB Lippincott, 1977:99.
15. Sigg K. Treatment of varicose veins by injection sclerotherapy: a method practiced in Switzerland. In: Hobbs JT, ed. The treatment of venous disorders. Philadelphia: JB Lippincott, 1977:113.
16. Belcaro V, Coen F. Pneumatic intermittent compression treatment of venous ulcerations caused by venous hypertension. In: Negus D, Jantet G, eds. Phlebology '85. London: Libbey, 1986:640–642.
17. Pappas CJ, O'Donnell TF Jr. Long-term results of compression treatment for lymphedema. J Vasc Surg 1992;16:555–564.
18. Keller WL. A new method of extirpating the internal saphenous vein and similar veins in varicose conditions: a preliminary report. NY Med J 1905;82:385.
19. Mayo HC. Treatment of varicose veins. Surg Gynec Obstet 1906;2:385.
20. Babcock WW. A new operation for the extirpation of varicose veins of the leg. NY Med J 1907;86:153.
21. De Takats G. Ambulatory ligation of the saphenous vein. JAMA 1930;94:1194.
22. De Takats G, Quillin L. Ligation of the saphenous vein. A report on 200 ambulatory operations. Arch Surg 1933;26:72–88.
23. De Takats G, Quint H. The injection treatment of varicose veins. Surg Gynec Obstet 1930;50:545.
24. McPheeters HO, Anderson JK. The injection treatment of varicose veins. 2d ed. Philadelphia: FA Davis, 1939:130–139; 164–173.
25. Lofgren EE. Treatment of long saphenous varicosities and their recurrence: a long-term follow-up. In: Bergan JJ, Yao JST, eds. Surgery of the veins. Orlando, FL: Grune & Stratton, 1985:285–299.
26. Cockett BF. The pathology and treatment of venous ulcers of the leg. Br J Surg 1955;43:260–278.
27. Schäfer K. The course, structure and passage through the fascia of the perforating veins. In: May R, Partsch H, Staubesan D. Eds. Perforating veins. Munich, Baltimore: Urban & Schwarzenberg 1981, p. 38.
28. Eger SA, Casper SL. Etiology of varicose veins from an anatomical aspect, based on the dissection of 38 adult cadavers. JAMA 1943;123:148–149.
29. Shah DM, Chang BB, Leopold PW, Corson JD, Leather RP, Karmody AM. The anatomy of the greater saphenous vein. J Vasc Surg 1986;3:273–283.
30. Large J. Surgical treatment of saphenous varices with preservation of the main great saphenous trunk. J Vasc Surg 1985;2:886–891.
31. Hanrahan LM, Keshesian GJ, Menzoian JO, et al. Patterns of venous insufficiency in patients with varicose veins. Arch Surg 1991;126:687–691.
32. Koyano K, Sakaguchi S. Selective stripping operation based on Doppler ultrasonic findings for primary varicose veins of the lower extremities. Surgery 1988;103:615–619.
33. Munn SR, Martin JB, MacBeth WAAG. To strip or not to strip the long saphenous vein? Br J Surg 1981;68:426–428.
34. Sutton H, Darke S. Stripping the long saphenous vein: pre-operative retrograde saphenography in patients with and without venous ulceration. Br J Surg 1986;73:305–307.
35. MacFarlane R, Godwin RJ, Barabos AP. Are varicose veins and coronary artery bypass surgery compatible? Lancet 1985;2:859.
36. McMullin GM, Coleridge-Smith PD, Scurr JH. Objective assessment of high ligation without stripping the long saphenous vein. Br J Surg 1991;78:1139–1142.
37. van Bemmelen PS, Bedford G, Beach K, Strandness DE. Quantitative segmental evaluation of venous valvular reflux with duplex ultrasound scanning. J Vasc Surg 1989;10:425–431.

38. van Bemmelen PS, Bedord G, Beach K, Strandness DE. Status of the valves in the superficial and deep venous system in chronic venous disease. Surgery 1991;109:730–734.
39. Nabatoff RA, Starck DCC. Complete stripping of varicose veins with the patient on an ambulatory basis. Am J Surg 1972;124:634–636.
40. Müller R. Traitment des varices par la phlebectomie ambulatoire. Bull Soc Fr Phleb 1966, 19:277–279.
41. Müller R. La phlebectomie ambulatoire. Phlebologie 1978;31:273–279.
42. Oesch A. Indikationen und Ergebnisse der ambulanten Varizentherapie. Therapeutische Umschau 1991;48:692–696.
43. Goren G, Yellin AE. Surgery for truncal varicose veins: the ambulatory stab avulsion phlebectomy for truncal varicose veins. Am J Surg 1991;161:166–174.
44. Goren G, Yellin AE. Invaginated actual stripping and stab avulsion (hook) phlebectomy: a definitive outpatient procedure for primary varicose veins. Amb Surgery 1994;2:27–35.
45. Baccaglini U, Spreafico G, Sorrentino P, et al. Outpatient surgery of varices of the lower limbs: experience of 2,568 cases at four universities. Int Angiol 1995;14:397–399.
46. Rivlin S. The surgical cure of primary varicose veins. Br J Surg 1975;62:913–917.
47. Varady Z. Die mikrochirurgische Phlebextraction. Vasomed Aktuell 1990;3:23–25.
48. Villavicencio JL, Collins GJ, Youkey JR, et al. Nonsurgical management of lower extremity venous problems. In: Bergan JJ, Yao JST, eds. Surgery of the veins. Orlando, FL: Grune & Stratton, 1985;335–356.

chapter 26

Chronic Venous Obstruction

Seshadri Raju

Chronic venous obstruction is predominantly postthrombotic. Occasionally, nonthrombotic causes may be involved, such as tumor compression or iliac vein compression syndrome by adjacent artery. A logical understanding of chronic venous obstruction has been impeded by lack of a suitable diagnostic tool for functional assessment. Unfortunately, ascending venography continues to be the mainstay for the diagnosis of venous obstruction in many institutions.

Although ascending venography yields morphologic information, it provides no reliable functional information. Functional collaterals may not be visualized and those that are visualized may not be adequately functional (1). Large and profuse collaterals appearing on venography have been shown to be poorly functional in many instances, presumably because of high resistance, kinks, or valves oriented against the direction of collateral flow. Conversely, hemodynamically sufficient collaterals are obviously present in many patients with normal distal venous pressures in the presence of axial venous obstruction, even though such collaterals may appear sparse and meager on venography (2). Outflow fractions obtained with occlusion plethysmography have been used for functional assessment of obstruction (3). Large experience gained with impedance plethysmography (see Chapter 7) indicates that this technique may be reliable and useful in acute venous obstruction. Its utility in chronic obstruction is open to question.

A significant component of distal venous pressure in performing occlusion plethysmography is provided by compliance pressure generated by distension of the distal venous tree following calf occlusion. Because outflow fraction is a volume measurement, following release of proximal calf occlusion, alterations in volume pressure relationships of the distal tree are likely to affect this measurement. An altered volume pressure relationship due to wall property changes following deep venous thrombosis is therefore likely to influence outflow fraction measurement, independent of any outflow obstruction that may coincidentally be present. Distal capacitance changes owing to the presence of organized thrombus or fibrosis may also affect outflow fraction measurement independent of postthrombotic obstruction. The entire relationship between these multiple variables with regard to their effect on outflow fraction measurements has not been clearly elucidated. Because many or all of these pathologic changes are present to a variable extent following deep venous thrombosis, a reduction in outflow fraction measurement in calf occlusion plethysmography suggests prior deep venous thrombosis, but does not necessarily show the presence of functional outflow obstruction (see Chapter 13).

A more reliable functional test of obstruction may be the measurement of arm/foot venous pressure differential (4). The presence of a differential greater than 4 mmHg indicates hemodynamic obstruction (Fig. 26.1). Not surprisingly, many patients with venographic obstruction will have a normal differential due to collateralization. Functional assessment of obstruction in these patients can be further refined by performing the reactive hyperemia test to assess the adequacy of collaterals present. Foot venous pressure in the recumbent patient is monitored before and after a 3-minute period of ischemic occlusion. A pressure elevation of less than 6 mmHg during the reactive hyperemia phase shows functionally ade-

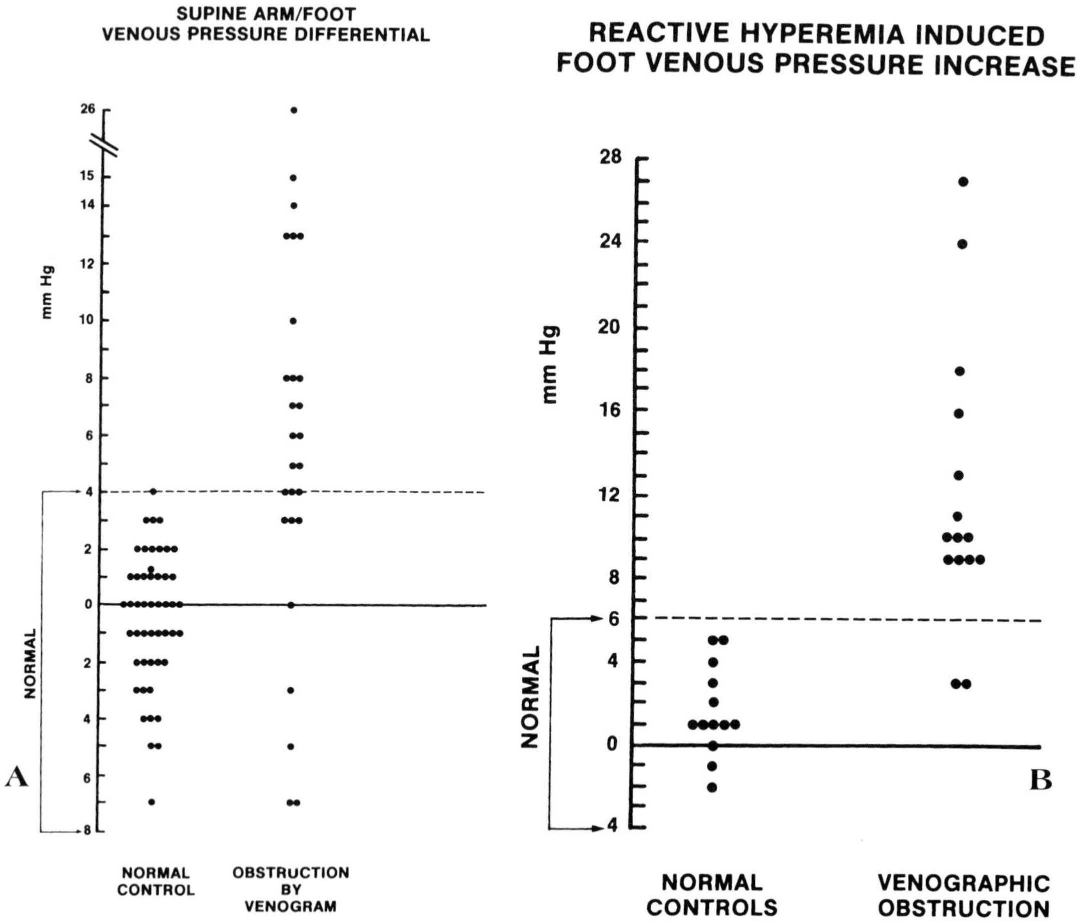

FIG. 26–1. Supine arm/foot venous pressure differential (**A**) and reactive hyperemia-induced foot venous pressure increase (**B**) in a group of "normal" and venographically obstructed limbs. By permission. Phlebology, McMillan Press Ltd. Hampshire, U.K. (1).

quate collateralization (Fig. 26.1). A greater than 6 mmHg elevation suggests that venous collaterals may be insufficient during periods of increased arterial inflow, such as during exercise. By performing both the reactive hyperemia test and the arm/foot venous pressure differential measurement, some interesting patterns of functional venous obstruction were derived and graded on this basis (Table 26.1). The grading system stratifies patients according to the functional adequacy of collaterals during rest and circulatory stress. Patients with grade IV obstruction show a significant arm/foot venous pressure differential with the paradoxical absence of expected foot venous pressure elevation (>6 mmHg) during reactive hyperemia. In such patients, the reactive hyperemia response is either muted or altogether absent. This phenomenon has been noted previously by others (5), but the precise mechanism is not understood (Fig. 26.2). The measurement of an arm/foot venous pressure differential and reactive hyperemia foot venous pressure elevation may be the most reliable test currently available for functional assessment of venous obstruction (3) (see Chapter 13). In a study comparing these tests with venography in 137 patients, no correlation was found between either the size and number of visualized collaterals or the hemodynamic grade of obstruction present (2). Therefore, venographic evaluation of obstruction can be misleading and is of little value in hemodynamic assessment. Obese patients with a normal venogram may have functional obstruction as demonstrated by arm/foot differential and reactive hyperemia test presumably because of vena cava compression by adiposity when the patient is recumbent. It is often stated that proximal obstruction in abdominal veins is likely to be functionally significant while femoral and crural obstructions are well-compensated. In a study of 127 venograms stratified by the grade of obstruction present, functionally severe obstructions were found at all anatomic levels (Fig. 26.3), although the incidence was clearly higher at more proximal levels. Predictably, venographic obstruction involving multiple anatomic levels appears to be functionally more severe than single level obstructions (2). Contrary to expectations, postexercise pressure on ambulatory venous pressure measurement was similarly elevated in functionally compensated and poorly compensated obstructions, and there were no significant differences be-

TABLE 26-1
GRADING OF OBSTRUCTION

		Arm/Foot Venous Pressure Differential (Normal <4 mmHg)	Reactive Hyperemia Foot Venous Pressure Elevation (Normal <6 mmHg)
Grade I†	Fully compensated	<4 mmHg	<6 mmHg
Grade II	Partially compensated	<4 mmHg	>6 mmHg
Grade III	Partially decompensated	>4 mmHg	>6 mmHg
Grade IV	Fully decompensated	>4 mmHg	<6 mmHg*

*Paradoxical response (see text).
†Since pressure parameters for both tests are normal, accurate diagnosis depends on Doppler and/or venography (see text).

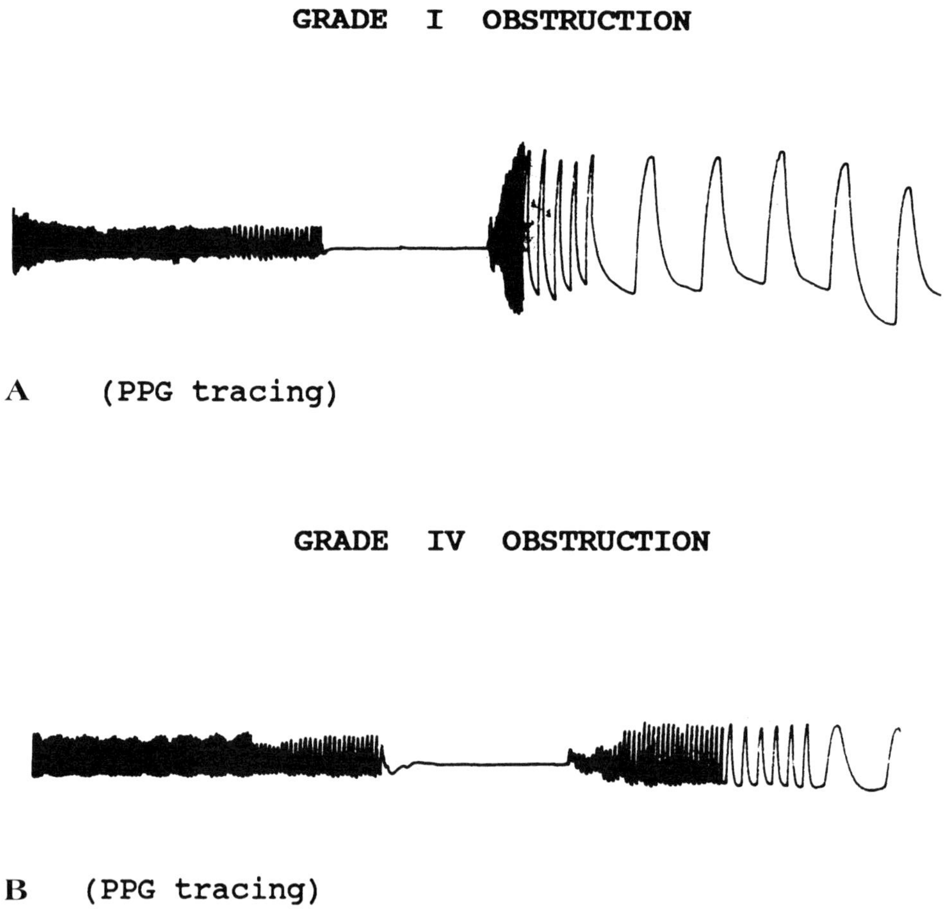

FIG. 26–2. **A** and **B**. Photoplethysmography tracing of digital arterial pulsations in a limb with grade I obstruction and another with grade IV obstruction, respectively. Classic reactive hyperemia response is evident in the former after release of ischemic cuff occlusion. This is absent in the latter. By permission J Vasc Surg (2).

tween the various grades of obstruction (Fig. 26.4). The presence of ambulatory venous hypertension in compensated obstructions (grades I and II) may be attributed in part to postthrombotic compliance changes in the calf venous pump that adversely affect postexercise pressure (see Chapter 12).

Combined obstruction and reflux is invariably an outcome of previous deep venous thrombosis (6). Functional assessment of patients with combined obstruction and reflux is difficult and in the main is empirically based on clinical experience. Skin ulceration and swelling can be caused by either obstruction or reflux pathology. When analyzed according to the associated grade of obstruction present, no difference in the incidence of stasis ulceration was noted (2). Likewise, the incidence of swelling was similar (about 70%) despite the grade of obstruction present (Table 26.2). These data suggest that associated reflux, either alone or combined with obstruction, plays a role in clinical manifestation of skin ulceration or swelling in these patients.

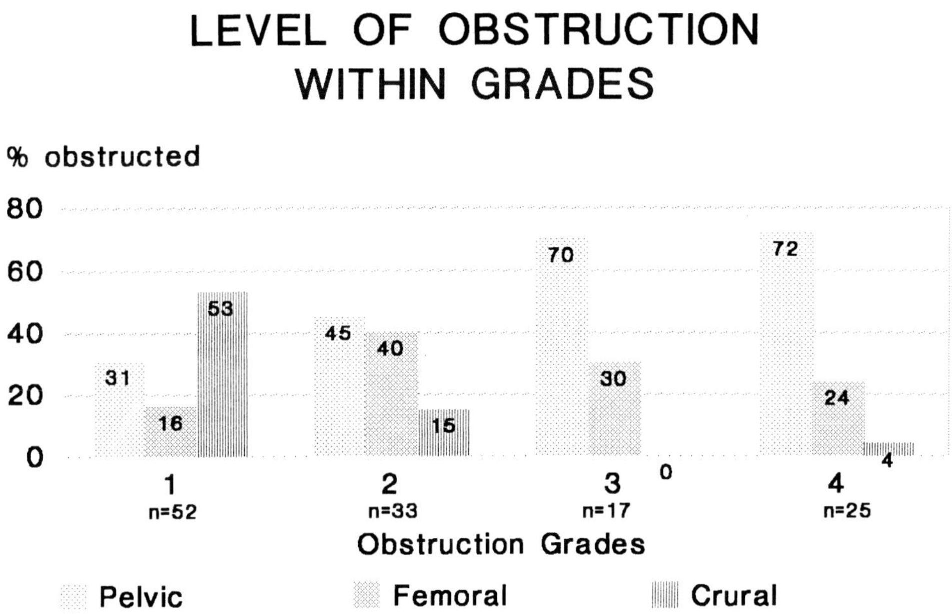

FIG. 26–3. Anatomic distribution of venous obstruction. Venograms were available for analysis in 127 of 137 limbs studied. By permission J Vasc Surg (2).

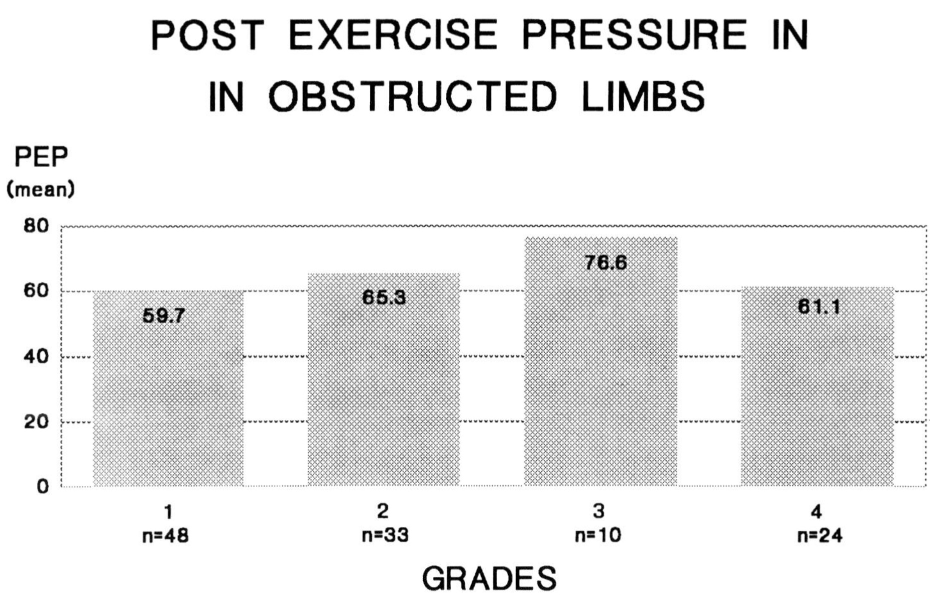

FIG. 26–4. Postexercise pressure in venous obstruction was elevated in all groups. There was no difference between the four grades of obstruction except for grade III with small numbers. By permission J Vasc Surg (2).

TABLE 26-2

INCIDENCE OF SKIN ULCERATION AND SWELLING IN VENOUS OBSTRUCTION

Obstruction Grade	No.	Incidence of Stasis Ulcer		Incidence of Swelling	
I	57	31%	NS	75%	NS
II	36	27%		80%	
III	17	5%		64%	
IV	27	30%		77%	

The association of reflux in this group of obstructed patients was studied by Valsalva foot venous pressure measurement and descending venography. A much higher Valsalva foot venous pressure elevation was found in ulcerated (7.6 mmHg $\pm$ 4.4 mmHg) compared with nonulcerated limbs (3.4 mmHg $\pm$ 2.0 mmHg; $P < 0.001$). Descending venography showed the incidence of reflux was also higher among ulcerated limbs compared with those without skin ulceration (77% vs. 35%) and the grade of reflux was higher than in the former group (2). These data support the clinical impression that stasis ulceration is predominantly a manifestation of reflux, even in the presence of coincident obstruction. Valsalva-based tests, including Valsalva foot venous pressure elevation, and descending venography are impeded by the presence of proximal venous obstruction. This is due to impedance to the transmission of the Valsalva impulse by the obstructing lesion and the data derived from these techniques probably understate the actual presence of reflux in ulcerated limbs (7). Skin ulceration can be cured by valve reconstruction techniques to abolish reflux even in the presence of coincident venous obstruction (see Chapter 23).

REFERENCES

1. Raju S. A pressure-based technique for the detection of acute and chronic venous obstruction. Phlebology 1988;3:207–216.
2. Raju S, Fredericks R. Venous obstruction: an analysis of one hundred thirty-seven cases with hemodynamic, venographic, and clinical correlations. J Vasc Surg 1991;14:305–313.
3. Neglén P, Raju S. Detection of outflow obstruction in chronic venous insufficiency. J Vasc Surg 1993;17:583–589.
4. Raju S. New approaches to the diagnosis and treatment of venous obstruction. J Vasc Surg 1986;4:42–54.
5. Rodbard S, Takeda Y, Takacs L. Post-occlusion "hyperemi": A study on a model. Quart J Exp Physiol 1969;54:346–365.
6. Johnson BF, Manzo RA, Bergelin RO, Strandness DE Jr. Relationship between changes in the deep venous system and the development of the postthrombotic syndrome after an acute episode of lower limb deep vein thrombosis: a one- to six-year follow-up. J Vasc Surg 1995;21:307–313.
7. Neglén P, Raju S. A comparison between descending phlebography and duplex Doppler investigation in the evaluation of reflux in chronic venous insufficiency: a challenge to phlebography as the "gold standard." J Vasc Surg 1992;16:687–693.

chapter 27

Vena Cava Syndromes

Peter Gloviczki and Eric Berens

Chronic obstruction of the superior or inferior vena cava is remarkably well-tolerated by most patients. Since extensive venous collateral circulation usually develops, the morbidity and mortality of caval obstructions are significantly less than those of similar pathology in the arterial system. Signs and symptoms of venous congestion depend mainly on the degree of venous hypertension that develops due to the venous outflow obstruction. Occasionally, patients may present with symptoms of cardiac failure because of inadequate venous inflow to the right heart. The clinical presentation and outcome are affected by the venous collateral circulation, the site and extent of caval obstruction, the duration and progression of an extrinsic compression or tumor invasion of the cava, and by the aggressive nature of a frequently present underlying malignant disease.

In this chapter, we review the etiology of caval obstructions and discuss the clinical presentation and evaluation of patients with superior and inferior vena cava syndromes of different origin. Since results of large vein reconstructions have significantly improved in the last decade, our attention focuses on surgical management of superior and inferior vena cava syndromes.

SUPERIOR VENA CAVA SYNDROME

Etiology

In 1757, William Hunter first described obstruction of the superior vena cava by a syphilitic aortic aneurysm (1). This etiology now is rare. In a review of the literature from 1934 to 1983, 85% of 1986 patients with superior vena cava syndrome had metastatic pulmonary or mediastinal malignancy (2). The most common tumor causing superior vena cava syndrome was metastatic adenocarcinoma of the lung. Benign causes were significantly less frequent. Mediastinal inflammation, including fibrosing mediastinitis or granulomatous fungal diseases such as histoplasmosis, account for most of the nonmalignant cases, particularly in the Mississippi River Valley and the upper Midwest region. Retrosternal goiter is another possible etiology. More recently, central venous catheters used for either hemodynamic monitoring, parenteral alimentation, or drug administration have become more common causes of superior vena cava obstruction (3, 4). In some patients, the superior vena cava thrombosis is idiopathic or it is related to an underlying deficiency of natural anticoagulants (antithrombin III, protein S, and protein C).

Clinical Presentation

The most frequent symptom of superior vena cava syndrome is the feeling of fullness in the head and neck that is more severe in the dependent position. Headache, somnolence, and dizziness may result from cerebral venous hypertension. Additional symptoms may include mental confusion, visual symptoms, dyspnea, orthopnea, or cough. Progressive swelling of the face and neck, palpebral edema, ecchymosis, and dilated jugular veins accompany cyanosis of the upper body. Extensive venous collaterals may develop in the chest wall. Death from superior vena cava syndrome is very rare and is usually preceded by convulsions and coma (5).

Diagnostic Evaluation

A careful clinical history with physical examination, routine laboratory tests, and chest roentgenogram frequently establishes the diagnosis of superior vena cava syndrome. Computer tomography with intravenous contrast has become the most important test in the evaluation of these patients. It should be done in every patient if tumor or benign fibrotic process is suspected. Fast computer tomography (Imitron scan) provides more details of the mediastinal structures.

In patients who are candidates for venous reconstruction, bilateral upper extremity venography should be performed to image the site and extent of the venous occlusion and to delineate the pathways of the venous collaterals (Fig. 27.1). In many of these patients, the azygos vein is the most important venous collateral. If the superior vena cava is obstructed central to the azygos vein, the direction of flow in the azygos vein is reversed and blood from the upper half of the body is drained by the azygos and hemiazygos system through lumbar veins into the inferior vena cava (Fig. 27.2). Since the internal jugular veins cannot be imaged with upper extremity venography in most patients, duplex scanning of the internal jugular veins is also done to confirm their patency. The presence of at least one patent internal jugular vein is necessary to plan venous reconstruction. Bronchoscopy, mediastinoscopy, thoracoscopy, or thoracotomy also may be necessary to provide tissue diagnosis of an underlying malignant disease.

Nonoperative Therapy

Conservative measures to alleviate symptoms of superior vena cava obstruction include elevation of the head, avoidance of a constricting garment or

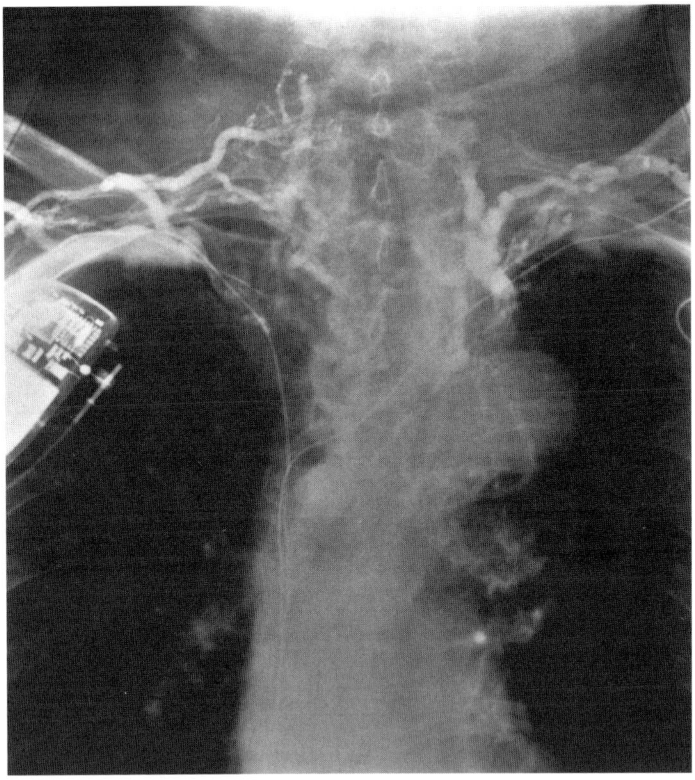

FIG. 27–1. Bilateral upper extremity venogram in a 38-year-old male patient demonstrates extensive superior vena cava and bilateral innominate vein thrombosis following placement of multiple pacemaker electrodes. Both internal jugular veins were patent on duplex scan.

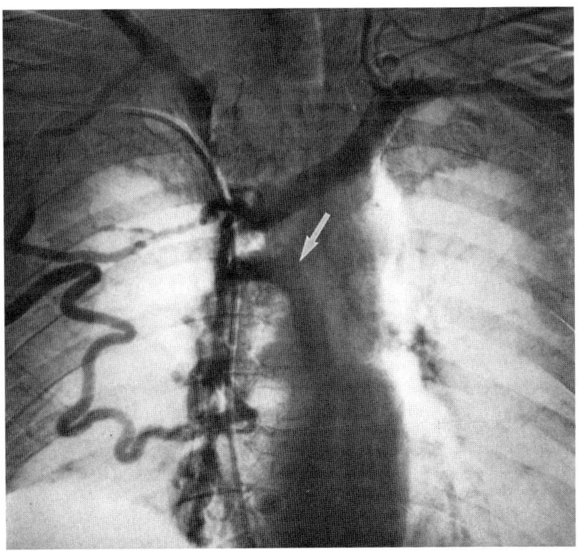

FIG. 27–2. Obstruction of the superior vena cava. There is retrograde flow in the azygos vein (*arrow*) that drains venous blood from the upper half of the body through lumbar collaterals into the inferior vena cava.

tight collar and the use of diuretics. Anticoagulation is effective to protect the venous collateral circulation. Thrombolytic treatment can be considered in benign acute superior vena cava syndrome that is caused by an intracaval catheter or by an underlying abnormality in blood coagulation. While symptoms of superior vena cava syndrome usually mark end-stage metastatic malignant disease, they frequently improve following irradiation or chemotherapy. Chen, et al., treated 42 patients with malignant superior vena cava syndrome using external beam radiotherapy and/or chemotherapy (6). Symptoms of superior vena cava syndrome resolved in 80% of the patients who underwent radiotherapy, with a mean interval of 4 weeks. A similar benefit of radiation or chemotherapy was noted by others (7).

In symptomatic patients with significant stenosis of the superior vena cava caused by malignant disease, an expandable intravascular wire stent can provide symptomatic relief.

Surgical Treatment

Indication. The ideal indication for superior vena cava replacement is persistent, symptomatic superior vena cava syndrome caused by benign disease. In our practice, caval reconstruction for benign disease has been performed for obstruction caused by mediastinal fibrosis, central venous instrumentation (long- and short-term venous catheters, pacemaker electrode, ventriculoatrial shunt), antithrombin III deficiency, and idiopathic venous thrombosis (4). Median sternotomy and caval reconstruction in patients with end-stage malignancy have been performed with success (8), although venous reconstruction in these patients is seldom indicated. Patients with malignant tumor should undergo reconstruction only if their life expectancy is more than 1 year. This group of patients may include those with lymphoma, thymoma, or metastatic medullary carcinoma of the thyroid gland (9). Dartevelle, et al., reported on a group of patients who had successful caval resection and reconstruction with resection of pulmonary and mediastinal malignant tumors (10).

Selection of Graft. For replacement of the superior vena cava or the innominate vein, autogenous spiral saphenous vein graft is our first choice. This graft was described in experiments by Chiu, et al., in 1974 (11), and it was Doty who introduced it in the clinical practice for superior vena cava obstruction (12). Our technique of preparing and implanting the spiral graft has been described in detail (4, 9, 13). The saphenous vein is removed from one or both lower extremities, depending on the length needed for caval bypass. The vein is opened longitudinally, valves are excised and the vein is wrapped around a 32- or 36-French polyethylene chest tube. The edges of the saphenous vein are approximated with running 6–0 or 7–0 monofilament nonabsorbable sutures (Figs. 27.3 and 27.4). The advantage of this graft material is that it is a nonthrombogenic autologous tissue. Potential disadvantages include the additional time (60–90 minutes) needed to prepare the graft and the fact that the length of the graft is limited by the availability of the saphenous vein.

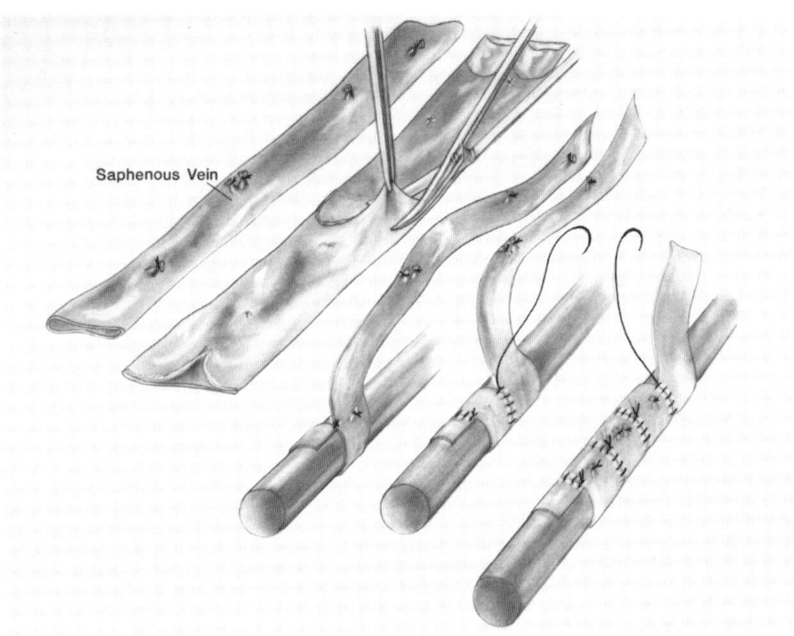

FIG. 27–3. Steps in the construction of a spiral vein graft using the greater saphenous vein. (Reproduced by permission from Gloviczki P, Pairolero PC. Venous reconstruction for obstruction and valvular incompetence. In: Goldstone J, ed. Perspectives in vascular surgery. St. Louis: Quality Medical Publishing Company, 1988:75–93.)

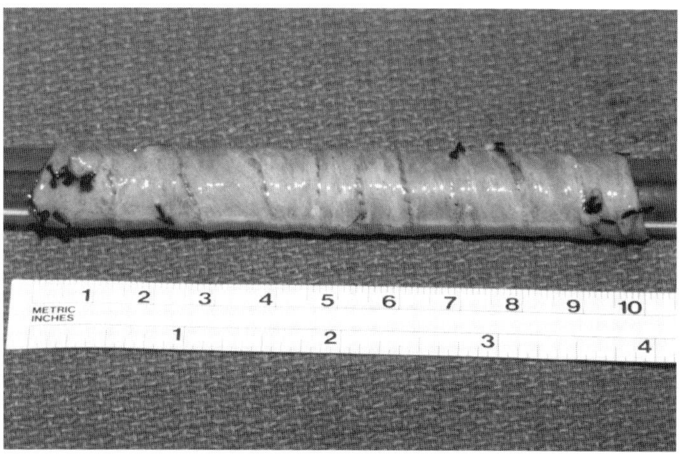

FIG. 27–4. Intraoperative photograph of a completed spiral saphenous vein graft. (Reproduced by permission from Gloviczki P, Roland CF, Elmore JR. Reconstruction of the vena cava with autogenous vein grafts. In: D'Addato M, Stella A, eds. Vein graft in vascular surgery. Bologna: Editoriale Grasso, 1991:220–230.)

Of the available autologous graft materials, greater saphenous vein, panel vein graft, autologous pericardium, and superficial femoral vein have been used to reconstruct the superior vena cava in a limited number of patients (14–18).

Of the currently available prosthetic materials, expanded polytetrafluoroethylene (PTFE) grafts with external ring support have given the best results for superior vena cava reconstruction (4, 9, 10, 19–25). It is a good alternative to spiral vein graft, especially if only a short segment of the superior vena cava must be replaced, or if the mediastinum is too tight and compression of the vein graft following closure of the sternum would be most likely (Fig. 27.5).

Surgical Technique. Superior vena cava reconstruction is performed using median sternotomy. If the internal jugular vein must be used for inflow, an oblique neck incision medial to the sternocleidomastoid muscle of the appropriate side is also done (Fig. 27.6). The mediastinum is exposed and biopsy or (if possible) resection of the tumor is performed before caval reconstruction. Following systemic anticoagulation with 5000 units of heparin, end-to-end or, rarely, end-to-side anastomosis is performed first with the jugular or innominate vein. The central anastomosis can be performed between the graft and the superior vena cava, although we prefer to anastomose the graft directly to the right atrial appendage. A partial occlusion clamp is placed on the appendage that is subsequently opened and the trabecular muscles are excised. The anastomosis is performed with 5–0 monofilament running sutures. Air is carefully flushed from the graft before reestablishing the circulation.

Postoperative anticoagulation is started 36–48 hours later with heparin and the patient is sent home on oral anticoagulation. Patients with spiral vein graft who have no underlying coagulation abnormality are maintained on Coumadin for only 3 months. Those with disturbances in the coagulation or those with ePTFE grafts usually benefit from lifelong anticoagulation.

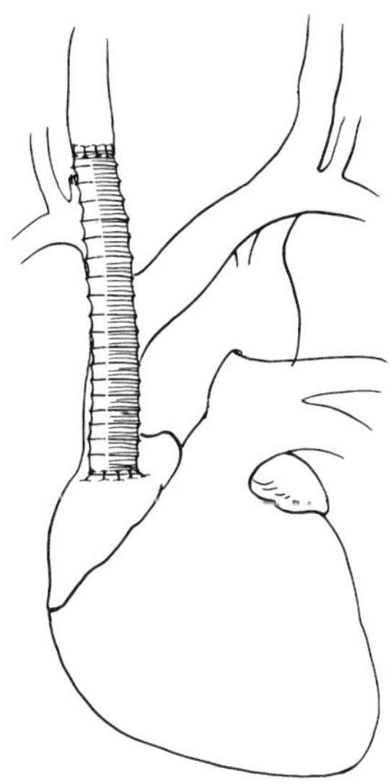

FIG. 27–5. Illustration of a right internal jugular vein-atrial appendage externally supported polytetrafluoroethylene graft.

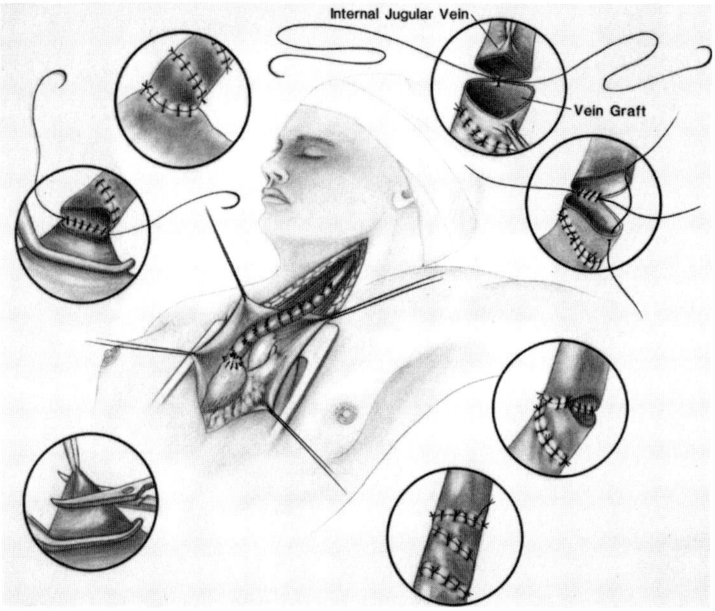

FIG. 27–6. Steps in performing a left internal jugular vein-right atrial bypass with a spiral vein graft. (Reproduced by permission from Gloviczki P, Pairolero PC. Venous reconstruction for obstruction and valvular incompetence. In: Goldstone J, ed. Perspectives in vascular surgery. St. Louis: Quality Medical Publishing Company, 1988:75–93.)

Results. Reconstruction of the occluded superior vena cava or innominate vein gives the most gratifying result of venous bypasses. Patency rate is very good, since the mean flow through the graft is usually high (mean: 1440 ml/mn; range: 750–2000 ml/mn) (9). Shorter grafts placed entirely within the mediastinum have a better chance of long-term patency than those with an anastomosis in the neck.

Doty, et al., reported on long-term results in nine patients who underwent spiral vein grafting for superior vena cava syndrome caused by benign disease (26). Seven of nine grafts remained patent during follow-up that extended from 1–15 years, and all but one of the patients became asymptomatic.

We recently reported our results in 12 patients who underwent superior vena cava reconstruction for benign disease (4). Of the nine patients who had spiral graft placement, seven had straight and two had bifurcated grafts implanted. All seven straight grafts were patent during a follow-up that extended up to 5 years after surgery (Fig. 27.7**A** and **B**). One limb of the bifurcated graft occluded early in both patients, but complete recanalization of the thrombosed limb was later observed in one. Six of the nine patients became asymptomatic, two had mild residual symptoms, and no significant improvement was noted in one.

Results with PTFE grafts implanted into the mediastinum in some series showed excellent patency. Dartevelle, et al., observed continued patency in 20 of 22 ePTFE grafts, with a mean follow-up of 23 months (10). Moore and Hollier observed no

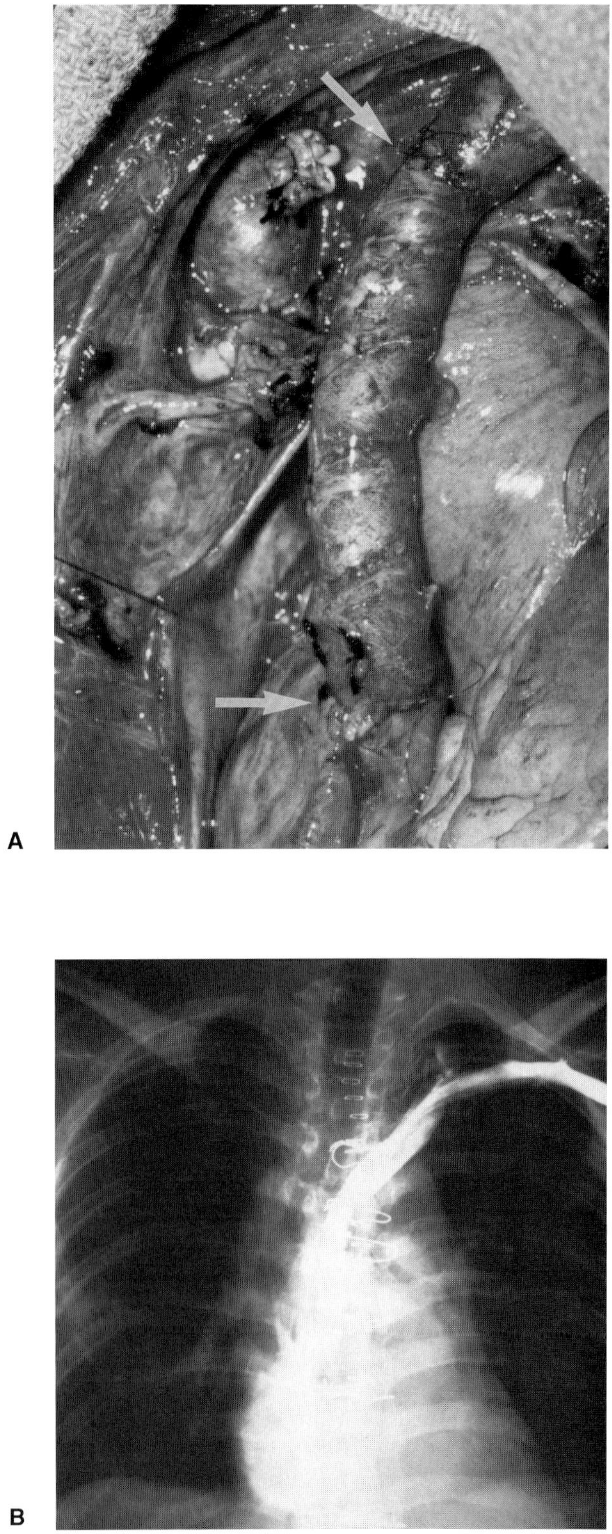

FIG. 27–7. **A.** Intraoperative photograph of a left innominate vein-atrial appendage spiral saphenous vein graft. *Arrows* indicate anastomoses. **B.** Postoperative venogram confirms widely patent spiral vein graft.

graft occlusion at a mean follow-up of 30 months among 10 patients who underwent large central vein reconstruction (27). In eight of these 10 patients, an additional arteriovenous fistula at the arm was used to increase flow and maintain patency. Reviewing other series from the literature, however, we found that patency of ePTFE grafts at 2 years was approximately 70% (9, 19–24). In our experience, some thrombus formation occurs even in patent PTFE grafts. This is a potential source of further thrombosis and failure of the graft. Because many patients with PTFE grafts need long-term anticoagulation and the primary patency rate of PTFE grafts is lower, spiral vein graft continues to be our first choice for superior vena cava replacement.

INFERIOR VENA CAVA SYNDROMES

Obstruction of the inferior vena cava may be the result of congenital abnormalities or acquired disease. Similar to patients with superior vena cava syndrome, the collateral circulation can be so extensive that even complete inferior vena caval obstruction can remain asymptomatic or cause only minimal disability.

The inferior vena cava has been anatomically divided into three distinct segments (28, 29). Segment I includes the infrarenal cava, segment II extends from the renal veins up to the hepatic veins while segment III is the suprahepatic vena cava, including all hepatic veins up to the level of the right atrium (Fig. 27.8). In segment I, the most frequent etiology of caval obstruction is spontaneous iliocaval

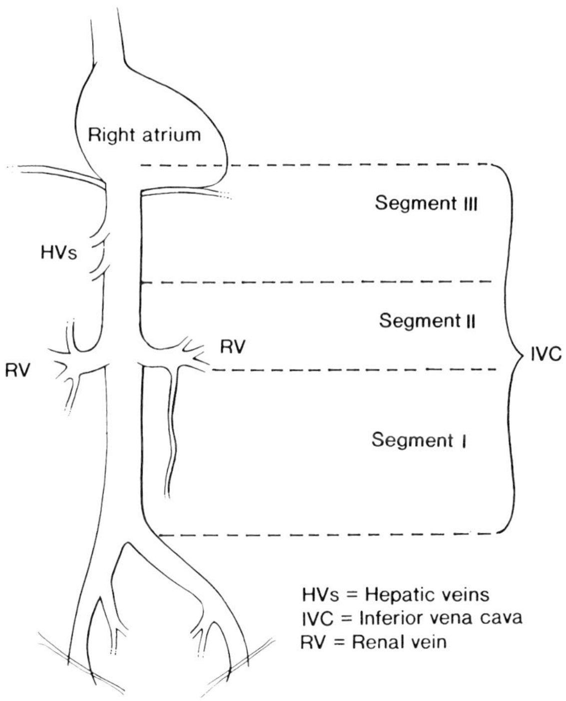

FIG. 27–8. Anatomic classification of the inferior vena cava: *Segment I* = infrarenal; *Segment II* = suprarenal; *Segment III* = suprahepatic.

venous thrombosis. In some patients, symptomatic caval occlusion develops after vena cava interruption performed for prevention of pulmonary emboli (4). In segment II, malignant tumors, most frequently renal cell carcinoma extending into the vena cava, cause obstruction of the caval lumen. In segment III, congenital anomalies, such as membranous occlusion or coarctation of the vena cava, with or without occlusion of the hepatic veins (Budd-Chiari syndrome) are the most frequent.

Since clinical presentation, patient evaluation and management of these conditions may differ considerably, the three most important inferior vena cava syndromes are discussed separately. While we focus our attention on chronic iliocaval venous thrombosis, we also discuss primary and secondary caval tumors and membranous occlusion or coarctation of the vena cava.

Chronic Iliocaval Thrombosis

Etiology. Chronic iliocaval venous thrombosis is the most frequent benign cause of obstruction of the infrarenal inferior vena cava. Caval thrombosis usually develops as progression of a spontaneous pelvic or iliofemoral deep venous thrombosis. It may also be the result of extrinsic iliocaval compression by

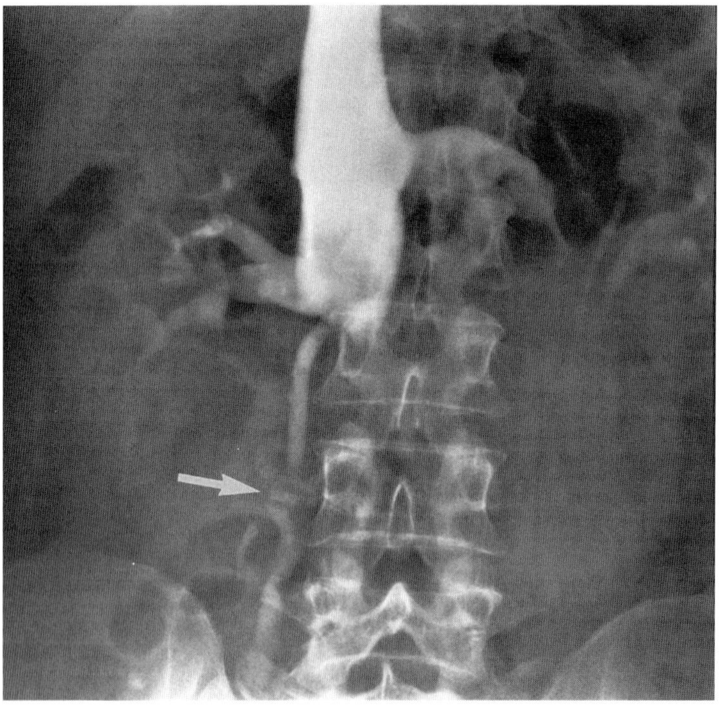

FIG. 27–9. Obstruction of the infrarenal inferior vena cava in a 30-year-old male patient with severe bilateral lower extremity chronic venous insufficiency. *Arrow* indicates site of the inferior vena cava clip.

the right common iliac artery, a tumor, or by retroperitoneal fibrosis. Iatrogenic inferior vena cava interruption for prevention of pulmonary emboli may result in complete caval obstruction (Fig. 27.9). A small, but definite, group of these patients develop symptoms of lower extremity venous hypertension. Because of the high flow through the renal veins, spontaneous iliocaval venous thrombosis rarely involves the suprarenal segment of the inferior vena cava.

Clinical Presentation. Symptoms of patients with caval obstruction depend on the development of venous collateral circulation. The main collaterals include the ascending lumbar, ovarian, vertebral, azygos, portal, and epigastric veins (Fig. 27.10). If the collateral circulation is inadequate, lower extremity chronic venous insufficiency develops. The clinical picture is characterized by bilateral leg swelling and bursting pain in the thighs after prolonged standing or, more frequently, after exercise. This "venous" claudication is a typical symptom in patients who develop venous hypertension on exercise due to significant venous outflow obstruction. Other typical signs of chronic venous insufficiency, such as stasis ulcer, pigmentation, induration, leg varicosity and stasis dermatitis, may

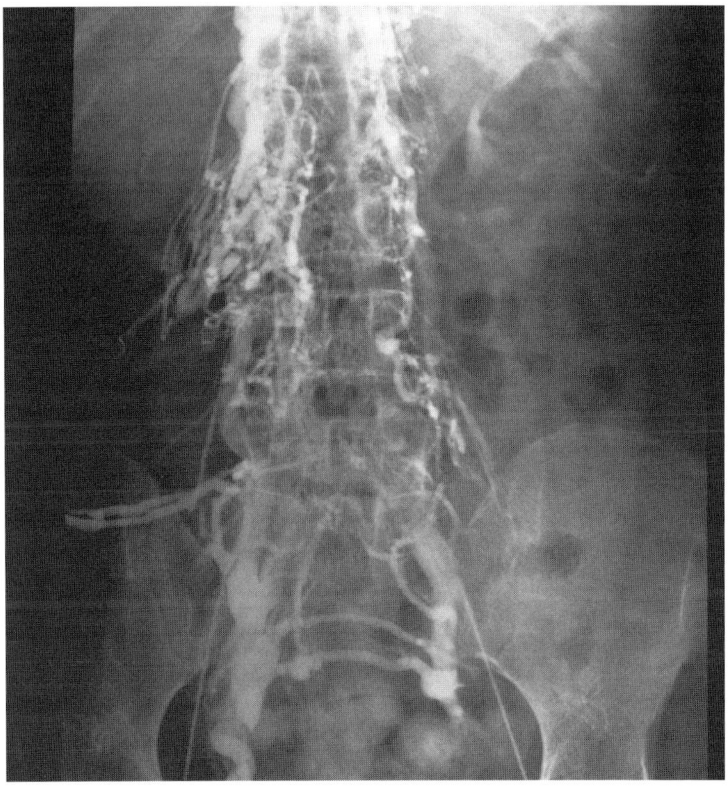

FIG. 27–10. Extensive bilateral pelvic and ascending lumbar collaterals in a 47-year-old female patient with spontaneous thrombosis of the entire infrarenal segment of the inferior vena cava.

also occur. In our experience, they are frequently markers of additional infrainguinal venous disease. The main cause of skin ulceration in these patients is usually not obstruction, but extensive valvular incompetence, as emphasized by Raju and Fredericks (30).

Evaluation of Patients. All patients with signs or symptoms of chronic lower extremity venous insufficiency should be thoroughly evaluated to determine the cause of the disease and plan appropriate treatment. A detailed history, including family history of venous disease, and physical examination, complemented with hand-held Doppler examination, provide correct clinical diagnosis in many patients. Noninvasive evaluation of the venous system using impedance, strain-gauge or air plethysmography can differentiate incompetence from venous outflow obstruction in most patients (see Chapter 13). Duplex scanning of the deep veins is used with increasing frequency to differentiate obstruction from incompetence and to separate primary from postthrombotic valvular incompetence. Data collected from the literature indicate that less than 15% of all patients with chronic lower extremity venous insufficiency have symptoms due to venous occlusive disease (31). Additionally, less than half of these have isolated proximal venous occlusion (32). If symptoms of proximal venous obstruction are present, computed tomography or magnetic resonance imaging of the abdomen and pelvis is mandatory to exclude tumor or extrinsic venous compression by a retroperitoneal process. Lymphoscintigraphy performed with technetium-labeled antimony trisulfide colloid differentiates lymphedema from venous edema with great accuracy (33). Mixed lymphatic and venous edema, however, occurs in patients with long-standing chronic venous insufficiency, as demonstrated by Collins, et al. (34).

Symptomatic patients who fail to respond to adequate conservative treatment are evaluated in more detail. Detailed imaging of the venous anatomy of the lower extremities, pelvis, and abdomen with contrast venography is essential before iliocaval reconstruction. Good visualization of inflow into the external or common iliac vein with a separate femoral injection (Fig. 27.11) is important, since a caval bypass should originate from the iliac rather than the femoral vein. Good quality imaging of the common femoral vein is also necessary, since a partially recanalized femoral vein may not be suitable for bypass. Lower extremity ascending venography, iliocavography and imaging of the suprarenal cava with brachial or axillary vein catheterization are performed.

It is important to remember that documentation of iliocaval obstruction by venography is not sufficient to proceed with surgical treatment. Additional evidence is needed to prove functional obstruction to venous flow. Raju and Fredericks analyzed different tests in 137 patients with venous obstruction (30). They found the arm/foot venous pressure differential and the reactive hyperemia test to be more accurate to determine significant obstruction than traditional venography or ambulatory venous pressure measurements. In our practice, femoral-central pressure gradient is determined in the supine patient. A minimum of 5 mmHg gradient is necessary before proceeding with caval reconstruction (4). A similar criterion is used by Gruss: if resting femoral pressure doubles after exercise, venous reconstruction is indicated (35).

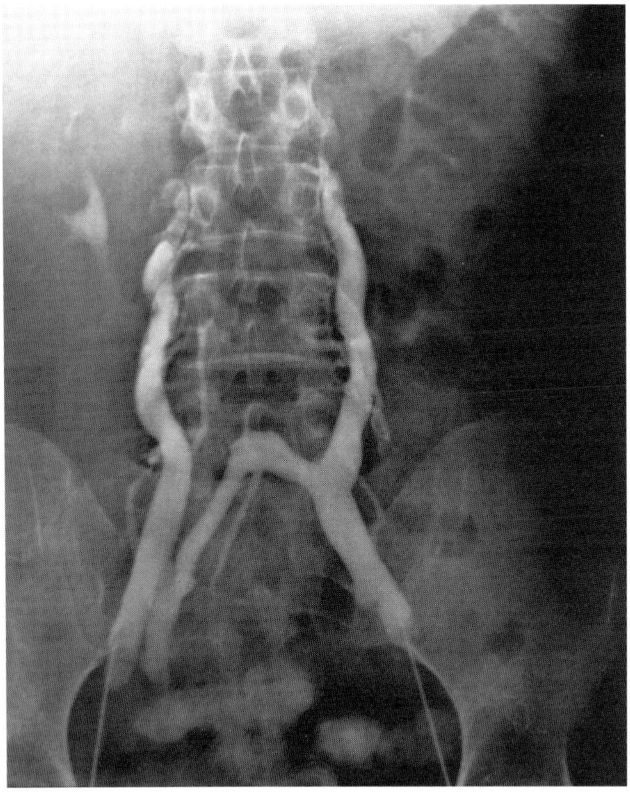

FIG. 27–11. Patent iliac veins fill large ascending lumbar collaterals in this patient with obstruction of the infrarenal inferior vena cava. The common iliac vein was suitable for inflow for an iliocaval bypass.

Nonoperative Therapy. Conservative management of chronic iliocaval thrombosis follows the same guidelines as treatment of lower extremity chronic venous insufficiency, which is discussed in detail in Chapter 15. In patients with proximal venous outflow obstruction, elastic compression alone may not control the symptoms and frequent elevation of the extremity even during the day may be necessary. However, conservative treatment is usually effective and surgical treatment is, fortunately, rarely needed. In good-risk patients with persistent severe leg swelling and pain, caval bypass now can be considered.

Surgical Treatment

Factors Affecting Outcome. Surgical intervention in patients with iliocaval thrombosis should be approached cautiously. Although the number of reports on patients with venous reconstruction for iliocaval thrombosis has increased in the last decade, the failure rate is still significant (4, 9, 36–41).

Patency of grafts implanted into the venous system is affected by several factors, including low venous flow, low venous pressure, the thrombogenic surface of the graft, and the frequently increased thrombotic potential of the patient (42). Significant infrainguinal venous disease decreases the chance of prolonged patency of proximal grafts. Schanzer, et al., found significant reflux in 60% of patients with deep venous occlusions (43). Because of low intraluminal pressure, external compression of a vein graft by the increased abdominal pressure or by the inguinal ligament may lead to early failure. In our clinical experience so far, ePTFE graft with external support has performed better for inferior vena cava grafts than has spiral vein graft (4, 9).

Venous flow through the graft may be diminished because of an already well-developed venous collateral circulation. The presence of a gradient in venous pressure, as mentioned earlier, confirms insufficient collateral circulation. If a gradient of 5 mmHg between the two sides of the venous occlusion cannot be demonstrated, we suggest conservative treatment.

Surgical Technique. We recently described in detail the technique of femorocaval and iliocaval bypasses (25). These operations should be carefully planned and perfectly executed. Short, large diameter ePTFE grafts with external ring or spiral support perform best. Unilateral, rather than bilateral, reconstruction is preferred (Fig. 27.12). The distal anastomosis, if possible, should be with the iliac rather than the femoral vein to avoid compression by the inguinal ligament and to result in a shorter graft. Exposure of the vena cava at the level of the renal vein should be done through a midline or subcostal incision using a transperitoneal approach. This is our preferred approach for short iliocaval grafts.

A distal arteriovenous fistula should be added to long iliocaval prosthetic grafts and to femorocaval grafts to increase flow and decrease chances of early failure (25). Earlier in our experience we ligated the fistula after 3–6 months. At present, we occlude it only if it is necessary because of evidence of cardiac failure, distal venous hypertension, or limb ischemia.

Some form of perioperative antithrombotic treatment is used by most surgeons during placement of a prosthetic graft in the venous system. For lower extremity venous reconstruction, the benefit of intermittent pneumatic compression pump in the perioperative period has been emphasized by Hobson, et al. (44). We give 5000 units of heparin intravenously before cross-clamping, and avoid protamine at the end of the procedure. Postoperatively, 500 ml of Dextran 40 is infused during the first 8 hours. Intravenous heparin is started in the operating room at a rate of 500 units per hour through a fine, polyethylene catheter introduced through a side branch of the greater saphenous vein and advanced up to the level of the distal vein graft anastomosis. The dose of heparin is gradually increased until full heparinization is achieved during the next 24 hours, obtaining an activated partial thromboplastin time 1.5–2 times normal. If extensive retroperitoneal dissection was required, full heparinization is delayed until 36 hours after the operation.

Results. In 1984, Dale was the first to successfully replace the iliocaval bifurcation with a bifurcated ePTFE graft (38). Raju, in 1986, reviewed the results of eight externally supported ePTFE grafts implanted for iliac vein thrombosis (40). Two of the eight grafts had long-term patency, with total symptomatic re-

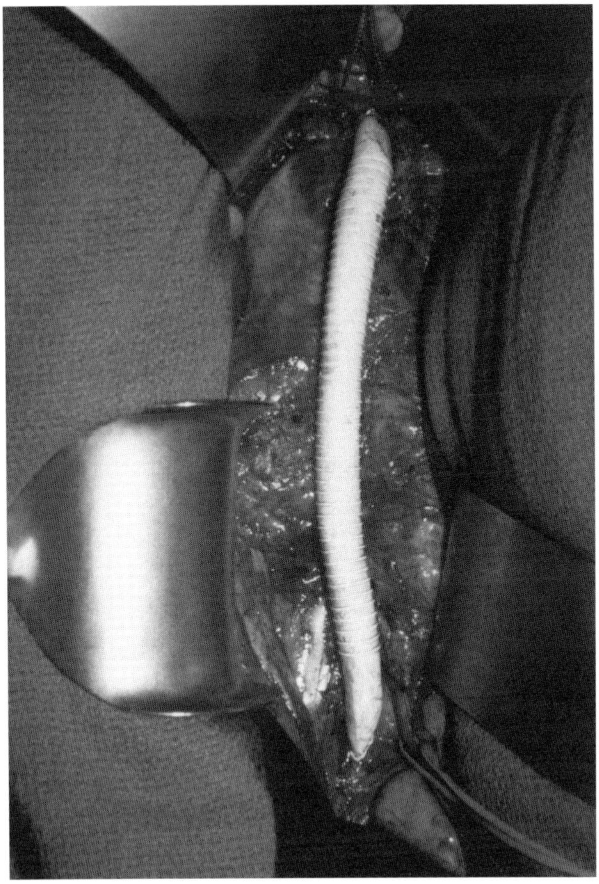

FIG. 27–12. Right iliac vein-inferior vena cava bypass. The site of the proximal anastomosis is at the level of the renal veins. An additional femoral arteriovenous fistula was performed. The patient is asymptomatic with a patent graft 1.6 years after reconstruction.

lief. We have recently reported on our results obtained in 15 patients who underwent inferior vena cava grafting for benign disease (4). Eleven of these patients had ePTFE graft placement, 10 for iliac or iliocaval venous thrombosis (Fig. 27.13**A** and **B**). A femoral arteriovenous fistula was used in eight patients. Seven of the 11 ePTFE grafts were patent at the last follow-up, which extended up to 5 years after surgery (median: 9 months). Six of the seven patients with patent grafts had no significant residual symptoms.

Iliocaval reconstruction in selected symptomatic patients with chronic venous occlusive disease has become possible. Long-term results, however, are still not available in a large number of patients to define the ultimate role of these procedures. Further attempts to improve patient selection and to decrease the thrombogenicity of prosthetic grafts for venous reconstructions are needed.

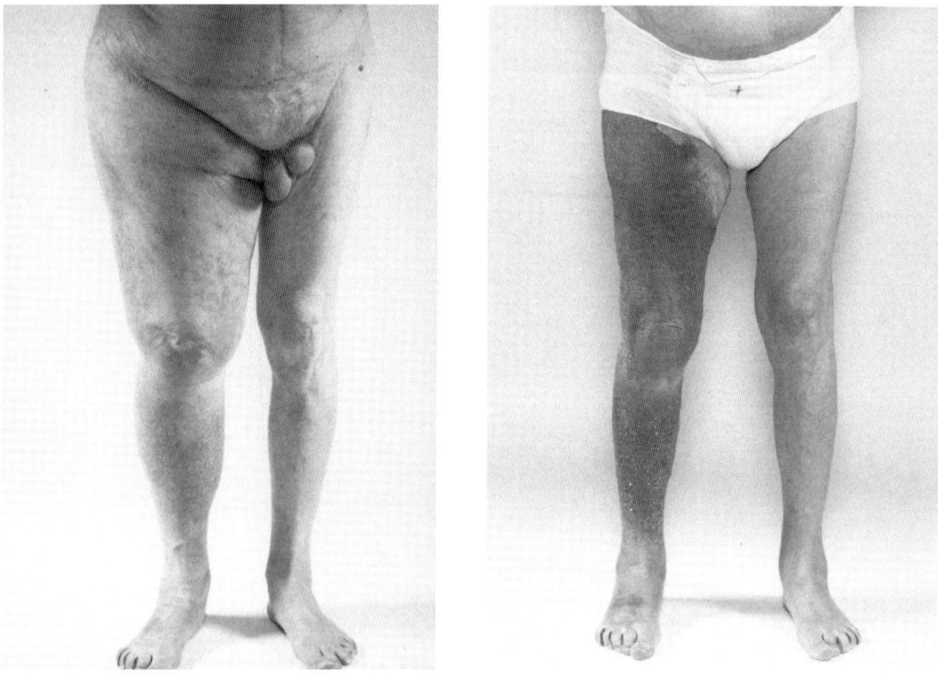

A B

FIG. 27–13. **A.** A 77-year-old male patient with severe swelling and venous claudication of the right lower extremity caused by iliac vein thrombosis. After 4 years of unsuccessful conservative treatment, the patient underwent iliocaval bypass. **B.** Photograph of the same patient 1 year after venous reconstruction. Excellent clinical result was obtained.

PRIMARY AND SECONDARY TUMORS OF THE INFERIOR VENA CAVA

Primary Leiomyosarcoma

Clinical Presentation. Leiomyosarcoma is the most common type of primary venous tumor. In a recent review of the literature that included 210 patients, we found invasion of the inferior vena cava in 127 cases (60%) (45). The disease was much more frequent among women than men and the average age at diagnosis was 55 years. The most frequent clinical signs or symptoms included a palpable mass (39–81%), back pain (69%), or abdominal pain (61%). Approximately one-fourth of patients with caval tumors may have hepatic vein obstruction resulting in portal hypertension or liver failure. If the suprarenal segment of the cava or the renal veins are invaded and the collateral circulation is not adequate, renal failure may develop. Among 13 patients with primary venous leiomyosarcoma who were treated at the Mayo Clinic in the last 35 years, only two complained of leg swelling (45).

Preoperative Imaging. Plain abdominal films are seldom helpful, but intravenous pyelography may identify displacement of the kidney or compression of the pelvis or ureter. Ultrasonography, computed tomography, and, more recently, magnetic resonance imaging have been used to localize the tumor and define its relation to the inferior vena cava. To plan venous reconstruction with tumor resection, we recommend preoperative contrast iliocavography in these patients.

Surgical Treatment. Wide local excision of the tumor with free margins is the only adequate treatment for primary venous leiomyosarcoma. Nephrectomy, cholecystectomy, or, rarely, partial hepatectomy may be necessary to perform complete resection of the tumor. If the suprarenal cava is invaded, resection with immediate caval reconstruction is necessary. Since only a portion of the caval wall is usually involved, direct lateral suture or closure with a patch can be done and prosthetic grafting is rarely needed. For the infrarenal segment, Kieffer, et al., advocate delayed reconstruction (28). We have performed resection with successful reconstruction of the infrarenal segment of the cava with ePTFE graft. We agree, however, that caval ligation at this level may be remarkably well-tolerated by many patients if there is no distal thrombotic disease.

Results. Primary leiomyosarcoma of the vena cava is a lethal disease. Median survival in our patients was 3.5 years (45). Of those eight patients who died, the tumor recurred in six. Survival in our material was not affected by tumor grade, size, or adjuvant treatment. A similar poor late survival of patients with primary caval tumors has been noted in other reviews as well (28, 29). The longest reported survival after resection of a primary leiomyosarcoma invading the inferior vena cava was 13 years (46). Earlier detection of the tumor because of more frequent use of abdominal imaging techniques is likely in the future. Wide local excision with selective venous reconstruction and careful postoperative follow-up provide the only chance of prolonged survival of these patients. Because of the poor prognosis, adjuvant radiotherapy and chemotherapy are offered to most patients following resection.

Renal Cell Carcinoma with Extension into the Vena Cava

Clinical Presentation. Renal carcinoma is the most frequent secondary tumor invading the inferior vena cava. Among 1850 patients operated on for renal cancer at the Mayo Clinic, Neves and Zincke found 54 patients (3%) with tumor extension into the vena cava (47). The presence of an abdominal mass, hematuria, and unexplained weight loss were the most frequent clinical features observed. Lower extremity swelling occurred in only three of the 54 patients.

Preoperative Evaluation. While ultrasound is excellent for screening and follow-up, magnetic resonance imaging has become the routine diagnostic test in our institution for renal cancer. This test identifies tumor thrombus in the cava with high accuracy. The advantage of magnetic resonance imaging over computed tomography has been emphasized by Myneni, et al. (48). In their study of 16 patients, magnetic resonance imaging was more accurate than computed tomography to determine the level of tumor extension in the cava, the involvement of the hepatic veins, and the invasion of the caval wall by the tumor. The gradient recall acquisition of steady-state (GRASS) imaging correctly identified the composition of thrombus in all eight patients studied and separated tumor from blood clot.

In addition to accurate preoperative imaging of the tumor, preoperative staging is most important, since the presence of local or systemic metastases are markers of poor prognosis and contraindicate extensive resection (47). In addition to the routine diagnostic workup, which includes liver function tests, chest roentgenogram, liver ultrasound, and bone scan (49), we perform computed tomography in all patients to search for pulmonary metastases.

Surgical Technique. Excision of renal carcinoma with extension into the vena cava is a challenging operation that requires expertise in vascular surgery. If the tumor extends into the right atrium, the help of a cardiac surgeon is also needed, since removal of these tumors requires profound hypothermia and cardiopulmonary bypass (50). If the tumor involves the suprarenal segment only, thoracotomy is not necessary for resection. The cava is clamped distal to the hepatic veins and the tumor thrombus is removed from a longitudinal cavotomy started at the renal veins. If the caval wall is invaded, it must be excised with a free margin. Direct closure is almost always possible and placement of a prosthetic graft (Fig. 27.14), as suggested by Katz, et al. (50), is rarely necessary. If the tumor extends into segment III, thoracolaparotomy and temporary cross-clamping of the suprahepatic inferior vena cava, with medial rotation of the liver, facilitate safe removal of all caval tumor.

Results. Perioperative mortality of these extensive operations is still significant, with early death in 9% of the patients in a series of 54 (47). The 5-year

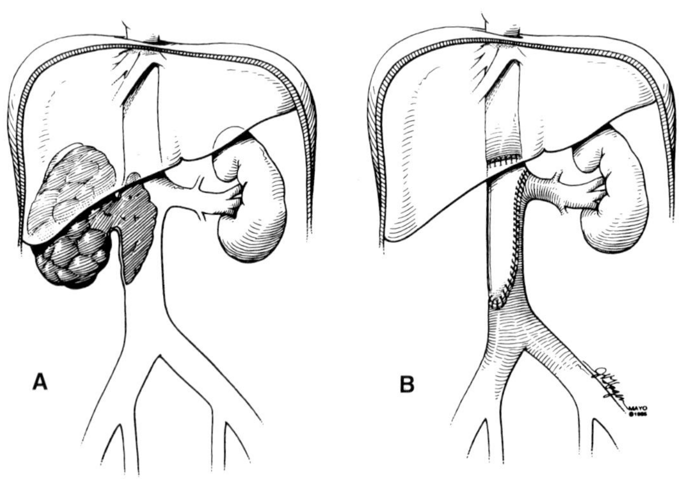

FIG. 27–14. A. Illustration of a right renal cancer invading the first and second segments of the inferior vena cava. **B.** Because of invasion of the caval wall, resection and graft placement was performed.

survival rate, however, in those patients without metastatic disease who had complete removal of the tumor was 68%. Chemotherapy or irradiation provides no significant benefit in this disease. Therefore, surgical excision with caval reconstruction continues to be the only effective method of treatment of renal cancer with caval extension in those patients who have no evidence of metastatic disease.

MEMBRANOUS OCCLUSION OF THE INFERIOR VENA CAVA

Clinical Presentation

Congenital membranous obstruction of the inferior vena cava at the level of the hepatic veins is the most frequent abnormality of the suprahepatic inferior vena cava (segment III). Symptoms of liver failure and portal hypertension dominate, and only some of the patients have persistent leg swelling. Severe lower extremity edema and venous claudication are rare. Caval occlusion can be associated with thrombosis of the hepatic veins (Budd-Chiari syndrome). In these patients, congestion of the liver may result in fibrosis and necrosis of the parenchyma, and portal hypertension and ascites develop (29). Without surgical treatment, death in the third or fourth decade of life is frequent because of liver failure or recurrent bleeding from esophageal varices (51).

Preoperative Evaluation. Laboratory tests may reveal liver or renal failure or abnormalities in nutrition and blood coagulation. Detailed imaging of the portal circulation with celiac and mesenteric arteriogram is performed. Ultrasound, computed tomography, and magnetic resonance imaging have been used to image the liver, the hepatic veins and the retrohepatic and suprahepatic inferior vena cava. Contrast cavography and direct venous pressure measurements are performed to image the cava, measure the gradient across the caval occlusion, and measure hepatic wedge pressures.

Surgical Treatment. Reports on individual cases or small series describe several types of cavoatrial bypasses for membranous occlusion of the cava (4, 29, 51–55) (Fig. 27.15**A-D**). Kieffer reported on his technique of placement of a short segmental interposition graft implanted after excision of the membranous portion of the suprahepatic inferior vena cava (29). We recently described in detail the technique of cavoatrial bypass performed through a right thoracotomy to expose the right atrium. The same exposure is used to proceed with a circumferential incision of the diaphragm to dissect the suprarenal cava after medial and anterior rotation of the liver (25). If the hepatic veins are thrombosed, cavoatrial bypass alone is not sufficient—portocaval or mesoatrial shunting is also needed.

Results. The largest experience with treatment of membranous occlusion of the vena cava comes from China. Wang, et al., implanted cavoatrial Dacron bypasses in 12 patients, nine of whom had improvement during a median follow-up of 1.5 years (54). Other surgical teams used ePTFE grafts, usually with external ring support (4, 29, 55). Kieffer, et al., recently reported their experience

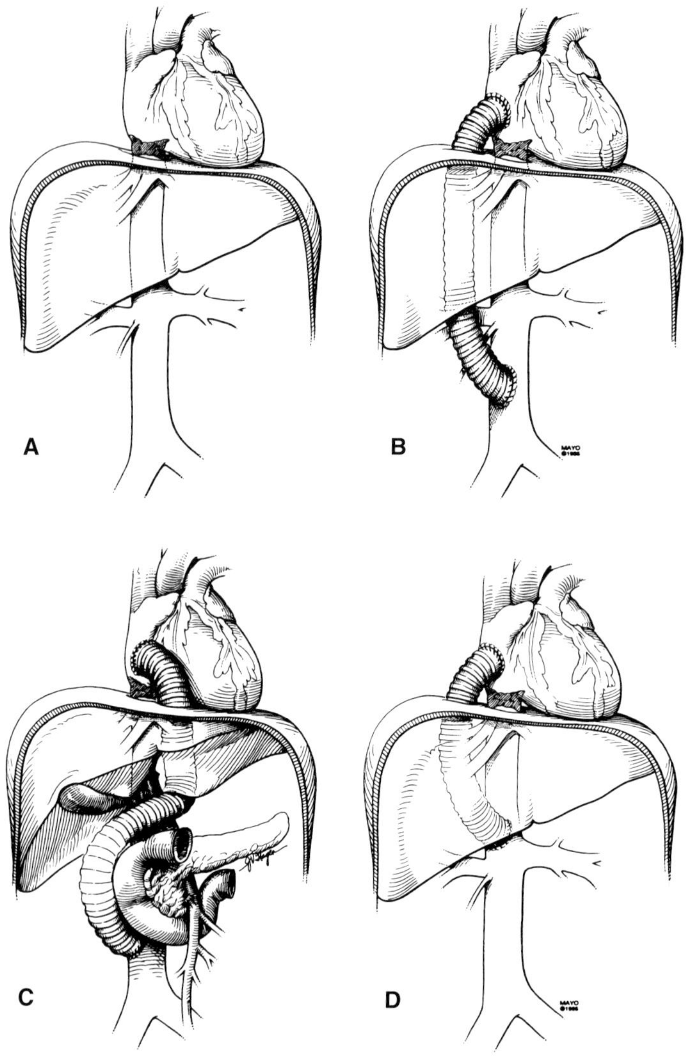

FIG. 27–15. A. Illustration of membranous occlusion of the suprahepatic inferior vena cava. **B.** Treatment with infrarenal inferior vena cava-right atrial expanded polytetrafluoroethylene graft. **C.** Inferior vena cava-right atrial graft placed in front of the hepatic pedicle and behind the left lobe of the liver. **D.** Suprarenal inferior vena cava-right atrial bypass. (Reproduced by permission from Gloviczki P, Hollier LH. Prosthetic replacement of the inferior vena cava. In: Kieffer E, ed. Surgery of the inferior vena cava and its branches. Paris: Expansion Scientifique Francaise, 1985:82–95.)

with six patients (29). Five had a patent bypass or interposition graft at a mean follow-up of 28 months after surgery. The short interposition graft, as suggested by Kieffer, appears to have the best chance of long patency. One such graft, which we implanted in a patient during orthotopic liver transplantation, has been patent

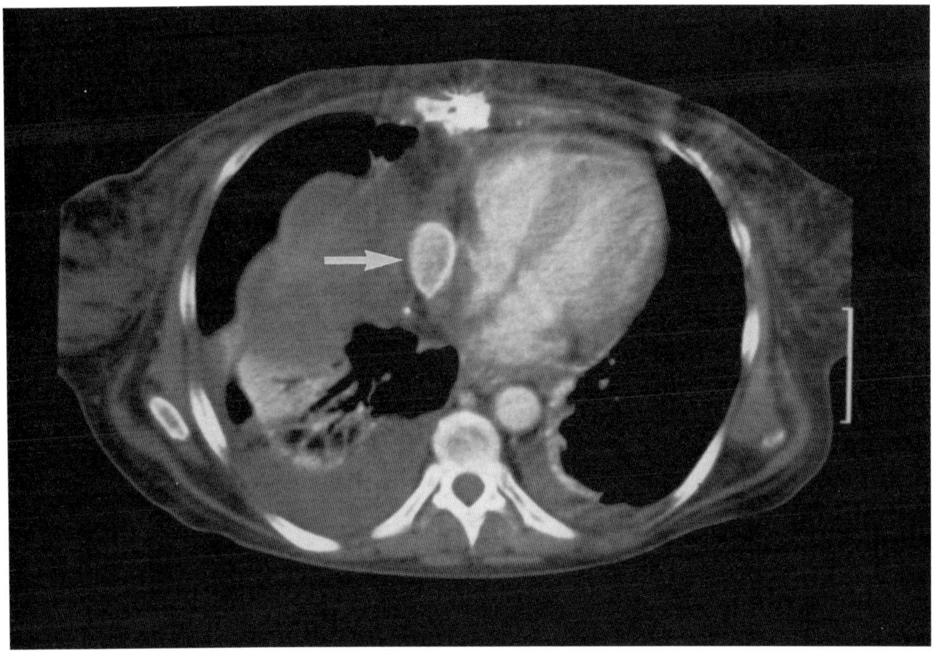

FIG. 27–16. Patent short cavoatrial interposition polytetrafluoroethylene graft (*arrow*) implanted during orthotopic liver transplantation. The graft has been patent for 5 years after surgery.

for 5 years (Fig. 27.16). Victor, et al., performed cavoatrial bypass in five patients. All five grafts were patent at the last follow-up, which extended up to 6 years after surgery (55).

The fate of the patient with membranous occlusion is determined by the extent of liver failure, the status of the hepatic veins, and the degree of portal hypertension. Orthotopic liver transplantation now offers hope to previously incurable patients with membranous occlusion of the vena cava associated with thrombosis of the hepatic veins and advanced liver failure.

REFERENCES

1. Hunter W. The history of an aneurysm of the aorta with some remarks on aneurysms in general. Med Obstet Soc Phys Lond 1757;1:323.
2. Ahmann FR. A reassessment of the clinical implications of the superior vena cava syndrome. J Clin Oncol 1984;4:961–969.
3. Sculier JP, Feld R. Superior vena cava obstruction syndrome: recommendations for management. Cancer Treat Rev 1985;12:209–218.
4. Gloviczki P, Pairolero PC, Toomey BJ, et al. Reconstruction of large veins for nonmalignant venous occlusive disease. J Vasc Surg 1992;16:750–761.
5. Bergan JJ, Yao JST. Indications for operations of the deep veins and vena cava. In: Greenhalgh RM, ed. Indications in vascular surgery. Philadelphia: WB Saunders, 1988:323–336.

6. Chen JC, Bongard F, Klein SR. A contemporary perspective on superior vena cava syndrome. Am J Surg 1990;160:207–211.
7. Yellin A, Rosen A, Reichert N, Lieberman Y. Superior vena cava syndrome. The myth—the facts. Am Rev Respir Dis 1990;141:1114–1118.
8. Doty DB. Bypass of superior vena cava: six years' experience with spiral vein graft for obstruction of superior vena cava due to benign and malignant disease. J Thorac Cardiovasc Surg 1982;83:326–338.
9. Gloviczki P, Pairolero PC, Cherry KJ Jr, Hallett JW Jr. Reconstruction of the vena cava and of its primary tributaries: a preliminary report. J Vasc Surg 1990;11:373–381.
10. Dartevelle PG, Chapelier AR, Pastorino U, et al. Long-term follow-up after prosthetic replacement of the superior vena cava combined with resection of mediastinal-pulmonary malignant tumors. J Thorac Cardiovasc Surg 1991;102:259–265.
11. Chiu CJ, Terzis J, MacRae ML. Replacement of superior vena cava with the spiral composite vein graft. Ann Thorac Surg 1974;17:555–560.
12. Doty DB, Baker WH. Bypass of superior vena cava with spiral vein graft. Ann Thorac Surg 1976;22:490–493.
13. Gloviczki P, Pairolero PC. Venous reconstruction for obstruction and valvular incompetence. In: Goldstone J, ed. Perspectives in vascular surgery. St. Louis: Quality Medical Publishing Company, 1988:75–93.
14. Benvenuto R, Rodman FSB, Gilmour J, Phillips AF, Callaghan JC. Composite venous graft for replacement of the superior vena cava. Arch Surg 1962;84:570–573.
15. Bass J Jr, Pan HC, Gottesman L. Superior vena cava syndrome: report of a new operative technique. J Int Med Assoc 1980;72:1105–1109.
16. Gladstone DJ, Pillai R, Paneth M, Lincoln JCR. Relief of superior vena caval syndrome with autologous femoral vein used as a bypass graft. J Thorac Cardiovasc Surg 1985;89:750–752.
17. Marshall WG Jr, Kouchoukos NT. Management of recurrent superior vena caval syndrome with an externally supported femoral vein bypass graft. Ann Thorac Surg 1988;46:239–241.
18. Zembala M, Kustrzycki A, Ostapczuk S, Dutkiewicz R, Hirnle T. Pericardial tube for obstruction of superior vena cava by malignant teratoma. J Thorac Cardiovasc Surg 1986;91:469–471.
19. Bergeron P, Reggi M, Jausseran J, et al. Our experience in superior vena cava surgery (in French). Ann Chir: Chir Thorac Cardiovasc 1985;39:485–491.
20. Herse B, Hannekum A, Hugel W, et al. Occlusion of the vena cava superior: an overview of therapeutic surgical options (in German). Chirurg 1986;57:565–572.
21. Herreros J, Glock Y, Fuente ADL, et al. The superior vena cava compression syndrome. Our experience of twenty six cases (in French). Ann Chir: Chir Thorac Cardiovasc 1985;39:495–500.
22. Masuda H, Ogata T, Kikuche K, Takagi K, Tanaka S. Total replacement of superior vena cava because of invasive thymoma: seven years' survival. J Thorac Cardiovasc Surg 1988;95:1083–1085.
23. Ricci C, Benedetti VF, Colini GF, Gossetti B, Mineo TC. Reconstruction of the superior vena cava: 15 years' experience using various types of prosthetic material. Ann Chir 1985;39:492–495.
24. Bardi K, Bouziri S, Jaafoura H, et al. Venous involvement in Takayasu's disease: does it exist? Ann Vasc Surg 1988;2:231–234.
25. Gloviczki P, Pairolero PC. Prosthetic replacement of large veins. In: Bergan JJ, Kistner RL, eds. Atlas of venous surgery. Philadelphia: WB Saunders, 1992:191–214.
26. Doty DB, Dory JR, Jones KW. Bypass of superior vena cava. Fifteen years' experience with spiral vein graft for obstruction of superior vena cava caused by benign disease. J Thorac Cardiovasc Surg 1990;99:889–895.

27. Moore WM Jr, Hollier LH. Reconstruction of the superior vena cava and central veins. In: Bergan JJ, Yao JST, eds. Venous disorders. Philadelphia: WB Saunders, 1991:517–527.
28. Kieffer E, Ruotolo C, Richard T, et al. Membranes and hypoplasia of the terminal inferior vena cava (in French). In: Kieffer E, ed. Surgery of the inferior vena cava and its branches. Paris: Expansion Scientifique Francaise, 1985:117–131.
29. Kieffer E, Bahnini A, Koskas F. Nonthrombotic disease of the inferior vena cava: surgical management of 24 patients. In: Bergan JJ, Yao JST, eds. Venous disorders. Philadelphia: WB Saunders, 1991:501–516.
30. Raju S, Fredericks R. Venous obstruction: an analysis of one hundred thirty-seven cases with hemodynamic, venographic, and clinical correlations. J Vasc Surg 1991;14:305–313.
31. O'Donnell TF Jr. Clinical diagnosis and classification of chronic venous insufficiency. In: Rutherford RB, ed. Vascular surgery. Philadelphia: WB Saunders, 1989:1504–1512.
32. Raju S, Fredericks RK. Late hemodynamic sequelae of deep venous thrombosis. J Vasc Surg 1986;4:73–79.
33. Gloviczki P, Calcagno D, Schirger A, et al. Non-invasive evaluation of the swollen extremity: experiences with 190 lymphoscintigraphic examinations. J Vasc Surg 1989;9:683–690.
34. Collins PS, Villavicencio JL, Abreu SH, et al. Abnormalities of lymphatic drainage in lower extremities: a lymphoscintigraphic study. J Vasc Surg 1989;9:145–152.
35. Gruss JD. Venous bypass for chronic venous insufficiency. In: Bergan JJ, Yao JST, eds. Venous disorders. Philadelphia: WB Saunders, 1991:316–330.
36. Hutschenreiter S, Vollmar J, Leoprecht H, Abendschein A, Rodl W. Reconstructive interventions of the venous system: clinical evaluation of late results using functional and vascular anatomic criteria. Chirurg 1979;50:555–563.
37. Husfeldt KJ. Venous replacement with Gore-Tex prosthesis. Experimental and first clinical results. In: May R, Weber J, eds. Pelvic and abdominal veins: progress in diagnostics and therapy. International Congress Series 550. Amsterdam: Excerpta Medica, 1981:249–258.
38. Dale WA, Harris J, Terry RB. Polytetrafluoroethylene reconstruction of the inferior vena cava. Surgery 1984;95:625–630.
39. Chan EL, Bardin JA, Bernstein EF. Inferior vena cava bypass: experimental evaluation of externally supported grafts and initial clinical application. J Vasc Surg 1984;1:675–680.
40. Raju S. New approaches to the diagnosis and treatment of venous obstruction. J Vasc Surg 1986;4:42–54.
41. Thorpe AC, Barker S, Burnand KG. Two cases of extra-anatomically bypassed inferior vena cava using polytetrafluoroethylene grafts with a concomitant distally placed arteriovenous fistula. Phlebology 1988;3:109–113.
42. Gloviczki P, Hollier LH, Dewanjee MK, et al. Experimental replacement of the inferior vena cava: factors affecting patency. Surgery 1984;95:657–666.
43. Schanzer H, Younis C, Train JS, Peirce II EC. Therapeutic implications of phlebographic obstruction in chronic venous stasis. J Cardiovasc Surg 1990;31:173–177.
44. Hobson RWI, Lee BC, Lynch TG, et al. Use of intermittent pneumatic compression of the calf in femoral venous reconstruction. Surg Gynecol Obstet 1984;159:284.
45. Dzsinich C, Gloviczki P, van Heerden JA, et al. Primary venous leiomyosarcoma: a rare but lethal disease. J Vasc Surg 1992;15:595–603.
46. Kalsbeck HL. Leiomyosarcoma of the inferior vena cava. Arch Chir Neerl 1974;26:35–40.
47. Neves RJ, Zincke H. Surgical treatment of renal cancer with vena cava extension. Br J Urol 1987;59:390–395.
48. Myneni L, Hricak H, Carroll PR. Magnetic resonance imaging of renal carcinoma with extension into the vena cava: staging accuracy and recent advances. Br J Urol 1991;68:571–578.

49. Vale JA, Hendry WF, Kirby RS, Whitfield HN, Lumley JSP. Diagnostic and surgical aspects of renal carcinoma with involvement of the inferior vena cava. Br J Urol 1991;68:345–348.
50. Katz NM, Spence IJ, Wallace RB. Reconstruction of the inferior vena cava with a polytetrafluoroethylene tube graft after resection for hypernephroma of the right kidney. J Thorac Cardiovasc Surg 1984;87:791–797.
51. Ahn SS, Yellin A, Sheng FC, Colonna JO, Goldstein LI, Busuttil RW. Selective surgical therapy of Budd-Chiari syndrome provides superior survival rates than conservative medical management. J Vasc Surg 1987;5:28–37.
52. Gloviczki P, Hollier LH. Prosthetic replacement of the inferior vena cava (in French). In: Kieffer E, ed. Surgery of the inferior vena cava and its branches. Paris: Expansion Scientifique Francaise, 1985:82–95.
53. Maillard JN, Elman A, Erlinger S, Sanguinetti J. Syndrome de Budd-Chiari par obstruction membraneuse de la veine cave inferieure. Traitement par anastomose mesenterico-cave et prothese cavo-auriculaire. Gastroenterol Clin Biol 1982;6:743–751.
54. Wang Z, Zhu Y, Wang S, et al. Recognition and management of Budd-Chiari syndrome: report of one hundred cases. J Vasc Surg 1989;10:149–156.
55. Victor S, Jayanthi V, Kandasamy I, Ratnasabapathy A, Adanagopalan N. Retrohepatic cavoatrial bypass for coarctation of inferior vena cava with a polytetrafluoroethylene graft. J Thorac Cardiovasc Surg 1986;91:99–105.

chapter 28

Axillary Subclavian Venous Thrombosis

John J. Bergan

> "... [A] regimental servant, 27 years old, previously healthy and very active, who was sent to me on April 25, 1855 by Mr. Bossey, on account of the condition of his right arm. This was swollen and when it hung down, had a feeling of weight and fullness as if the blood could not return from it. The arm was indeed about a quarter or a third larger than the other; but its chief enlargement felt as if due to a great muscular development."

So begins the description of a case of subclavian venous thrombosis, treated more than 100 years ago by Sir James Paget (1). Paget continues with a description of the therapy which included a milk diet, six leeches, and three grains of mercury with chalk. The patient did improve and then an attack of scarlatina developed, during which time "all signs of the infection of the arm disappeared." In light of present knowledge, we can guess that thrombolysis occurred and this was triggered by the severe viral infection. In this fashion, present-day lytic therapy is anticipated by accurate observations of an experienced clinician. Thus, does medical science advance.

> In June 1989, a 27-year-old man presented to the emergency room of a metropolitan Southern California hospital, describing marked swelling of his right arm and numbness and tingling on the radial aspect of the forearm and hand. Marked venous distension was seen over the arm, shoulder, and forearm. Treatment consisted of immediate heparinization, conversion to Coumadin, and long-term anticoagulation. Very little change in the arm swelling occurred. The patient experienced persistent paresthesias and pain on minor effort such as showering or driving an automobile. Ultimately, occupational retraining was required and the patient remained partially disabled 3 years after the acute event.

These two cases, treated more than 130 years apart, illustrate many of the features of axillary-subclavian venous thrombosis. They emphasize lack of progress in defining acceptable treatment to prevent disability in young persons afflicted with the condition. The marked disability demonstrated by the modern case justifies analysis of the problem and a discussion of therapeutic options available in this modern era. These are the subject of this chapter.

HISTORIC OVERVIEW

Paget's case, referred to earlier, was included in a publication of a series of lectures delivered by Sir James Paget prior to 1875. There were, in fact, two cases included in these lectures which Sir James termed "gouty phlebitis." The third case to appear in publication was von Schroetter's description of a subclavian venous thrombosis occurring during labor in the right arm of a healthy painter (2). The eponym Paget-Schroetter's syndrome was given to this condition by E.S.R. Hughes in his 1949 scholarly, monograph-like analysis of the problem (3).

A more inclusive term, thoracic outlet syndrome, was coined by Peet and the Mayo group in 1956 (4) (Fig. 28.1). Perhaps thoracic inlet syndrome would be a more accurate term for venous symptoms. The neuroarterial components imply outflow while veno-occlusive manifestations are due to inflow. However, present usage includes all components of neural, arterial, and venous symptoms within a single term, thoracic outlet syndrome. There is no need for another term, no matter how accurate.

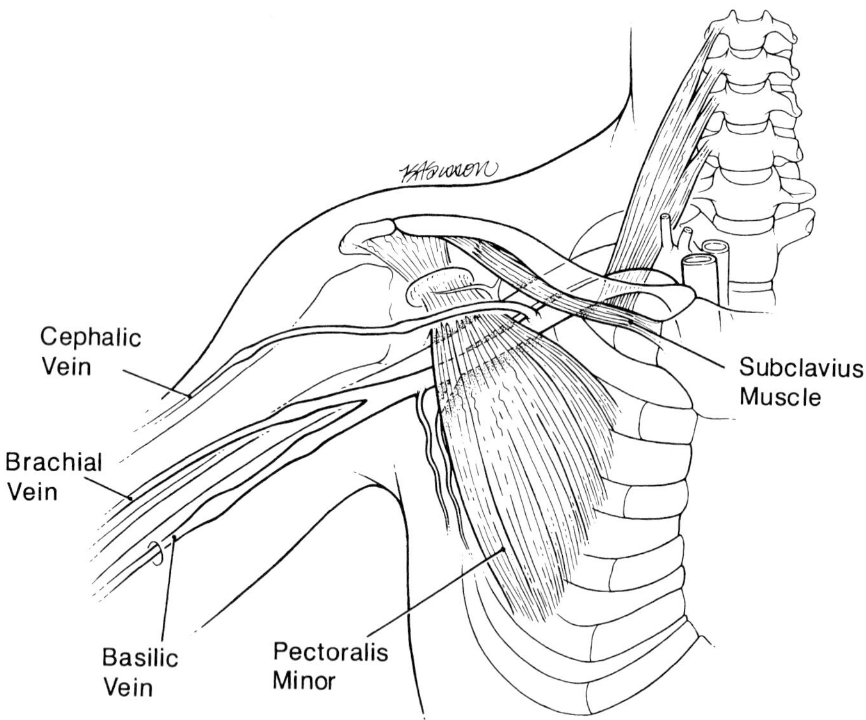

FIG. 28–1. This diagram depicts the anatomy of the thoracic outlet and emphasizes the venous structures. Note the relationship of the scalenus anticus muscle to the vein and artery, the proximity of the clavicle, and the subclavius muscle and the rib to the vein. Also note the entry of cephalic and basilic veins into the axillary subclavian axis and the prominence of the pectoralis minor in relationship to the underlying neurovascular structures.

TABLE 28-1

ANATOMIC CAUSES OF AXILLARY-SUBCLAVIAN VENOUS THROMBOSIS*

Clavicle—first rib	Pectoralis minor muscle
Subclavius muscle—first rib	Costocoracoid ligament
Costoclavicular ligament	Humeral head
Anterior scalene muscle	Prevenous phrenic nerve

*Mechanism is chronic, subclinical, and intermittent compression which produces scarring, narrowing, and eventual thrombosis. Incidence: 4–7% of manifestations of thoracic outlet compression.

Other shoulder syndromes do appear in the nomenclature. These include hyperabduction syndrome (1951) (5), cervical rib syndrome (1906) (6), scalenus anticus syndrome (1935) (7), first rib syndrome (1910) (8), costoclavicular syndrome (1943) (9), and the little known subcoracoid-pectoralis minor syndromes of Wright (1945) (10). Those are of academic, not clinical, importance. Of greater clinical interest is the syndrome of intermittent venous compression (1951) (11, 12), which may precede axillary-subclavian thrombosis (Table 28.1).

Therapy of venous occlusion of the axillary-subclavian axis has followed historically the therapy of neurovascular compression. Cervical and first rib resection had been proposed (5, 8) and scalenus anticus resection performed even before heparin and Coumadin anticoagulation became routine. Venous thrombectomy was advocated after 1970 (13) and was improved by addition of the Fogarty balloon catheter to the vascular armamentarium (14) (Table 28.2). It was natural to expect lytic therapy to be tried (15) after this became available.

Surgical therapy in addition to conventional decompressions by cervical, first rib, and scalenus resections has included clavicular resection (16), balloon dilatation (17), and direct venous reconstruction (18).

Massive edema and other stigmata of severe venous stasis have been noted after venous thrombosis in patients with a functioning arteriovenous access fistula,

TABLE 28-2

SIGNS AND SYMPTOMS OF AXILLARY-SUBCLAVIAN VENOUS THROMBOSIS*

- Swelling
- Pain
- Cyanosis
- Venous distension
- Decreased temperature (arm and hand)
- Tenderness, hypersensitivity (arm and hand)

*Asymptomatic venous occlusion occurs frequently. Intermittent venous occlusion may occur without thrombosis.

and venous reconstruction has been found useful in these cases (19). When such reconstructions have failed, spiral vein grafting has been employed (20) and endoluminal stents are now under consideration (21).

THEORY OF ETIOLOGY

In America, the pioneer vascular surgeon Rudolph Matas, writing in the early 1930s, summarized the first 50 years of recorded experience with axillary-subclavian venous thrombosis (22). He pointed out that in those days of lack of precise diagnosis, only 74 cases were described. Even in Great Britain, where Sir James described the condition in 1875, only 17 cases had been reported by 1933.

Although a great deal of attention was paid to the condition in Europe in those early days, the English-speaking medical community contributed very little knowledge to the subject. Only P.S. Lowenstein's report from St. Louis (23) emerges to give insight into the cause of the condition.

Observers of subclavian axillary venous thrombosis before the 20th century gave accurate reports. They advanced theories regarding etiology that remain today. Von Schroetter's original view (2) was that sudden stretching and compression trauma was the chief cause of the phlebitis. That opinion held for the next 20 years, when predisposing elements of the condition began to emerge. Although others contributed to this knowledge, it was Lowenstein's paper (23) that incited the greatest interest in the English language surgical community. This emphasized overstretching and contusion of the axillary vein between the clavicle, first rib, costocoracoid ligament, and subclavius muscle. In England, Gould and Patey laid special stress on the subclavius muscle and pointed out that when the muscle was stretched with the arm in the abducted position, trauma was transmitted to the vein, which might incite endophlebitis and thrombosis (24).

Today, it is recognized that intermittent venous occlusion presents all of the findings of the thrombotic syndrome without the organic occlusion (12). Leriche held that such symptoms were the result of vasomotor reflexes originating in the perivenous sympathetic nerve fibers. These, he said, caused profound venous spasm. It was acknowledged that trauma might incite such spasm and produce the manifestations of edema, venous engorgement, and diffuse swelling without organic occlusion. Leriche's influence is evidenced by the reports of relief of the condition by excision of the injured venous segment.

Matas showed extraordinary wisdom when he summarized characteristics of the syndrome. He observed that effort thrombosis affected the upper extremity almost exclusively, that the dominant arm was affected 2½ times more often than the nondominant arm, that it was a predominantly male disease, and that it was a lesion peculiar to the vigorous youth or to middle-aged sound and vigorous individuals.

Within Hughes' review of 320 cases in world literature from 1875 to 1948 is an accurate summary of major findings (3), including an accurate depiction of clinical presentation of symptomatic patients. Hughes pointed out that the incidence is at a maximum in people under 24 years of age; males are more frequently affected (78%); the right arm was reported to be involved in 66%; and swelling of the arm is often the first symptom, but pain, discomfort, or discoloration may appear quickly. The onset may be quite sudden and reaches a maximum in 24–48 hours. The whole arm and shoulder become involved in a firm, nonpitting swelling largely due to interstitial fluid accumulation. A bluish discoloration of the arm is an almost constant feature. Superficial veins, particularly those about the anterior aspect of the shoulder and chest, are visibly distended. Among the neurologic findings are paresthesias and even pruritus.

Weaknesses of a retrospective literature review may be owing to absence of technology that clarifies manifestations of the condition, e.g., Hughes' contentions, "it is doubtful whether nonfatal pulmonary embolism has ever occurred" and "the opposite arm is rarely involved." Such dogmatism derives from each previous author's description of his cases. This, in turn, depends upon available technology to define clearly the pathologic processes. Ventilation/perfusion (V/Q) scans, phlebography, pulmonary arteriography, and other modern contributions all modify interpretation of prior observations.

Because of the accuracy of Lowenstein's anatomic study (23), it is well to quote his final paragraph. He says, ". . . marked abduction or extension (throwing backward) of the arm, probably together with lateral rotation, produces a pronounced pressure by the costocoracoid ligament (furthered by the subclavius muscle) on the extended axillary vein with resultant changes in the vascular endothelium sufficient to cause an axillary thrombosis."

MODERN ETIOLOGY AND PROGNOSIS

Little can be added to the exact anatomic observations of early workers interested in this entity. However, a great deal has changed in the practice of medicine. This has markedly altered the incidence and etiology of axillary-subclavian venous thrombosis. Parenteral alimentation, pacemaker wires, and dialysis access are obvious examples of change in etiology of subclavian thrombosis. Also, contraceptive therapy increases the incidence of thromboembolic events. This risk is limited to current users, is unaffected by duration of use, and is lowest in patients taking pills with less than 50 μg of estrogen (49). Even epidemiologic studies can now be relied upon for clarifying etiology and developing strategies of prophylaxis and treatment. Bergqvist's study in Malmo is an example of this. Studying only patients with pulmonary embolism, he discovered that in 24 cases, major embolism emanated from thrombi around central venous catheters, many of which were placed in the axillary-subclavian axis (26).

Accurate modern diagnosis of pulmonary embolism has confirmed that pulmonary embolism occurs after axillary-subclavian venous thrombosis. In Torrance, California, 14 patients were examined, five of whom demonstrated pulmonary embolization confirmed by arteriogram, ventilation perfusion scans, and arterial blood gas abnormalities (27). These 14 patients are typical of modern patients with symptoms of axillary-subclavian venous thrombosis. They provide a sad commentary on hazards of modern life. In these patients, the causes of thrombosis were effort (3), trauma (3), drug abuse (4), underlying neoplastic disease (3), and congenital venous malformation (1).

An important contrast to that report is a 1988 publication that provides accurate epidemiologic information from the city of Malmo (28) , where one hospital serves all 240,000 inhabitants. The report describes all patients who underwent arm phlebography for suspected deep venous thrombosis during a 15-year period. Of 296 patients who had arm phlebography; 165 phlebograms were normal, 11 showed compression of the vein without thrombosis, and 120 had thrombosis. Of these, 73 (61%) were primary thromboses and 47 (39%) were secondary. In primary thrombosis, 66 were spontaneous, seven with effort, seven with anticonception medication, and 13 with earlier thromboembolic events. Among secondary venous thromboses were 29 indwelling catheters or pacemaker electrodes, 13 malignancies, two injections of irritant compounds, and 3 miscellaneous. None of the 73 patients with primary thrombosis had a fatal pulmonary embolus, and only one patient had symptoms mimicking pulmonary embolus. In contrast, in patients with secondary thrombosis, three had a fatal pulmonary embolus (6.4%) and another had contributory pulmonary embolus verified at autopsy.

None of the patients in this series had to change occupation due to arm disability. It is unclear from the wording of the report whether primary or secondary axillary-subclavian venous thrombosis produced a higher degree of moderate or mild symptomatology. The low incidence of morbidity and late symptomatology is strikingly at variance with other clinical observations.

TERMINOLOGY

Many terms implying etiology of this condition have been applied in the past. In particular, many forms of effort have been described to cause thrombosis. However, it is best to keep terminology as simple as possible. Therefore, present practice calls for the terms primary and secondary to be used. This primary and secondary classification was suggested by Crowell in 1960 (29) and is increasingly useful in defining the natural history of the condition. Primary implies no antecedent trauma such as placement of a venous line. This should include intermittent venous occlusion without thrombosis as the clinical findings are identical. Secondary types include the many traumatic, infectious, chemical, and coagulopathy-induced forms of venous occlusion.

NATURAL HISTORY

Natural history of axillary-subclavian occlusion has been very difficult to elucidate. Patients seen in the hospital represent only a fraction of patients who actually experience the occlusion. Perhaps the most important early modern study was that of Coon and William from the early 1960s (30). That study is flawed by the fact that only patients who were hospitalized were included. Therefore, patients with lesser symptomatology did not receive consideration. The authors' conclusion that anticoagulant therapy decreased morbidity has been perpetuated throughout the modern era.

Further perpetuation of these authors' observations and conclusions is seen in a subsequent Harvard study, similarly flawed. That report included an observation that residual disability appears in 74% of patients (31). Commentary on that paper, presented to the 1970 meeting of the International Cardiovascular Society, included DeWeese's opinion regarding aggressive employment of thrombectomy on six extremities; claviculectomy was helpful in exposing the vessel, and all patients so treated became asymptomatic despite the fact that half of the operated veins were shown to be closed on subsequent phlebography. Tilney prophetically observed: "I think . . . this condition will be seen with increasing frequency with the use of indwelling venous lines and with the use of subclavian vein catheters for long-term parenteral nutrition."

Supporting these observations are those of Campbell, et al., reporting from the University of California at San Diego (32). They wisely summarized their observations thusly: "chronic morbidity was more dependent upon etiology than on initial treatment. Thrombosis secondary to intimal injury caused no persistent symptoms, . . . effort thrombosis was intermediate [in severity], and . . . all of those with obstruction secondary to extrinsic compression had easy fatigability. The majority also had concomitant swelling, pain, and prominent collaterals."

Subsequent experience has emphasized the fact that intimal injury is an important cause of axillary-subclavian venous thrombosis in the modern era.

A very radical viewpoint was expressed by a group in Rio de Janeiro (33), who stated, "there was edema and functional impairment of the arm in all cases."

Other observations add minor information. Daskalakis and Bouhoutsos observed that "intermittent compression of the subclavian and axillary veins seems to be a clinical entity. It appears to precede thrombosis" and "cases with persistent symptoms but no venous thrombosis may have a pre-venous or accessory phrenic nerve" (34). That observation confirms that of E.S.R. Hughes in 1949.

Many students of this condition believe that secondary venous thrombosis does not often cause symptoms. When it does, they respond to brief anticoagulation (35). In contrast are observations that conclude that extrinsic obstruction, when causing the problem (primary thrombosis), allows only 50% of the patients to be symptom-free in the long term. This suggests that patients with severe symptoms are those with primary thrombosis, persistent obstruction, and little or no recanalization.

Against all these observations of morbidity following axillary-subclavian venous thrombosis is the report referred to previously from Malmo (28), which differs greatly from other reports from England and America. The Malmo experience is important because the material was not selected. The Swedish observers noted that ". . . in our unselected material, none of the patients were reported to have to change occupation due to disability of the arm. Moderate pain restricting daily activity in some way was found in five patients (4%) and mild discomfort with occasional swelling of the arm and increased tiredness in certain positions was noted in 26 patients (22%). The mean follow-up time for our material is long (8 years) and no patient was lost to follow-up." Although there are a few American observations that support those conclusions, the majority opinion from England and America emphasizes prolonged morbidity of the condition.

SPECIAL CIRCUMSTANCES

There are special forms of secondary axillary-subclavian venous thrombosis which demand attention. Among these is the particular group of patients with vascular access through subclavian vein cannulation and patients with surgically constructed upper extremity arteriovenous fistulas being used for hemodialysis in whom axillary-subclavian venous thrombosis develops. Treatment of such problems is difficult because the access site may represent the patient's last remaining available access. If this is true, ligation of the arteriovenous fistula is not a desirable solution to the problem.

Today, patients with very severe chronic venous insufficiency of the upper extremity are often found to have a proximal occlusion and a distal arteriovenous fistula. In these patients, massive edema and even cutaneous ulcerations are commonplace. The edema interferes with safe puncture of the dialysis fistula and the chronic infection of stasis ulcerations endangers the prosthetic portion of the fistula. In this circumstance, Schwab, et al. (36), advocated balloon dilatation of proximal venous stenosis. In that report, 100% of the dilatations were successful. Only 2 of 11 recurred, and these were successfully retreated. In contrast is a more typical report (37), in which 16 axillary venous dilatations were performed with initial success in 12. However, at 6 months, patency was 50% and at 1 year, only 40%. The authors state, "our experience has taught us that while axillary-subclavian vein lesions are technically easy to dilate, virtually all the stenoses will recur."

PRESENT-DAY EXPERIENCE

Upper and lower extremity venous thromboses are similar in one important aspect—that the thrombosis may be present without symptoms or clinical signs. For this reason, thrombosis, particularly around indwelling catheters and pacemaker wires, may go unnoticed. Despite this, clinically recognized and, therefore, symptomatic axillary-subclavian venous thrombosis is being increasingly identified. The etiology has shifted, however. In primary care hospitals, secondary causes of subclavian thromboses predominate (Table 28.3). Central lines for chemotherapy, fluid infusion, and dialysis are important in this regard. The malignant state also contributes, in part, because of a malignancy-associated coagulopathy and also because tumor treatment may require a central line for venous access.

TABLE 28-3

PRESENT-DAY ETIOLOGY OF AXILLARY-SUBCLAVIAN VENOUS THROMBOSIS

	Chicago (38)	Malmo (28)	Akron (39)
Primary	7	73	6
Secondary	58	47	27
Dialysis	6	—	—
Central line	12	29	13
Malignancy*	40	13	8
Other	—	5	6

*With and without indwelling catheters for chemotherapy and/or prior central lines.

TABLE 28-4

CLINICAL FINDINGS IN PATIENTS WITH PHLEBOGRAPHY-PROVEN UPPER EXTREMITY VENOUS THROMBOSIS*

	Primary (73)	Secondary (47)
Pain	54%	43%
Venous distension	45%	23%
Erythema	16%	4%
Cyanosis	10%	0%
Fever	5%	2%
Edema	96%	98%

*Modified from Lindblad B, Tengborn L, Bergqvist D. Deep vein thrombosis of the axillary-subclavian veins: Epidemiologic data, effects of different types of treatment, and late sequelae. Eur J Vasc Surg 1988;2:161–165.

Fortunately, secondary axillary-subclavian venous thrombosis presents a relatively benign course (Table 28.4). A summation of nine prospective studies in which 152 cases of subclavian venous thrombosis were identified in 539 patients undergoing subclavian venous catheterization suggests that nearly one-third of patients sustain subclavian occlusion. Of these 152 cases, 127 were totally asymptomatic. As Table 28.4 indicates, the clinical manifestations are mild in symptomatic cases in comparison to cases of primary thrombosis.

DIAGNOSTIC MODALITIES

Table 28.5 displays the currently available methods of corroborating clinical diagnosis of axillary-subclavian venous thrombosis. Following clinical evaluation, phlebography is advocated because this allows immediate treatment of the condition. However, this is true only for primary venous thrombosis without intrinsic cause. When secondary axillary-subclavian venous thrombosis is sus-

TABLE 28-5

DIAGNOSTIC MODALITIES IN AXILLARY-SUBCLAVIAN VENOUS THROMBOSIS

Clinical examination*	Venous pressure measurement
Phlebography*	MR angiogram (phlebogram)
Doppler examination	
Duplex scanning	Impedance phlebography

*Lower extremity venous thrombosis is suspected on clinical examination and confirmed by duplex scans. Upper extremity thrombosis is suspected by clinical examination but best confirmed by phlebography which leads directly to treatment by lytic agents. Duplex examination may be less sensitive than MR angiography.

pected, confirmation of diagnosis can be obtained by Doppler or duplex venous examination. As lytic therapy will usually not be considered in such a situation, the noninvasive techniques are more attractive than phlebography. Magnetic resonance imaging is probably more sensitive than duplex scan in the diagnosis of upper limb venous abnormalities, and it may be used preferentially in the future. However, at this time the ultrasound examinations are less expensive and are widely available. Follow-up phlebography is appropriate when duplex examination does not correlate with clinical presentation. Similarly, if computed tomographic scanning is indicated for other reasons, such scanning with contrast infusion will confirm the presence of an axillary-subclavian venous thrombosis. The findings of deep venous thrombosis on computerized tomography are well-known and familiar to radiologists and surgeons alike.

Venous pressure measurements have been advocated by some, and the performance of venous pressure measurements can be done during phlebography with the patient doing the shoulder bracing maneuver. Perhaps venous pressure determinations and associated phlebography are of greatest use in diagnosis of intermittent or nonthrombotic venous obstruction. In such a situation, positional phlebography with the arm abducted to 90° with or without hyperabduction, shoulder bracing in the military position will be useful. Abnormal phlebograms can be obtained in such provocative positions in normal and asymptomatic people. However, in patients exhibiting the intermittent symptomatology of nonthrombotic axillary-subclavian venous occlusion and in whom an abnormal phlebogram is obtained, such results will be important.

Impedance phlebography (IPG) has been advocated by some, but at this time can be looked upon as a step toward more accurate diagnosis by imaging techniques. Experience in the lower limb indicates that IPG may be less reliable in chronic venous obstruction. Therefore, the diagnosis of axillary-subclavian venous thrombosis is suspected on physical examination and confirmed by imaging modalities; and, if lytic therapy is indicated, the imaging modality of choice is direct phlebography.

THERAPEUTIC SUGGESTIONS

Because secondary axillary-subclavian venous thrombosis is not usually symptomatic, the vast majority of patients with indwelling lines and pacemakers do not experience symptomatology of venous thrombosis or other manifestations of venous insufficiency. However, patients who exhibit clinical signs of upper extremity venous thrombosis due to a foreign body within the axillary-subclavian axis demand treatment. Choices of treatment include anticoagulation to prevent propagation of the thrombus and/or removal of the foreign body with or without lytic therapy. Clearly, symptoms dictate need for treatment and the type of treatment to be given. It is in this situation that lytic therapy is usually undesirable. Furthermore, interventional therapy with balloon angioplasty is usually unsuccessful also. Neither is surgical decompression of the thoracic outlet appropriate. Therefore, treatment of the acute stage of central line-induced subclavian thrombosis should begin with removal of the cause of the occlusion. Anticoagulation with systemic heparin may be added if clinical findings are troublesome. Lytic therapy should be instituted in rare situations of limb threat.

As suggested in the report from Malmo, primary axillary-subclavian venous thrombosis also may not require vigorous therapy. However, until that report is confirmed by other observations, aggressive therapy should be strongly considered. Permanent upper extremity disability from axillary-subclavian venous thrombosis is only too real. The afflicted patient has a markedly restricted earning capacity and chance for full enjoyment of life. If such a patient is seen within 8 days of the onset, the following program can be initiated promptly.

After venographic confirmation of the thrombosis, the guidewire is passed through the thrombus and the infusion catheter placed just distal to the thrombosis. The guidewire is removed and lytic therapy begun. Initiation of lytic therapy does not require bolus administration of the agent. Instead, 50,000–100,000 units of urokinase is infused per hour. A low-dose heparin prophylaxis of pericatheter thrombosis is initiated in a separate site at the rate of 250–500 units of heparin per hour. Repeat phlebogram at intervals is useful in monitoring efficacy of therapy. Heparin anticoagulation is continued after lysis is achieved and also when no lysis is obtained. Oral anticoagulation with Coumadin is given for 12–24 weeks.

Prior to removal of the therapeutic infusion catheter, phlebography should be done in neutral and provocative positions. Special attention should be given to the vein beneath the pectoralis minor as well as the vein under the clavicular head.

During administration of oral prothrombin depressant therapy, a decision can be made regarding decompression of the thoracic outlet. If lytic therapy is unsuccessful and persistent thrombosis is present, little is to be gained from first rib resection. If a persistent venous spur remains following successful lytic therapy, such decompression may be elected. At this time, there are insufficient factual data to allow a definitive opinion about the benefits of rib resection following successful lytic therapy. If surgical decompression is elected, simple scalenus anticus resection will not be sufficient. The underlying pathogenetic problem is the clavicular head-subclavius muscle combination in proximity to the anterior end of the first rib. If first rib resection is elected, this should not be done through the supraclavicular approach. The portion of first rib which compresses the axillary vein is under the clavicle and cannot be resected supraclavicularly. Therefore, surgical decompression inevitably will require a transaxillary first rib resection with very careful attention to the anterior aspect of the rib in immediate proximity to the subclavian vein.

Unsuccessful lysis of the subclavian thrombus or anticoagulant therapy alone without lytic therapy may leave the patient with residual symptoms of venous insufficiency. It is in this situation that thoracic outlet decompression is most controversial. Advocates of first rib resection argue that venous collaterals are decompressed and the patient is improved.

There is little logic to such an argument and even less physiologic proof. Until such proof is available, first rib resection should not be done. Instead, it should be considered only for those patients in whom lytic therapy has been successful or in treatment of symptomatic, intermittent venous compression without occlusion. Balloon dilation of residual stenosis after lytic therapy has been disappointing. Even the most successful of initial results have been followed by restenosis, probably because extrinsic pressure is unaffected by intraluminal dilatation. The utility of percutaneously placed expandable stents in this context is untested.

Chronic Subclavian Venous Obstruction

Patients disabled by subclavian venous obstruction may be candidates for direct venous reconstruction (40). Two options are available: venous bypass or endovenectomy and venoplasty. Venous bypass has been done by turning down the distal end of the jugular vein and performing a single axillary-jugular venovenous anastomosis. Also, use of cephalic vein and free saphenous vein transplants have been reported.

Endovenectomy after medial clavicular resection has much theoretic appeal for persons truly disabled. The adjacent jugular vein serves as a near-ideal patch and clavicular resection produces no disability and little cosmetic deformity.

Direct venous reconstruction of the axillary-subclavian axis has been disappointing, however. Neither autogenous reconstructions nor use of prosthetic grafts have been done enough to be classified as reliably successful. When success has been obtained, it has commonly been in association with a distal arteriovenous fistula (see Chapter 27). An example of this is the patient on hemodialysis in whom it is necessary to preserve the access site. A proximal venous reconstruction allows this. Jain and Smejkal have even reported successful reconstruction after a primary graft failure in such a situation. This was accomplished by use of a spiral vein graft (20).

REFERENCES

1. Paget J. Clinical lectures and essays. London: Longmans, Green & Company, 1875.
2. Von Schroetter L. Erkankungender gefasse. In: Nothnagel H, ed. Handbuch der Pathologie und Therapie. Vienna: Holer, 1884.
3. Hughes ESR. Venous obstruction in the upper extremity (Paget-Schroetter's syndrome): a review of 320 cases. Int Abs Surg 1949;88:89–127.
4. Peet AM, Henriksen JD, Anderson TP, et al. Thoracic outlet syndrome. Mayo Clin Proc 1956;31:281–287.
5. Beyer JA, Wright IS. The hyperabduction syndrome. Circulation 1951;4:161–172.
6. Murphy JB. The clinical significance of cervical ribs. Surg Gynecol Obstet 1906; 3:514–520.
7. Ochsner A, Gage M, DeBakey M. Scalenus anticus (Naffziger) syndrome. Am J Surg 1906;28:669–695.
8. Murphey T. Brachial neuritis caused by pressure of first rib. Aust Med J 1910; 15: 582–585.
9. Falconer MA, Weddel G. Costoclavicular compression of the subclavian artery and vein. Lancet 1943;2:539–544.
10. Wright IS. The neurovascular syndrome produced by hyperabduction of the arms. Am Heart J 1945;29:1–19.
11. McClerry RS, Kesterson JE, Kirtley JA, et al. Subclavius and anterior scalene muscle compression as a cause of intermittent obstruction of the subclavian vein. Ann Surg 1951;133:588–602.

12. Adams JT, DeWeese VA, Mahoney EB, et al. Intermittent subclavian vein obstruction without thrombosis. Surgery 1968;63:147–165.
13. DeWeese JA, Adams JT, Gaiser DL. Subclavian venous thrombectomy. Circulation 1970;16(Suppl 2):158.
14. Inahara T. Surgical treatment of "effort" thrombosis of the axillary and subclavian veins. Am J Surg 1968;34:479–483.
15. Becker GJ, Holden RW, Rabe FE, et al. Local thrombolytic therapy for subclavian and axillary vein thrombosis. Radiology 1983;149:419–423.
16. Lord JW Jr. Critical reappraisal of diagnostic and therapeutic modalities for thoracic outlet syndromes. Surg Gynecol Obstet 1989;168:337–340.
17. Fankuchen EI, Neff RA, Collins RA, et al. Urokinase perfusion for axillary-subclavian vein thrombosis. Cardiovasc Intervent Radiol 1984;7:90–93.
18. Jacobson JH, Haimov M. Venous revascularization of the arm. Surgery 1977;81:599–604.
19. McCready RA, Hyde GL, Schwartz RW, et al. Massive upper extremity edema following vascular access surgery. Ann Vasc Surg 1988;2:75–78.
20. Jain KM, Smejkal R. Use of spiral vein graft to bypass occluded subclavian vein. J Cardiovasc Surg 1988;29:572–573.
21. Jakob H, Maass D, Schmeidt W, et al. Treatment of major venous obstruction with an expandable endoluminal spiral prosthesis. J Cardiovasc Surg 1989;30:112–117.
22. Matas R. Primary thrombosis of the axillary vein caused by strain. Report of a case with comments on diagnosis, pathogeny, and treatment of this lesion in its medicolegal relations. Am J Surg 1934;24:642–666.
23. Lowenstein PS. Thrombosis of the axillary vein. An anatomic study. JAMA 1924;82:854–857.
24. Gould EP, Patey DH. Primary thrombosis of the axillary vein: a study of 8 cases. Br J Surg 1928;16:208–212 (cited by Matas [22]).
25. Vessey M, Mant D, Smith A, et al. Oral contraceptives and venous thromboembolism: findings in a large prospective trial. Br Med J 1986;29:226.
26. Bergqvist D, Lindblad B. A 30-year survey of pulmonary embolism verified at autopsy: an analysis of 1,274 surgical patients. Br J Surg 1985;72:105–108.
27. Harley DP, White RA, Nelson RJ, et al. Pulmonary embolism secondary to venous thrombosis of the arm. Am J Surg 1984;147:221–224.
28. Lindblad B, Tengborn L, Bergqvist D. Deep vein thrombosis of the axillary-subclavian veins: epidemiologic data, effects of different types of treatment, and late sequelae. Eur J Vasc Surg 1988;2:161–165.
29. Crowell DL. Effort thrombosis of the subclavian and axillary vein. Ann Int Med 1960;52:1337–1343.
30. Coon WW, William PW III. Thrombosis of axillary and subclavian veins. Arch Surg 1967;94:657–662.
31. Tilney NL, Griffith HJG, Edwards EA. Natural history of major venous thrombosis of the upper extremity. Arch Surg 1970;101:792–796.
32. Campbell CB, Chandler JG, Tegtmeyer CJ, et al. Axillary, subclavian, and brachiocephalic vein obstruction. Surgery 1977;82:816–826.
33. Brochner G, Rojas M, Armas AJ, et al. Axillary-subclavian venous thrombosis. J Cardiovasc Surg 1989;30:108–111.
34. Daskalakis E, Bouhoutsos J. Subclavian and axillary vein compression of musculoskeletal origin. Br J Surg 1980;67:573–576.
35. Donayre CE, White GH, Mehringer SM, et al. Pathogenesis determines late morbidity of axillosubclavian vein thrombosis. Am J Surg 1986;152:179–184.
36. Schwab SJ, Quarles D, Middleton JP, et al. Hemodialysis-associated subclavian vein stenosis. Kidney Intern 1988;33:1156–1159.

37. Glanz S, Gordon DH, Lipkowitz GS, et al. Axillary and subclavian stenosis: percutaneous angioplasty. Radiology 1988;168:371–373.
38. McCarthy WJ, Vogelzang RJ, Bergan JJ. Changing concepts and present day etiology of upper extremity venous thrombosis. In: Bergan JJ, Yao JST, eds. Venous disorders. Philadelphia: WB Saunders, 1990:407–420.
39. Hovattas MC, Wright DJ, Fenton AH, et al. Changing concepts of deep venous thrombosis of the upper extremity. Surgery 1988;104:561–567.
40. Saunders RJ, Haug CE. Management of subclavian vein obstruction. In: Bergan JJ, Kistner RL, eds. Atlas of venous surgery. Philadelphia: WB Saunders, 1991:255–272.

SUGGESTED READING

Aziz S, Straehley CJ, Whelan TJ Jr. Effort-related axillosubclavian thrombosis. Am J Surg 1988;152:57–61.

Druy WM, Trout HH, Giordano JM, et al. Lytic therapy in the treatment of axillary and subclavian vein thrombosis. J Vasc Surg 1985;2:821–827.

Fraschini G, Jadeja J, Lawson M, et al. Local infusion of urokinase for the lysis of thrombosis associated with permanent central venous catheters in cancer patients. J Clin Oncol 1987;5:672–678.

Jackson NJ, Nanson EM. Intermittent subclavian vein obstruction. Br J Surg 1961;49:303–306.

Jones JC, Balkcom IL, Worman RK. Pulmonary embolus after treatment for subclavian-axillary vein thrombosis. Postgrad Med 1987;82:244–249.

Kunkel JM, Machleder HI. Treatment of Paget-Schroetter syndrome: a staged, multidisciplinary approach. Arch Surg 1989;124(10):1153–1158.

Landercasper J, Gall W, Fischer M, et al. Thrombolytic therapy of axillary-subclavian venous thrombosis. Arch Surg 1987;122:1072–1075.

Prescott SM, Tikoff G. Deep venous thrombosis of the upper extremity: a reappraisal. Circulation 1979;59:350–355.

Roos DB. Thoracic outlet syndromes: update 1987. Am J Surg 1987;154:566–573.

Sanders RJ, Raymer S. The supraclavicular approach to scalenectomy and first rib resection: description of technique. J Vasc Surg 1985;2:751–756.

Stevenson IM, Parry EW. Radiological study of the aetiological factors in venous obstruction of the upper limb. J Cardiovasc Surg 1975;16:580–585.

Sullivan KL, Minken SL, White RI Jr. Treatment of a case of thromboembolism resulting from thoracic outlet syndrome with intra-arterial urokinase infusion. J Vasc Surg 1988;7:568–571.

Swinton NW, Edgett JW Jr, Hall RJ. Primary subclavian-axillary vein thrombosis. Circulation 1968;38:737–745.

Theiss W, Wirtzfeld A. Fibrinolytische Behandlung von akuten und subakuten Thrombosen der tiefen Venen des Schultergurtels. DMW 1982;107:933–936.

Wurtz A, Quandalle P, Lemaitre L, et al. Innominate vein compression syndrome. Br J Surg 1989;76:575–576.

Zimmerman R, Harenberg J, Gerhardt P. Urokinase therapy of subclavian-axillary vein thrombosis. Klin Wochenschr 1981;59:851–856.

chapter 29

Investigation of Lymphedema

Hugo Partsch

DEFINITION AND CLASSIFICATION

Lymphedema is defined as tissue swelling due to a failure of lymph drainage. Based on etiology, lymphedema can be divided into primary (idiopathic) and secondary lymphedema. Hereditary forms are called Nonne-Milroy's disease for the congenital and Meige's syndrome for the type which starts at puberty. The praecox form occurs predominantly in females with onset in the second and third decades. Lymphedema tardum occurs, by definition, after the age of 35.

From a practical standpoint, malignant diseases should be ruled out in every patient older than 35 years of age who has lymphedema. Nonmalignant causes for secondary lymphedema include trauma, surgical removal of lymph nodes, radiotherapy, and infections including invasion with *Wuchereria bancrofti* (filariasis) (1–3).

CLINICAL DIAGNOSIS

The diagnosis of lymphedema can be suspected on clinical grounds in the majority of cases. However, with mild or initial stages, or when mixed with venous obstructions and lipedema, diagnostic difficulties may occur.

Elephantiasis with involvement of the entire limb is easily recognized. Firm and nonpitting edema, limited folding of the skin (Stemmer's sign), deepened natural skin-folds, and hyperkeratosis with papillomatosis are typical features (Fig. 29.1).

Mild forms of lymphedema with distal distribution often pose a difficult diagnostic challenge. Unilateral swelling of the back of a foot with slightly increased skin markings and thickened skin folds of the toes which prevent pinching of skin, particularly at the base of the second toe, are often misdiagnosed. In such cases, supplementary investigative procedures are essential.

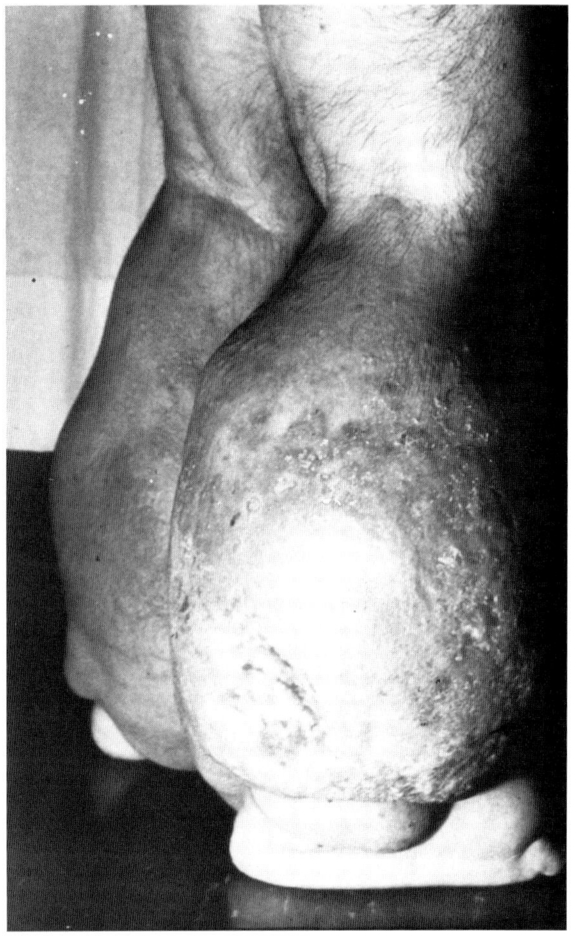

FIG. 29–1. Massive lymphedema tardum (elephantiasis).

Quantitative Lymphoscintigraphy

Today isotope lymphography is the most appropriate method for routine diagnosis of lymphedema (4–7). The essential function of the lymphatic system of transporting such large molecules back to the vascular compartment can be tested by introducing labeled proteins or colloids into the tissue. This method reveals functional information rather than anatomic details.

External scintillation detection using a gamma camera is usually performed in the region of the injection depots (radiocolloid uptake into lymphatics), in the extremity (transit in the large collectors), and over the regional lymph nodes (storage of the colloid).

Based on more than 20 years of experience with different kinds of isotope lymphography studies (6, 8–10), the following methodologic recommendations can be made:

1. Since lymph transport is mainly affected by muscular activity, a standardized stress test is an essential prerequisite for quantitative data.
2. The prefascial lymph transport should be studied after subcutaneous injection

of the tracer. Intracutaneous injection does not permit unequivocal demarcation between lymphedema and normals.
3. The subfascial lymph transport should be studied after intramuscular tracer-injection.
4. Measurement of the clearance rate of the tracer from the depot does not always distinguish between healthy subjects and lymphedema patients.
5. Quantification of storage rates over the regional lymph nodes is not reliable without taking into account the different distances between the lymph nodes and the detector.

Mostbeck and coworkers have described a method which permits exact measurement of lymph node uptake as a percentage of the dose administered, using a combination of transmission and emission scintigraphy (9, 10).

Method. The patient is irradiated with a ^{57}Co area source which allows the regional absorption to be calculated. This is followed by the subcutaneous (interdigital webs) or intramuscular (dorsal lower leg) injection of 1 mCi ^{99m}Tc-labeled microcolloid (Nanocoll), after which the patient walks for 15 minutes on a horizontal treadmill at a speed of 3.2 km/h. Emission scintigraphy is then performed with ventral and dorsal views.

Lymph node storage can be calculated as a percentage of the dose from the geometrical mean of these two frames and the correction matrix of the transmission scintigraphy.

Results. Pertinent results are illustrated in Figure 29.2. As can be seen, intracutaneous tracer injection does not allow a differentiation between healthy persons and lymphedema patients. Subfascial lymph transport is extremely reduced in patients with lymphedema, as well as patients with a postthrombotic syndrome (PTS). Figure 29.3 shows an example. One advantage of this quantitative method over traditional technique is that subclinical forms of lymphedema can also be detected (Fig. 29.4).

Using the quantitative method, one can show that erysipelas (cellulitis) is preceded by a disturbed lymph flow in the majority of the cases (11).

Studies with isotopic lymphography in patients with chronic venous insufficiency (12, 13) can be summarized as follows:

There is a statistically significant increase in prefascial lymph transport (lymph node storage rates) after tracer injection into dermatosclerotic skin areas of the lower leg;

A decrease in prefascial lymph transport with tracer injection into the border of an ulcer and in cases with recurrent erysipelas; and

A decrease in subfascial lymph transport (intramuscular tracer injection) in patients with deep vein thrombosis and with postthrombotic syndrome (PTS).

Indirect Lymphography

The development of new contrast media enables us to opacify skin lymphatics by injecting these dyes intradermally. Although anatomic information

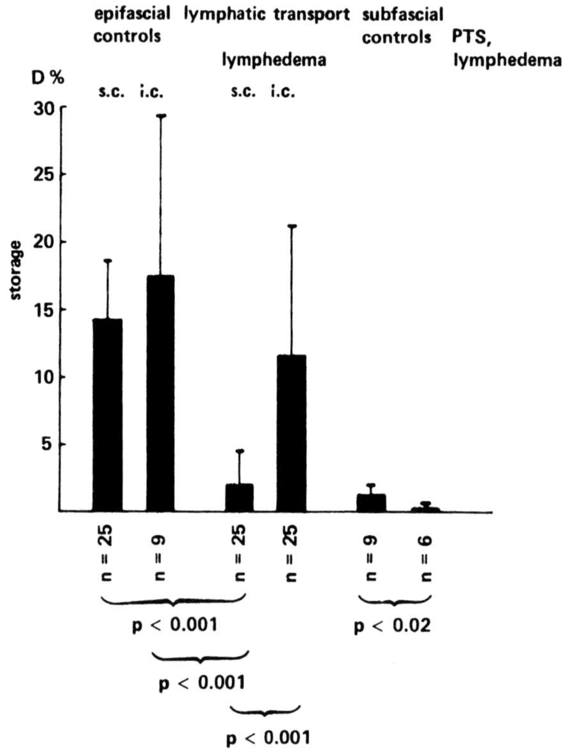

FIG. 29–2. Storage rates (percentile activity of injected dosage) in the inguinal lymph nodes in different groups of patients.

about deep lymphatics and lymph nodes is not obtained, this method does give a valuable picture of the local dermal lymphatics and provides important clues about the lymph drainage of the limb as a whole.

Method. Nonionic, water-soluble, dimeric, hexaiodinated contrast agents such as Iotasul or Iotrolan are infused by a motor pump (0.12 ml/min) subepidermally using thin, butterfly needles with a total amount of 2–4 ml per

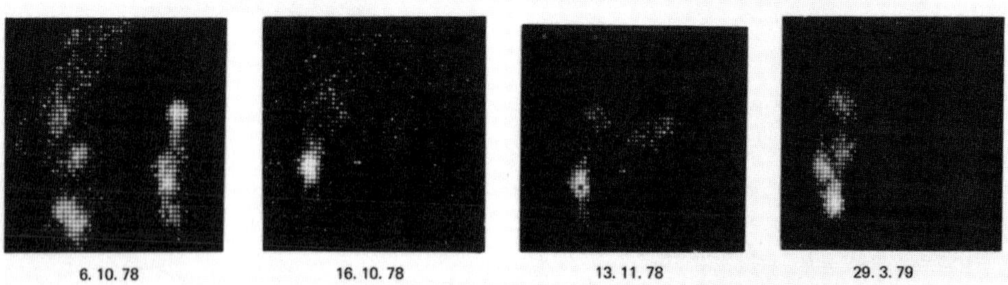

FIG. 29–3. Lymph node scanning in a patient suffering from recurrent erysipelas on his left lower leg. *6.10.78* = First acute signs; *16.10.78* = Reduced lymph drainage on the left side; *13.11.78* = Slight improvement. *29.3.79* = A new attack in January 1979 again severely reduced lymph transport (no visible lymph nodes on left side).

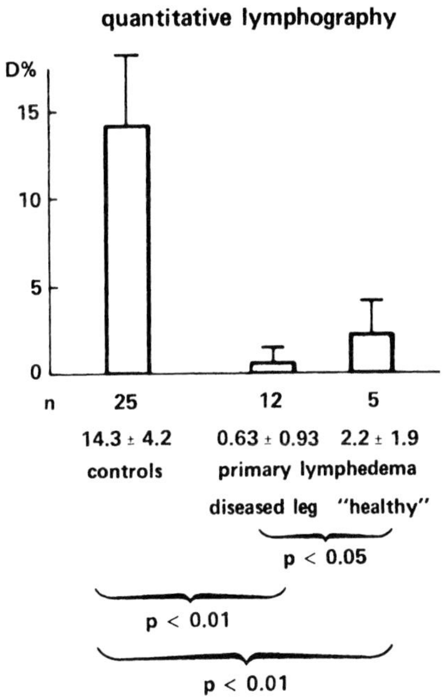

FIG. 29–4. By quantitative isotopic lymphography it can be demonstrated that in patients with primary lymphedema there is a statistically significant reduction in lymph transport in the diseased leg and also in the "normal" appearing contralateral leg.

injection site. It is essential that the tip of the needle be situated in the uppermost part of the dermis, resulting in a bluish, glassy-appearing wheal. Under normal conditions, lymphatics begin to fill after a few minutes. This can be observed by an image converter and documented on mammography films at 5-minute intervals.

Results. The infused contrast medium forms growing depots which taper into peripheral lymph collectors of normal skin. These collectors can be followed for about 10–30-cm length on average. Under pathologic circumstances, retrograde flow of the contrast medium leads to a filling of small skin lymphatics ("dermal backflow"), which constitutes the "precollector" part of the dermal lymphatics.

In lymphedematous skin, four different patterns can be observed:

Type I: No lymphatics can be demonstrated. Instead the contrast medium spreads in a cuff-like pattern obviously marking the adventitial space of blood vessels. This feature is found especially in congenital lymphedema.

Type II: Type II is characterized by a dense network of small precollector skin lymphatics and by rather sparse lymph collectors. This pattern is found mainly in patients with peripheral lymphedema praecox and tardum (Fig. 29.5).

Type III: Precollector skin lymphatics and lymph collectors are both enlarged, possibly due to proximal obstruction. Patients with lymphedematous involvement of the entire limb tend to show this constellation.

Type IV: Neither precollector lymphatics nor collectors can be found. This pattern can be seen due to "die-back" of lymphatics in the presence of proximal abnormalities. Technical problems in patients with extremely dense and thick skin can also yield a similar picture.

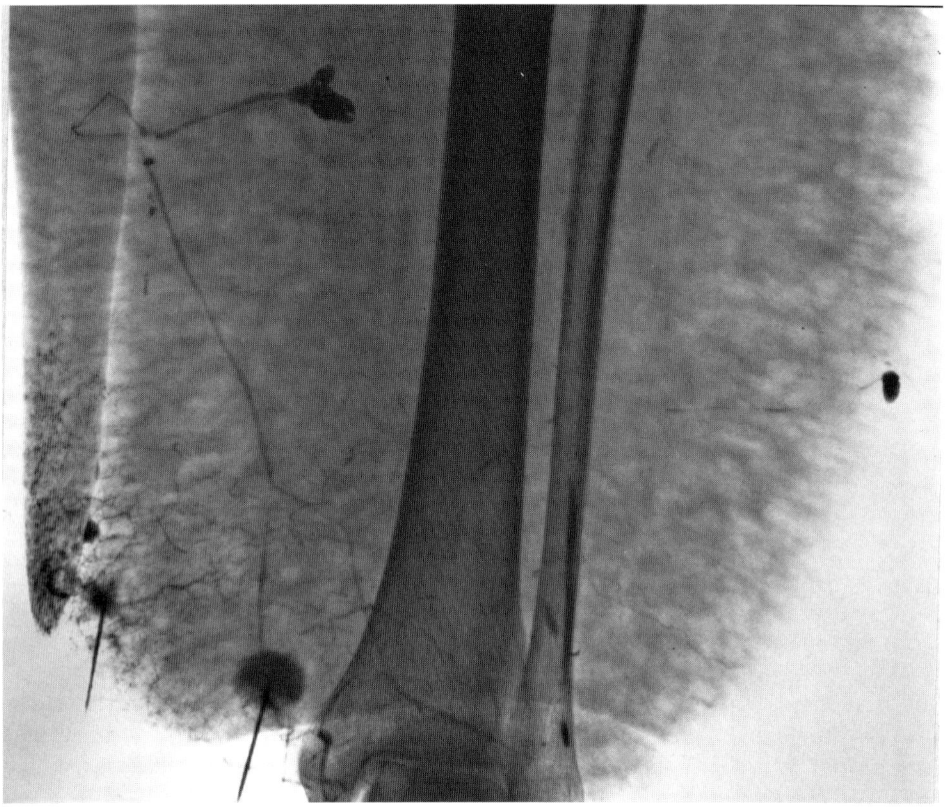

FIG. 29–5. Indirect lymphography in the patient in Figure 29.1. After subepidermal dye injection, dermal backflow and venous drainage can be shown. Only a few lymph collectors are opacified.

This indirect lymphography technique has allowed us to recognize unique lymphatic patterns not only in the lymphedema of limbs (17), but also in lipodermatosclerosis of the lower leg due to chronic venous insufficiency (13), in cases of stasis papillomatosis (18), and in lipedema (16). For example, infusing the contrast medium into the dermatosclerotic area of the distal lower leg caused by venous incompetence leads to an opacification of wide prefascial lymph collectors. At the same time, the precollector lymphatics are filled by dermal backflow as a sign of valvular incompetence of the skin lymphatics. They are irregularly shaped, fragmented, and show extravasation of the dye into the tissue (Fig. 29.6).

These findings are indicative of microlymphangiopathy in the skin caused by venous incompetence and are comparable with the results obtained with microlymphangiography (19). The wide and well-filled lymph collectors correlate with an increased prefascial lymph transport demonstrated by isotopic lymphography in the presence of venous hypertension. No lymphatics can be filled by injecting the dye into the border of a venous ulcer. Lipedema, which is often confused with lymphedema, shows a very characteristic and quite specific pattern—in the region of the leg edema the depot of the contrast medium shows a flame-shaped structure (Fig. 29.7). The collectors display a tortuous configuration. Indirect lymphography on the dorsum of the foot, which is free from edema, shows a normal pattern.

Practical Application. Indirect lymphography is similar in principle to the traditional patent blue test. However, details of lymphatic drainage of the skin can be demonstrated with much higher accuracy. Regional lymph nodes are only rarely opacified and the technique is not suited to the direct assessment of proximal lymphatics and lymph nodes. However, this method may be helpful in excluding patients from proximal shunting operations. When peripheral skin lymphatics are absent (type I), and also when pathologic changes are mainly confined to the distal dermal lymphatics (type II), lymphatic bypass surgery does not appear sensible. When extensive peripheral changes (type IV) have occurred due to

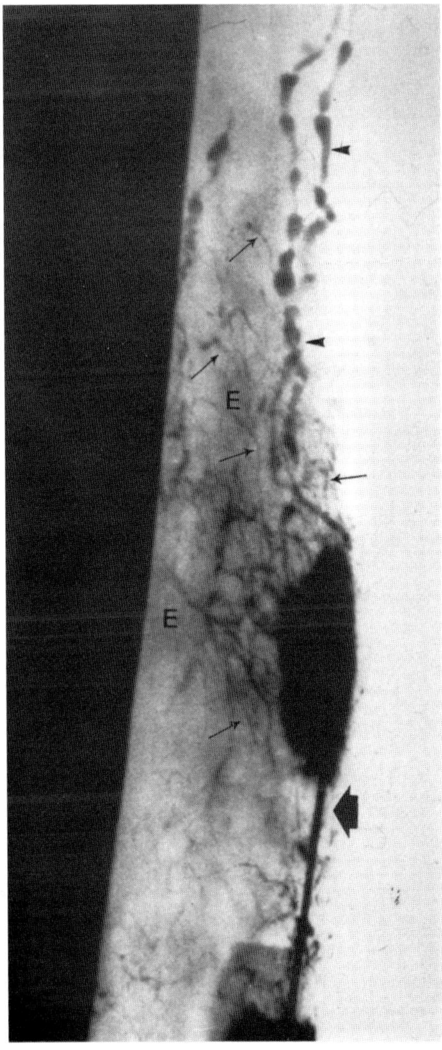

FIG. 29–6. Indirect lymphography in the region of lipodermatosclerosis. The *thick arrow* points to the injection needle. The *medium-sized arrows* point to large collectors, which show increased contractions, and the *thin arrows* point to smaller lymphatics filled by retrograde flow ("dermal backflow"). *E* indicates extravasation of the dye.

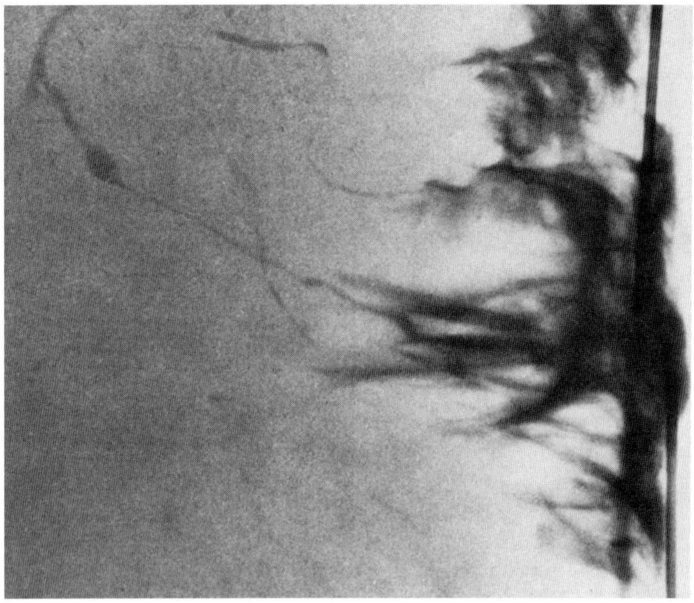

FIG. 29–7. Flame-like distribution of the contrast medium depot in lipedema.

proximal disease, results of surgery such as shunting procedures can be expected to be poor. Indirect lymphography may thus be useful for routine diagnosis and is complementary to isotopic lymphography.

Fluorescence Microlymphangiography

The superficial lymphatic capillary network of the skin can be seen under the vital microscope by subepidermal injection of fluorescing macromolecules (dextran coupled to fluorescein-isothiocyanate = FITC-dextran). Morphology and extent of tracer propagation within the dermal lymphatic network can be assessed by video analysis (20). Diminution or obstruction of more proximal lymphatics results in the visualization of an extensive network owing to cutaneous reflux and horizontal flow through incompetent skin lymphatics. In some cases of primary lymphedema, a total aplasia of initial skin lymphatics has been demonstrated. Microlymphangiopathy with extravasation of the dye can be shown in skin areas altered by chronic venous insufficiency (19). At the present time, the practical application of this method is limited, mainly due to the lack of easy availability of the necessary equipment.

Patent Blue Test and Direct Lymphangiography

Intravital dyes such as patent blue have been used for some time to delineate subcutaneous lymphatics prior to direct cannulation for x-ray lymphography. Since the dye injection provides information regarding the local clearance of the dye by the area lymphatics, it can be of value for detecting lymphatic abnormalities. An injection of 0.1–0.5 ml of an 11% aqueous solution of patent blue is made into the first and third interdigital webs of the foot or into an area of interest intra- or subcutaneously. From the extent and the pattern of distribution of the dye, conclusions may be drawn regarding the existence of dermal backflow and leakage into tissue. However, it must be stressed that there is a considerable overlapping between pathologic and normal findings (21).

The direct method of x-ray lymphography (22) is performed by cannulating a lymph collector marked by patent blue injection and by infusion of 5–20 ml contrast medium into the cannulated duct. Oily contrast media are no longer used to obtain optimal information about the lymph nodes. Since such agents may damage the already sparse lymphatics, their use is contraindicated in patients with primary lymphedema. Fat embolism leading to pulmonary dysfunction is a well-recognized complication of the oily agents used in the past for this purpose. Water-soluble media are safer and provide sufficient contrast for diagnosis, especially if xeroradiograms are taken (23).

Direct lymphography utilizing the newer water-soluble media can no longer be recommended as a tool for routine diagnosis of lymphedema. It should be restricted to cases in which specific questions concerning a radiotherapeutic or surgical intervention cannot be answered by ultrasound or computer tomography alone.

SUMMARY

In clinical practice the diagnosis of lymphedema can be established by isotope lymphography. Other investigative techniques such as indirect lymphography, microlymphangiography, and patent blue test may add useful information in certain cases. Direct lymphography should be restricted to answering very specific questions for choice and assessment of therapeutic interventions in selected cases.

REFERENCES

1. Földi M. Insufficiency of lymph flow. In: Földi M, Casley-Smith JR, eds. Lymphangiology. Stuttgart: Schattauer, 1983:195–213.
2. Olszewski WL. Clinical picture of lymphedema. In: Olszewski WL, ed. Lymph stasis: pathophysiology, diagnosis and treatment. Boca Raton, FL: CRC Press, 1991:347–377.
3. Casley-Smith JR. Discussion of the definition, diagnosis and treatment of lymphedema (lymphostatic disorder). In: Casley-Smith JR, Piller NB, eds. Progress in lymphology. Proceedings of the Xth International Congress of Lymphology. South Australia: University of Adelaide Press, 1985:1–16.
4. Zum Winkel K, Sheer KE. Scintigraphic and dynamic studies of the lymphatic system with radiocolloids. Minerva Nucl 1965:390–397.
5. Hauser W, Atkins AL, Richards P. Lymph nodes scanning with ^{99m}Tc sulfur colloid. Radiology 1969;92:1369–1373.
6. Lofferer O, Mostbeck A, Partsch H. Nuklearmedizinische Diagnostik von Lymphtransportstörungen der unteren Extremitäten. Vasa 1972;1:94–101.

7. Cluzan R, Pecking A. Radionuclide lymphography. In: Olszewski WL, ed. Lymph stasis: pathophysiology, diagnosis and treatment. Boca Raton, FL: CRC Press, 1991:398–408.
8. Haid H, Lofferer O, Mostbeck A, Partsch H. Die Lymphkinetik beim postthrombotischen Syndrom unter Kompressionsverbänden. Med Klin 1968;63:754–759.
9. Mostbeck A, Lofferer O, Kahn P, et al. Quantitative lymphographie. In: Höfer R, Bergmann H, eds. Radioaktive Isotope in Klinik und Forschung. Wien: Egermann, 1984;16:489–498.
10. Mostbeck A, Kahn P, Partsch H. Quantitative lymphography in lymphoedema. In: Bollinger A, Partsch H, Wolfe JHN, eds. The initial lymphatics. New York: Thieme-Stratton, 1985:123–130
11. Stöberl Ch, Partsch H. Erysipel und Lymphödem—Ei oder Henne? Z Hautkr 1987;62:56–62.
12. Partsch H. Lymphangiopathie bei chronischer Veneninsuffizienz. Phlebol Proktol 1984;13:85–89.
13. Partsch H, Urbanek A, Wenzel-Hora, B. Dermal lymphangiopathy in chronic venous incompetence. In: Bollinger A, Partsch H, Wolfe JHN, eds. The initial lymphatics. New York: Thieme-Stratton, 1985:178–187.
14. Partsch H, Wenzel-Hora BI, Urbanek A. Differential diagnosis of lymphedema after indirect lymphography with Iotasul. Lymphology 1983;16:12–18.
15. Partsch H, Urbanek A, Wenzel-Hora BI. The dermal lymphatics in lymphoedema visualized by indirect lymphography. Br J Dermatol 1984;110:431–438.
16. Partsch H, Stöberl Ch, Urbanek A, Wenzel-Hora BI. Clinical use of indirect lymphography in different forms of leg edema. Lymphology 1988;21:152–160.
17. Partsch H, Bollinger A. Regionale Hypoplasie dermaler Lymphgefässe—eine neue Variante des kongenitalen Lymphödems. Wien Klin Wochenschr 1986;98:704–708.
18. Stöberl Ch, Partsch H. Lymphostatische Stauungspapillomatose. Hautarzt 1988;39:441–446.
19. Franzeck UK, Isenring G, Bollinger A. Lymphatic microangiopathy in chronic venous insufficiency. In: Bollinger A, Partsch H, Wolfe, JHN eds. The initial lymphatics. New York: Thieme-Stratton, 1985:171–177.
20. Bollinger A, Jäger K, Sgier F, Seglias J. Fluorescent microlymphography. Circulation 1981;64:1195–1200.
21. Brunner U, Pouliadis G. Dye test in primary and secondary lymphedema. In: Bollinger A, Partsch H, Wolfe JHN, eds. The initial lymphatics. New York: Thieme-Stratton, 1985:131–137.
22. Kinmonth JB. Lymphangiography in man. Clin Sci 1952;2:13–20.
23. Bruna J. Computerized tomography, xeroradiography, lymphography, and xerolymphography in diagnosis of lymph stasis. In: Olszewski WL, ed. Lymph stasis: pathophysiology, diagnosis and treatment. Boca Raton, FL: CRC Press, 1991:412–432.

chapter 30

Congenital Vascular Malformations of Venous Predominance: Klippel-Trenaunay Syndrome

J. Leonel Villavicencio

Several congenital vascular malformations present clinically with varicose veins, a cutaneous portwine stain, and giantism. Even though congenital malformations are present in a relatively small percentage of patients attending vascular clinics, the severity of the clinical manifestations and the magnitude of the problem are challenging. The management of the different types of anomalies associated with congenital vascular malformations requires knowledge of the pathophysiology involved, common sense, experience, and a multidisciplinary approach.

The most common vascular malformations observed in the vascular clinic are the Klippel-Trenaunay (KTS), Parkes-Weber, and Maffucci syndromes. Hemangiomas may or may not be present with these syndromes. The presence of hemangiomas usually requires careful examination of their size, nature, location, and associated symptoms. Management depends on the patient's age, the histologic nature of the lesion, and the severity of the symptoms. Hemangiomas are often found in the Maffucci syndrome and less frequently in Parkes-Weber syndrome or KTS. On occasion, a hemangioma may thrombose spontaneously and as a result produce acute symptoms that require prompt medical attention.

The clinical syndrome that was described by Klippel and Trenaunay in 1900 (1) was a congenital vascular anomaly with capillary portwine stain, varicose veins, and limb hypertrophy occurring in association (Fig 30.1). Since that time, almost 15,000 cases have been reported. Nonetheless, there is still confusion regarding the nomenclature, cause, and management of this clinical entity (2, 3). A condition akin to KTS was described by Parkes-Weber (4) in 1907. He reported a similar, but clinically distinct, group of patients with varicose veins, limb hypertrophy, and the presence of hemangiomas with a definite pulsation and thrill. This report was the first description of the clinical condition subsequently known as the Parkes-Weber syndrome (4).

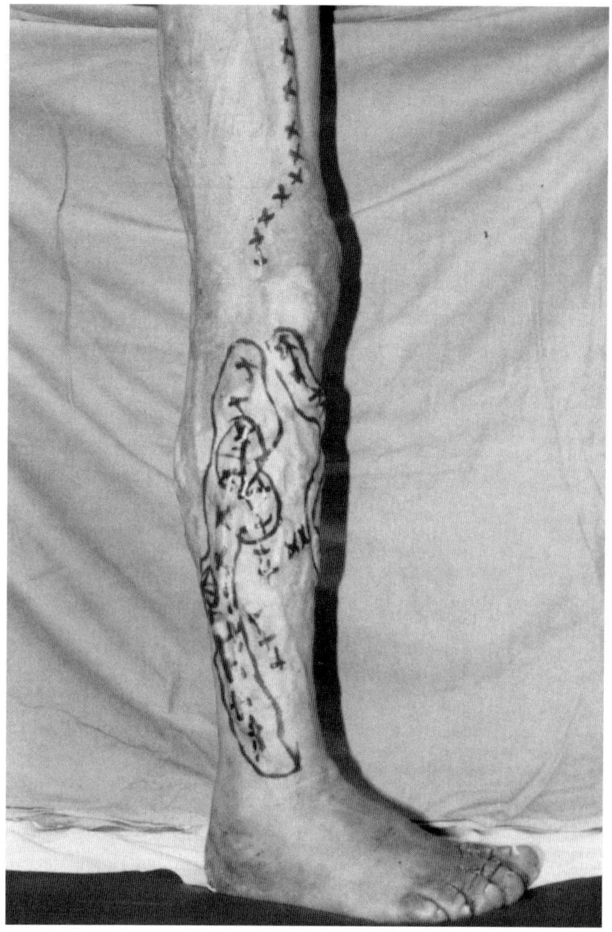

FIG. 30–1. Klippel-Trenaunay syndrome. A capillary portwine stain, varicose veins, and limb hypertrophy without clinically detectable arteriovenous fistulae, occur in association in the syndrome described by Klippel and Trenaunay in 1900. (Reproduced by permission from Villavicencio JL. Treatment of varicose veins associated with congenital vascular malformations. In: Bergan JJ, Goldman MP, eds. Varicose veins and telangiectasias. Diagnosis and treatment. St. Louis: Quality Medical Publishing Company, 1993:332.)

Although both syndromes are clinically similar, the differences between KTS and Parkes-Weber are probably a matter of degree. The clinical distinction hinges on the absence of clinically detectable arteriovenous fistulas in KTS that are evident in the Parkes-Weber syndrome. The natural history of congenital arteriovenous fistulas and their sequelae highlight their importance in Parkes-Weber syndrome and have made their treatment the natural focus of management. The absence of clinically detectable arteriovenous fistulas in KTS has left the management of this condition without a clear focus. However, recent investigations with radioactive isotopes have allowed the detection of previously subclinical arteriovenous fistulas (5, 6). The findings of arteriovenous fistulas in a small percentage of patients with KTS further blur the distinction between the two syndromes (7). As experience with KTS has grown, it has become evident that this condition may be associated with angiomatous involvement of other organ systems, including the eye, gastrointestinal tract, bladder, and external genitalia (8–11). Dargeon (12) described a child with a bladder hemangioma who also had unilateral lower extremity hypertrophy and a portwine skin malformation. Kuffer, et al. (13), reported the association of visceral angiomas and thrombocytopenia in KTS. Hendry and Vinnicombe (14) reviewed 31 patients with bladder hemangiomas; 10 patients (31%) were younger than 20 years, and two had KTS. Bladder hemangioma is present in 3–6% of all patients with KTS.

As often happens in congenital vascular malformations, more than one system is often involved in the process. Involvement of the lymphatic system has been frequently described in KTS (15, 16). Lymphoscintigraphic anomalies of the lymphatic flow have been reported by our group and others in patients with KTS (17). Additionally, KTS has been reported in association with the Sturge-Weber syndrome, in which a vascular stain is present on the upper face and ipsilateral leptomeninges (18, 19). It seems likely that these clinical syndromes may have a common cause and may be regional manifestations of the same genetic disorders (20).

The cause of the anomalies observed in KTS is controversial. Servelle (15) stated that the changes seen in this syndrome were the sequelae of obstruction. He based his assumptions on the phlebographic demonstration of venous obstruction. On the other hand, Baskerville, et al. (21), reported that most patients had no impairment of venous drainage and suggested that a mesodermal abnormality occurring during fetal development led to the maintenance of microscopic arteriovenous fistulas, which resulted in the clinical syndrome. More recently, a theory was advanced suggesting that KTS was the result of either (a) a half chromatid mutation of the zygote before fertilization or (b) an early somatic mutation that allows survival of the cells by mosaicism, but produces a lethal gene preventing its transmission (20). The sporadic occurrence of KTS, its equal sex incidence, the variation in severity, and the relative rarity of generalized involvement are consistent with this theory. Genetic mutation could account for the spectrum of diseases known as the syndromes of KT, Parkes-Weber, and Sturge-Weber.

The surgical management of KTS and Parkes-Weber syndrome has been extensively discussed and is the subject of controversy. In the presence of active arteriovenous fistulas in a severely symptomatic patient, the decision to proceed with therapeutic embolization or to intervene surgically is less subject to controversy than in a patient whose main clinical manifestations are giantism and sequelae of chronic venous hypertension. Servelle operated on 786 patients with KTS since 1945 (15). He found that elongation of limbs was invariably noted. Varicose veins were present in 36% of the cases, and a cutaneous portwine stain was present in only 32% of the patients. It is interesting that, based on his phlebographic studies, Servelle demonstrated anomalies of the popliteal vein in 51% of his cases, the superficial femoral vein in 16%, the popliteal and femoral veins in 29%, and the iliac veins in 3%, with inferior vena cava involvement in only 1%. Servelle considered that deep venous obstruction was the primary cause, and that surgery directed to the abnormal superficial varicosities could worsen the patient's condition by increasing the outflow obstruction. Other authors also have cautioned against surgery on this basis (22, 23).

DIAGNOSTIC CONSIDERATIONS

Diagnosis begins with a careful clinical examination. The presence of giantism, varicose veins, and a portwine stain malformation usually located on the lateral aspect of the limb is strongly suggestive of the diagnosis of KTS. We have noted considerable variation in the extension and location of the portwine stain. It may occupy the entire length and usually the lateral aspect of one or more limbs or it may be present only in isolated areas of the extremity. Often the portwine stain is the background of large bulging veins (Fig. 30.2). A lateral marginal venous collector, which is a remnant of a fetal vein, often can be observed in these patients (Fig. 30.3) (24).

Symptomatic patients in whom the diagnosis of KTS or Parkes-Weber syndrome is suspected must undergo a number of invasive and noninvasive vascular tests. Bidirectional Doppler examination is used to assess reflux at the saphenofemoral or saphenopopliteal junctions, reflux of the abnormal marginal vein, and perforator incompetence. Duplex scanning is extensively utilized to evaluate the whole venous system and any anomaly that might be present. Strain-gauge plethysmography is valuable in the evaluation of obstruction of the venous outflow and venous capacitance. To assess the importance and contribution of the large lateral collecting vein in the venous outflow of the limb, strain gauge plethysmog-

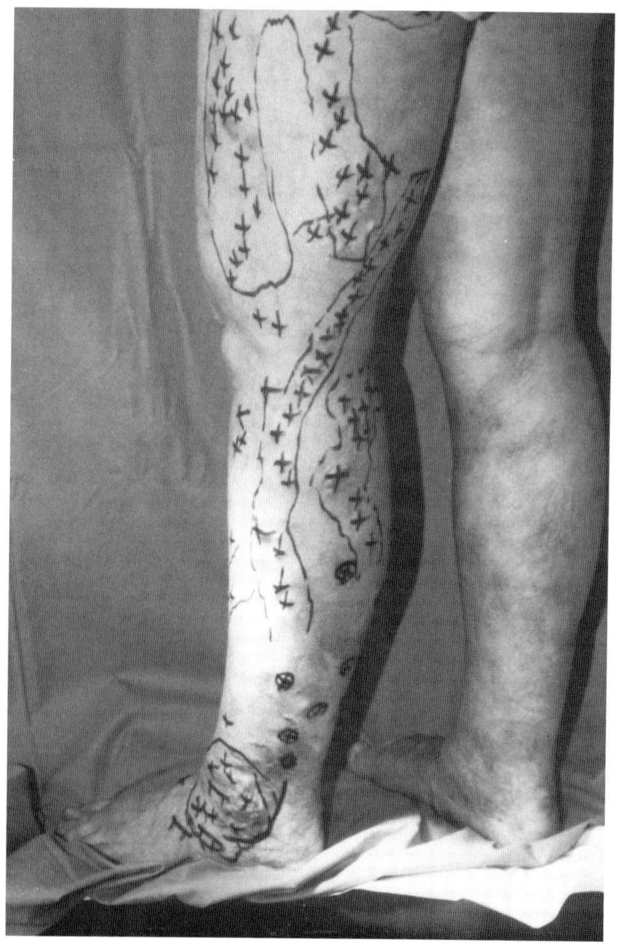

FIG. 30–2. The classic location of the portwine stain is on the lateral aspect of the entire extremity. However, several variations are possible. Large varices can be seen bulging over the area covered by the capillary malformation. (Reproduced by permission from Villavicencio JL. Treatment of varicose veins associated with congenital vascular malformations. In: Bergan JJ, Goldman MP, eds. Varicose veins and telangiectasias. Diagnosis and treatment. St. Louis: Quality Medical Publishing Company, 1993:332.)

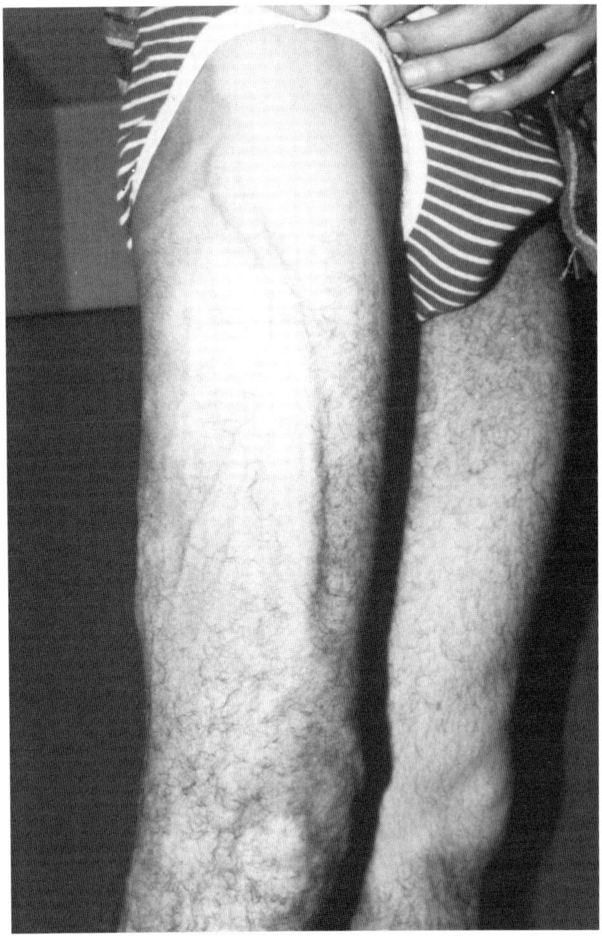

FIG. 30–3. A large lateral collector (vena marginalis) draining into the iliac system is present in this young man with Klippel-Trenaunay syndrome. The trunk contained competent valves and had large perforators.

raphy readings should be repeated with compression of the entire large lateral collector shortly before the thigh cuff is deflated. A pattern of venous outflow obstruction is observed if the lateral vein collector plays an important role in the venous outflow of the limb. Photoplethysmography is used to document venous refilling time and to provide an index of venous reflux.

Both ascending and descending phlebography, as well as selective varicography, are important for the diagnosis. Varicography is useful in localizing the point of entrance of the abnormal lateral collector into the deep system and in demonstrating the anatomy of the area (Fig. 30.4). Descending phlebography provides information on the valvular system and the degree of competence or incompetence. Twenty-four percent of the patients in our series had avalvulia and the contrast material traveled from the groin to below the knee with ease. Ascending phlebography demonstrates the distribution of the collector systems, the presence of the perforators, and specifically provides information on the degree of aplasia or hypoplasia of the deep venous system (Fig. 30.5). A word of caution about the phlebographic technique and the interpretation of the films is in order. Due to

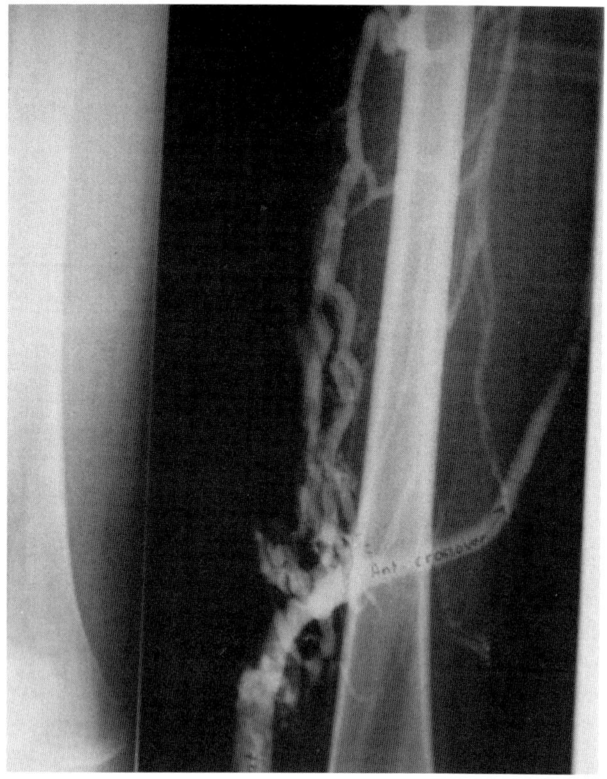

FIG. 30–4. Ascending phlebography and varicography demonstrate the lateral collector crossing anteriorly toward the greater saphenous vein. A plexiform network of varicosities containing large perforators can be seen over the lateral aspect of the thigh. (Reproduced by permission from Villavicencio JL. Treatment of varicose veins associated with congenital vascular malformations. In: Bergan JJ, Goldman MP, eds. Varicose veins and telangiectasias. Diagnosis and treatment. St. Louis: Quality Medical Publishing Company, 1993:333.)

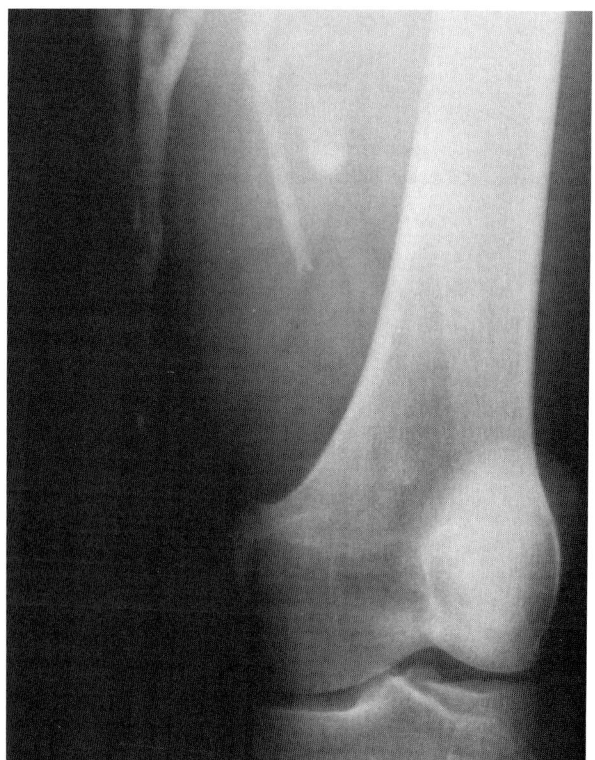

FIG. 30–5. Complete agenesis of the popliteal vein in a 32-year-old man. A large portion of the deep venous system was substituted by the large lateral collector which can be seen in this phlebogram. Competent valves are observed in the lateral collector.

the large capacity of the venous bed of the superficial system of patients with KTS, the contrast media may not appear in the deep system. This will give an erroneous impression of aplasia or hypoplasia of the deep system, and the patient may be denied surgical treatment for this reason. When poor deep venous filling is encountered despite the injection of large volumes of contrast media (>200 ml), the procedure should be repeated after compression of the large superficial venous system has been achieved with elastic stocking or elastic bandages.

Serial arteriography or digital computerized arteriography should be performed in search of arteriovenous fistulas. A small percentage of patients with KTS have "hypoactive" arteriovenous fistulas detected with isotopic techniques (25, 26). Both computer tomography (CT) and magnetic resonance imaging (MRI) have been used in selected patients to assess the extent of the venous malformation. The MRI studies enhance the diagnosis of atresia of the inferior vena cava or the pelvic veins and display the distribution of the malformations in the soft tissues in a superb manner. Sequences of T2-weighting with second echo enhance the venous imaging and have been very useful in demonstrating the presence of intrathoracic hemangiomas. The T1 sequences are helpful in showing venous malformations or plexuses of veins either in the muscles or in the subcutaneous tissues. MRI also provides information on the presence or absence of deep venous system, the localization of the abnormal lateral collectors and the degree of enlargement of the extremity (27) (Fig. 30.6). In patients with suspected Parkes-

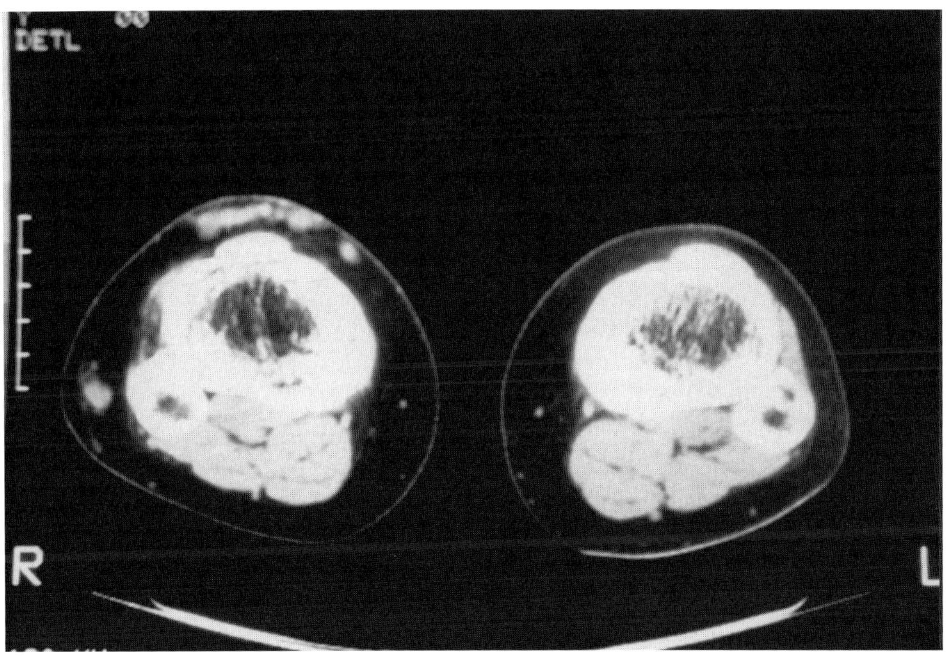

FIG. 30–6. Magnetic resonance imaging of the lower extremities of a patient with Klippel-Trenaunay syndrome. The right lower leg is larger than the left and a large lateral collector can be observed. Other varicosities can be seen in the subcutaneous tissue. MRI is especially useful in demonstrating the magnitude of the involvement of the soft tissues, the location of hemangiomas, and the presence of abnormal vessels.

Weber syndrome, angiography may demonstrate the presence, magnitude, and location of arteriovenous connections. This information is essential in guiding the interventional radiologist in planning the therapeutic embolization of the arteriovenous fistulas. Surgical ligation of most of the arterial branches of the main arterial trunks of the extremities, or "skeletization," as described by Malan and Puglionisi (28) and Vollmar and Voss (29) is now rarely performed.

To assess concomitant malformations, cystoscopy, sigmoidoscopy, and other specialized studies should be performed.

At our institution, we have studied 42 cases of KTS during the last 13 years. Patient ages ranged from 3 days to 65 years. There were 15 males and 27 females. The disease was localized to a single lower extremity in 30 cases, bilateral lower extremities in six, and to the lower and upper extremities of the same side in six.

Table 30.1 summarizes the clinical findings in our series. A portwine stain, varicose veins, and the presence of a lateral vein collector were present in the majority of our patients. Leg ulcers were present in 12% of the cases and were particularly refractory to treatment. Ulcer healing took place promptly after compression sclerotherapy of the surrounding large varices. Fifty-five percent of the patients had hemangiomas distributed in the chest or extremities (Fig. 30.7).

In Table 30.2 are shown the concomitant anomalies found in our series. Twelve percent of our patients had either aplasia or hypoplasia of a major deep venous trunk (Fig. 30.5). Fifty percent of patients with KTS had venous aneurysms and only 1.5% had episodes of thromboembolism. This is in contrast with the relatively high incidence of thromboembolic phenomena reported in some European series (29, 30). Avalvulia was observed in 24% of our patients. This finding correlates with the massive reflux observed in these cases and with the characteristic arteriographic-like phlebogram.

MANAGEMENT

Traditionally, compression therapy, leg elevation, and sclerotherapy have been the only forms of management offered to patients with KTS. These methods are valuable and should be recommended to all patients. However, some patients

TABLE 30-1

CONGENITAL VASCULAR MALFORMATIONS: KLIPPEL-TRENAUNAY SYNDROME CLINICAL FINDINGS (42 CASES)

	No.	%
Portwine stain	39	93
Varicose veins	40	95
Lateral marginal vein	39	90
Phlebangiomas	23	55
Limb hypertrophy	35	83
Leg ulcers	5	12

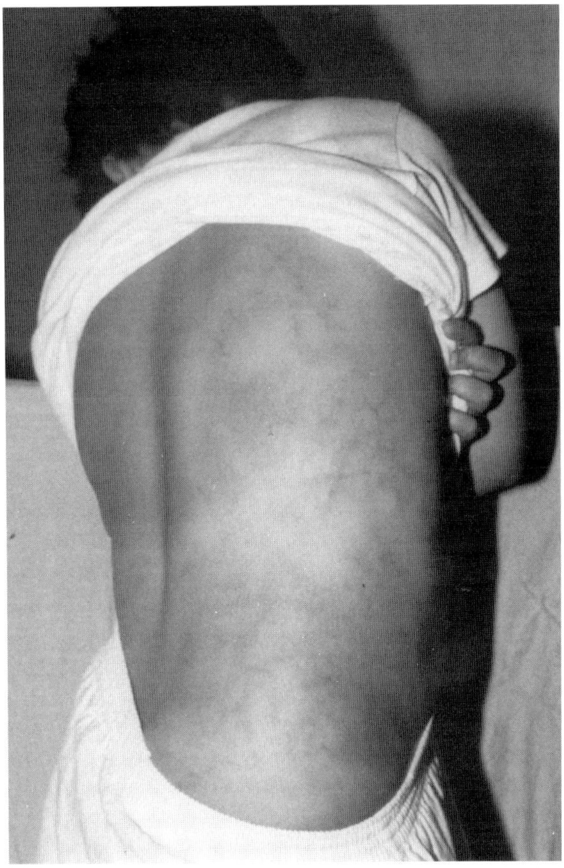

FIG. 30–7. A large hemangioma can be observed on the lateral aspect of the thorax of this child. Often hemangiomas have an intrathoracic component. They may spontaneously thrombose, producing severe clinical manifestations that require prompt medical attention.

suffer from severe symptoms that do not respond to conservative treatment. In this group, surgical treatment must be considered. Surgical excision of the large superficial venous trunks in KTS has been condemned by some authors (29) who have observed worsening of the venous hypertension after excision of the super-

TABLE 30-2

CONGENITAL VASCULAR MALFORMATIONS: KLIPPEL-TRENAUNAY SYNDROME CONCOMITANT ANOMALIES (42 CASES)

	No.	%
Deep veins aplasia/hypoplasia	5	12
Avalvulia	10	24
Large perforators (incompetent)	22	52
Venous aneurysms	21	50
Intrapelvic/intrathoracic phlebangiomas	8	19
Gastrointestinal bleeding	1	2.3

ficial venous plexuses. However, surgery must be considered and planned on the basis of both the patient's symptoms and the results of the noninvasive and invasive diagnostic investigations. When duplex scanning or phlebographic examination has demonstrated a patent deep venous system, we have not hesitated in performing extensive excision of the large varicose clusters and hemangiomatous masses including the grossly dilated lateral venous collector. Ligation and division of the large incompetent perforators that are routinely present along the anomalous venous trunks and the posterior and medial aspects of the calf must be performed (Fig. 30.8). If hypoplasia and/or obstruction of the deep venous system has been diagnosed, this extensive surgical procedure should not be performed. In our experience, the most common problems necessitating intervention are frequent and copious bleeding from skin varicosities or superficial hemangiolymphangiomas, nonhealing venous ulceration, gross deformity impairing lifestyle, pain and edema, recurrent thrombophlebitis, and acute thrombosis of hemangiomas.

In 614 operated cases, Servelle (15) found these deep venous anomalies: (a) compression of the popliteal vein in 71% of the cases, with a perivenous sheet involving the whole length of the vein in approximately 15% of the patients; (b)

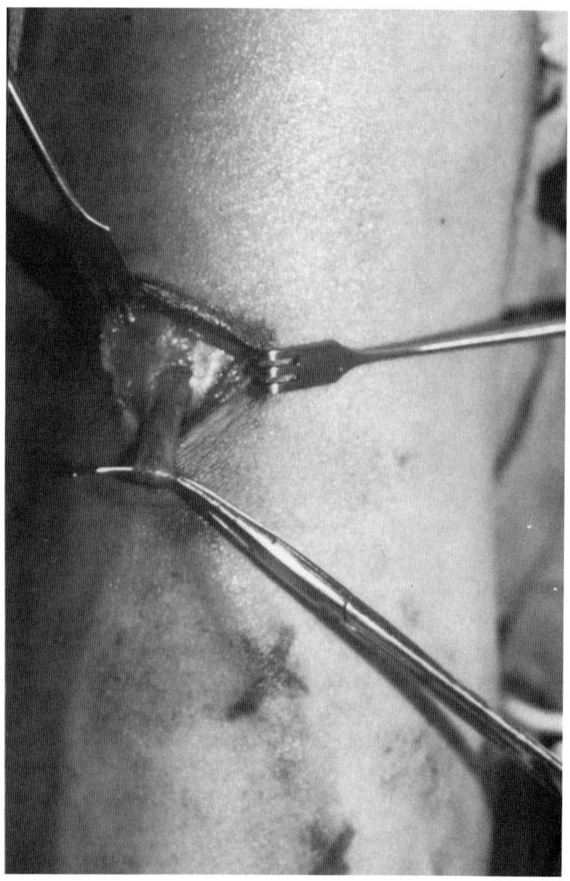

FIG. 30–8. A large perforator is clearly demonstrated in this patient with Klippel-Trenaunay syndrome and greatly dilated superficial venous trunks. (Reproduced by permission from Villavicencio JL. Treatment of varicose veins associated with congenital vascular malformations. In: Bergan JJ, Goldman MP, eds. Varicose veins and telangiectasias. Diagnosis and treatment. St. Louis: Quality Medical Publishing Company, 1993: 335.)

agenesis or hypoplasia of the popliteal vein in 7% of the cases; (c) compression of the femoral vein in 54% of the cases, with a complete perivenous sheet in 2%; and (d) hypoplasia and complete agenesis of the femoral vein in 40% and 3% of the cases, respectively. Servelle recommended venolysis and resection of all the compressing fibrous bands along the entire length of the vein. He reported that the veins are restored to almost normal caliber after this operation. We have been able to confirm Servelle's observation in three cases. A perivenous fibrous sheet was found around the popliteal vein in 2 patients and in the superficial femoral vein in one.

SURGICAL MANAGEMENT

Preoperative Marking

Preoperative marking is the single most important technical step in surgery of the superficial venous system (Fig. 30.9). The examiner must have experience and a thorough knowledge of anatomy, physiology, and pathophysiology. Inadequate preoperative marking is not usually listed as a causative factor

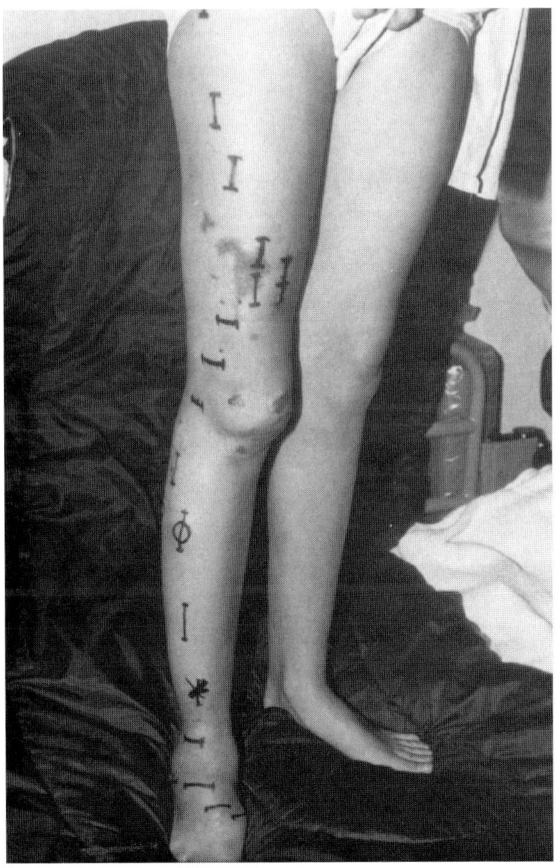

FIG. 30–9. Preoperative marking is the single most important technical step in surgery of the venous system. Areas of perforators, large varicose clusters, hemangiomas, and areas where surgical incisions should be placed are carefully marked. In this patient, a large knee hemangioma was also resected. (Reproduced by permission from Villavicencio JL. Treatment of varicose veins associated with congenital vascular malformations. In: Bergan JJ, Goldman MP, eds. Varicose veins and telangiectasias. Diagnosis and treatment. St. Louis: Quality Medical Publishing Company, 1993:335.)

in recurrent varicose veins. However, an improperly and carelessly marked extremity represents an invitation for recurrence.

Preoperative marking must be performed as follows:

1. The patient must have the extremity washed daily with antiseptic soap and water for at least 3 days immediately preceding surgery.
2. The extremity and pubis should be carefully shaved before marking. This is especially important in hirsute patients.
3. Marking should be done before the administration of any preanesthetic medication. Tracing the veins requires the patient to be standing on a platform under a good source of illumination. The patient should not be drowsy.
4. Marking should be done with a water-resistant marker, so that it will not come off during skin preparation.
5. Each surgeon develops his/her own technique for marking by using different signs and tracings to identify perforators and clusters of veins. For this reason, surgery must be performed by the surgeon who marks the patient (in teaching centers, the senior surgeon must be present during marking and must assist the resident or fellow with the operation). An effort should be made to locate the point of entrance of the lateral venous collector into the deep system, since this point varies considerably.

The policy of selective "segmental excision" of the superficial venous system with division and ligation of incompetent perforators should be followed. The "classic stripping" of venous trunks is not recommended. General anesthesia is utilized in all cases. A pneumatic tourniquet has been employed in 80% of our patients in whom extensive varicosities were present. After emptying the venous bed with an Esmarch rubber bandage, the tourniquet is inflated at 250–300 mmHg and the bandage removed. The mean surgical time has been 57 minutes. The procedure involves the segmental resection of the abnormal lateral collector vein and its ligation at the point of entrance into the deep system. Segmental excision is safer than stripping because of the large size of the veins and their tributaries. Indeed, venous aneurysms have been encountered in most patients. These require identification and excision to prevent postoperative bleeding and hematomas. Once the large incompetent perforators have been ligated and divided, the clusters of veins can be excised through small incisions. Whenever possible, crochet hook excision of the superficial clusters of varicose veins should be done to diminish postoperative scarring, even though the cosmetic aspect of the management is not of particular concern to patients suffering from disfiguring malformations. It is of interest that only 2 of the 17 patients that have been operated on for KTS were found to have incompetence of the long saphenous system. These patients underwent long saphenous excision to a point just below the knee. Superficial venous clusters and venous dilatations can be excised easily in the bloodless field provided by the pneumatic tourniquet. Cavernous hemangiomas or superficial hemangiolymphangiomas have been excised in 25% of our patients (Fig. 30.10). In patients with extensive abnormalities, it is wise to stage the surgical procedures to obtain optimal results. Staging was performed in our series in 11 of 17 cases. In the postoperative period, external compression with elastic hosiery is strongly recommended for an indefinite period.

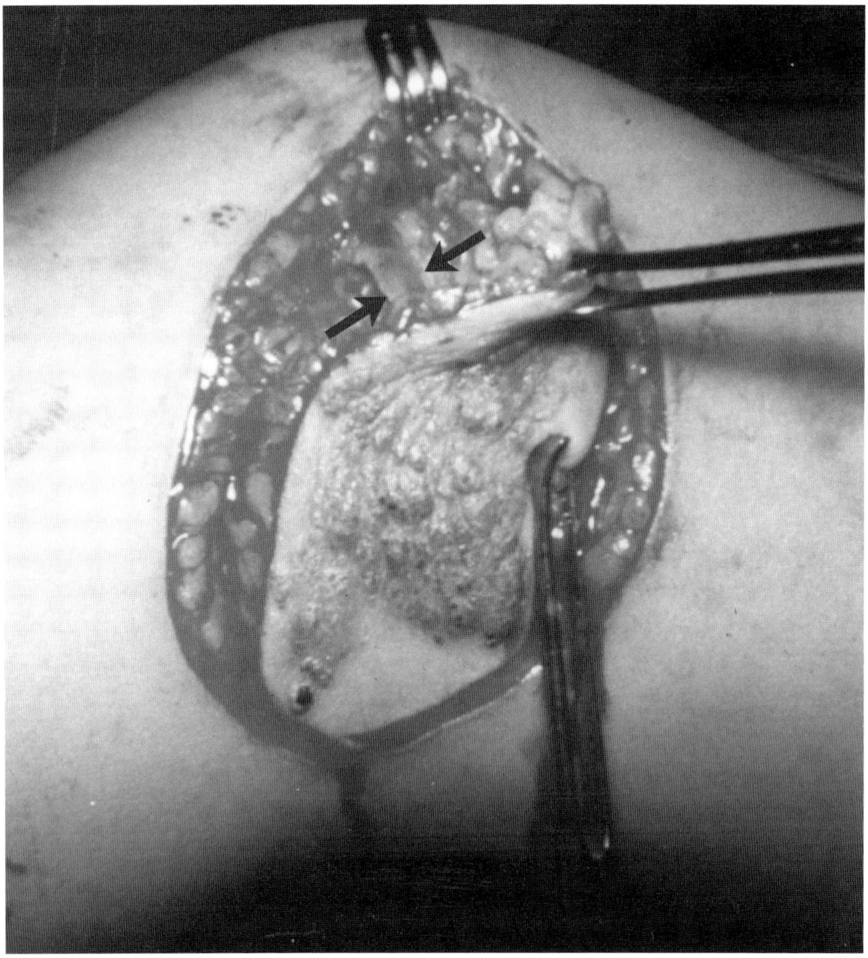

FIG. 30–10. Cavernous hemangiomas or superficial hemangiolymphangiomas such as illustrated in this photograph bleed frequently and should be excised. (Reproduced by permission from Villavicencio JL. Treatment of varicose veins associated with congenital vascular malformations. In: Bergan JJ, Goldman MP, eds. Varicose veins and telangiectasias. Diagnosis and treatment. St. Louis: Quality Medical Publishing Company, 1993:338.)

Sclerotherapy plays an important role in the management of KTS and should begin 2 months after surgery, once the postoperative ecchymosis has disappeared. This form of treatment must be used in association with surgery in patients with intractable symptoms. Sclerotherapy should be utilized to maintain the patient free of symptoms and should be repeated as often as necessary.

If the principles of management delineated above are followed, an excellent functional outcome should be expected. Surgery is largely a containment exercise to palliate symptoms. Cure cannot be achieved. No patient's condition, however, has worsened as a result of the extensive resection of superficial veins. The surgical procedures performed in our series of 17 patients are listed in Table 30.3. No patient had recurrent bleeding, all ulcerations healed, and the mean patient's satisfaction index was 3 (1 = not satisfied; 2 = moderately satisfied; 3 = satisfied; and 4 = very satisfied).

Table 30.4 shows the percentages of patients submitted to surgery in some important series. It should be noted that not every patient afflicted with KTS needs surgery. Most patients can be controlled with conservative measures and the prudent use of sclerotherapy and compression. Vollmar has been particularly reluctant to operate on patients with KTS, and his policy is reflected in an incidence of only 19.2% of patients operated on. This is in contrast to the more aggressive approach observed in other European and American series in which the percentage of patients submitted to surgery is higher (15, 30–32).

SUMMARY

Surgery of the superficial veins in patients with KTS has been controversial because it was believed to result in acute venous hypertension, secondary to obstruction. However, the results of our series do not support this belief. Superficial venous surgery may have been unsuccessful in the past for a number of reasons, the most obvious of which is the presence of venous obstruction secondary to deep venous aplasia or hypoplasia. In such a situation, severe venous hypertension results and venous gangrene has been reported. Adequate demonstration of a hemodynamically sound deep venous system is a crucial prerequi-

TABLE 30-3

CONGENITAL VASCULAR MALFORMATIONS: KLIPPEL-TRENAUNAY SYNDROME SURGICAL PROCEDURES IN 17 PATIENTS*

	No.	%
Excision of large varices and perforator ligation	17	100
Greater saphenous stripping	1	2.3
Excision of lateral collector	17	100
Excision of phlebangiomas	9	21.4
TMT amputation	3	7.1
Subfascial procedures (Cockett)	3	7.1
Excision of venous aneurysms	5	12
Lysis of superficial femoral vein	1	2.35
Lysis of popliteal vein	2	4.7
Resection of intestinal malformation	1	2.35
Skin grafting	4	9.5

*Surgery was staged in 11 patients. Postoperative sclerotherapy was performed in 15 cases.

TABLE 30-4

CONGENITAL VASCULAR MALFORMATIONS: KLIPPEL-TRENAUNAY SYNDROME INCIDENCE OF ASSOCIATED LESIONS

Author	Patients	Nevus %	Varices %	Hypertrophy	Abnormal Deep Veins	DVT	Surgery
Browse (30)	49	38/96	49/100	36/73%	33%*	20%	38/77%
Gloviczki (31)	144	137/95	134/93	134/93%	6/5%	3.5%	76/52%
Villavicencio (32)	42	39/93	40/95	35/83%	5/12%**	1.5%	17/40%
Servelle (15)	768	251/32	282/36	100%	313/51%	N/A	614/78%
Vollmar (29)	83	100	100	100%	94%	8/16 (50%)	16/19.2%

*Phlebographic anomalies of pelvic veins.
**Phlebographic anomalies of 17 operated patients.

site to superficial venous surgery. Additionally, superficial surgery sometimes has been inappropriately directed toward removal of the long and short saphenous systems. We found varicosities of the saphenous trunk in only two of 17 operated cases. All patients had documented perforator vein incompetence, often in communication with the large lateral collector. Perforator ligation and division should be an integral part of the treatment program. Because of the large diameter of the incompetent perforator veins, stripping of any venous trunks in patients with KTS should not be done because of the risk of profuse bleeding or postoperative hematomas. Instead, segmental excision is the procedure of choice. Patients with intractable symptoms who have a patent deep venous system should be treated with an aggressive surgical policy directed toward the elimination of reflux to the superficial system and the excision of the dilated venous clusters and hemangiomatous masses. The management of the severe lymphatic anomalies and gross deformities often observed in patients with KTS should be an integral part of the treatment of this syndrome. Prevention of scoliosis in young patients should be carried out by epiphysial stapling of the larger extremity (33, 34). The treatment of diffuse congenital vascular malformations must be a multidisciplinary endeavor in which different specialties participate in the treatment of these unfortunate patients.

REFERENCES

1. Klippel M, Trenaunay P. Du noevus variqueux et osteo-hypertrophique Arch Gen Med (Paris) 1900;185:641–672.
2. McKusick VA. Mendelian inheritance in man: catalogues of autosomal dominant, autosomal recessive and X-linked phenotypes. 10th ed. Baltimore: Johns Hopkins University Press, 1992:643–644.

3. Vollmar J. Zur Geschichte und Terminology der Syndrome nach FP Weber and Klippel Trenaunay. Vasa 1974;3:231–241.
4. Parkes-Weber F. Angioma formation in connection with hypertrophy of limbs and hemihypertrophy. Br J Dermatol 1907;19:231–235.
5. Bollinger A, Vogt B, Luthy E, Hegglin R. Flow measurement in patients with multiple arteriovenous fistulae of the extremity. Helv Med Acta 1976;33:76–87.
6. Haimovici H, Sprayregen S. Congenital microarterio-venous shunts: angiographic and Doppler ultrasonographic identification. Arch Surg 1986;121:1065–1070.
7. Bourde C. Classification des syndromes de Klippel-Trenaunay et de Parkes-Weber d'apres les donnees angiographiques. Ann Radiol 1974;17:153–160.
8. O'Connor PS, Smith JL. Optic nerve variant in the Klippel-Trenaunay-Weber syndrome. Ann Ophthalmol 1983;10:131–137.
9. Gloviczki P, Hollier L, Telander RL. Surgical implications of Klippel-Trenaunay-Weber syndrome. Ann Surg 1983;197:353–362.
10. Hall BD. Bladder hemangiomas in the Klippel-Trenaunay-Weber syndrome. N Engl J Med 1971;285:1032–1033.
11. Tjaden BL, Buscema J, Haller JA, Rock JA. Vulvar congenital dysplastic angiopathy. Obstet Gynecol 1990;75:552–554.
12. Dargeon HW. Tumors of childhood. New York: Paul B. Hoeber, 1960:367.
13. Kuffer FR, Starzynski TE, Girolami A, et al. Klippel-Trenaunay syndrome, visceral angiomatosis and thrombocytopenia. J Pediatr Surg 1968;3:65–72.
14. Hendry WF, Vinnicombe M. Hemangioma of the bladder in children and young adults. Br J Urol 1971;43:309.
15. Servelle M. Klippel-Trenaunay syndrome: 768 operated cases. Ann Surg 1985;201:365–373.
16. Baskerville PA, Ackroyd JS, Lea Thomas M, Browse NL. The Klippel-Trenaunay syndrome: clinical radiological hemodynamic features and management. Br J Surg 1985;72:232–236.
17. Collins PS, Villavicencio JL, Abreu SH, et al. Abnormalities of lymphatic drainage in lower extremities: a lymphoscintigraphic study. J Vasc Surg 1989;9:145–152.
18. Stewart G, Farmer G. Sturge-Weber and Klippel-Trenaunay syndromes with absence of inferior vena cava. Arch Dis Child 1990;65:546–547.
19. Furakawa T, Igata A, Toyokkura Y, Ikeda S. Sturge-Weber and Klippel-Trenaunay syndrome with nevus of ota and ito. Arch Dermatol 1970;102:640–645.
20. Happle R. Lethal genes surviving by mosaicism. A possible explanation for sporadic birth defects involving the skin. J Am Acad Dermatol 1987;16:899–906.
21. Baskerville PA, Ackroyd JS, Browse NL. The etiology of the Klippel-Trenaunay syndrome. Ann Surg 1985;202:624–627.
22. Lindenhauser SM. The Klippel-Trenaunay syndrome. Ann Surg 1965;162:303–314.
23. Vollmar J, Vogt K. Angiodysplasie und Skeletsystem. Chirurg 1976;47:205.
24. Vollmar J, Voss EU. Vena marginalis lateralis persistens-die vergessene Vene der Angiologen. Vasa 1979;8:192–202.
25. Partsch H, Lofferer O, Mostbeck A. Shuntvolumsbestimmung bei gemischten Angiodysplasien der Extremitaten. Wien Klin Wschr 1973;85:544–547.
26. Partsch H, Lofferer O, Mostbeck A. Zur Diagnostik von arteriovenosen Fisteln bei Angiodysplasien der Extremitaten. Vasa 1975;4:288–295.
27. Stanson AW, Breen JF. Computed tomography and magnetic resonance imaging in venous disorders. In: Gloviczki P, Yao JST, eds. Handbook of venous disorders: guidelines of the American Venous Forum. New York: Chapman & Hall Medical, 1996:190–232.
28. Malan E, Puglionisi A. Congenital angiodysplasias of the extremities. I: Generalities and classification. Venous dysplasias. J Cardiovasc Surg 1964;5:87–130.

29. Vollmar J, Voss EU. Chir der kongenitalen Angiodysplasien. Langenbecks Arch Chir 1978;347:255–259.
30. Browse NL, Burnand KG, Thomas ML. The Klippel-Trenaunay syndrome. In: Browse NL, Burnand KG, Thomas ML, eds. Diseases of the veins: pathology, diagnosis and treatment. London: Edward Arnold, 1988:609–625.
31. Gloviczki P, Stanson AW, Stickler G, et al. Klippel-Trenaunay syndrome: the risks and benefits of vascular intervention. Surgery 1991:110–400.
32. Villavicencio JL. Treatment of varicose veins associated with congenital vascular malformations In: Bergan JJ, Goldman MP, eds. Complex problems involving varicose veins. Part 4. Varicose veins and telangiectasias. St Louis: Quality Medical Publishing Company, 1993:329–342.
33. Blount WP, Clarke GR. Control of bone growth by epiphysial stapling: a preliminary report. J Bone Surg 1949;31A:464–477.
34. Phemister DB. Operative arrestment of longitudinal growth of bones in the treatment of deformities. J Bone Surg 1933;15:1–15.

chapter 31

Diagnosis and Treatment of the Pelvic Venous Disorders: Pelvic Congestion and Pelvic Dumping Syndromes

J. Leonel Villavicencio, David Gillespie, Silke Durholt, Emmanouil Pikoulis, and Norman M. Rich

HISTORICAL BACKGROUND

Pelvic pain in women has been recognized by numerous clinicians in the past and has been the subject of a large number of reports in the medical literature. Richet described a case of tubo-ovarian varicocele in 1857 (1). His report triggered the interest of other investigators in Europe and America who recognized the association of dyspareunia with vulval varices and postintercourse pelvic discomfort. Puzzled by the bizarre manifestations of the pelvic complaints, numerous hypotheses and theories on the cause of the syndrome have been proposed by gynecologists and other specialists. During the 1890s and the early part of the 20th century, physicians did not have the sophisticated diagnostic tools currently available, and their "etiologic guesses" were based on astute clinical observations, occasional surgical findings, and, often, plain speculation without objective proof. An excellent review of the various causes of chronic pelvic pain was published by Hobbs (2). Symptoms of dyspareunia, pelvic discomfort or pain, vulval and pelvic congestion, and other manifestations of the pelvic congestion syndrome have been attributed to underdeveloped sexual organs stressed during intercourse (3), varicosities of the broad ligaments (4), disorders of the pelvic venous circulation with or without pelvic varices, and vulval congestion (5). Pelvic varices have been classified as primary and secondary. The latter are the sequelae of parametritis, pelvic peritonitis, and other pathologic pelvic processes (6, 7).

The term pelvic congestion syndrome was coined by Taylor, who, in 1949, published several important papers. Taylor reported 105 cases of women with pelvic pain, dyspareunia, and vulvar congestion with or without vulval varices (8–11). He believed that the symptoms were of psychosomatic origin, even though he acknowledged the importance of abnormal circulation and secondary frigidity. A great step forward in the understanding of the disease occurred with the publications of Ahlberg (12–14), Chidekel (15, 16), Thomas, et al. (17), Craig and Hobbs (18), and Dixon and Mitchell (19). The radiologic studies of these investigators demonstrated the pelvic venous circulation by injections of radiopaque dye directly into the uterus, the clitoral vein, and the vulval varices (varicography). Of particular importance in the understanding of the disturbed hemodynamic mechanisms of the pelvic venous circulation were the renal phlebographic studies of Ahlberg. He demonstrated reflux of the ovarian vein and filling of some pelvic visceral veins after the injection of contrast media into the renal vein of the upright patients. The technique has been refined and used extensively in the investigation of the pelvic congestion syndrome by Hobbs (2), Lechter (20–22), Gomez (23, 24), and others. Our group has shown that there is clinical and phlebographic correlation between the presence of varices of the vulva, posterior thigh, and the pelvic congestion syndrome with insufficiency of the internal iliac venous system (pelvic dumping syndrome) (25).

PELVIC VENOUS SYSTEM: GENERAL CONSIDERATIONS

The pelvic venous system is formed by two separate venous plexuses which drain the blood from the visceral and the parietal territories. The pelvic venous system drains into three main collector systems: the internal iliac vein, the ovarian, and the hemorrhoidal. The internal iliac trunk is single in approximately 73% of the cases and double in 27%. It joins the external iliac vein at the level of the promontory and has an internal diameter between 12–15 mm. When the internal iliac vein is formed by a single trunk, it collects blood from its two main venous territories: the parietal and the visceral. The parietal is formed by the superior and inferior gluteal, the sacral and iliolumbar, the obturator, and the hemorrhoidal veins. The visceral tributaries are formed by the vesical, vaginal, uterine, internal pudendal, and rectal plexuses.

When the internal iliac vein is formed by two separate trunks, usually the anterior trunk receives most of the visceral branches, and the posterior trunk, the parietal tributaries. The ovarian vein is formed by five separate trunks which drain the venous territories of the parametrium, cervix, mesosalpinx, and the pampiniforme plexus. These venous plexuses form the ovarian vein, which may have 2–3 trunks initially and becomes a single trunk at the level of L4. Its diameter is approximately 3.1 mm and increases with pregnancies. The right ovarian vein drains directly into the inferior vena cava and, occasionally, into the right renal vein. The left ovarian drains into the left renal vein. Variations are very common in the number of trunks and in the site of drainage. The vein has two or three valves, which are incompetent in 47% of the women. During pregnancy, the entire pelvic venous system increases considerably in size and it is not unusual to observe an ovarian vein that triples its original diameter. The increase in venous volume and the hormonal factors that are in effect during pregnancy facilitate the distension and dilatation of the venous system, particularly in patients with a family history of varicose veins. The scarcity of valves in the pelvic veins favors a free and abundant crossover circulation (25).

Dodd and Wright stated that "varicose veins of the vulva are an embarrassing form of varicosity which is distressing mentally and physically." Varicose veins occurred in about 8% of all pregnant women referred to an antenatal vein clinic, and vulval varices were diagnosed in 23.3% of pregnant women suffering from varicose veins (26). Often the varicosities remain after delivery and tend to progress with subsequent pregnancies (17). Why do vulvar varices and symptoms of pelvic congestion syndrome occur? In some cases, it has been possible to show the presence of massive gonadal reflux by retrograde phlebography. In others, incompetence of the internal iliac vein and its tributaries (internal pudendal, obturator and gluteal veins) has been demonstrated by Doppler and selective internal iliac retrograde phlebographic studies (25); and, in a few, obstruction of the ovarian vein outflow by compression of the left renal vein by the superior mesenteric artery (Nutcracker syndrome) has resulted in clear symptoms of pelvic congestion with development of large perirenal and ovarian varices similar to the male varicocele (27) (Fig. 31.1). In many cases, however, the etiology remains unclear.

ANATOMIC CONSIDERATIONS

The current textbooks of descriptive and topographic anatomy and related publications offer a detailed description of the location and distribution of

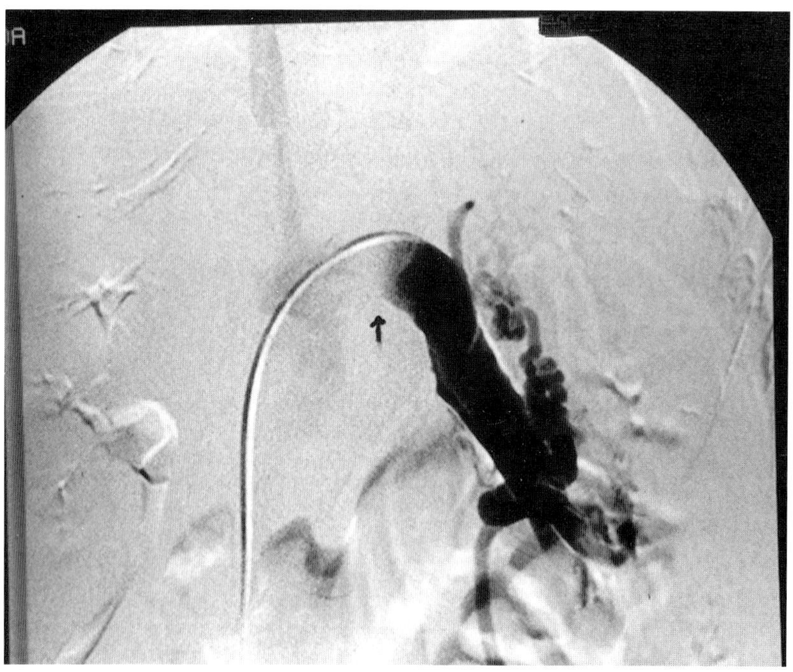

FIG. 31–1. Retrograde phlebography of the left renal vein in a case of "Nutcracker syndrome." Perirenal varices are clearly observed. The *arrow* shows the site of obstruction of the renal vein by the superior mesenteric artery.

valves in the veins of practically every anatomic territory with the exception of the internal iliac vein (28–33). Fabricius Ab Aquapendente, anatomist of the famed Padua School of Anatomy, made the most precise anatomic description of the venous valves in his De Venarum Ostiolis published in 1603 (34). His eight anatomic plates constitute the most beautiful printed artwork of his time and are living testimony of his patient and accurate observations that began in 1574. Fabricius failed to recognize the true function of the valves when he wrote: "Valves are present, so to speak, as intelligent doorkeepers of the many parts, to prevent escape of the nutriment downwards, until the parts above have acquired their fitting share of it." Fabricius did not describe the valves in the internal iliac veins.

Sappey, in his extensive and detailed work, also did not describe valves in the internal iliac system (35). Alfred Houze de L'Aulnoit, disciple of Sappey, wrote in his exemplary thesis "Recherches Anatomiques et Physiologiques sur les Valvules des Veines" (36): "Valves are exceptionally found in the common, external and internal iliac veins." In 1854, de L'Aulnoit described valves in the tributaries of the internal iliac vein but not in its trunk, and made an insightful and profound observation when he stated that the valves in the spermatic vein were incompetent and might be "the cause of varicocele"!

Dodd and Cockett, in their classic book, stated: "Valves are not described in the trunk of the internal iliac vein, but are said to be present in its peripheral tributaries. In a few postmortems, we have examined the internal iliac veins but we saw no valves. Quain's Anatomy (1892), states it has not valves" (37).

The paucity of information in the medical literature regarding the valvular anatomy of the internal iliac vein and its tributaries stimulated us to dissect 82 iliac venous system specimens in 42 human cadavers (29 men, 13 women). We also sought to gain information on the relationship between the pelvic dumping syndrome and the anatomy of the region (25). Each specimen contained common, external, and internal iliac veins including the tributaries of the latter. We recorded the anatomic variations of the internal iliac vein trunk and the location of the valves in the complete iliac venous system, including 485 tributaries of the internal iliac veins. We excluded five specimens that were not suitable for analysis. The internal iliac vein drained into the external iliac venous system by means of a single trunk in 73% of the specimens and by two well-formed and separated trunks in 27%. One specimen (1.2%) had a well-developed valve in the common iliac vein. The external iliac vein had one valve in 26.2% of the specimens. The right external iliac vein had three times as many valves as the left. The internal iliac vein had valves in 10% of its main trunk and there were valves in the 485 tributaries dissected. The scarcity of valves in the pelvic veins has led us to consider that varicose veins in the vulva or elsewhere develop not only because of valvular insufficiency, but also because of genetic structural venous wall anomalies which may become evident during the hormonal and hemodynamic changes occurring during pregnancy. It is recognized that there is a large increase in pelvic flow during pregnancy and that the femoral vein dilates to more than twice its normal size. Under these conditions the valve cusps separate and become incompetent (38).

The analysis of the gross anatomical variations of the internal iliac vein trunk revealed two completely separated venous trunks in 27% of all specimens (Fig. 31.2). This finding was most frequently observed in the female specimens. In some

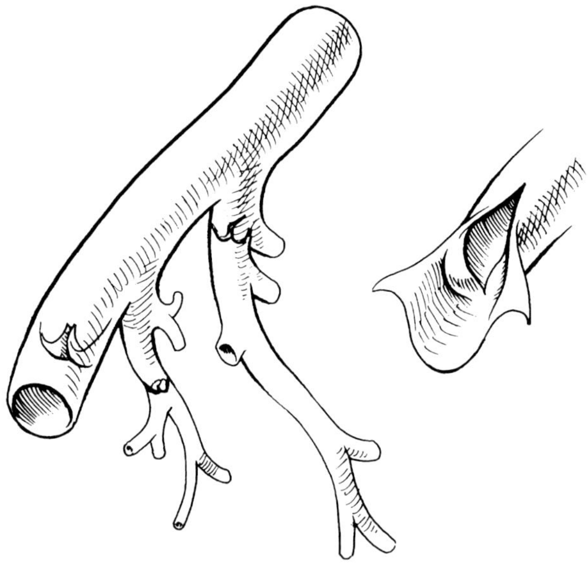

FIG. 31–2. Artist rendition of a specimen of external and internal iliac veins demonstrating a double internal iliac trunk. Ostial and parietal valves are illustrated. Valves were present in 27% of the cadaver specimens. Drawing by Gary Wind.

specimens, one trunk received the blood from the visceral tributaries and the other from the parietal branches. This information should be relevant for the radiologist who is trying to catheterize selectively the internal iliac vein trunk, since both trunks may need to be visualized to elucidate the source of venous reflux. The existence of double trunks and the presence of valves in the internal iliac trunks may explain the technical difficulties experienced by Dixon and Mitchell (19) in their attempts to demonstrate reflux from the iliac veins into areas of vulval varicosities.

The parietal valve encountered in the external iliac vein in about one-third of all specimens is worthy of discussion. Our observations revealed that the right external iliac had almost three times as many valves as the left. The scarcity of valves in the left external iliac leaves the saphenofemoral area of a relatively large number of patients without protection against the high thoracoabdominal pressures. This anatomic finding may offer objective support to the reported higher incidence of varicose veins in the left lower extremity. On the other hand, it is important to keep in mind the absence or presence of this valve during the interpretation of reflux at the saphenofemoral junction. A competent external iliac valve will disguise an incompetent saphenofemoral junction when the Doppler probe is placed on the saphenous trunk and the patient is asked to perform a Valsalva maneuver.

Clinical Presentation

There are at least four well-recognized syndromes originating from disorders of the pelvic venous circulation:

1. The "pelvic dumping syndrome," or insufficiency of the gonadal veins, which in multiparous women may reach considerable size and carry a large volume of blood (Fig. 31.3).
2. Insufficiency of the internal iliac vein and its tributaries. In this situation, large varicose veins develop in the territories of the hypogastric vein, such as the internal pudendal, obturator and gluteal veins (Fig. 31.4). Gluteal varices appear usually after the second pregnancy in absence of incompetence of the gonadal veins (Fig. 31.5). Hemorrhoids and vulval varices are a common finding in patients with insufficiency of the internal iliac vein.
3. A syndrome of obstruction to the flow of the left ovarian vein by compression of the left renal vein by the superior mesenteric artery (Nutcracker syndrome) (39, 40). Large perirenal varices and tortuous ovarian and pelvic varicosities are commonly observed in the phlebographic studies (Fig. 31.1). Additionally, in the presence of clinical symptoms, a gradient of 10 mmHg or more between the inferior vena cava and the left renal vein is diagnostic of this syndrome.
4. Vulval varices in absence of symptoms of pelvic congestion.

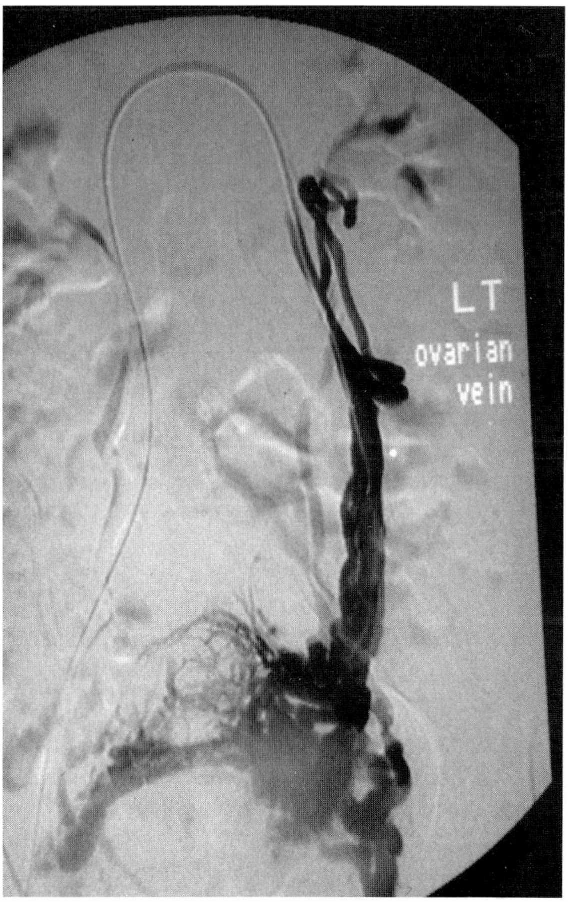

FIG. 31–3. Retrograde gonadal phlebography demonstrating large left ovarian vein. Several trunks form this vessel. Reflux of contrast material can be observed in the pelvis.

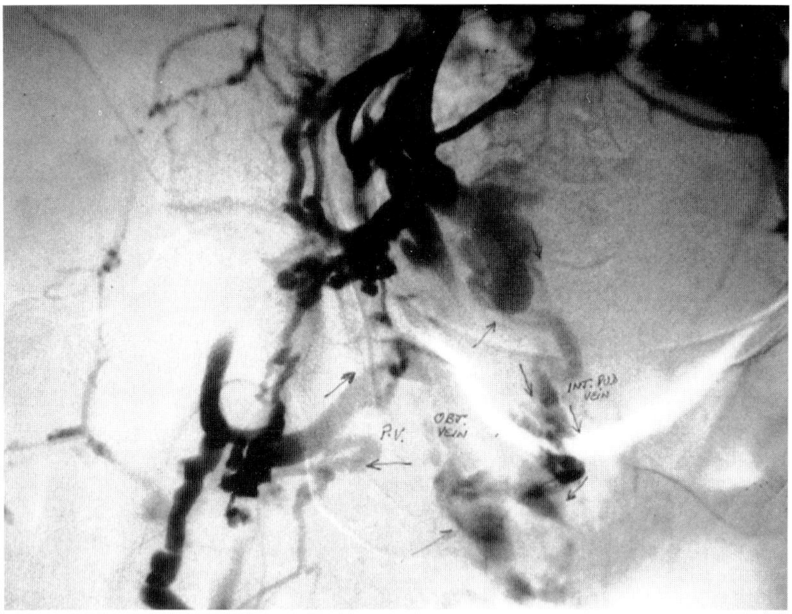

FIG. 31–4. Retrograde internal iliac vein catheterization. The catheter is in the iliac vein and the incompetent tributaries connecting with the vulvar varices are clearly seen. The connections at the saphenofemoral junction, the obturator, and internal pudendal veins were opacified by hand injection at the mouth of the internal iliac vein. There was no incompetence of the gonadal veins.

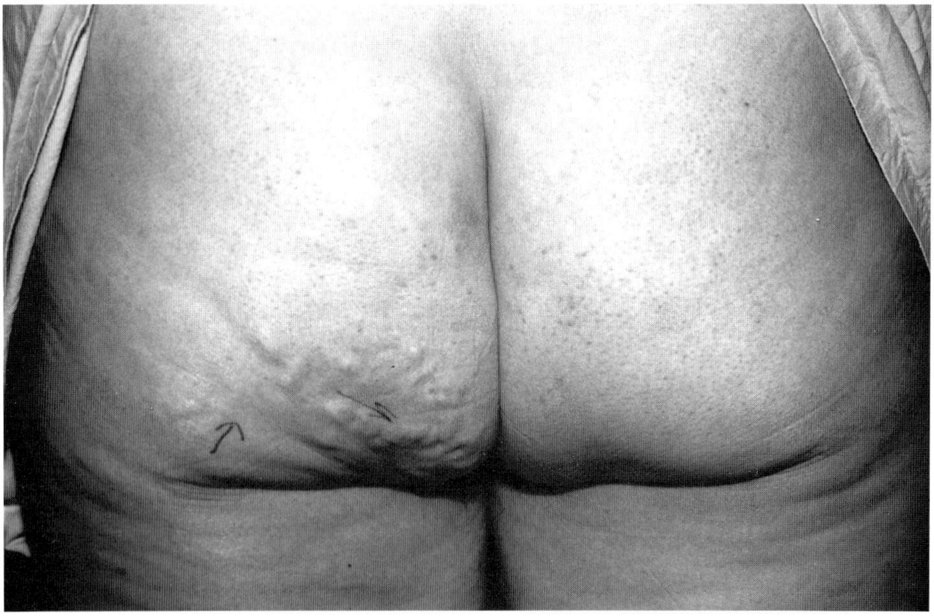

FIG. 31–5. Patient with a mass of gluteal varices. Retrograde phlebography (Fig. 31.7) demonstrated connection with the internal iliac vein. There was no incompetence of the gonadal veins. She had retroperitoneal ligation of incompetent trunks followed by sclerotherapy. She has been asymptomatic for 8 years.

Varicose veins of the lower extremities are found in nearly 50% of patients with pelvic varices. In some cases, their distribution may suggest pelvic venous insufficiency since they appear in the territory of the tributaries of the internal iliac vein such as the gluteal, sciatic, obturator, and internal pudendal veins. Varicosities on the posterior, posteromedial and proximal inner third of the thigh are almost always related to pelvic venous insufficiency. In a small group of patients, pelvic insufficiency is manifested through the connections of the internal iliac vein tributaries with the deep and superficial external pudendal veins and may give the equivocal impression of saphenofemoral incompetence.

The four syndromes described may produce two main groups of symptoms: (a) symptoms of pure pelvic venous congestion without vulval varices and (b) symptoms of vulval varices with or without pelvic congestion.

Pelvic venous congestion symptoms will be more common in cases of obstruction to the venous outflow of the gonadal veins (Nutcracker syndrome), as well as in patients with massive ovarian vein reflux in the presence of competent internal iliac vein tributaries. Symptoms include chronic pelvic pain; slight to severe pelvic discomfort that increases during menstruation and prolonged standing; dyspareunia; and postcoital distress. There are signs of bladder irritability such as dysuria and increased micturition without evidence of urinary infection. Because of the problems involved in diagnosis and the nature of the symptoms, these patients may develop secondary frigidity and become depressed, and, on occasion, psychotic and suicidal (41–45).

Vulval varices are an unsightly and embarrassing form of varicosities that may be present with or without symptoms of pelvic congestion (Fig. 31.6). Patients

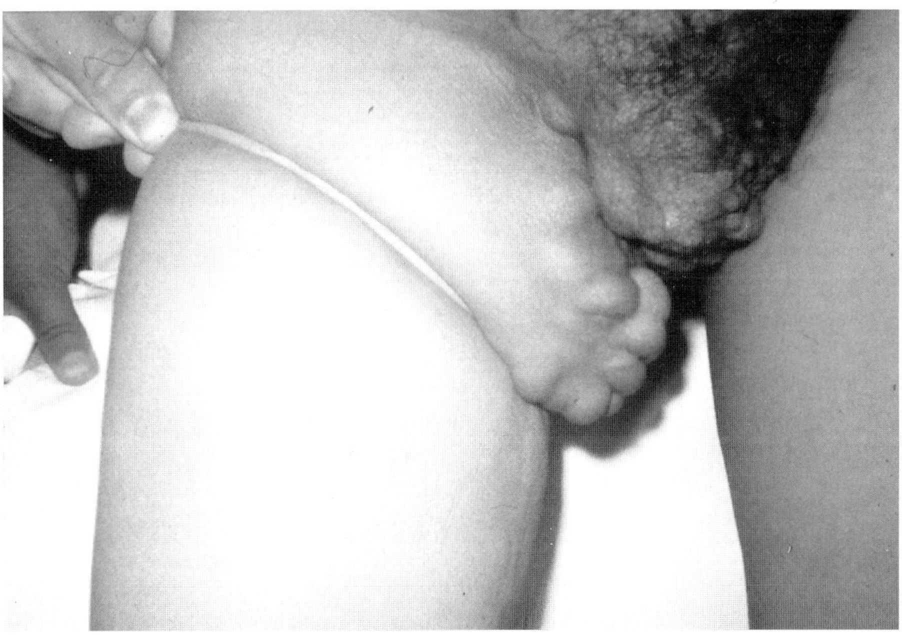

FIG. 31–6. Disfiguring varices of the vulva. The patient had massive reflux (pelvic dumping syndrome) toward the distal thigh and knee. The tourniquet demonstrates control of the distal varices. (Courtesy of Dr. Luis Sigler.)

complain of tenderness and congestion of a dilated mass of varicose veins often associated with the menses and resolving after the menstrual period. There is fear of rupture and occasionally they either rupture or thrombose (46). They are often due to incompetence of the parietal (gluteal, obturator, iliolumbar) or visceral (vaginal, uterine, vesical, paracervical, hemorrhoidal, internal pudendal) tributaries of the internal iliac vein. Figure 31.7 illustrates a symptomatic patient with massive phlebographic gluteal reflux and absent gonadal vein reflux. Patient complaints were confined to a painful tender mass during sitting or prolonged standing and postcoital discomfort. It seems that in these cases, the pelvic reflux has only "local" manifestations. However, some authors describe large vulvar varices resulting from massive reflux of greatly dilated incompetent ovarian veins and consider this source of reflux as the most important cause of vulvar varices (2, 21, 22). We believe that the most severe cases of vulvar varices, with chronic pelvic pain and lifestyle-impairing symptoms, are the consequence of a combination of gonadal and internal iliac venous insufficiency in association with genetic, hormonal, hemodynamic, and psychologic factors which play roles of varying magnitude.

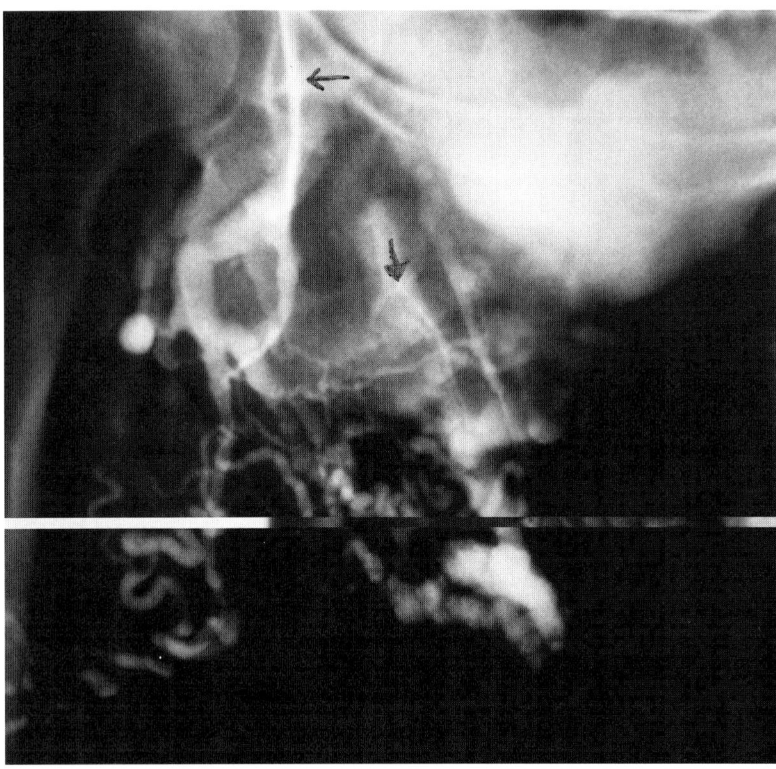

FIG. 31–7. Retrograde phlebography of the internal iliac vein. The catheter is seen (*upper arrow*) in the internal iliac vein at the origin of the gluteal trunks. This study corresponds to the patient of Figure 31.5. Connections with branches of the saphenous vein can be observed in the *lower left* of the photograph.

Diagnosis

Most patients are referred by the gynecologist to the vascular surgeon with a history of chronic pelvic pain, vulval varices, and varicose veins of the lower extremities. A frequent complaint is the presence of a tender mass or lump, palpable in the lower part of the vulva, and especially noticeable while standing or sitting for prolonged periods. Usually, the gynecologist has thoroughly investigated the patient to rule out endometriosis, chronic pelvic inflammatory disease, polycystic ovaries, and urinary and bowel disease. Next, the disorders of the pelvic venous circulation that may cause chronic pain should be investigated.

The analysis of 42 patients treated in our service for symptomatic pelvic varices revealed that all patients were multiparous with a mean of 3.1 pregnancies (range: 2–5) and a mean age of 31.9 years (range: 20–45 years). The majority of patients were in the 31–40-year age group and had noticed the onset of pelvic varices during the second pregnancy. There were two patients in whom symptomatic pelvic varices appeared after the fourth pregnancy. Eighteen patients had associated lower extremity varicose veins. In addition to pelvic varices, 11 patients had chronic pelvic pain and severe symptoms of pelvic congestion. Among them, there were three women with mesoaortic compression of the left renal vein (Nutcracker syndrome) and obstruction to the ovarian vein outflow. The remaining 31 patients had various degrees of symptomatic vulvar varices.

Physical Examination. We identified three main clinical patterns of distribution of vulval varicosities which are closely related to the insufficient venous territories: (a) anterior aspect of pubis, clitoris, vulva, and labia majora (territories of the round ligament and obturator vein); (b) inner thigh and posterior half of the vulva and often the vagina (internal pudendal and gonadal veins); and (c) gluteal and posteromedial aspect of the thigh (gluteal, internal pudendal, and sciatic veins). Vulval varices are often in connection with the internal saphenous and femoral veins through anastomosis with the deep and superficial external pudendal veins (Fig. 31.4). In this manner, varices of the vulva may drain its large pelvic venous load into the internal saphenous vein and its tributaries (pelvic dumping syndrome). One may clearly observe the vulvar varices in continuity with varicose veins of the anteromedial or posteromedial aspects of the thigh and knee. Retrograde phlebography with selective ovarian or internal iliac vein injection may often fill varices at the level of the distal thigh and knee. The appearance of varicosities over the upper third and posterior aspect of the thigh is characteristic of incompetence of the pelvic veins through their gluteal and ischiatic tributaries. Hemorrhoids were present in 87% of our patients.

Noninvasive Investigations

Doppler Examination. With the patient in the upright position and the body weight placed on the opposite limb, a 9-MHz bidirectional Doppler probe is placed directly over the mass of dilated vulval veins. A loud venous reflux during Valsalva maneuver is evidence of incompetence of the investigated territory. The study is repeated over different areas of varicosities. Competence of the saphenofemoral junction is tested by placing the Doppler probe on the saphenous trunk

5 cm distal to the saphenofemoral junction while the patient performs a Valsalva maneuver. A loud reflux is heard if the external iliac valve and the saphenofemoral junction are incompetent. If no reflux is heard, the test is repeated with distal thigh or calf compression-release. Prolonged reflux will be heard upon release if the saphenous trunk is incompetent. Vulval reflux was present in 23 of the 31 patients with vulval varices and in 6 of the 11 patients with vulval varices and predominant symptoms of pelvic congestion. Saphenofemoral junction incompetence was documented in 10 of the 18 patients with varicose veins of the limb.

Pelvic Imaging. Pelvic ultrasound and Doppler examination of patients with chronic pelvic pain who were suspected of having venous congestion was reported by Hodgson, et al. (47). In their patient, pelvic ultrasound scan revealed predominantly distended varicose veins in the pelvis. The diagnosis of pelvic varices was confirmed by selective gonadal phlebography which showed large ovarian veins with pelvic varicosities. This patient did not have vulval or limb varicosities. The patient was symptom-free after long sections of the ovarian veins were removed. Graeme Richardson from Australia has been able to image the pelvic veins and diagnose pelvic varices with color-flow duplex ultrasound. We have found difficulties in reproducing his experience. In a prospective study, transvaginal ultrasound was proved to compare favorably with transabdominal ultrasound for gynecologic diagnosis (48). It is possible that the full bladder required for abdominal ultrasound distorts the appearance of dilated veins by compression. A transvaginal probe is well tolerated and the proximity of the uterus and ovaries allows higher imaging resolution. Stones, et al. (49), studied 14 patients with pelvic pain, venographic evidence of congestion, and transabdominal ultrasound findings of dilated veins of more than 4.5 mm in diameter. They were able to observe vasoconstriction in the diameter of pelvic varicose veins in response to intravenous dihydroergotamine, and concluded that transvaginal ultrasound can identify dilated pelvic veins and assist in the diagnosis of pelvic congestion.

Invasive Investigations. Laparoscopy has been used extensively in the diagnosis of gynecologic, urologic, and oncologic conditions. Ovarian varicocele and dilated masses of varicose veins can be seen and the diagnosis of pelvic varices can be made objectively. Rundqvist, et al. (50), performed laparoscopy in 13 of 15 women with chronic pelvic vein. In 11 patients, pelvic varices were diagnosed and later confirmed by selective left renal phlebography. Laparoscopy has been increasingly used to investigate the etiology of pelvic pain. If pelvic varices are identified, retrograde phlebography is indicated (51–53).

Phlebography. Visualization of the pelvic venous system is essential in the diagnosis and modern management of the severely symptomatic patient with a presumptive diagnosis of pelvic congestion syndrome and vulval varices. This has been accomplished through different routes during the last 50 years. Each route follows the drainage pathways of the selected site. Intraosseus phlebography through the trochanter or iliac crest will demonstrate the iliac system and its parietal tributaries. Its use is limited in the diagnosis of pelvic varices. Transuterine phlebography has been extensively utilized in the past (16, 54–56). It can demonstrate the uterine, broad ligament and ovarian varicosities. The studies are reported using a scoring system based on the classification of Kaupilla (56). The scored features are the diameter of the ovarian vein, the rate of disappearance of the contrast media and the congestion of the ovarian venous plexus. The drawbacks of the technique are the discomfort that patients experience with the pressure injection of the dye, and the risk of perforation of the uterus, which occurred in 6 of 50 patients in one series (55).

Vulval Varicography. This method has been extensively used by Mitchell (19), Hobbs (2), Craig (18), Thomas (17), Kennedy (58), and others. The technique consists of the injection of 15–25 ml of a nonionic contrast media into the vulval varices after cannulation of a suitable vein. We have used this technique either alone or in combination with retrograde phlebography in 12 of 42 patients with vulvar varices. It produces an excellent visualization of the drainage pathways of the pelvic varices. It is especially useful when retrograde phlebography fails to visualize the source of reflux.

Retrograde Selective Gonadal-Internal Iliac Phlebography and Cineangiography. Retrograde gonadal phlebography is performed using the Seldinger technique through the common femoral vein. The left ovarian vein is selectively catheterized as it drains into the renal vein. Based on our recent experience with mesoaortic compression of the left renal vein in three patients with pelvic congestion syndrome, it is suggested that venous pressures at the inferior vena cava and the left renal vein be routinely measured to investigate gradient. The right ovarian vein is then catheterized using special Sidewinder catheters (I, II, or III) (58). This vein is more difficult to catheterize since it drains directly into the inferior vena cava. Lechter reported variations in the site of drainage of the gonadal veins in 22% of 100 cadaver dissections (59). Once the ovarian vein is catheterized, nonionic, low osmolality, iodinated contrast dye is injected after tilting the patient into a semierect position. The patient must remain in this position until the pelvic veins are visualized. The use of cineangiography has made possible the visualization of the passage of the contrast media as it refluxes down to the pelvic veins, filling the vulval varices and, occasionally, the lower extremity varicosities This technique has the important advantage that one can identify the stream of dye as it refluxes into the different pelvic venous territories and, if necessary, it is possible to slow down the scene to analyze the venous connections. As the catheter is withdrawn, the internal iliac veins are selectively catheterized. Our experience with this method has been quite satisfactory. Conversely, Lechter (59), Kennedy (58), and Dixon (19) have reported failures. This may be explained by the lessons learned during the cadaver dissection of 82 iliac venous systems (25). We learned that one of every three specimens had two separate independent internal iliac venous trunks (Fig. 31.2). In these cases, each trunk must be selectively catheterized. The vulval varices may drain into one of the trunks and spare the other. We also learned that one of the anatomic variations of the internal iliac vein is drainage of the trunk directly into the vena cava (parallel external and internal iliac veins). Finally, we also learned that the internal iliac vein has an ostial/parietal valve in 10.3% of the specimens dissected. Failure to visualize the connections of the internal iliac vein with vulval varices may be due to the catheter being placed at the external iliac or just at the mouth of the internal iliac veins. The catheter must be inserted at least 3–4 cm into the vein and, if possible, even further down (Fig. 31.7). In this manner, we have been able to demonstrate the connections of the vulvar varices with named internal iliac vein tributaries (Fig. 31.4). The connections between the vulval varices and the internal iliac vein tributaries were clearly demonstrated by vulval varicography by Thomas, et al. (17). Failure to show the vulvar connections by selective internal iliac vein catheterization of its trunk and tributaries may be due to: (a) catheterization of the wrong trunk, or (b) insufficient insertion of the catheter into the internal iliac trunk. The most important source of reflux are the gonadal veins. For these reasons, a complete study of the pelvic venous syndromes should include both gonadal and internal iliac selective opacification. In some questionable cases, we have added vulval varicography following the technique described by Thomas.

We performed 44 phlebographic studies in 42 patients with vulval varices. In seven patients, the magnitude of the symptoms did not merit the study. Varicography of vulvar varices was performed in 12 patients. In four, it was in addition to retrograde phlebography; and in eight, it was a single study. There was a group of 11 patients with predominant symptoms of pelvic congestion and moderate vulvar varices who had selective gonadal phlebography. Three of them had mesoaortic renal vein compression with perirenal varices and large ovarian varicosities (Fig. 31.8). A gradient of at least 10 mmHg was present between the

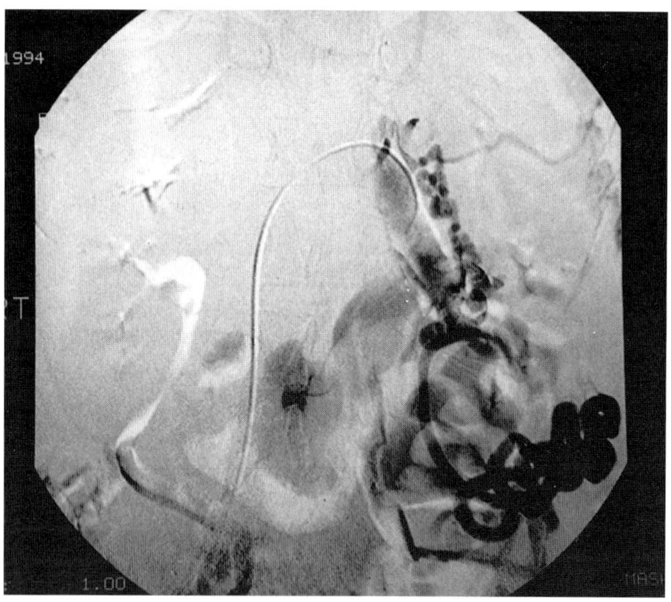

FIG. 31–8. Renal and gonadal phlebography in a patient with "Nutcracker syndrome." Large convoluted ovarian varices can be seen in the *lower right* corner of the photograph. Perirenal and ureteral varices are visible. There is no flow of contrast material into the inferior vena cava. (Courtesy of Dr. Bradley W. Dick, Suburban Hospital, Radiology Department, Bethesda, MD.)

inferior vena cava and the left renal vein with the patient upright at 70°. The gradient decreased to 1–2 mmHg when the patient leaned forward. Twelve of 18 patients with associated varicose veins of the lower extremities had ascending phlebography for localization of perforators and clarification of the anatomy of the saphenous vein, which was found duplicated in four cases. The remaining patients had selective retrograde phlebography of the gonadal and/or internal iliac vein. Of interest is a group of patients with no gonadal reflux and varices of the parietal tributaries of the internal iliac vein (gluteal, obturator) (Fig. 31.7). The phlebographic studies provided information on the reflux pathways of the pelvic venous plexuses and the connections of the vulvar varices with the iliac and/or gonadal systems. We identified four phlebographic reflux patterns: gonadal, internal iliac vein tributaries, saphenofemoral-pudendal, and a mixed pattern. The identification of the vulvar connections, and the analysis of the clinical, noninvasive, and invasive studies performed were essential in selecting the type of therapeutic approach.

Treatment

The management of the clinical manifestations of the pelvic venous disorders depends on the severity of the symptoms. Pelvic pain is difficult to ascertain. The perception of pain varies among people, and the frustration of women with unexplained abdominal pain increases their anxiety and depression. Severe pelvic pain in association with documented ovarian and vulvar varicosities requires surgical treatment. On the other hand, there are patients with a mild chronic dull ache in the pelvis associated with moderate vulval varicosities. The judgment of the clinician will determine the type of treatment.

Conservative Management. It is known that most women with chronic pelvic pain have a history of abnormal emotional development that produces symptoms leading to anxiety and depression, often complicated with sexual maladjustment . They are taking larger quantities of medication and have more hospital referrals than patients with proved organic disease (51). For these reasons, psychotherapy should be carefully considered in some of these patients. However, it would be unwise to refer a patient to a psychotherapist before ruling out a pelvic problem that could have surgical solution (61). Gynecologists have treated conservatively the pelvic congestion syndrome with the administration of various drugs. Loffredo recommends treatment with antibiotics and nonsteroid anti-inflammatory and phlebotonic drugs such as gingko and extract of horse chestnut (62). Beard has utilized the intravenous administration of dihydroergotamine, which produces a decrease in the caliber of the pelvic varices and reduces the intensity of the pain (44, 63). Hormonal therapy to suppress the ovarian function has been utilized by Reginald (64) and Hegenscheid (61), who obtained relief of the pain as long as the ovarian function was suppressed. Marhic (65, 66) utilized the rheologic drug Troxerutin in the treatment of 60 women with vulvar varices and pelvic pain. He found that high dosages of this drug produced significant relief in the group of treated patients as compared with a placebo group.

Vulvar varices during pregnancy are treated essentially with special compression garments (67–70).

Sclerotherapy and Embolization. Vulval varices can be injected with different concentrations of sclerosing agents, depending on the vein size. The small veins can be injected with 1% Sotradecol (67) or 2% Variglobine (70, 71). Hobbs (2) recommends 3% Sotradecol in small amounts (0.25 ml). Wallois recommends the use of 1% Sotradecol or 0.5% Aethoxysklerol (72). In our series of patients, we have used sclerotherapy in combination with the extraperitoneal ligation of the incompetent tributaries of the internal saphenous vein. This procedure is usually performed after the surgical phase has been completed. Sclerotherapy as a single procedure has been performed in cases of small pelvic varicosities with minimal symptoms. We have used Sotradecol 1% or 2% Aethoxysklerol.

Sclerotherapy has been also utilized by Thon in the treatment of varicocele after percutaneous catheterization of the spermatic vein (27). His group performed percutaneous retrograde sclerotherapy of the insufficient spermatic vein in 802 patients with left-sided idiopathic varicocele. The procedure was not feasible for anatomic and technical reasons in 20% of 989 patients with varicocele. A recurrence rate of 10% was reported. In women, attempts to eliminate the reflux from the ovarian vein by nonsurgical methods include embolization with balloons and coils. Edwards, et al., reported the successful treatment of a patient with pelvic congestion syndrome by ovarian vein embolization (73). Steel coils of 3-mm diameter were embolized in the ovarian vein tributaries and 5-mm coils were placed above their confluence. The patient remained asymptomatic 6 months after embolization. Phlebography performed 1 month after embolization demonstrated complete occlusion of both ovarian veins with absence of reflux into the ovarian venous plexus. Detachable balloons have been utilized to occlude the spermatic vein in men and the ovarian in women (61, 74). Fifty-two varicoceles were treated in 50 patients by occlusion of the spermatic vein using detachable balloons 1–2 mm in diameter. Satisfactory occlusion was achieved in all patients, and only one recurrence was noted at 8 months of follow-up. Similar results were reported by Stoesslein (75, 76) and Mitchel (77).

Surgical Treatment

Local Excision of Vulval Varicosities. Local excision through several small incisions at the labia majora, gluteal region, and other sites of pelvic varices has been performed by our group, as well as by other investigators (2, 19, 67–69, 78). Local excision is indicated in patients with threatening rupture during pregnancy and in patients with moderate-sized pelvic varicosities. It has been performed by our group as an isolated procedure in five patients and in combination with surgery of the varicose veins of the lower extremities in patients with associated venous insufficiency. In varices of the lower extremity, removal of the superficial varicosities without treatment of the source of reflux will result in recurrence. The same is true in cases of severe gonadal and/or internal iliac vein insufficiency where only the external varicosities are removed. Sclerotherapy or local excision of residual pelvic varicose veins after the extraperitoneal resection of the gonadal veins and ligation of the internal iliac vein tributaries has produced long-term relief of symptoms in 95% of our patients with a mean follow-up period of 12.6 years (range: 2.5–19 years).

Operative Technique. Under general anesthesia, a 15-cm long incision is carried out at a midpoint between the pubis and the umbilicus toward the tip of the 12th rib. The internal and external oblique muscles are divided following the direction of the skin incision. The transversus abdominis muscle is incised following the direction of its fibers. In a thin patient, the muscle-splitting incision may prove to be a good alternative. However, the latter requires more retraction and results in more postoperative discomfort. The properitoneal fat and peritoneum lie directly under the transversus muscle and are bluntly dissected and retracted medially. As the dissection progresses, the retroperitoneal structures will come into view. The ovarian vein can be easily identified as a large vessel formed by one to three venous trunks. The vein becomes a single trunk as it nears its termination in the renal vein in the left or the inferior vena cava in the right. After identifying the ureter, a 10–15-cm long segment of vein is excised. In patients with documented reflux of the internal iliac vein tributaries, the iliac vessels are identified and exposed. The internal iliac vein and its branches are identified and carefully dissected. Mobilization of the external iliac artery facilitates exposure of the vein and its parietal tributaries, especially the gluteal veins. The incompetent internal iliac vein tributaries are interrupted with metallic clips. The most frequent sources of reflux have been the obturator, internal pudendal, and gluteal veins. The obturator vein runs toward the obturator foramen and is superior and lateral to the internal pudendal vein. The latter is deeper and medial to the obturator vein. The ligating clips should be placed as close as possible to the pelvic wall. The gluteal trunk runs laterally and posteriorly. Preoperative phlebographic identification of these vessels is essential. Due to the abundant connections between the two sides, bilateral gonadal vein resection is recommended. Dissection of the internal iliac vein tributaries in the contralateral case is carried out only if vulval connections have been identified. Following closure and dressing of the abdominal wounds, the patient is placed in the lithotomy position and the bulging vulval varices are injected with a sclerosant agent. We have used 1% Sotradecol or 2% Aethoxysklerol. Surgery for associated varicose veins of the lower extremities is staged if the varices are extensive. Moderate varicosities may be treated during the same operative session. A two-team approach in these cases shortens considerably the operating time. A compressive bandage and special pads are placed over the injected area. Early ambulation is strongly encouraged. The most common postoperative discomfort is in the area of the injected vulvar varices. The thrombosed mass of varicosities becomes inflamed and very tender over a period of several days. Packed ice and appropriate analgesics usually control the symptoms. The mass gradually decreases in size in the course of 3–4 months. Once the refluxing points have been surgically eliminated, sclerotherapy is highly successful in the pelvic area as it is in the lower extremities.

NUTCRACKER SYNDROME AS A CAUSE FOR OVARIAN VEIN OBSTRUCTION AND PELVIC CONGESTION SYNDROME

In our series, we recognized three patients with symptoms of pelvic congestion syndrome, perirenal varices and greatly dilated ovarian, ureteral, and pelvic varicosities. Patients complained of pelvic pain localized to the left hypochondrium and extending toward the tip of the gluteal area. Pain was described as deeply seated and severe. Vulval varicosities were small. Two patients had saphenofemoral insufficiency and varicose veins which had been operated elsewhere. The third patient had no vulvar or lower extremity varices. Microscopic hematuria was present in only two patients. CT scanning and magnetic resonance imaging showed compression of the left renal vein between the aorta and the superior mesenteric artery. Descending iliac phlebography was suggestive of pelvic varicosities with competent internal iliac vein tributaries. Renal and gonadal phlebography demonstrated large perirenal, ureteral, and ovarian varicosities. The contrast material did not flow into the vena cava, staying for a prolonged period in the renal vein, and demonstrating an area of compression by the superior mesenteric vein (Fig. 31.9). This compression syndrome has been reported in males as a cause of varicocele and in females as producing ovarian congestion (79, 80). The most common manifestations are hematuria and renal and ureteral varicosities. Left flank pain irradiating toward the left gluteal area in female patients with symptoms of pelvic congestion syndrome should alert the physician to the possibility of obstruction to the gonadal outflow (81–85). Diagnosis is made by gonadal retrograde phlebography with determination of renocaval pullback pressures. In normal patients, the renocaval pressure gradient should be 0–1 mmHg (86). In our patients, gradients ranged from 8–12 mmHg. One patient was oper-

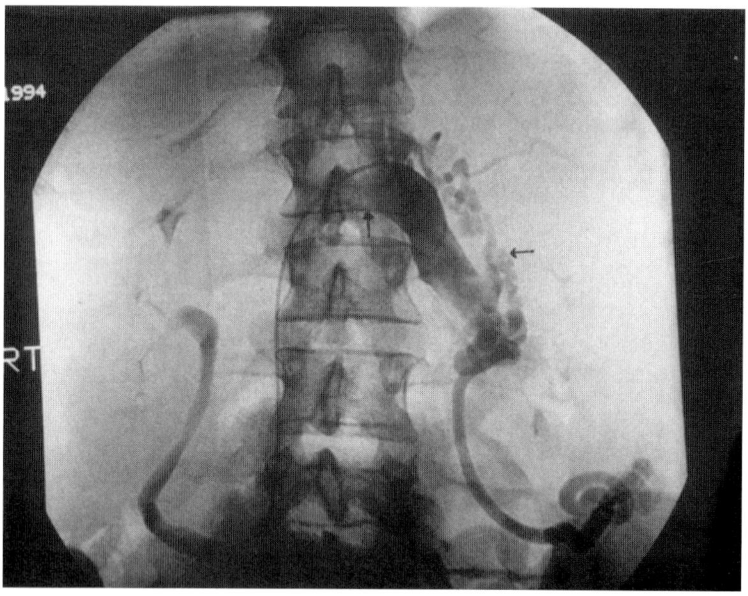

FIG. 31–9. Obstruction of the left renal vein at the site of the *upper arrow* by the superior mesenteric artery. Renal and ureteral varices are a consequence of the outflow obstruction. There was a 12 mmHg cavorenal gradient. This patient was operated on by Dr. Hugh Trout using a sleeve of reinforced Gore-Tex as described in the text. She remained asymptomatic 16 months after surgery. (Courtesy of Dr. Bradley W. Dick, Suburban Hospital, Radiology Department, Bethesda, MD.)

ated on following the technique described by Barnes (39) and was symptom-free 16 months after surgery.

SUMMARY

In our series of 42 patients, the analysis of the clinical symptoms and the results of the noninvasive and radiologic examinations were essential in selecting the type of therapeutic approach:

(a) Patients with mild clinical symptoms and small vulvar varicosities. This group was treated by local excision and sclerotherapy. Local excision of vulval varicosities as an isolated procedure was performed in five patients. It was performed in combination with varicose vein surgery of the lower extremities in seven other patients who also had mild gonadal vein enlargement. Intraoperative sclerotherapy was performed in all patients to complete the treatment. The long-term results of local excision are good if there are no further pregnancies and if the pelvic reflux is not significant. In this group, there were two recurrences in patients with further pregnancies.

(b) Patients with predominant symptoms of pelvic congestion syndrome and small vulvar varicosities. There were 11 patients in this group. Retrograde renal phlebography showed significant gonadal reflux without insufficiency of the internal iliac vein in eight patients and mesoaortic obstruction with large varices of the left ovarian vein in three (nutcracker syndrome). One was operated upon and was described earlier. The other two have not been operated on. The remaining eight patients were submitted to a combined bilateral retroperitoneal excision of the gonadal veins and sclerotherapy of the vulvar varices. Six patients are asymptomatic. One has mild recurrent symptoms and the other had no relief.

(c) Patients with large, painful masses of vulvar varices and lifestyle-impairing symptoms were submitted to a combined retroperitoneal approach followed by sclerotherapy as described in the operative technique. Ligation of the incompetent internal iliac vein tributaries as a single procedure was performed in 11 patients. In eight other patients, it was done in association with gonadal vein excision. Sclerotherapy of the vulvar varicose clusters was performed after closing the abdominal incisions. There were two recurrences in patients with ligation of the internal iliac vein tributaries performed as a single procedure.

The mean follow-up period in this series is 12.6 years (range: 2.5–19 years). An overall 87.5% of good long-term results is due to the careful selection of patients for each therapeutic approach. Other forms of treatment, such as embolization of the incompetent tributaries of the internal iliac vein or the ovarian vein, should be carefully considered either alone or as a supplement to surgery. The endovascular technology is advancing at an accelerated pace, and less invasive therapeutic approaches will undoubtedly be evaluated in a not too distant future. Obstruction to the ovarian vein outflow by mesoaortic renal vein compression should be kept in mind in patients with suggestive clinical history and phlebographic findings of renal and ovarian varicosities.

REFERENCES

1. Richet NA. Traite practique d'anatomie medico-chirurgicale. Paris: E. Chamerot, Libraire Editeur, 1857.
2. Hobbs JT. The pelvic congestion syndrome. Practitioner 1976;216:529–540.
3. Freund WA. Die Tubo-ovarialis Varicocele. Gynäk Klinik 1885;I:203.
4. Cotte G. Les troubles functionelles de l'appareil genital de la femme. Paris: Masson et Cie, 1928.
5. Schubert G. Die Bedeutung der Varicocele der Frau. Abl Gynäk 1922;46:1643.
6. Emge LA. The surgical treatment of varicose veins of the female pelvis. JAMA 1925;85:1690–1693.
7. Fothergill WE. Varicocele in the female. Br Med J 1921;ii:925–926.
8. Taylor HC Jr. Vascular congestion and hyperemia: the effect on function and structure in the female reproductive organs. Part I. Physiological basis and history of the concept. Am J Obstet Gynecol 1949;57:211–230.
9. Taylor HC Jr. Vascular congestion and hyperemia: the effect on function in the female reproductive organs. Part II. Clinical aspects of the congestion-fibrosis syndrome. Am J Obstet Gynecol 1949;57:637–653.
10. Taylor HC Jr. Vascular congestion and hyperemia: the effect on function in the female reproductive organs. Part III. Etiology and therapy. Am J Obstet Gynecol 1949;57: 654–668.
11. Taylor HC Jr. Pelvic pain based on a vascular autonomic nervous disorder. Am J Obstet Gynecol 1954;67:1177.
12. Ahlberg NE, Bartley O, Chidekel N. Retrograde contrast filling of the left gonadal vein. Acta Radiol 1965;3:385–92.
13. Ahlberg NE. Circumference of the left gonadal vein, an anatomical and statistical study. Acta Radiol 1965;3:503–512.
14. Ahlberg NE. Right and left gonadal veins, an anatomical and statistical study. Acta Radiol 1966;4:1–9.
15. Chidekel N. Female pelvic veins demonstrated by selective renal phlebography with particular reference to pelvic varicosities. Acta Radiol 1968;193:1–20.
16. Chidekel N, Edlundh KO. Transuterine phlebography with particular reference to pelvic varicosities. Acta Radiol 1968;7:1–12.
17. Thomas ML, Fletcher EWL, Andress MR, Cockett FB. The venous connections of vulval varices. Clin Radiol 1967;18:313–317.
18. Craig O, Hobbs JT. Vulval phlebography in the pelvic congestion syndrome. Clin Radiol 1974;25:517–525.
19. Dixon JA, Mitchell WA. Venographic and surgical observation in vulvar varicose veins. Surg Gynecol Obstet 1970;131:458–464.
20. Lechter A. Pelvic varices: treatment. J Cardiovas Surg 1985;26:111.
21. Lechter A, Alvarez A, Lopez G. Pelvic varices and gonadal veins. Phlebologie 1987;2:181–188.
22. Lechter A. Pelvic and vulval varices: pelvic congestion syndrome. In: Bergan JJ, Goldman MP, eds. Varicose veins and telangiectasias. St Louis: Quality Medical Publishing Company, 1993:353–369.
23. Gomez ER, Villavicencio JL, Lepage P, Coffey JA, Salander JM, Rich NM. The transpelvic approach in the management of pelvic varices: an anatomical-clinical correlation. Abstract European-American Symposium on Venous Diseases, Washington DC, March 1987.
24. Gomez ER, Villavicencio JL, Coffey JA, Rich NM. Pathogenesis and surgical management of varicose veins of the vulva and upper thigh: the internal iliac venous insuffi-

ciency syndrome. In: Veith FJ, ed. Current problems in vascular surgery. St Louis: Quality Medical Publishing Company, 1990:141–142.
25. Lepage PA, Villavicencio JL, Gomez ER, Sheridan MN, Rich NM. The valvular anatomy of the iliac venous system and its clinical implications. J Vasc Surg 1991;14:687–683.
26. Dodd H, Wright HP. Vulval varices in pregnancy. Br Med J 1959;I:831–832.
27. Thon WF, Sigmund G, Bahren W, Steinmann J. Perkutane Sklerotherapie bei-vena-testikularis-Insuffizienz. Akt Urol 1986;17:240–243.
28. Toldt C. An atlas of human anatomy. 2nd ed. Vol. II. New York: The MacMillan Co., 1944:672–677.
29. Anson BJ. An atlas of human anatomy. Philadelphia: WB Saunders, 1950:379–399.
30. Pernkopf E. Atlas of topographical and applied human anatomy. Vol II. In: Ferner H, ed. Philadelphia: WB Saunders, 1980:301–323.
31. Sobotta. Atlas of human anatomy. Vol 2. In: Hild WJ, ed. Blood vessels of pelvic viscera in the female. 10th Engl. ed. Baltimore: Uban and Schwarzenberg, 1983:204–222.
32. Testut R, Jacob O. Pelvic veins. In: Tratado de anatomia topografica. Vol. II. 8a ed. Chap. 6. Barcelona: Salvat, 1977:387–388.
33. Laufman H. Surgical anatomy of the venous system. In: Laufman H, ed. The veins. Austin, TX: Silvergirl, Inc., 1986:14–24.
34. Aquapendente FA. De venarum ostiolis (1603). (Franklin KJ, trans.) Springfield, IL: Charles C Thomas, 1933.
35. Sappey PhC. Traite d'anatomie descriptive. First Vol. Paris: V Masson (Ed), 1850:572.
36. De l'Aulnoit AH. Recherches anatomiques et physiologiques sur les valvules des veines. Paris: Thesis, 1854.
37. Dodd H, Cockett FB. Surgical anatomy of the veins of the lower limb. In: Dodd H, Cockett FB, eds. The pathology and surgery of the veins of the lower limb. London: Churchill & Livingstone, 1976:47.
38. Tamvakopoulos SK. Non-invasive estimation of the lower limb venous dynamics in pregnant women [Abstract 02.3]. Proceedings of the IV European American Symposium on Venous Diseases, Washington, DC, March 1987.
39. Barnes RW, Fleisher HL, Redman JF, Smith JW, Harshfield DL, Ferris EJ. The Nutcracker syndrome. J Vasc Surg 1988;8:415–421.
40. Burihan E, Ikeda S, Baptista-Silva JCC, Francisco J Jr, Freitas. Pelvic varices: evaluation by duplex ultrasonography-pelvic phlebography and surgery; case report. Phlebology '95. Negus D, Janjet G, Coleridge-Smith PD, et al., eds. Phlebology 1995;(Suppl 1):1033.
41. Gomez J, Dally P. Psychologically mediated abdominal pain in surgical and medical outpatient clinics. Br Med J 1977;i:1451–1453.
42. Magni G, Salmi A, Leo D, Ceola A. Chronic pelvic pain and depression. Psychopathology 1984;17:132–136.
43. Duncan CH, Taylor HC. A psychosomatic study of pelvic congestion. Am J Obstet Gynecol 1952;64:1–12.
44. Beard RW, Highman JW, Pearce S, Reginald PW. Diagnosis of pelvic varicosities in women with chronic pelvic pain. Lancet 1984;ii:946–949.
45. Pearce S, Beard RW. Chronic pelvic pain. In: Broome A, Wallace L, eds. Psychology and gynecological problems. London: Tavistock Publishers, 1984:95–116.
46. Veltman LL, Ostergard DR. Thrombosis of vulvar varicosities during pregnancy. J Obstet Gynecol 1972;39:55–56.
47. Hodgson TJ, Reed MW, Peck RJ, Hemingway AP. Case report: the ultrasound and Doppler appearances of pelvic varices. Clin Radiol 1991;44:208–209.
48. Tessler FN, Schiller VL, Perrella RR, Sutherland ML, Grant EG. Transabdominal versus endovaginal pelvic sonography: prospective study. Radiology 1989;170:553–556.

49. Stones RW, Raw T, Rogers V, Fry R, Beard RW. Pelvic congestion in women: evaluation with transvaginal ultrasound and observation of venous pharmacology. Br J Radiol 1990;63:710–11.
50. Rundqvist E, Sandhol, LE, Larsson G. Treatment of pelvic varicosities causing lower abdominal pain with extraperitoneal resection of the left ovarian vein. Ann Chir Gynaecol 1984;73:339–341.
51. Beard RW, Reginald PW. Pelvic pain in women. Br Med J 1986;293:1160–1162.
52. Hobbs JT. The pelvic congestion syndrome. Br J Hosp Med 1990;43:200–206.
53. Sevilla ME. La varicocele. Pathologie commune aux deux sexes. Phlebologie 1993;46:81–87.
54. Topolanski-Sierra R. Pelvic phlebography. Am J Obstet Gynecol 1958;76:44–45.
55. Murray E, Comparato M. Uterine phlebography. Am J Obstet Gynecol 1968;102: 1088–1093.
56. Kaupilla A. Uterine phlebography with venous compression. A clinical and roentgenological study. Acta Obstet Gynecol Scand 1970;49:33–34.
57. Zak K, Holy J, Prochazka J, Koristek V, Weber I. Beitrag zur Diagnose und Therapie der varizen des kleinen Beckens und der Varicocele pelvina. Gynaecologia 1969;167:426–429.
58. Kennedy A, Hemingway A. Radiology of ovarian varices. Br J Hosp Med 1990;44:38–43.
59. Lechter A, Lopez G, Martinez C, Camacho J. Anatomy of the gonadal veins: a reappraisal. Surgery 1991;109:735–739.
60. Schobinger RA. Iliofemoral dumping syndrome [Abstract]. V European American Symposium on Venous Diseases. Vienna, Austria, November 1990.
61. Hegenscheid F, Schubert M. Beckenvenenvarikosis-einetherapiebare Ursache des chronischen Unterbauchsmerzes der Frau. Zentralbl Gynaecol 1990;112:1157–1162.
62. Loffredo V. Aspects cliniques et examens complementaires dans les etats congestifs pelviens. Rev Fr Gynecol Obstet 1991;86(2bis);191–194.
63. Reginald PW, Beard RW. Intravenous dihydroergotamine to relieve pelvic congestion with pain in young women. Lancet 1987;ii:351–353.
64. Reginald PW, Adams J. Medroxyprogesterone acetate in the treatment of pelvic pain due to venous congestion. Br J Obstet Gynaecol 1989;96:1148–1152.
65. Marhic C. Efficacite clinique et rheologique de la troxerutine en gynecologie obstetrique. Rev Fr Gynecol Obstet 1991;86:191–4.
66. Marhic C. Varicose vulvaire de la grossesse. Rev Fr Gynecol Obstet 1991;86:184–186.
67. Nabatoff RA. Management of varicose veins during pregnancy. Obstet Gynecol 1970;36:928–934.
68. Sumner DS. Venous dynamics—varicosities. Clin Obstet Gynecol 1981;24:743–760.
69. Ouvry PA, Davy A. Les varices vulvaires. Phlebologie 1991;44:375–380.
70. Zelikovski A. Varicosities of uncommon site: therapeutic aspects. Int Surg 1981;66:73–77.
71. Marmasse J. Varices in pregnant women. Legs and vulva. Treatment. Phlebologie 1981;34:89–104.
72. Wallois P. Les varices vulvaires. Le point de vue du phlebologue. Phlebologie 1989;42:451–454.
73. Edwards RD, Robertson IR, MacLean AB, Hemmingway AP. Case report: pelvic pain syndrome/successful treatment of a case by ovarian vein embolization. Clin Radiol 1993;47:429–431.
74. White RI, Kaufman SL, Barth KH, Kadir S, et al. Occlusion of varicoceles with detachable balloons. Radiology 1981;139:327–334.
75. Stoesslein F, Schildhaus J. Neuer abloesbarer Ballon zur therapeutischen Gefaessembolisation. Radiol Diagn 1984;25:525–432.
76. Stoesslein F. Materialien und Indikationen zur transversalen perkutanen Embolisation. Radio Diagn 1984;25:507–512.

77. Mitchel SE, White RI, Mura DR. Long-term follow-up of percutaneous balloon occlusion of varicocele. 71st Scientific Assembly and Annual Meeting of Radiological Society of North America, November 1985.
78. Rasmussen OO, Hammington B. Postpartum persisting pudendal varicose veins—effect of local excision. Vasa 1987;16:352–353.
79. Vassilev I. Etude radiographique de la veine spermatique gauche au cours des varicoceles idiopathiques. Press. Med 1962;70:704.
80. Chait A, Matasar KW, Fabian CE, Mellins HZ. Vascular impressions on the ureters. Am J Roentgen Rad Ther 1971;3:729–749.
81. de Schepper A." Nutcracker" fenomeen van de vena renalis en veneuze pathologie van de linker nier. J Belge Radiol 1972;55:507–511.
82. Pastershank SP. Left renal vein obstruction by a superior mesenteric artery. J Can Assoc Radiol 1974;25:52–54.
83. Stewart BH, Reiman G. Left renal venous hypertension "nutcracker" syndrome. Managed by direct reno-caval reimplantation. Urology 1982;20:365–369.
84. Sacks BA, Gomori J, Lerner M, Masters R, DeWolf W. Left renal vein hypertension in association with the nutcracker phenomenon. Cardiovasc Intervent Radiol 1981;4:253–255.
85. Beckman CF Abrams HL. Idiopathic renal vein varices: incidence and significance. Radiology 1982;143:649–652.
86. Beinart C, Sniderman KW, Tamura S, Vaughan ED Jr, Sos TA. Left renal vein to inferior vena cava pressure relationship in humans. J Urol 1982;127:1070–1071.

section V

Deep Venous Thrombosis

chapter 32

Diagnosis of Deep Venous Thrombosis: Diagnostic Versus Surveillance Testing

Anthony J. Comerota

Most physicians today acknowledge that the signs and symptoms of acute deep venous thrombosis (DVT) are nonspecific and that the clinical diagnosis is unreliable. Therefore, an accurate diagnosis of DVT is essential in order to treat this potentially lethal and frequently morbid disease.

Ascending phlebography has been shown to be highly sensitive and specific and has been accepted as the "gold standard" for the diagnosis of DVT. Phlebography, however, is invasive, causes patient discomfort, is associated with allergic reactions and renal toxicity, cannot be performed in pregnant women, and cannot be repeated frequently. Because of its intrinsic morbidity, which includes severe local tissue destruction if dye extravasation occurs and the fact that it can cause postphlebographic thrombosis, alternative forms of accurate diagnosis are highly desirable.

A variety of diagnostic methods have been introduced during the past two to three decades in an attempt to overcome the disadvantages of phlebography (1). This review addresses the most commonly used noninvasive techniques which have generally been recognized as the most reliable.

Impedance plethysmography (IPG) and phleborheography (PRG) are noninvasive tests that have been refined to the degree that reported diagnostic sensitivities exceed 90% (2–5). Previous investigators indicated that normal results of noninvasive studies were associated with a low risk of venous thromboembolic complications (2, 6, 7), suggesting that such tests could be used to replace ascending phlebography. These studies, however, conflict with the data reported by others that document high false negative and high false positive rates (8, 9). The latter reports seriously questioned the diagnostic reliability of the noninvasive tests and generated concerns on the part of referring physicians as to how to integrate the results of the noninvasive tests with patient care. At Temple University Hospital, we noticed an unacceptably low sensitivity for detecting proximal venous thrombosis with IPG and PRG compared to our experience in

Cincinnati, which was previously reported (5). We also observed that the noninvasive tests and phlebography were being performed more frequently on asymptomatic patients at high risk for DVT, namely those undergoing total joint replacement, compared to our previous experience. As we attempted to resolve the difference in our results compared to the results of others, it became evident that most centers reporting excellent diagnostic sensitivities and predictive values were evaluating symptomatic patients. Therefore, we thought there could be a difference in the results of the noninvasive tests when evaluating symptomatic patients compared to those who are asymptomatic but at high risk for DVT. If this were true, it should reflect a difference in the distribution of clots in these two patient groups and differences in the magnitude of clots, as well as differences in occlusive thrombi versus nonocclusive thrombi.

Noninvasive studies have continued to develop and evolve toward direct imaging techniques. Venous duplex imaging (VDI) has been studied and appears superior to hemodynamic tests for deep venous thrombosis (10, 11). The question remained, however, did venous duplex imaging have the same limitations of the hemodynamic noninvasive studies when applied to those asymptomatic patients at high risk for DVT? Color-flow duplex scanning then emerged as the newest technological advancement in the noninvasive evaluation of vascular disease, and has recently been applied to the study of venous disease (12, 13). It was expected that further improvements in diagnostic sensitivity and predictive values would be provided by the addition of color. To put the noninvasive methods of the diagnosis of acute DVT into proper perspective, a number of important questions must be answered:

1. Does patient selection influence diagnostic reliability of noninvasive hemodynamic testing for DVT?
2. Is there a difference in the incidence of DVT in symptomatic patients compared to asymptomatic patients at high risk for DVT?
3. Is there a difference in the location of thrombi in these two patient groups?
4. Is there a difference in the magnitude of thrombi in these two patient groups?
5. Does the addition of ^{125}I-fibrinogen uptake improve diagnostic sensitivity enough to make the noninvasive results of symptomatic and asymptomatic patients comparable?
6. Is the diagnostic reliability of venous duplex imaging (VDI) superior to that of hemodynamic testing for acute DVT?
7. Does the addition of color flow scanning improve the sensitivity and predictive values compared to conventional venous duplex imaging?

Two consecutive, prospective analyses were performed to determine whether patient selection influenced diagnostic reliability and whether the incidence of DVT was different in symptomatic compared to asymptomatic patients. In the first study, a prospective analysis of 351 patients having IPG, PRG, ^{125}I-fibrinogen uptake testing (RFUT), and ascending phlebography was performed (14). All patients had at least one noninvasive diagnostic test and ascending phlebography during the same 24-hour period. All patients were categorized into one of three groups on the basis of their ascending phlebogram. Those without evidence of DVT were categorized as normal, those with isolated calf vein thrombosis as B/K and patients with proximal vein thrombosis (whether or not calf vein throm-

TABLE 32-1

IMPEDANCE PLETHYSMOGRAPHY COMPARED WITH PHLEBOGRAPHY (N = 308)

	Overall	Diagnostic		Surveillance	p Value
SPEC	85% (119/140)	81% (66/81)	vs	90% (53/59)	NS
SENS	49% (83/168)	71% (69/97)	vs	20% (14/71)	<0.0001
A/K	68% (79/116)	83% (68/82)	vs	32% (11/34)	<0.0001
B/K	8% (4/52)	7% (1/15)	vs	8% (3/37)	NS
−PV	58% (119/204)	70% (66/94)	vs	48% (53/110)	<0.005
+PV	80% (83/104)	82% (69/84)	vs	70% (14/20)	NS

SPEC = specificity; SENS = sensitivity; −PV = negative predictive value; +PV = positive predictive value.

bus was present) as A/K. By convention, all patients with thrombus in the popliteal vein were considered to have proximal (A/K) DVT, even if the clot was limited to the distal popliteal vein, below the knee joint. Patients who had symptoms of acute deep venous thrombosis had the noninvasive studies to confirm the clinical suspicion of acute DVT, and these patients were classified as the "diagnostic group." Those patients who were asymptomatic but at high risk for postoperative DVT because they were orthopedic surgical patients undergoing total hip replacement had noninvasive studies as part of a surveillance program. Therefore, these patients were classified as the "surveillance group."

The results of IPG compared with phlebography are shown in Table 32.1 and the results of the PRG compared with phlebography are shown in Table 32.2. While the PRG appears to be a more sensitive test than IPG, both analyses demonstrate that these hemodynamic tests are significantly more sensitive in detecting blood clots in symptomatic patients than in asymptomatic patients. The sensitivity for the diagnosis of acute DVT is unacceptably low for both tests when they are used to evaluate asymptomatic patients as part of a surveillance program.

TABLE 32-2

PHLEBORHEOGRAPHY COMPARED WITH PHLEBOGRAPHY (N = 302)

	Overall	Diagnostic		Surveillance	p Value
SPEC	78% (116/134)	81% (65/80)	vs	94% (51/54)	<0.05
SENS	59% (99/168)	78% (82/105)	vs	27% (17/63)	<0.0001
A/K	78% (88/113)	92% (79/86)	vs	33% (9/27)	<0.0001
B/K	20% (11/55)	16% (3/19)	vs	22% (8/36)	NS
−PV	63% (116/185)	74% (65/88)	vs	53% (51/97)	<0.001
+PV	85% (99/117)	85% (82/97)	vs	85% (17/20)	NS

SPEC = specificity; SENS = sensitivity; −PV = negative predictive value; +PV = positive predictive value.

TABLE 32-3

COMPARISON OF THE PHLEBOGRAPHIC RESULTS BETWEEN PATIENT GROUPS

Location	Diagnostic (N = 212)	Surveillance (N = 139)	p Value
No thrombi	(94/212) 44%	(63/139) 45%	NS
A/K	(99/212) 47%	(36/139) 26%	<0.0001
B/K	(19/212) 9%	(40/139) 29%	<0.0001

Insight as to why the results are so different between these two patient groups might be obtained by analysis of the phlebographic characteristics of the thrombi; that is, the distribution of the thrombi and the magnitude of occlusion. These data are listed in Tables 32.3 and 32.4, respectively. Although there is no difference in the incidence of DVT between patient groups, there is a significant difference in the percentage of patients with proximal (AK) thrombi in the diagnostic group (84%: 99/118) compared with those in the surveillance group (47%: 36/76) ($p < 0.001$). We would intuitively expect that occluding thrombi in the deep venous system would create hemodynamic abnormalities, and therefore would more likely cause symptoms, whereas nonoccluding thrombi would not alter venous return and would likely remain asymptomatic. Available phlebograms in patients with A/K thrombi were reviewed to determine whether the clot was occluding or nonoccluding (Table 32.4). Eighty-four percent of AK thrombi in the diagnostic group (58/69) were occluding versus 23% in the surveillance group (7/31) ($p < 0.0001$). The distribution of thrombi in other reports evaluating diagnostic and surveillance patients is listed in Table 32.5. The distribution and magnitude of DVT in any surveillance group will depend upon the frequency and efficacy of DVT prophylaxis administered.

To put these noninvasive data into perspective with those obtained by other investigators, the results of patients evaluated with phlebography and impedance plethysmography are listed in Table 32.6. The sensitivities of detecting proximal DVT (A/K thrombi) are remarkably consistent. Following a single IPG test, a sensitivity of 80–90% can be expected in patients in the diagnostic group. If sequential IPGs (or other noninvasive testing) are performed prior to obtaining confirmatory phlebography, one can expect the sensitivity for proximal DVT detection

TABLE 32-4

OCCLUDING VERSUS NONOCCLUDING THROMBI IN PATIENTS WITH PROXIMAL DEEP VENOUS THROMBOSIS (N = 100)

	Diagnostic (N = 69)	Surveillance (N = 31)	p Value
Occluding	84% (58/69)	23% (7/31)	<0.0001
Nonoccluding	16% (11/69)	77% (24/31)	<0.0001

TABLE 32-5

INCIDENCE AND DISTRIBUTION OF THROMBI OF PATIENTS WITH DEEP VENOUS THROMBOSIS (BY PHLEBOGRAPHY). PATIENT ANALYZED ACCORDING TO SYMPTOMATIC (DIAGNOSTIC GROUP) AND ASYMPTOMATIC (SURVEILLANCE GROUP) PRESENTATION

	Diagnostic		Surveillance		
Author (ref).	**Comerota (14)**	**Hull (15)**	**Comerota (14)**	**Hull (16)**	**Paiement (17)**
Total no.	**212**	**274**	**139**	**310**	**554***
DVT Present	56% (118/215)	42% (114/274)	55% (76/139)	35% (109/310)	34% (190/554)
DVT A/K	46% (99/212)	28% (78/274)	28% (36/139)	20% (63/310)	13% (73/554)
DVT B/K	9% (19/212)	13% (36/274)	29% (40/139)	15% (46/310)	21% (117/554)
Normal	44% (94/212)	58% (160/274)	45% (63/139)	65% (201/310)	66% (364/554)

*Includes 17 patients with bilateral venograms (3%).
DVT = deep venous thrombosis
A/K = proximal DVT defined as thrombi located in the popliteal vein or a more proximal vein.
B/K = infrapopliteal (calf) vein thrombosis.

to improve by 10–15% (6). When the IPG (or other hemodynamic tests such as PRG) is performed for surveillance purposes, uniformly poor sensitivities have been observed.

The timing of postoperative phlebography in the surveillance group is important when assessing the magnitude of thrombi. The shorter the interval between operation and postoperative phlebography, the more likely one is to diagnose calf vein thrombosis and nonoccluding thrombi. Of the patients reported in Table 32.7, 94% had the phlebogram performed within 7 postoperative days. The effect of

TABLE 32-6

RELIABILITY OF NONINVASIVE STUDIES FOR THE DIAGNOSIS OF ACUTE DEEP VENOUS THROMBOSIS. COMPARISON OF THE RESULTS OF PRG AND IPG WHEN USED IN SYMPTOMATIC (DIAGNOSTIC) PATIENTS AND ASYMPTOMATIC (SURVEILLANCE) PATIENTS

	Symptomatic Patients (Diagnostic)			Asymptomatic Patients (Surveillance)		
	PRG	IPG		PRG	IPG	
Author (ref).	**Comerota (14) (N = 185)**	**Comerota (14) (N = 178)**	**Wheeler (3)* (N = 2394)**	**Comerota (14) (N = 117)**	**Comerota (14) (N = 130)**	**Paiement (17) (N = 937)**
SENS (prox DVT)	92%	83%	94%	33%	32%	12%
SPECIFICITY	81%	81%	95%	94%	90%	99%
+ PRED VALUE	85%	82%	88%	85%	70%	47%
− PRED VALUE	74%	70%	97%	53%	48%	92%

*Pooled data (12 reports).

TABLE 32-7

HEMODYNAMIC ABNORMALITIES OF PROXIMAL THROMBI BY PATIENT GROUP (N = 94)

IPG/PRG*	Diagnostic (N = 69)	Surveillance (N = 25)	p Value
Neither +	3% (2/69)	58% (13/25)	<0.001
One +	97% (67/69)	48% (12/25)	<0.001
Both +	74% (51/69)	20% (5/25)	<0.001

*Note: All patients had IPG and PRG and phlebography in the same 24-hour period.

^{125}I-fibrinogen on improving the sensitivity of diagnosing postoperative DVT is appreciated by examining the data in Tables 32.8 and 32.9. The RFUT significantly improves overall sensitivity as well as the sensitivity of diagnosing AK and BK thrombi for both IPG and PRG. Because of the false-positives associated with the RFUT, the specificity is reduced compared to that obtained by the noninvasive test alone. Likewise, the negative predictive value of the combination of tests is significantly better than that of either IPG or PRG alone. Although adding the IPG or PRG to the RFUT appears to improve the sensitivity for detecting AK thrombi compared with the RFUT alone, this difference is not significant.

To determine whether patient selection influences the results of the combination of tests (IPG plus RFUT) the surveillance data in the current series were compared with both diagnostic and surveillance data published previously by Hull, et al. (15, 16), and with surveillance data reported by Paiement, et al. (17) (Table 32.10). Similar observations were made with the results of the combination of tests as with the noninvasive tests alone. The RFUT plus IPG had significantly better sensitivity when used in symptomatic patients compared to asymptomatic patients in an intensive surveillance program (Table 32.10). The same trend is observed with the combination tests compared to the IPG alone. There is signifi-

TABLE 32-8

COMBINED IMPEDANCE PLETHYSMOGRAPHY AND ^{125}I-FIBRINOGEN UPTAKE TEST VERSUS PHLEBOGRAPHY (N = 111)

	RFUT alone	IPG alone	IPG + RFUT	p Value*
SPEC	71% (39/55)	91% (50/55)	67% (37/55)	<0.005
SENS	73% (41/56)	16% (9/56)	77% (43/56)	<0.0001
A/K	63% (15/24)	25% (6/24)	71% (17/24)	<0.001
B/K	81% (26/32)	9% (3/32)	81% (26/32)	<0.0001
−PV	72% (39/54)	52% (50/97)	74% (37/50)	<0.005
+PV	72% (41/57)	64% (9/14)	71% (43/61)	NS

*Significance of difference between IPG alone and IPG plus RFUT.

TABLE 32-9

COMBINED PHLEBORHEOGRAPHY AND ^{125}I-FIBRINOGEN UPTAKE TEST VERSUS PHLEBOGRAPHY

	RFUT alone	PRG alone	PRG + RFUT	p Value*
SPEC	74% (37/50)	94% (47/50)	68% (34/50)	<0.001
SENS	70% (37/53)	26% (14/53)	77% (41/53)	<0.0001
A/K	52% (11/21)	33% (7/21)	67% (14/21)	<0.05
B/K	81% (26/32)	22% (7/32)	84% (27/32)	<0.0001
−PV	70% (37/53)	55% (47/86)	74% (34/46)	<0.01
+PV	74% (37/50)	82% (14/17)	72% (41/57)	NS

*Significance of difference between PRG alone.

cantly better sensitivity in the diagnostic patients compared to those in the surveillance group.

A second prospective study was performed to determine whether the same limitations occurred with venous duplex imaging as with the hemodynamic tests for DVT (18). This study evaluated VDI, PRG (the most sensitive hemodynamic test), and ascending phlebography within the same 24-hour period. The results are shown in Table 32.11. The overall sensitivity of VDI is 96% (51/53) compared to 55% (29/53) for the PRG ($p < 0.001$). Venous duplex imaging detected 100% (44/44) of AK thrombi compared to 66% (29/44) detected by PRG ($p < 0.001$). It is interesting to note that VDI detected 78% (7/9) of BK thrombi compared to 0% (0/9) detected by PRG ($p < 0.001$). Although the positive predictive value and specificity between the two noninvasive tests were not different, the negative predictive value was significantly better for VDI.

The data reported here indicate that there are significant differences in the ability of noninvasive tests to accurately diagnose DVT in patients who have symptoms compared to asymptomatic patients in surveillance programs. Patient se-

TABLE 32-10

COMPARISON OF IPG + ^{125}I-FIBRINOGEN UPTAKE TESTS DONE FOR SURVEILLANCE VERSUS DIAGNOSIS OF DEEP VENOUS THROMBOSIS

	Diagnostic	Surveillance		
Author (ref)	Hull (15)	Hull (16)	Comerota (14)	Paiement (17)
SPEC	95% (154/160)	93% (140/150)	67% (37/55)*	94% (708/751)
SENS	90% (103/114)	46% (50/109)*	77% (43/56)*	46% (95/206)
A/K	100% (78/78)	48% (30/63)*	71% (17/24)*	23% (17/73)
B/K	69% (25/36)	43% (20/46)*	81% (26/32)	59% (78/133)
−PV	93% (152/163)	93% (140/150)	74% (37/50)*	87% (708/810)
+PV	93% (103/111)	70% (140/199)*	71% (43/61)*	69% (82/124)

*Indicates that difference compared to diagnostic testing is significant $p < 0.01$.

TABLE 32-11

VENOUS DUPLEX IMAGING AND PHLEBORHEOGRAPHY COMPARED TO ASCENDING PHLEBOGRAPHY

All patients (N = 110)			
	VDI	*PRG*	*p Value*
Sensitivity			
All	96% (51/53)	55% (29/53)	$p < 0.001$
A/K	100% (44/44)	66% (29/44)	$p < 0.001$
B/K	78% (7/9)	0% (0/9)	$p < 0.001$
Pos. pred. value	93% (51/55)	83% (29/35)	N.S.
Specificity	93% (53/57)	89% (51/57)	N.S.
Neg. pred. value	96% (53/55)	68% (51/75)	$p < 0.001$
Diagnostic Patients (N = 72)			
	VDI	*PRG*	*p Value*
Sensitivity			
All	98% (43/44)	61% (27/44)	$p < 0.001$
A/K	100% (37/37)	73% (27/37)	$p < 0.01$
B/K	86% (6/7)	0% (0/7)	$p < 0.01$
Pos. pred. value	91% (43/47)	82% (27/33)	N.S.
Specificity	86% (24/28)	79% (22/28)	N.S.
Neg. pred. value	96% (24/25)	56% (22/39)	$p < 0.001$
Surveillance Patients (N = 38)			
	VDI	*PRG*	*p Value*
Sensitivity			
All	89% (8/9)	22% (2/9)	$p < 0.05$
A/K	100% (7/7)	29% (2/7)	$p < 0.05$
B/K	50% (1/2)	0% (0/2)	N.S.
Pos. pred. value	100% (8/8)	100% (2/2)	N.S.
Specificity	100% (29/29)	100% (29/29)	N.S.
Neg. pred. value	97% (29/30)	81% (29/36)	N.S.

lection has a profound influence on the diagnostic sensitivity of hemodynamic testing, and these tests are unreliable when used in surveillance programs. That being the case, noninvasive studies relying on hemodynamic principles cannot determine the true incidence of postoperative DVT, even when combined with the RFUT. Binder RFUT is no longer available in the United States for clinical use. Therefore, anatomic studies continue to be a necessary requirement for a complete surveillance program after total joint replacement. These data indicate that noninvasive hemodynamic testing is inadequate as an endpoint for generating reliable epidemiologic data. Additionally, studies evaluating the efficacy of DVT prophylaxis cannot use hemodynamic tests to determine whether DVT exists, and therefore will continue to require anatomic studies as an endpoint.

The reason for these observations is that there is a significant difference in the location of thrombi as well as the magnitude of thrombi in these two patient groups. Patients in the surveillance program had more BK thrombi and nonoccluding thrombi than symptomatic patients, as mentioned previously. This makes intuitive sense, since thrombi which do not affect venous hemodynamics are unlikely to create symptoms (except for pulmonary emboli).

Venous duplex imaging did not show the same limitations as the hemodynamic tests for DVT. There was no difference in those patients evaluated in the surveillance group compared to those in the diagnostic group. VDI detected 100% of proximal (A/K) thrombi in both diagnostic and surveillance groups and 78% (7/9) of all isolated below knee thrombi. VDI was significantly more sensitive than PRG for detecting both above knee and below knee thrombi ($p < 0.001$) and, importantly, the negative predictive value of VDI was significantly higher than that for PRG ($p < 0.001$). VDI reliably diagnosed nonocclusive and infrapopliteal thrombi, thereby offering superior epidemiologic and natural history capability in patients with acute DVT. Based upon these observations, it appears that VDI offers superior noninvasive diagnostic acumen without the limitations of traditional hemodynamic techniques. In experienced vascular laboratories, VDI may be more sensitive than even ascending phlebography. This is most certainly true when all patients requiring diagnostic evaluation are considered, since some patients are excluded from phlebography owing to access problems, contrast toxicity or allergic reactions. VDI may become the new diagnostic standard for deep venous thrombosis.

Whether the addition of color to venous duplex improves diagnostic sensitivity remains to be shown. A recent report by Sumner, et al. (19), failed to show that color-flow scanning improved diagnostic sensitivity. Importantly, experience with venous duplex imaging and a good gray scale instrument significantly improved sensitivity in patients in a surveillance program. Sumner's report underscores the importance of experience with the technique and good instrumentation. One cannot assume that excellent results can be obtained with all instruments, nor can one assume that instruments are interchangeable. Additionally, the dedication of the physician interpreting the exam and the ability and persistence of the technologist performing the examination are the keys to reproducibly good results.

REFERENCES

1. Comerota AJ, Knight LC, Maurer AH. The diagnosis of acute deep venous thrombosis: noninvasive and radioisotopic techniques. Ann Vasc Surg 1988;4:406–424.
2. Hull RD, Hirsh J, Carter CJ, et al. Diagnostic efficacy of impedance plethysmography for clinically suspected deep vein thrombosis. Ann Internal Med 1985;102:21–28.
3. Wheeler HB, Anderson FA. The diagnosis of venous thrombosis by impedance plethysmography. In: Bernstein EF, ed. Noninvasive diagnostic techniques in vascular disease. 3rd ed. St. Louis: CV Mosby, 1985:755.
4. Cranley JJ. Phleborheography. In: Kempczinski RF, Yao JST, eds. Practical noninvasive vascular diagnosis. 2nd ed. Chicago: Year Book Medical Publishers, 1987:438–463.
5. Comerota AJ, Cranley JJ, Cook SE, et al. Phleborheography—a 10 year experience. Surgery 1982;91:573–581.

6. Huisman MV, Buller HR, Cate JV, Vreeken J. Serial impedance plethysmography for suspected deep venous thrombosis in outpatients. N Engl J Med 1986;314:823–828.
7. Stallworth JM, Plonk GW, Horne JB. Negative phleborheography, clinical follow-up in 593 patients. Arch Surg 1981;116:795–797.
8. Vaccaro P, Van Aman M, Miller S, Fochman J, Smead WL. Shortcomings of physical examination and impedance plethysmography in the diagnosis of lower extremity deep venous thrombosis. Angiology 1987;38(3):232–235.
9. Young AE, Henderson BS, Phillips DA, Couch NP. Impedance plethysmography: its limitations as a substitute for phlebography. Cardiovasc Radiol 1978;1:233–239.
10. Comerota AJ, Katz ML. The diagnosis of acute deep venous thrombosis by duplex venous imaging. Semin Vasc Surg 1988;1:32–39.
11. Elias A, Le Corff G, Bouvier JL, Benichou M, Serradimigni A. Value of real-time B-mode ultrasound imaging in the diagnosis of deep vein thrombosis of the lower limbs. Int Angiol 1987;6:175–182.
12. Persson AV, Jones C, Zide R, Jewell ER. Use of the triplex scanner in diagnosis of deep venous thrombosis. Arch Surg 1989;124:593.
13. Mattos MA, Londrey GL, Leutz DW, et al. Color flow duplex scanning for the surveillance and diagnosis of acute deep venous thrombosis. J Vasc Surg 1992;15:366–376.
14. Comerota AJ, Katz ML, Grossi RJ, et al. The comparative value of noninvasive testing for diagnosis and surveillance of deep vein thrombosis. J Vasc Surg 1988;7:40–49.
15. Hull R, Hirsh J, Sackett DL, et al. Replacement of venography in suspected venous thrombosis by impedance plethysmography and ^{125}I-fibrinogen leg scanning. Ann Int Med 1981;94:12–15.
16. Hull RD, Raskob GE, Gent M, et al. Effectiveness of intermittent pneumatic leg compression for preventing deep vein thrombosis after total hip replacement. JAMA 1990;17:263.
17. Paiement G, Wessinger SJ, Waltman AC, Harris WH. Surveillance of deep vein thrombosis in asymptomatic total hip replacement patients. Am J Surg 1990;155:400–404.
18. Comerota AJ, Katz ML, Greenwald LL, Leefmans E, Czeredarczuk M, White JV. Venous duplex imaging: should it replace hemodynamic tests for deep venous thrombosis? J Vasc Surg 1990;11:53–61.
19. Mattos MA, Londrey GL, Leutz DW, Hodgson KJ, Ramsey DE, Barkmeier LD, Stauffer ES, Spadone DP, Sumner DS. Color-flow duplex scanning for the surveillance and diagnosis of acute deep venous thrombosis. J Vasc Surg 1992 Feb;15(2):366–75; discussion 375–6.

chapter 33

Vena Caval Interruption and Filters

Lazar J. Greenfield and Thomas A. Whitehill

Deep venous thrombosis (DVT) continues to be a clinically challenging disorder with an annual incidence of 300,000–600,000 episodes that lead to at least 50,000 deaths per year from pulmonary embolism (1). The emphasis in the management of acute DVT is balanced between control of the primary thrombosis and effective prevention of associated life-threatening pulmonary embolism, as well as survival for those in whom such emboli occur. Venous thrombotic disease can readily be managed by effective anticoagulation in the majority of patients, as can most associated pulmonary thromboembolisms. However, under circumstances in which anticoagulation either cannot be used or fails to protect the patient, there is a well-accepted indication for mechanical protection at the level of the inferior vena cava.

Historically, surgical approaches have evolved from ligation, plication, and the application of clips to the permanent caval filter devices introduced transvenously by either the jugular or femoral vein. Early surgical efforts to prevent recurrence of pulmonary embolism were directed at the common femoral vein, which was ligated bilaterally. The next approach was ligation of the inferior vena cava below the renal veins, which added the adverse effect of a sudden reduction in cardiac output (2). This deleterious effect, which could be lethal in the presence of increased pulmonary vascular resistance coupled with stasis sequelae and recurrent embolism through dilated collateral veins, led to efforts to compartmentalize the vena cava by means of sutures, staples, and external clips so as to provide filtration without causing occlusion (3, 4). Despite promising early patency data, high rates of caval occlusion were identified after relatively short follow-up periods. Additionally, these techniques added the morbidity associated with general anesthesia and laparotomy.

Since 1968, the experience gained with early transvenous endovascular filters has helped to define the performance criteria expected of a safe and effective filtration device. These criteria include (a) ease of insertion into the proper position under local anesthesia, (b) effective protection against further embolism, (c) maintenance of long-term caval patency, (d) stability of position over time, and (e) lack of any tendency toward caval wall penetration or erosion.

INDICATIONS FOR VENA CAVAL FILTER PLACEMENT

Currently accepted indications for inferior vena caval filter insertion include (a) documented deep venous thrombosis (DVT) or pulmonary embolism (PE) with a recognized contraindication to anticoagulation, (b) recurrent pulmonary embolism despite adequate anticoagulation, (c) bleeding complications requiring that anticoagulation therapy be discontinued, (d) patients who have undergone pulmonary embolectomy, and (e) patients who have had failure of another form of caval interruption demonstrated by recurrent thromboembolism. Case-selective or relative indications include (f) adjunctive use in the presence of iliofemoral thrombosis with a 5-cm or longer free-floating tail, (g) presence of septic pulmonary embolism, (h) chronic pulmonary embolism in a patient with pulmonary hypertension and cor pulmonale, and (i) adjunctive use in a patient with significant cardiopulmonary disease who would not tolerate any recurrent thromboembolism.

Long-term favorable experience with Greenfield vena caval filters has led some authors to further liberalize the indications for filter insertion. Recent recommendations for caval filtration include routine DVT prophylaxis in cancer patients and high-risk general surgical patients, general use in older or pregnant women with DVT and/or PE instead of anticoagulation, and general prophylactic use instead of anticoagulation (5, 6). Additional studies will be required, however, to determine whether these indications are appropriate and whether the risk of anticoagulation outweighs the risk of filter placement alone. At the present time, we recommend continued primary use of appropriate anticoagulation to control the underlying thrombotic disorder in patients who are eligible for anticoagulant therapy.

STAINLESS STEEL GREENFIELD FILTER

The standard for performance of transvenous vena caval filters remains the stainless steel Greenfield filter (SGF) for which complete long-term follow-up experience is available, since the device was introduced in 1972 (7). The Greenfield filter was developed to maintain caval patency after trapping emboli and to preserve prograde caval flow, avoiding stasis and facilitating lysis of the trapped emboli (Fig. 33.1). The cone-shaped filter is 4.6 cm long from apex to base, the latter formed by its six legs which provide for caval fixation by means of small recurved hooks. The spacing between the legs is 2 mm at the apex of the cone and a maximum of 6 mm at the base when the device is expanded, dependent on inferior vena cava (IVC) size. The spacing between limbs is such that the filter effectively traps most emboli 3-mm or greater in diameter. The conical geometry allows for progressive vertical central filling while maintaining circumferential blood flow, thus avoiding progressive venous thrombosis, caval obstruction, and venous hypertension. When thrombus fills the filter to 70% of its depth, only 49% of the cross-sectional area is blocked. Experience has shown that there is no increase in distal venous pressure until 80% of the filter is filled with clot, at which point more than 64% of the cross-sectional area is blocked (8). These design features result in the very high patency rates and minimal incidence of stasis sequelae noted

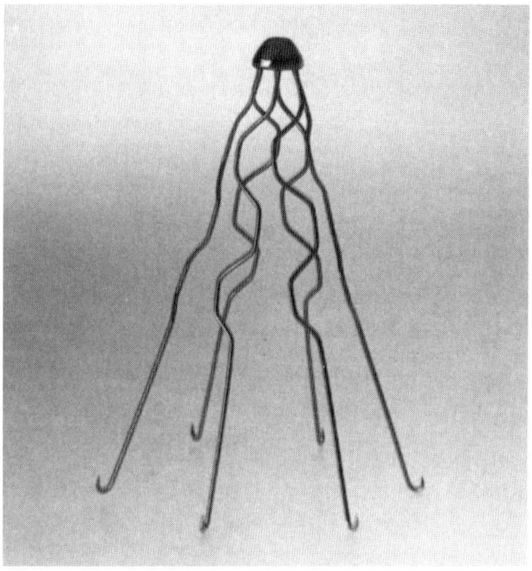

FIG. 33–1. The original stainless steel Greenfield filter (SGF) introduced in 1972 for mechanical protection against pulmonary thromboembolism.

in long-term follow-up. Additionally, an unexpected result of flow preservation has been the evidence that progressive lysis of the trapped thrombus occurs over time.

The SGF has been reported to show a 4% rate of recurrent embolism over a 12-year period of observation in 469 patients and a long-term filter patency rate of 98% (9). Similar results have been obtained in other follow-up series with long-term patency rates in excess of 95% (10, 11). The results with suprarenal filter placement are quite comparable with a 100% patency rate in the 22 patients studied in the series of 69 filters so placed since 1976 (12). Over a period of years, 9% of the stainless steel filters can be seen to move slightly in a distal direction, which is presumably a gravitational effect (13).

The patency rate of the Greenfield filter is not dependent on prolonged anticoagulation, and the termination of anticoagulant therapy is dictated by the patient's underlying thrombotic disorder. The notably few associated complications include misplacement due to premature discharge or inaccurate fluoroscopic control of the carrier, rare limb penetration of the cava, or filter limb fracture. Although it is possible to retrieve a misplaced device, misplacements into the renal, hepatic, or iliac veins have not caused functional problems. The only functional consequence of misplacement below the diaphragm may be inadequate filtration of caval flow. This unusual problem is easily remedied by placement of a second filter. Intracardiac misplacement may produce tricuspid valve dysfunction or arrhythmias, which are the indications for filter removal. Various techniques have been reported for filter retrieval transvenously or it may be removed operatively.

Because of reliable preservation of caval patency, the filter has adapted well to a variety of unusual clinical problems, i.e., suprarenal inferior vena caval and superior vena caval placements. The filter has also been a useful adjunct in the successful management of septic thrombophlebitis. This is possible because preserved prograde venous flow though the filter permits in vivo sterilization of any infected thrombus within it by parenteral antibiotic treatment (14).

Technical Considerations for Filter Insertion

The procedure should be performed under optimal fluoroscopy. This can be achieved in the operating room with a C-arm fluoroscope if the patient is not obese, or in the radiology suite where better imaging can be obtained in the obese patient. A preoperative venacavogram should be obtained and available for review at the time of insertion. Operative insertion is usually undertaken via the jugular vein which can be exposed under local anesthesia. The patient should be positioned with a small folded towel between the shoulder blades to extend the neck. With the head turned to the left, a short transverse incision is made over the base of the sternocleidomastoid muscle to allow separation of the sternal and clavicular heads of the muscle in order to expose the underlying jugular vein. Once a 4–5-cm length of jugular vein is exposed, it can be controlled by twill tape proximally and a vascular clamp distally, taking care not to injure the vagus nerve. The filter carrier system, previously checked and filled with heparinized saline, is loaded with the filter and the plunger system locked securely. The guidewire should be removed from the carrier system to allow it to be positioned in the inferior vena cava prior to introduction of the carrier unit. Although a large loop floppy J-wire is provided with the unit, it is often easier to use a straight 0.035-inch standard guidewire instead. The guidewire is introduced into the jugular vein through a No. 15 Jelco needle and the twill tape secured. The guidewire is advanced under fluoroscopic guidance and directed through the right atrium into the inferior vena cava as far as the bifurcation.

The radiographic diameter of the vena cava should be measured with correction for magnification, which can be as much as 25–30%. Very large vena cavas (>30 mm in diameter) may be found in patients with right heart failure. In these patients, it is safer to introduce separate filters into each iliac vein. Fortunately, the vena cava is narrower in the anteroposterior diameter than in the transverse diameter, which provides an additional measure of security for fixation. Once the guidewire is positioned in the inferior vena cava below the level of the renal veins, the external stiff end of the guidewire is introduced retrograde through the carrier if one is dealing with the standard 24 Fr system (Fig. 33.2). The newer titanium Greenfield filter (TGF) can also be used with this exposure and its dilator-sheath system is described in the next section. The sheath provides a protected route for the filter-carrier system to the level of insertion, obviating the risk of premature discharge of the filter. With either system, the puncture hole in the jugular vein is enlarged by a short transverse incision and then either the carrier or the dilator-sheath system is inserted into the vein and passed down to the level of L2–L3. If the operator is using the dilator-sheath system, the dilator should be withdrawn once the sheath is in the infrarenal inferior vena cava, but not if the sheath is in the thorax where negative pressure might allow air embolism to occur. The TGF preloaded carrier is then inserted into the sheath until it is seen to completely exit the distal intravascular sheath at the desired level of filter introduction. Use of the standard stainless steel carrier follows a similar path over the guidewire to the level of L2–L3.

At this point, the stylet is unlocked and the stainless steel carrier is gradually retracted until the filter springs open at the appropriate level in the vena cava. The introducer system and guidewire should then be withdrawn with no further

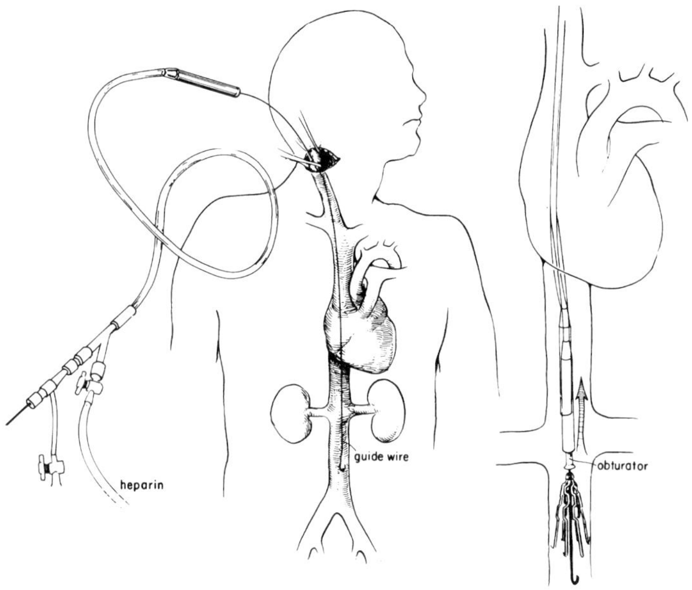

FIG. 33–2. Technique of insertion of the SGF using a guidewire for positioning the carrier and for axial centering of the filter at discharge. (Reproduced by permission from Greenfield LJ, Stewart JR, Crute S. Improved technique for insertion of Greenfield vena cava filter. Surg Gynecol Obstet 1983;156:217–219.)

attempts to manipulate the filter. Any delay in positioning the filter with the carrier can be associated with thrombus formation inside the carrier; therefore, heparinized saline should be used to flush the system through the attached Luer-Lok connection either periodically or continuously. Contrast medium can also be injected, if necessary, to verify filter position as well as its proximity to any thrombus that might be in the inferior vena cava. Thrombus within the vena cava should not be allowed to contact the filter since this could lead to propagation of thrombus through the filter and above the level of mechanical protection. If thrombus does extend to the level of the renal veins, or if the distal inferior vena cava is thrombosed, the filter should be inserted at the level of T12, above the level of the renal veins. Following removal of the carrier system and guidewire, the venotomy is closed with 5–0 monofilament suture and the wound closed without drainage after assuring hemostasis. A follow-up abdominal radiograph is obtained to confirm the position of the filter. Often there is a discrepancy between the fluoroscopic image and that of the abdominal radiograph due to slight parallax of the fluoroscopic image (15).

ALTERNATIVE FILTER DEVICES

Percutaneous insertion of devices designed to provide effective filtration of thromboemboli in the vena cava offers a number of potential advantages for the patient including reduction in discomfort, savings of time, and decreased cost, owing to the use of the radiology suite rather than the operating room (16). Insertion is made possible by use of the Seldinger technique, which allows the percutaneous insertion of progressively larger dilators over a Teflon-coated guidewire and a sheath. Enlarging the skin incision permits tract expansion either by balloon or dilators to allow the insertion of a larger sheath. Percutaneously-inserted caval devices are customarily placed through the right femoral approach, but they may be inserted through the neck by way of the jugular vein. The latter route is less desirable because of the risk of air embolism.

Initial efforts at percutaneous introduction of the standard 24 Fr carrier system of the SGF required a very large sheath (26 Fr) and prolonged compression of the insertion site; this resulted in a 30–40% incidence of insertion site venous thrombosis (17). This led to the enthusiastic proliferation of many innovative devices that can be inserted percutaneously by radiologists using a smaller-diameter delivery system in an effort to retain the advantage of percutaneous insertion while minimizing the incidence of insertion site venous thrombosis (Fig. 33.3). Despite the insertion of large numbers of these alternative filter devices, it has been difficult to obtain accurate follow-up information in order to compare their effectiveness (Table 33.1).

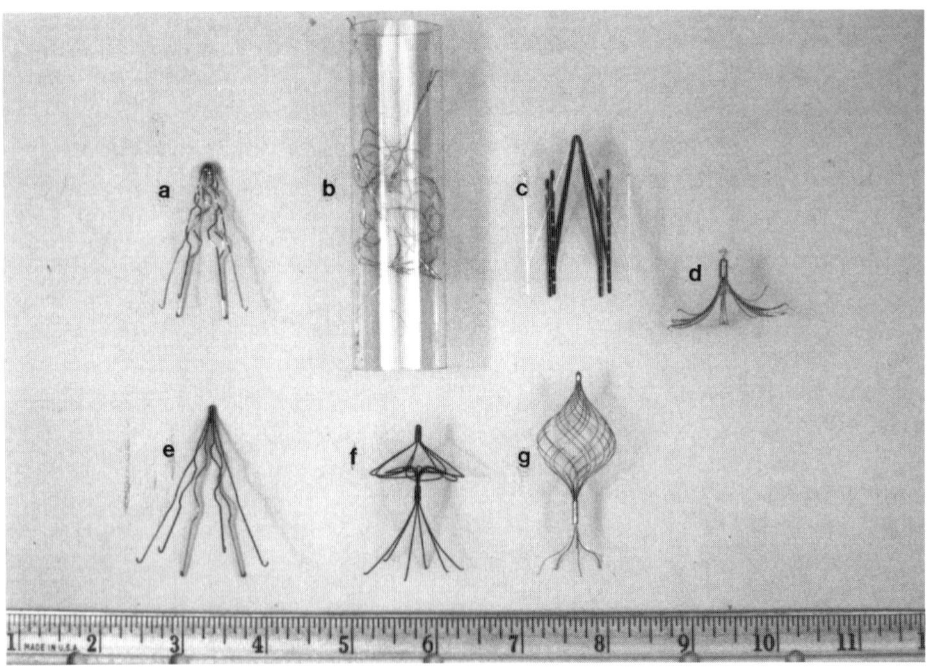

FIG. 33–3. Comparison of vena caval filter devices which have been tested clinically: *a,* SGF; *b,* Bird's Nest filter; *c,* VenaTech filter; *d,* Amplatz filter; *e,* original titanium Greenfield filter; *f,* Nitinol filter; and *g,* Gunther filter. (Reproduced by permission from Stein PD. Venous disorders. Philadelphia: WB Saunders, 1991:556.)

TABLE 33-1

COMPARISON OF INFERIOR VENA CAVAL FILTERS

Filter	Greenfield SS	Greenfield Titanium	VenaTech	Bird's Nest	Simon Nitinol
Evaluation	Registry (1988)	Clinical trial (1991)	Clinical trial (1990)	Clinical trial (1988)	Clinical trial (1990)
Duration	12 years	30 days	1 year	6 months	6 months
Number	469	186 (123 at FU)	97 (77 at FU)	568 (440 at 6 months)	224 (102 at FU)
Recurrent PE	4%	3%	2%	2.7% (33–67% in subset with OBJ, FU)	4% based upon those who had follow-up
Caval patency	98%	100%	92%	97%	81%
Filter patency	98%	Not reported	63% without thrombus	81%	Not reported
Insertion site DVT	41% (percutaneous)	8.7%	23%	"Few" none OBJ.	11%
Migration	35% >3mm	11% >9mm	14% >10mm	9% with original model	1.2% of those with FU
Penetration	Not reported	1%	Not reported	Not reported	0.6% of those with FU
Misplacement	4%	0%	Not reported	Not reported	Not reported
Incomplete opening	Not reported	2%	6%	Not reported	Not reported
Means of Follow-up	Pelvic scan, x-ray, noninvasive vascular exam	PE, x-ray, CT, (noninvasive vascular exam 2 sites)	Objective data are variable by site (cavagram, duplex, CT, x-ray)	Phone interview, objective data random & available for 40/440	Clinical, x-ray, lab

Bird's Nest Filter

In 1984, Roehm, et al., reported the use of a percutaneously placed intracaval device which consisted of four stainless steel wires preshaped into a crisscrossing array of nonmatching bends (18). Placement of such a complex array was intended to provide multiple barriers to thromboemboli. Each of these wires is 25 cm long, 0.18 mm in diameter, and ends in a strut which is connected to a fixation hook. One strut is Z-shaped so that a pusher wire can be attached. As initially described, the device was preloaded into an 8 Fr Teflon catheter. Initial problems with proximal migration of this model led to redesign of the struts in 1986 using a stiffer 0.46-mm wire in an attempt to improve fixation. This modification required a concomitant increase in diameter of the catheter system to 12 Fr. During placement of this modified device, the pusher is used to set the first group of hooks into the caval wall; the wires are then extruded with the goal of closely packing the formed loops into a 7-cm long segment of infrarenal vena cava (Fig. 33.3). Finally, the second group of hooks is pushed into the caval wall. The pusher is then disengaged by unscrewing it from the filter and the catheter is withdrawn. Purported, but unproved, advantages of this device include (a) the ability to trap smaller emboli by virtue of the tighter meshing of wires, (b) the configuration avoids the need for intraluminal centering, (c) the ability to accommodate to cavas as large in diameter as 40 mm, (d) the possibility that wires may be able to occlude nearby collaterals, and (e) the lack of radially-oriented struts, thereby limiting the tendency toward caval wall penetration.

A series of 481 patients was reported in 1988 (19). Only 37 patients with the filter in place 6 months or longer had been studied by vena cavography or ultrasound, so long-term data are limited. Of these patients, seven (19%) had an occluded cava. Three patients underwent pulmonary angiography for suspicion of recurrent embolism, which was confirmed in 1 case (3%). As indicated earlier, the original model showed a troublesome tendency to migrate proximally in spite of what appeared to be adequate placement. This problem was encountered in five patients and resulted in the death of one, who, 10 days after placement, was found to have the filter embedded within a massive pulmonary embolus. In a later series of 32 patients accumulated using the modified strut version, three instances of proximal migration were encountered. Two of these occurred within 24 hours of placement and were successfully corrected by angiographic manipulation. The third instance was not detected until 6 months after insertion, at which point the filter could not be repositioned from the right heart where it had become embedded (20). Additional testing is now in progress after subsequent modifications to the fixation hooks.

Amplatz Filter

The Amplatz filter, also introduced in 1984, is a cone-shaped stainless steel device designed to be positioned in the vena cava in an inverted position (21). Pronged loops are designed to limit caval wall penetration to 2 mm to prevent injury to pericaval structures. It is also designed to be retrievable by means of another hook at its apex (Fig. 33.3).

A series of 52 patients in whom the device has been used has been reported (22). Mean follow-up of 11 months revealed one documented recurrent PE (2%) and caval occlusion in 9 of 42 patients (21%) examined for its presence. This suggests that the Amplatz filter may trap clot more efficiently, but its denser arrangement of wires may encourage a higher rate of caval thrombosis. Of concern is the finding that thrombus formation in the apex of the filter, which is on its proximal or cardiac side, was demonstrable venographically in 9 of 34 patients (25%). Additionally, larger trapped thrombi were noted in four (12%), of which two had propagation beyond the filter. In one of these individuals, thrombus was observed on both sides of the device and pulmonary embolism was found at subsequent autopsy. Two patients required Greenfield filter placement above the original Amplatz filter. Despite these findings, the authors of the report felt that apical thrombus was not likely to result in embolism.

The finding of one insertion site venous thrombosis (3%) is similar to that reported in other filter series using 12 Fr catheters. Distal migration and tilting were seen in one patient each during the follow-up period. No evidence of proximal migration was observed. The apical hook aided in repositioning a misplaced device in one patient at the time of insertion. Additionally, retrieval of filters 1–16 days after placement was performed in five of eight patients who were considered candidates for temporary filtration because of short-term contraindication to anticoagulation. Two of these five subsequently showed evidence of intramural changes suggestive of local hemorrhage. The time required for retrieval ranged from 20 minutes to 2 hours, and the difficulties encountered during the procedure varied widely. While these results indicate retrievability is indeed possible, its actual benefit remains questionable since a filter that has remained patent during the period of greatest thrombotic risk should be able to remain in place indefinitely without any long-term sequelae. This device was withdrawn from the market in 1991.

Nitinol Filter

Nitinol is a nickel-titanium alloy that can be drawn into a straight wire which, although pliable when cooled, will rapidly transform into a previously imprinted rigid shape upon warming to body temperature. Although a filter composed of this alloy was initially described in 1977, the preliminary results of a multicenter clinical trial testing it were not available until 1989 (23). The filter design makes use of a 28-mm dome of eight overlapping loops below which six diverging legs form a cone (Fig. 33.3). Each leg has end hooks designed to engage the caval wall. Insertion requires that iced normal saline be continuously infused through a 9 Fr delivery system. During placement, the cooled filter wire is rapidly advanced by the feeder pump and discharged from the storage catheter. The filter purportedly then instantly reshapes into its predetermined configuration and locks into place.

Of the 103 placements recorded in the initial multicenter trial, detailed information on only 44 subjects is available. During a limited follow-up period, two patients sustained recurrent pulmonary embolism (5%). In one individual, thrombus propagating above the filter was seen on venacavography. There were seven cases of confirmed vena caval occlusion and two cases suspected on the basis of clinical findings, for an overall caval occlusion rate of 18%. Five (11%) had stasis sequelae. Insertion site thrombosis was seen in 5 of 18 patients studied by ultrasonography (28%). Proximal migration was noted in one instance.

A more recent update on the use of this device in 224 patients indicates that of the 102 individuals followed and the 65 in whom 6-month follow-up evaluations have been completed, four patients experienced recurrent embolism (4%) with one fatality (1%). Additionally, there were 20 documented caval occlusions (20%)

to which the author added three deaths as a result of massive caval thrombosis (3%) (24). These findings raise concerns that the Nitinol alloy and/or the filter design may be thrombogenic.

Vena Tech Filter

The Vena Tech filter, introduced in 1986, is a stamped cone-shaped filter made of Phynox, a material with properties similar to the alloy Eligiloy that is used in temporary cardiac pacing wires. The filter cone consists of six angled radial prongs, each connected to a hooked stabilizing strut; this array is designed to center and immobilize the device within the vena cava (Fig. 33.3). It is generally inserted via a right internal jugular approach by means of a 12 Fr catheter system which is positioned over a guidewire. After the filter is pushed through the entire length of the insertion catheter, it is released into place by quickly withdrawing the catheter.

The initial reported experience was from France, where the design was introduced as the "LGM" filter (25). In a series of 100 patients, the indication for filter placement was thromboembolism in 77%, prophylaxis in iliocaval thrombosis in 13%, and contraindication to anticoagulation in 9%. As a result, most patients remained on anticoagulation after placement. In 100 attempted insertions, all percutaneously via the jugular route, 98 filters were discharged and 82 were positioned correctly. Eight filters had a 15° or greater tilt, five did not open completely, and both these difficulties occurred in another three cases, for a 16% rate of malposition. The authors comment that many of these instances were early in their experience and may be operator-dependent. Recurrent PE was seen in two patients (2%), both of whom had incompletely opened filters. One year follow-up demonstrated seven caval occlusions (8%). Twenty-nine percent of patients had lower extremity edema in spite of using support stockings. Migration of the device, both proximally to the renal veins (4%) and distally to the iliac veins (9%), was observed. Another small series reported a 2.5% incidence of recurrent embolism and an occlusion rate of 8% (26). There was a 13% rate of either tilting or incomplete opening and a similar rate of distal migration. A more recent experience with this filter has shown an occlusion rate of 22% (27). Breakage of stabilizer struts has also been reported in individual cases (28). This experience is surprising, given that the addition of struts was intended to promote centering and avoid any tendency for the device to tilt.

Gunther Filter

The Gunther filter, described in 1987, was another device designed for temporary or permanent percutaneous placement. This filter, consisting of a helix of wires with an inverted cone above it, was designed to be inserted in an inverted position (Fig. 33.3). It was tested solely in Europe on a preliminary basis. Initial experience revealed a 7% caval occlusion rate and a 70% incidence of migration, particularly in the caudal direction (29, 30). Proximal migration into the right ventricle has also been observed (31). Caval penetration by the struts was seen in two of a series of nine patients in whom it was used. These individuals subsequently developed recurrent embolism from thrombus propagating through a clotted filter basket. A high incidence of perforation during retrieval attempts emphasized that major difficulties were encountered in a limited experience with this device and it was withdrawn from the market.

TITANIUM GREENFIELD FILTER

The most recent development in the Greenfield filter is the modified hook titanium Greenfield filter (TGF-MH) which is inserted using a 12 Fr introducer through a 14 Fr sheath (Fig. 33.4). Its conical shape is similar to that of the SGF, but it is 8 mm wider at the base and 0.5 cm taller (Fig. 33.5). The behavior of ti-

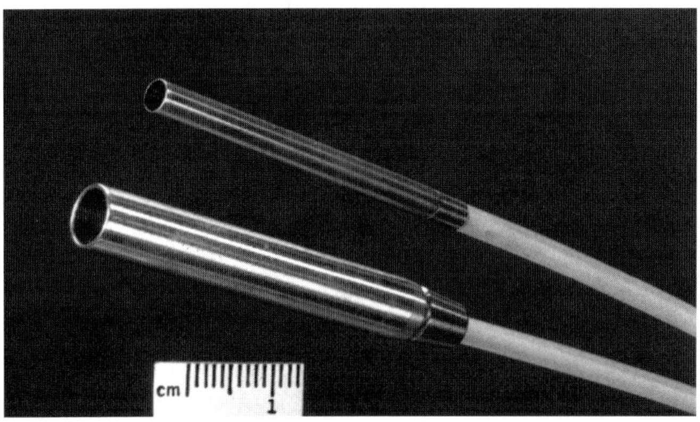

FIG. 33–4. Comparison of the carriers used for the available models of the Greenfield filter: *above,* the 12 Fr carrier for the TGF-MH; and *below,* the 24 Fr carrier for the SGF.

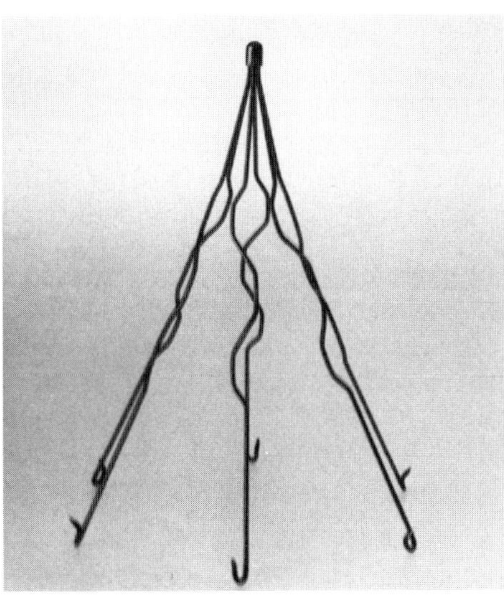

FIG. 33–5. The modified hook titanium Greenfield filter (TGF-MH) is shown with recurved hooks set at an angle of 80° for stabilization without full penetration of the vena cava.

tanium in the tissues and its thrombogenicity in the circulation have been studied. It remains as inert as stainless steel in the tissue and there is no evidence of any additional thrombogenicity. Mechanical properties of the TGF have been tested extensively and it shows remarkable resistance to flexion fatigue and induced corrosion (32). Because this filter is sufficiently elastic to allow it to be folded into the 12 Fr carrier, modification of the original hook design was necessary to improve filter stabilization in the cava against both upward and downward vectors of force. This modified hook design has reduced the incidence of filter migration and caval penetration found with the hook design of the original titanium filter (33, 34). This filter can be inserted through either the jugular or femoral vein, but usually the femoral vein is preferred for ease of entry. The TGF can also be inserted at the time of laparotomy either through a pursestring suture in the vena cava or through a small venous tributary. Under these circumstances, fluoroscopy is not required because the proper position of the carrier can be established by palpation and the filter discharged at the appropriate level.

Filter Insertion Technique

Under local anesthesia, a 4-mm stab incision is made over the right femoral vein, which is entered with a thin-wall needle that allows passage of a 0.035-inch guidewire. The guidewire is passed into the upper reaches of the inferior vena cava after which the dilator-sheath system is introduced and passed into the inferior vena cava. The dilator is withdrawn and the preloaded carrier is passed under fluoroscopic control through the sheath to the desired level of filter placement. If resistance is encountered at the level of the common iliac vein as it angles out of the pelvis, the sheath and carrier should be advanced together; this will usually facilitate passage. Once the carrier is seen to exit the sheath, the base of the sheath should be secured to the carrier and the filter tip positioned at the desired level of introduction. Both the carrier catheter and sheath are retracted as a unit to release the filter. After filter discharge, the carrier and sheath are withdrawn and gentle pressure is applied to the insertion site. An additional advantage to the use of the sheath-carrier is that any premature discharge of the filter would result in filter discharge into the sheath rather than into the patient. The filter is also preloaded into the carrier system, obviating concern about crossed limbs. The delivery system differs from that of the stainless steel version in that a guidewire is not used for axial stabilization of the filter during insertion. This may result in some early tilting of the filter and occasional asymmetry of the legs if the sheath-carrier is displaced against the wall of the vena cava; however, subsequent alignment of the legs of the filter has been seen on most follow-up radiographs.

Clinical Experience

Experience with the TGF-MH is obviously limited since the device has only recently been approved by the FDA. The initial prospective multicenter trial showed that filter insertion was successful in 181 of 186 patients (97%); placement of the remainder was precluded only by unfavorable anatomy (35). All but two of the insertions were performed percutaneously. At the time of insertion, incomplete opening was seen in 2% but was readily corrected by guidewire manipulation in each of them. Leg asymmetry was seen in 5%, but there was no association between this asymmetry and either recurrent embolism or penetration of the wall of the cava. Filter apex perforation of the vena cava at the time of insertion occurred in one patient and there was misplacement of one filter into a lumbar vein in another patient. No clinical sequelae were seen in either patient, although a second filter was inserted in each patient. The only complication noted in the series was a hematoma at the insertion site in one patient. Initial follow-up data were obtained from all participating institutions at 30 days and showed minimal filter movement in 11%; there was no significant proximal migration. CT scans were obtained when the diameter of the base of the filter was seen to have enlarged greater than 5 mm. There was evidence of penetration of the wall of the vena cava in only one case (0.8%), with no clinical sequelae. Long-term follow-up experience will be necessary to confirm that the performance of the TGF-MH is equivalent to the SGF, but it is obvious that this new device has made filter insertion easier, less expensive and less invasive to accomplish.

SUMMARY

There is considerable ingenuity in the number of devices now available for clinical use as vena caval filters. The primary objective, to provide a safe and effective device for permanent implantation, should lead to continued evolution of materials and design. The standard for comparison, however, should remain the stainless steel Greenfield filter. The present concern regarding the percutaneous insertion of the SGF overlooks the fact that it can be inserted quite safely at operation with the patient under local anesthesia with minimal morbidity. It seems clear that advances in percutaneous techniques will make this the obvious choice for the future, but the safety and efficacy of the conical design of the Greenfield filter suggest that a new design may not be needed.

In the overall management of the patient with thrombotic disease, it is imperative to understand that any filtration device plays only a small role and it is incumbent upon the physician who treats the patient to assume the responsibility for the management and long-term follow-up of the underlying disorder.

REFERENCES

1. Consensus Development Panel. Prevention of venous thrombosis and pulmonary embolism. JAMA 1986;256:744–749.
2. Nasbeth DC, Moran JM. Reassessment of the role of inferior vena cava ligation in thromboembolism. N Engl J Med 1965;273:1250.
3. DeMeester TR, Rutherford RB, Blazek JV, et al. Plication of the inferior vena cava for thromboembolism. Surgery 1967;62:56.
4. Lindenauer SM. Prophylactic staple plication of the inferior vena cava. Arch Surg 1973;107:669.

5. Cohen JR, Tenenbaum N, Citron M. Greenfield filter as primary therapy for deep venous thrombosis and/or pulmonary embolism in patients with cancer. Surgery 1991;109:12.
6. Fink JA, Jones BT. The Greenfield filter as primary means of therapy in venous thromboembolic disease. Surg Gynecol Obstet 1991;172:253.
7. Greenfield LJ, McCurdy JR, Brown PP, et al. A new intracaval filter permitting continued flow and resolution of emboli. Surgery 1973;73:599.
8. Schroeder TM, Elkins RC, Greenfield LJ. Entrapment of sized emboli by the KMA-Greenfield intracaval filter. Surgery 1979;83:435.
9. Greenfield LJ, Michna BA. Twelve year clinical experience with the Greenfield vena caval filter. Surgery 1988;104:706.
10. Chimochowski GE, Evans RH, Zarins CK, et al. Greenfield filter versus Mobin-Uddin umbrella: the continuing quest for the ideal method of vena caval interruption. J Thorac Cardiovasc Surg 1980;79:358.
11. Gomez GA, Cutler BS, Wheeler HB. Transvenous interruption of the inferior vena cava. Surgery 1983;93:612.
12. Greenfield LJ, Cho K, Proctor M, et al. Late results of suprarenal Greenfield vena cava filter placement. Arch Surg 1992;127:969–973.
13. Messmer JM, Greenfield LJ. Greenfield caval filters: long-term radiographic follow-up study. Radiology 1985;156:613–618.
14. Peyton JWR, Hylerman MB, Greenfield LJ, et al. Comparison of the Greenfield filter and vena caval ligation for experimental septic thromboembolism. Surgery 1983;93:533.
15. Greenfield LJ. Technical considerations for insertion of vena caval filters. Surg Gynecol Obstet 1979;148:422.
16. Hye RJ, Mitchell AT, Dory CE, Freischlag J, Roberts AC. Analysis of the transition to percutaneous placement of Greenfield filters. Arch Surg 1990;125:1550.
17. Glanz S. Gordon DH, Kantor A. Percutaneous femoral insertion of the Greenfield vena cava filter: incidence of femoral vein thrombosis. Am J Roent 1987;149:1065.
18. Roehm JOF Jr, Gianturco C, Barth MH, et al. Percutaneous transcatheter filter for the inferior vena cava: a new device for treatment of patients with pulmonary embolism. Radiology 1984;150:255.
19. Roehm JOF Jr, Johnsrude IS, Barth MH, et al. The bird's nest inferior vena cava filter: progress report. Radiology 1988;168:745.
20. McCowan TC, Ferris EJ, Keifsteck JE, et al. Retrieval of dislodged bird's nest inferior vena caval filters. J Intervent Radiol 1988;3:179.
21. Lund G, Rysavy JA, Salomonowitz E, et al. A new vena caval filter for percutaneous placement and retrieval: experimental study. Radiology 1984;152:369–372.
22. Epstein DE, Darcy MD, Hunter DW, et al. Experience with the Amplatz retrievable vena cava filter. Radiology 1989;172:105.
23. Simm M, Athanasoulis CA, Kim D, et al. Simon nitinol inferior vena cava filter: initial clinical experience. Radiology 1989;172:99.
24. Dorfman GS. Percutaneous inferior vena caval filters. Radiology 1990;174:987.
25. Ricco JB, Crochet D, Sebilotte P, et al. Percutaneous transvenous caval interruption with the "LGM" filter: early results of a multicenter trial. Ann Vasc Surg 1988;3:242.
26. Maquin P, Fajadet P, Railhac N, et al. LGM and Gunther: two complementary vena cava filters. Radiology 1989;173:476.
27. Millward SF, Marsh JI, Peterson RA, et al. LGM (VenaTech) vena cava filters: clinical experience in 64 patients. J Vasc Interv Radiol 1991;2(4):429–433.
28. Awh MH, Taylor FC, Lu CT. Spontaneous fracture of a Vena Tech inferior vena caval filter. Am J Roent 1991;157:177.
29. Gunther RW, Schild H, Hollman JP, Vorwerk D. First clinical results with a new caval filter. Cardiovasc Intervent Radiol 1987;10:104–108.

30. Fobbe F, Dietzel M, Korth R, et al. Gunther vena caval filter: results of long-term follow-up. AJR 1988;151:1031.
31. Johnson SG, Pickford M, Wilkins RA. Migration of a Gunther filter to the right ventricle. J Intervent Radiol 1988;3:33.
32. Greenfield LJ, Savin MA. Comparison of titanium and stainless steel Greenfield vena caval filters. Surgery 1989;106:820.
33. Greenfield LJ, Cho KJ, Pais SO, Van Aman M. Preliminary clinical experience with the titanium Greenfield vena caval filter. Arch Surg 1989;124:657.
34. Greenfield LJ, Cho KJ, Tauscher JR. Evolution of hook design for fixation of the titanium Greenfield filter. J Vasc Surg 1990;9:345.
35. Greenfield LJ, Cho KJ, Proctor M, et al. Results of a multicenter study of the modified hook titanium Greenfield filter. J Vasc Surg 1991;14:253.

chapter 34

Venous Thrombectomy

B. Eklöf and P. Neglén

BACKGROUND

There are three modalities of treatment for deep venous thrombosis: anticoagulation, thrombolysis, and thrombectomy. The objectives of any therapy for extensive venous thrombosis are to (a) prevent fatal pulmonary embolism (PE) and proximal extension of the thrombus; (b) avoid progression of the disease, which can lead to phlegmasia cerulea dolens, venous gangrene, and limb loss; and (c) prevent the later postthrombotic (PT) sequelae by preservation of the venous outflow and functional valves (1).

The risk for developing PE and its subsequent mortality and morbidity increases with the proximity of the thrombus in the venous system (2). In patients with calf vein thrombosis, less than 5% have symptomatic PE, although 29–40% have evidence of pulmonary embolism by lung scanning (3, 4). Approximately 9–18% of patients with iliofemoral venous thrombosis have been found to have scan/angiography-verified symptomatic PE (5–7) and an additional 25–36% of cases have asymptomatic, but scan-positive, emboli (6, 7). When the inferior vena cava (IVC) is involved, the symptomatic PE rate increases to 23–34% of patients (8–11), and the scan-positive rate to 63% (11).

Anticoagulation with heparin was already prevalent in the 1930s; dicoumarol came into use a decade later. In the late 1950s enzymatic thrombolysis was introduced and clinically evaluated. Despite the anticoagulant treatment, 4% of cases with iliofemoral deep vein thrombosis (DVT) had recurrence of PE within 1 month (7, 12) and 18% had recurrence following IVC thrombus (10). Other investigators have shown no further scan-positive PE in patients with IVC thrombosis, or in those with iliofemoral DVT, 10 days after initiating anticoagulant treatment (8, 9).

Killewich, et al. (13), described the "natural course" of DVT treated with anticoagulation and found 14% early extension (<7 days) and 19% late extension (30–160 days). Heparin infusion usually provides immediate symptomatic relief of swelling and pain, possibly due to its anti-inflammatory effect. The main disadvantage is that lysis of the thrombus depends on the endogenous fibrinolytic mechanisms and requires weeks to months. It often leads to incomplete recanalization and frequently results in destruction of the venous valves involved in the thrombotic process (14). Thus, anticoagulant treatment is of less value than thrombolytic therapy in prevention of the postthrombotic syndrome.

Thrombolytic therapy appears then to be the logical solution to the problem, as it may induce early lysis of the thrombus with preservation of normal venous valve function. A long-term significant functional benefit is observed if the thrombus is completely lysed. However, examination of pooled data from randomized prospective studies shows that significant or complete lysis occurred in only 47% of patients receiving thrombolytic therapy within 3 days of onset of symptoms (vs. 6% following anticoagulation) (14). It is likely that the delicate valve cusps are destroyed within 3–5 days so the lysis must be quick and complete. The dilemma is to select patients with fresh thrombus for fibrinolytic therapy, since there are no objective methods to determine the age of the thrombus.

Our own experience with standard dosage of streptokinase (SK) therapy in 47 patients revealed that only 2 of 35 (6%) patients had normal vein function after 29 months (15). Additionally, severe complications were encountered during the SK treatment, including spontaneous rupture of intraabdominal organs with life-threatening bleeding (16). There are only a few reports with long-term follow-up comparing heparin versus SK in the development of postthrombotic sequelae. Two studies reported superior results with SK treatment (17, 18), while a third demonstrated no difference between the two treatment groups (19). Severe postthrombotic syndrome occurred in approximately 30% of patients during a follow-up period of 5.7 years.

A major disadvantage for the SK treatment is the number of contraindications, which reduce its availability as a treatment alternative. Porter found that only 15% of DVT patients in his clinical practice presented within 3 days of onset of symptoms and had no contraindications (14). Others have reported a high incidence of contraindications (between 24–80%) (20–23). Problems also arise with iliofemoral thrombosis, with a large amount of clot often extending from below the knee to the common iliac vein. Interface with the blood-borne enzyme is limited or nonexistent. Although induced thrombolysis would appear to be the treatment of choice for extensive DVT, the many contraindications, the potential risks, and the doubtful long-term results convinced us to turn to the surgical alternative in carefully selected patients with acute iliofemoral venous thrombosis.

The first thrombectomy (TE) of a leg vein was ascribed to Läwen in 1938 (24), the same year in which Dos Santos described phlebography (25), Gregoire showed that DVT of the lower limb may lead to phlegmasia cerulea dolens (26), and Haimovici (27) described its further progress to venous gangrene. During the 1950s and early 1960s, several enthusiastic reports on clinical success of venous thrombectomy were published in the United States (28–30). The development of the Fogarty catheter greatly facilitated removal of the thrombus (31). Mavor and Galloway showed a 61–79% improvement of patency of the thrombectomized iliac vein (32). However, the Lansing and Davis report in 1968 (33), a 5-year follow-up of Haller and Abrams material (30), halted the enthusiastic wave of thrombectomy and the procedure was abandoned by most surgeons in the United States and Europe. During the 1970s surgical thrombectomy was revived in continental

Europe (34). Inspired by a report from Jean Kunlin (35) on the use of a temporary arteriovenous fistula (AVF) to improve outcome of venous reconstructive surgery, we performed our first iliofemoral TE with a temporary AVF in Lund, Sweden, in 1974. Our personal experience with this surgical procedure now comprises 203 patients: Lund, Sweden (1974–1978) 70 patients; Helsingborg, Sweden (1978–1981) 31 patients; and Kuwait (1981–1990) 102 patients. Based on this experience and the results reported by others, we propose that venous thrombectomy with temporary AVF is the method of choice for treatment of an acute iliofemoral venous thrombosis.

SELECTION OF PATIENTS FOR THROMBECTOMY

The patient should be in reasonable health with normal life expectancy and rehabilitation potential. Elderly patients (>70 years of age), patients with metastatic malignant disease or severe arteriosclerotic disease, or those unable to walk prior to the onset should not be operated on. The thrombus should be less than 7 days old.

SURGICAL TREATMENT

To plan the surgical intervention, to avoid intraoperative complications, and to optimize the results, it is absolutely necessary to delineate the full extent of the thrombus prior to surgery. Duplex Doppler study will document thrombosis with high accuracy below the inguinal ligament, but can rarely determine the exact level of the tail of the thrombus. A femoral phlebogram from the contralateral side is usually required to achieve this purpose (Fig. 34.1). When the diagnosis is established, heparin infusion is started.

Prophylactic antibiotics are given to reduce the rate of wound infection (36). Surgery is performed under general anesthesia with endotracheal intubation. PEEP (10 cm H_2O) is added during manipulation of the thrombus to prevent intraoperative embolization. The involved leg and abdomen are prepared.

A longitudinal incision is made in the groin to expose the long saphenous vein (LSV), which is followed to its confluence with the common femoral vein (CFV). The anterior wall of the CFV is exposed, avoiding dissection of the lateral and posterior walls. The vein is not encircled. Proximal and distal control are maintained by external pressure using a sponge on a stick. The superficial femoral artery 3–4 cm below the femoral bifurcation is dissected free in preparation for the construction of an arteriovenous (AV) fistula. When the dissection is completed, heparin (5000 IU) is given intravenously.

A transverse venotomy is made on the CFV just above the confluence. A No. 8–10 venous Fogarty thrombectomy catheter is passed through the thrombus into the vena cava. The balloon is inflated and withdrawn. The maneuver is repeated until no more thrombotic material is extracted (Fig. 34.2). With the balloon inflated in the common iliac vein, a suction catheter is introduced to the level of the internal iliac vein to evacuate thrombi from this vein.

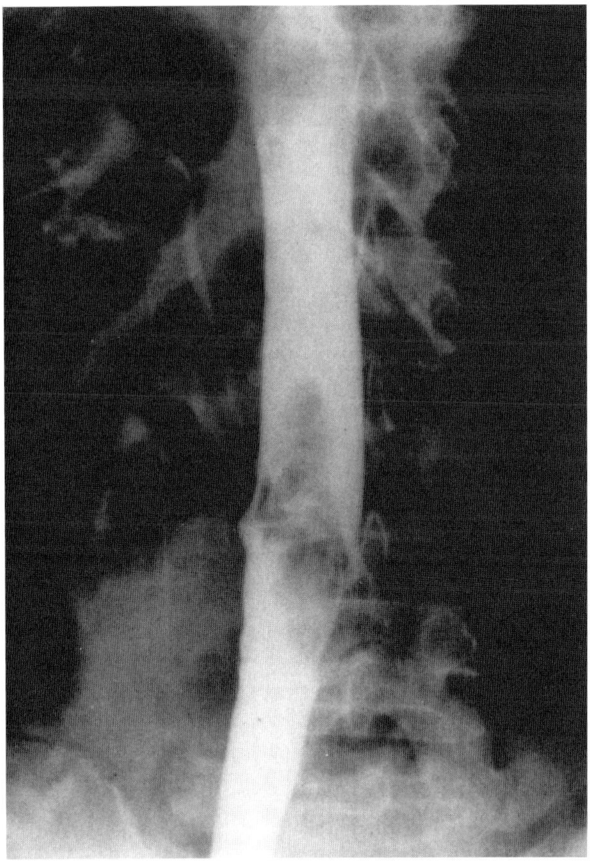

FIG. 34–1. A femoral phlebogram from the contralateral side of a swollen leg shows a free-floating thrombus tail in the inferior vena cava.

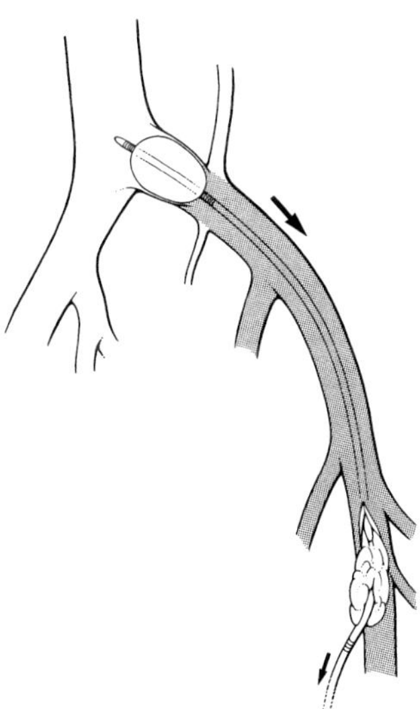

FIG. 34–2. A venous Fogarty thrombectomy catheter size No. 8/10 is inserted into the common femoral vein and passed through the thrombus into the vena cava. The balloon is inflated and thrombotic material is extracted. (Reproduced by permission from Eklöf B, Juhan C, Neglén P. Iliofemoral thrombectomy and temporary arteriovenous fistula. In: Bergan JJ, Kistner RL, eds. Atlas of venous surgery. Philadelphia: WB Saunders, 1992:223–231.)

Backflow is not a reliable sign of clearance since a proximal valve in the external iliac vein is present in 25% of patients (37), preventing retrograde flow in a cleared vein. On the other hand, excellent backflow can originate from the internal iliac vein and its tributaries, despite residual occlusion of the common iliac vein. Therefore, an intraoperative completion phlebogram is mandatory. An alternative is the use of an angioscope which enables removal of residual thrombus material under direct vision (38).

The distal thrombus is removed by manual massage of the leg, starting at the foot. The Fogarty catheter can sometimes be gently advanced in retrograde fashion. The aim is to remove all fresh thrombi from the leg.

The venotomy is closed with continuous Prolene suture and an AV fistula is created using the long saphenous vein or a branch, anastomosing it end-to-side to the superficial femoral artery (Fig. 34.3). A prosthetic sleeve (4-mm diameter) applied to the venous side of the AV fistula may help to limit the fistula's size and avoid hypertension and congestive heart failure. The sleeve is useful later to close the fistula percutaneously. The sleeve will retain 6- or 8-mm coils or balloons introduced percutaneously for thrombosis of the fistula.

The use of a cell saver device minimizes the use of bank blood. An intraoperative phlebogram (or angioscopy) is performed to assure complete clearance of the clot from the iliocaval segment. A suction drain is applied for 24 hours and the wound closed in layers.

In cases of phlegmasia cerulea dolens or venous gangrene, we begin the operation with fasciotomy of the calf compartments in order to decrease the compartments' pressure and reestablish arterial circulation. If there is an extension of the thrombus into the IVC, the cava is approached transperitoneally through a right subcostal incision. The IVC is exposed by deflecting the duodenum and ascending colon medially. An Adams-DeWeese partial-occlusion clip is applied just below the renal veins. The cava is opened and the thrombus is removed (Fig. 34.4). If the iliofemoral segment is involved, the operation is continued in the groin

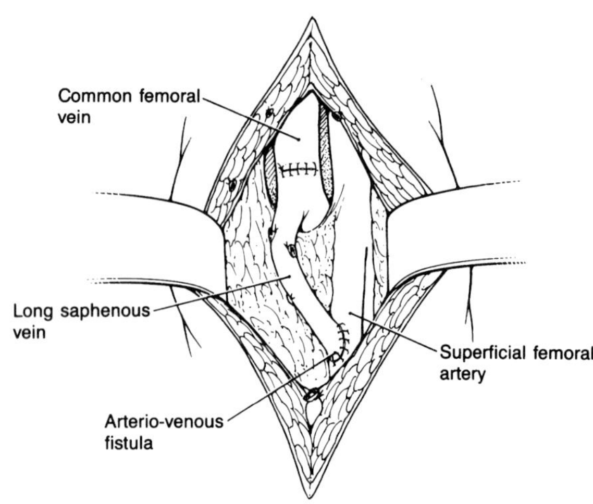

FIG. 34–3. After thrombectomy the transverse venotomy is closed with a continuous Prolene suture and an AV fistula created, using the long saphenous vein or its branch and anastomosing it end-to-side to the superficial femoral artery, i.e., below the level of the profunda artery. (Reproduced by permission from Eklöf B, Juhan C, Neglén P. Iliofemoral thrombectomy and temporary arteriovenous fistula. In: Bergan JJ, Kistner RL, eds. Atlas of venous surgery. Philadelphia: WB Saunders, 1992:223–231.)

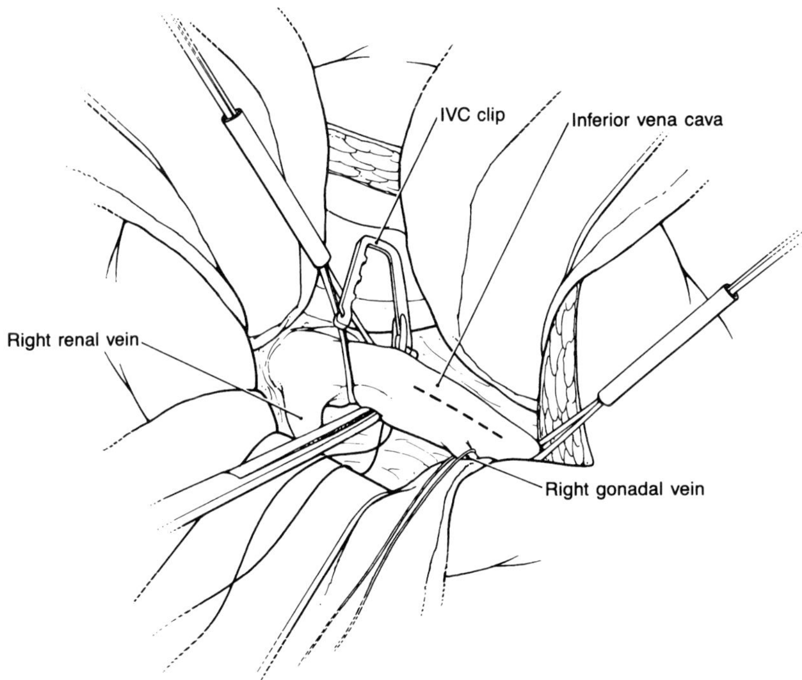

FIG. 34–4. The inferior vena cava is exposed transperitoneally by deflecting medially the duodenum and ascending colon. An Adams-DeWeese partially occluding clip is applied just below the renal veins. The cava is opened longitudinally and the thrombus is removed. (Reproduced by permission from Eklöf B, Juhan C, Neglén P. Iliofemoral thrombectomy and temporary arteriovenous fistula. In: Bergan JJ, Kistner RL, eds. Atlas of venous surgery. Philadelphia: WB Saunders, 1992:223–231.)

as described earlier. When complete thrombectomy is achieved, the caval clip can be removed before closure of the abdomen. When laparotomy is contraindicated in high-risk patients, a caval filter of the Greenfield or Günther type can be introduced before thrombectomy to protect against pulmonary embolism.

Heparin is continued for at least 5 days postoperatively. Warfarin is started the first postoperative day and continued for 6 months. The patient is ambulatory, wearing a compression stocking, the day after the operation. In cases in which early reocclusion of the thrombectomized iliac vein results in a severely compromised venous outflow from the leg, and clinical signs of phlegmasia cerulea dolens develop, immediate insertion of a synthetic femorofemoral crossover bypass graft should be considered if the distal veins are patent. Quick reestablishment of venous outflow and relief of stasis in the leg may prevent retrograde extension of thrombus and subsequent valve insufficiency (39). The patient is usually discharged on the 10th to 12th postoperative day to return after 6 weeks for closure of the AV fistula.

Complications

Mortality. One of the reasons that venous thrombectomy was abandoned in the 1960s was its high perioperative mortality secondary to pulmonary embolism. Haller and Abrams (30) reported a mortality of 9%; two-thirds of the deaths were related to pulmonary embolism. Although surgery is still not without risk, results have improved owing to the present pre- and postoperative precautions. In our series, two patients died (1% mortality). One patient succumbed in acute respiratory failure due to chronic pulmonary fibrosis. Autopsy did not reveal fresh pulmonary emboli. The other patient had cirrhosis of the liver, which was not detected preoperatively. The patient died on the 32nd postoperative day of complications of anticoagulation.

Morbidity

Pulmonary Embolism. In our series, there was no fatal pulmonary embolism in the perioperative period. It is of utmost importance to obtain a preoperative phlebogram to determine extension of the thrombus into the inferior vena cava. When present, there is risk that the caval thrombus may break off during manipulation with the Fogarty catheter (Fig. 34.1). We do not use a separate balloon catheter to occlude the inferior vena cava but routinely ask the anesthetist to apply PEEP during the operative manipulation of the thrombotic vein. In a randomized study (7), we found positive perfusion scans at admission in 45% of all patients; additional defects were seen in 11% of cases after conservative treatment, whereas in the thrombectomized group the incidence was 20%. Mavor and Galloway (32) demonstrated that an incomplete clearance of the thrombus in the iliac vein increased the incidence of rethrombosis and pulmonary embolism. In our series, no additional lung perfusion defects developed after the first postoperative week following thrombectomy with temporary AV fistula. Because the fistula effectively prevented rethrombosis, we may assume that the fistula was instrumental in reducing the incidence of postoperative pulmonary embolism.

Other postoperative complications were infrequent (33). Early rethrombosis of the iliac vein occurred in 11% (Table 34.1). (There was 89% patency!)

ROLE AND CLOSURE OF THE ARTERIOVENOUS FISTULA

The objectives of a temporary AVF are to increase the velocity of blood flow in the thrombectomized segment; to prevent immediate rethrombosis; to allow time for healing of the endothelium; and to promote development of collaterals in the event of incomplete clearance or immediate rethrombosis of the iliac segment. Closure of the fistula is performed after 6–10 weeks.

Experimental studies indicate that reendothelialization (40) following thrombosis is nearly complete within 4 weeks after surgical thrombectomy. Thus, it appears that the temporary fistula should be retained for at least 4 weeks. The fis-

TABLE 34-1

EARLY PATENCY OF THE ILIAC VEIN FOLLOWING THROMBECTOMY WITH TEMPORARY ARTERIOVENOUS FISTULA

Author	Year	No. of Patients	Patent Iliac Vein (%)
Delin, et al.	1982	13	85
Plate, et al. (21)	1984	31	87
Piquet, et al. (42)	1985	92	80
Einarsson, et al. (23)	1986	51	88
Kniemeyer (46)	1987	157	90
Juhan, et al. (22)	1987	42	93
Vollmar, et al. (43)	1989	93	82
Neglén, et al. (6)	1991	48	89
Total		527	87

tula may be closed surgically under local anesthesia; however, closure of the fistula may be technically quite difficult (20). The new percutaneous technique of AV fistula closure developed by Endrys is easier than traditional closure methods and is now favored over surgical closure (41). Through a puncture of the femoral artery on the contralateral side, a catheter is inserted and positioned at the fistula level. Occlusive devices, such as detachable balloons or coils that result in thrombosis of the fistula, can be introduced through the catheter. If a prosthetic sleeve has been applied to the venous side of the fistula, accurate placement without risk of embolization of the device becomes easier. At the time of the fistula closure, performance of an arteriovenogram to evaluate the patency of the iliac and caval veins is of prognostic value. More than 10% of patients have been shown to have residual venous stenosis despite initial successful surgery (Fig. 34.5). A transvenous percutaneous angioplasty with stenting can be performed immediately under the protection of the AVF, which is retained for another 4 weeks.

Results of Thrombectomy Plus an Arteriovenous Fistula

Early Results. Most early reports of clinical results after thrombectomy were based mainly on clinical outcome alone without phlebography. Table 34.1 shows the reported patency of the iliac vein <3 months after removal of the thrombus using an AV fistula. Among 527 patients compiled from the various reports, an aggregate average patency rate of 87% results. Einarsson, et al., reported that arteriovenography performed on 60 legs confirmed venous patency after thrombectomy at the same rate (23). In Piquet's material, all patients had an extension of the thrombus into the inferior vena cava and an Adams-DeWeese clip was applied in addition to thrombectomy (42). A temporary fistula was utilized

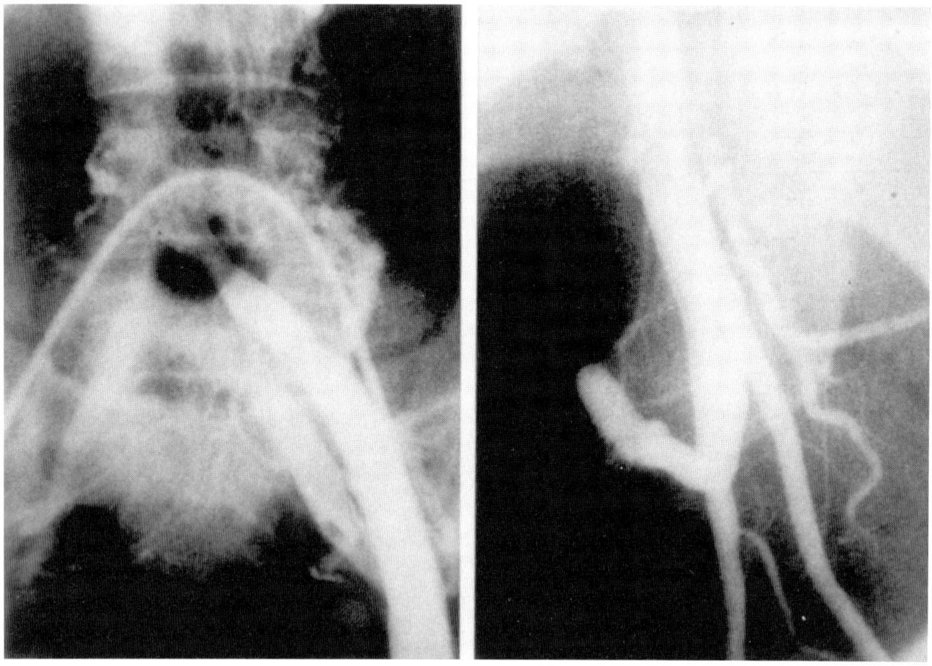

FIG. 34–5. Angiography before closing the AV fistula reveals stenosis of the common iliac vein (*left*). Arteriogram after placement of balloon shows complete obliteration of the AV fistula and normal arterial morphology (*right*). (Reproduced by permission from Neglén P, Al-Hassan H, Endrys J, Nazzal M, Christenson J, Eklöf B. Iliofemoral venous thrombectomy followed by percutaneous closure of the temporary arterio-venous fistula. Surgery 1991;110:493–499.)

in 59% of the cases. In the group of 27 patients with excellent patency of the iliocaval vein, 21 had a fistula. Vollmar (43) confirms the advantage of the AV fistula, showing 82% patency in 93 patients with a temporary fistula compared to 54% in 26 patients without it.

Long-Term Follow-up Results. There are only a few studies on long-term results after thrombectomy performed with an adjunctive AV fistula (Table 34.2). Because development of the postthrombotic syndrome can take many years, reports of clinical "success" in many published series may be premature in that the follow-up is relatively short.

In Plate's randomized study, a significant difference in persistence of symptoms between operated and nonoperated patients was found (7% vs. 42%, respectively) (21). Moderate leg swelling, secondary varicose veins, and venous claudication were observed more frequently in the nonsurgical group. In Plate's report, 37% of the operated patients were free of symptoms at 5-year follow-up compared to 18% in the nonsurgical group (44). Table 34.3 shows the "long-term"

TABLE 34-2

THE FREQUENCY OF CLINICAL SUCCESS (I.E., ASYMPTOMATIC PATIENTS WITH NO SIGNS OF POSTTHROMBOTIC SYNDROME) AT 6–60 MONTHS FOLLOW-UP AFTER THROMBECTOMY WITH TEMPORARY ARTERIOVENOUS FISTULA

Author	Year	No. of Patients	Follow-up (months)	Clinical Success (%)
Poilleux, et al.	1975	27	—	78
Plate, et al. (21)	1984	31	6	42
Piquet, et al. (42)	1985	82	51	51
Einarsson, et al. (23)	1986	55	10	75
Kniemeyer (46)	1987	37	36	62
Juhan, et al. (22)	1987	36	12–48	93
Winter, et al. (38)	1989	100	12	64
Plate, et al. (44)	1990	19	60	37
Neglén, et al. (6)	1991	37	24	83
Total		424		65

results of iliac patency in several series. The average patency rate in these 289 patients was 76%. Radionucleotide phlebography in Plate's randomized study showed a patent iliac vein in 71% in the surgical group at 5 years, compared to 30% in the conservative group (44).

TABLE 34-3

THE PATENCY RATE OF THE ILIAC VEIN AT 6–60 MONTHS FOLLOW-UP AFTER THROMBECTOMY WITH TEMPORARY ARTERIOVENOUS FISTULA

Author	Year	No. of Patients	Follow-up (months)	Patent Iliac Vein (%)
Plate, et al. (21)	1984	31	6	76
Piquet, et al. (42)	1985	57	39	80
Einarsson, et al. (23)	1986	58	10	61
Juhan, et al. (22)	1987	36	12–48	93
Törngren, et al.*	1988	54	19	54
Plate, et al. (44)	1990	19	60	77
Neglén, et al. (6)	1991	34	24	88
Total		289		76

*Swedenborg, J., Törngren S. Is there a place for surgical thrombectomy in venous thrombosis? Acta Chir Scand. Suppl 548; 1988. Proc. of 1st Joint Meeting of the Swedish and British Angiology Societies. Eds Farrell B, Norgren L, Tooke J. The Almqvist & Wiskell Periodical Co. Stockholm, Sweden, p. 38.

TABLE 34-4

THE INCIDENCE OF PATENT AND COMPETENT FEMOROPOPLITEAL VEIN SEGMENTS AT 6–60 MONTHS FOLLOW-UP AFTER THROMBECTOMY WITH TEMPORARY ARTERIOVENOUS FISTULA

Author	Year	No. of Patients	Follow-up (months)	Competence (%)
Plate, et al. (21)	1984	31	6	52
Einarsson, et al. (23)	1986	53	10	42
Kniemeyer (46)	1987	157	43	45
Plate, et al. (44)	1990	14	60	36
Neglén, et al. (6)	1991	34	24	46
Total		289		44

Table 34.4 shows the "long-term" valvular competence and reflux of the femoropopliteal segment following thrombectomy combined with fistula. Among the collected total of 289 patients, an average of 44% had patent and competent valves in the femoropopliteal segment. It is vital to preserve these valves and retain a normal calf pump function to prevent the development of the postthrombotic syndrome. Plate, et al., found patent and competent valves in the femoropopliteal segment in 52% in the surgical group compared with 26% in the conservatively treated group at 6 months (21). Browse, et al., predicted that the incidence of the postthrombotic syndrome would not differ between the groups after 5 years (45). However, Plate, et al., found a decreased incidence of severe postthrombotic syndrome 5 years after surgery and more pronounced venous hypertension among patients treated with anticoagulants only. The thrombectomized patients had a significant reduction in ambulatory venous pressure (AVP), improved venous emptying as demonstrated by plethysmography, and better calf pump function with less reflux measured by foot volumetry. Taking in account the results of all functional tests at the 5-year follow-up, 36% of the operated patients had a normal venous function compared to 11% of those treated conservatively (44). Kniemeyer (46), Einarsson (47), and Neglén, et al. (6), have reported similar results. An interesting difference in Kniemeyer's technique is the more distal placement of the temporary fistula.

Results of Thrombectomy Without Arteriovenous Fistula

Table 34.5 lists the clinical results after thrombectomy without an AV fistula. In several studies, however, adjunctive measures such as local infusion of thrombolytic agents, ligation of the superficial femoral vein, and postoperative local heparin infusion were utilized. In 2437 thrombectomies, the average clinical success was 76% (range from 6% (33) to 100% (48, 49)). Period of follow-up and the definition of clinical success have widely varied among the studies. Few authors have followed their patients with phlebography or studies of venous function. Kistner

TABLE 34-5

THE FREQUENCY OF CLINICAL SUCCESS AT FOLLOW-UP AFTER THROMBECTOMY WITHOUT ARTERIOVENOUS FISTULA

Author	Year	No. of Patients	Follow-up (months)	Clinical Success (%)
Mahorner, et al. (28)	1957	11	15	64
Haller, et al. (30)	1963	34	18	76
Bradham, et al. (54)	1964	13	early	100
DeWeese	1964	31	24	68
Fontaine, et al.	1965	72	>12	83
Hafner, et al.	1965	41	42	98
Kaiser, et al.	1965	49	36	65
Smith	1965	18	17	78
Britt	1966	19	early	42
Fogarty, et al. (31)	1966	21	22	86
Little et al.	1966	19	early	95
Wilson, et al.	1967	39	early	39
Lansing, et al. (33)	1968	17	60	6
Bertelsen	1969	15	early	87
Mavor, et al. (32)	1969	110	96	89
Mavor, et al. (32)	1969	54	36	95
Edwards, et al.	1970	61	54	80
Johansson, et al.	1973	21	24	19
Senn, et al.	1973	130	early	75
Baumann	1976	44	early	80
Matsubara, et al.	1976	17	6	67
Stephens	1976	16	late	75
Denck	1977	123	late	85
Lindhagen, et al. (48)	1978	21	6	77
Lindhagen, et al. (48)	1978	12	12	100
Hortsch, et al.	1979	21	early	86
Kistner, et al. (50)	1979	58	12–60	84
Kistner, et al. (50)	1979	19	60–96	83
Kistner, et al. (50)	1979	19	96–132	89
Nadjabat, et al.	1979	63	12	94
Proven, et al.	1979	12	<96	67
Goto, et al. (49)	1980	43	46	100
Metz, et al.	1980	52	36	80
Andriopoulos, et al.	1982	134	28	80
Röder, et al. (52)	1984	45	5	77
Röder, et al. (52)	1984	30	120	67
Shinoya, et al.	1989	43	late	85
Vollmar, et al. (43)	1989	26	52	54
Husfeldt, et al.	1991	900	—	80
Paquet, et al.	1991	44	60	76
Total		2437		76

published the results of thrombectomy combined with ligation of the superficial femoral vein in 1979 (50). Follow-up of 57 patients after 49 months with phlebography confirmed patency of the iliac vein in 75%. The philosophy behind ligation of the superficial femoral vein was to avoid early pulmonary embolism and the severe postthrombotic syndrome secondary to reflux in the deep venous system. In a recent follow-up after more than 15 years, the approach seems to be valid (51).

An interesting finding in some reports on thrombectomy without AV fistula is the early rethrombosis of the iliac vein in 21–37% (32, 48, 52), which should be compared with 11% when a temporary fistula is used (Table 34.1).

POSTTHROMBOTIC SYNDROME

One of the main objectives of an aggressive approach to the treatment of DVT is to preserve venous patency and normal valves, thereby avoiding the development of the postthrombotic syndrome. With anticoagulant treatment alone, resolution and recanalization of the thrombus is often incomplete and results in destruction of valves. Only 30% of iliac vein segments remain open and severe reflux invariably occurs 5 years later (53). The venous hypertension leads to postthrombotic sequelae in 66–82% of patients (17, 54), with a severe form in which venous claudication or venous ulcers develop in one-third of cases with time (54, 55). Thus, conservative treatment of iliofemoral venous thrombosis with anticoagulation alone is not an optimal method.

Following thrombectomy, 65% of patients remain free of the postthrombotic syndrome (Table 34.2). Iliac vein patency averages 76% (Table 34.3) with observation times ranging from 6–60 months. Preservation of patency and valvular competence in the femoropopliteal segment averages 44% (Table 34.4). In the prospective randomized study performed by Plate, et al. (21, 44), almost one-third of the patients had expired between the 6-month and 5-year follow-up because of the advanced age in the material and the frequent concomitant malignant disease. This renders proper statistical analysis inconclusive, but the results showed a favorable trend with the use of thrombectomy. At 5-year follow-up, 37% of surgically treated patients were asymptomatic compared to 18% in the conservative group. Radionuclide phlebography of the iliac vein showed a patency of 77% and a normal iliac vein in 71% in the surgical group compared with 30% in the conservative group. In the early follow-up, twice as many thrombectomized cases had preserved valves (52% vs. 26%), and valve reflux was four times less common than in cases conservatively treated (9% vs. 37%, respectively). Observations after 5 years indicate that there is a higher risk to develop venous hypertension after conservative treatment; and if all tests for reflux, obstruction, and calf pump function are taken together, 36% of the operated patients had a normal venous function compared to 11% of the conservatively treated patients.

Indications for Surgery

The most logical way to treat thromboembolic venous disease is by induced thrombolysis. Unfortunately, approximately 50% of patients presenting with acute iliofemoral venous thrombosis have contraindications for this treatment. Thrombectomy combined with a temporary AV fistula appears to give superior results compared with anticoagulant treatment. The results of surgery have improved because of better preoperative management and surgical technique, with special precautions in patients with extension of the thrombus into the IVC. The use of intraoperative phlebography or phleboscopy to demonstrate clearance of the iliac vein and creation of the temporary AV fistula will decrease the risk of early rethrombosis. The new technique of percutaneous closure of the AV fistula with a detachable balloon has simplified the procedure. Until results of a prospective study comparing surgery with thrombolysis are at hand, thrombectomy with a temporary AVF is our method of choice in the treatment of selected patients with acute iliofemoral venous thrombosis.

REFERENCES

1. Raju S, Fredericks RK. Late hemodynamic sequelae of deep venous thrombosis. J Vasc Surg 1986;4:73–79.
2. Mavor GE, Galloway JMD. The iliofemoral venous segment as a source of pulmonary emboli. Lancet 1967;22:871–874.
3. Yao JST, Henkin RE, Bergan JJ. Venous thromboembolic disease. Arch Surg 1974;109:664–670.
4. Kistner RL, Ball JJ, Nordyke RA, Freeman GC. Incidence of pulmonary embolism in the course of thrombophlebitis of the lower extremities. Am J Surg 1972;124:169–176.
5. Norris CE, Greenfield LJ, Herrman JB. Free-floating iliofemoral thrombus. A risk of pulmonary embolism. Arch Surg 1985;120:806–808.
6. Neglén P, Al-Hassan H, Endrys J, Nazzal M, Christenson J, Eklöf B. Iliofemoral venous thrombectomy followed by percutaneous closure of the temporary arterio-venous fistula. Surgery 1991;110:493–499.
7. Plate G, Ohlin P, Eklöf B. Pulmonary embolism in acute iliofemoral venous thrombosis. Br J Surg 1985;72:912–915.
8. Farber SP, O'Donnell TF Jr, Deterling RA, Millan VG, Callow AD. The clinical implications of acute venous thrombosis of the inferior vena cava. Surg Gynecol Obstet 1984;158:141–144.
9. Girard P, Hauuy MP, Musset D, Simonneau G, Petitpretz P. Acute inferior vena cava thrombosis. Early results of heparin therapy. Chest 1989;95:284–291.
10. Radomski JS, Jarrell BE, Carabasi RA, Yang SL, Koolpe H. Risk of pulmonary embolus with inferior vena cava thrombosis. Am Surg 1987;53:97–101.
11. Neglén P, Nazzal MMS, Al-Hassan HK, Christenson JT, Eklöf B. Surgical removal of an inferior vena cava thrombosis. Eur J Vasc Surg 1992;6:78–82.
12. Girard P, Mathieu M, Simonneau G, et al. Recurrence of pulmonary embolism during anticoagulant treatment: a prospective study. Thorax 1987;42:481–486.
13. Killewich LA, Bedford GR, Beach KW, Strandness DE Jr. Spontaneous lysis of deep venous thrombi: rate and outcome. J Vasc Surg 1989;9:89–97.
14. Porter JM, Taylor LM. Current status of thrombolytic therapy. J Vasc Surg 1985;2:239–249.
15. Albrechtsson U, Andersson J, Einarsson E, Eklöf B, Norgren L. Streptokinase treatment of deep venous thrombosis and the post-thrombotic syndrome. Follow-up evaluation of venous function. Arch Surg 1981;116:33–37.
16. Eklöf B, Gjöres JE, Lohi A, Staszkiewicz W, Norgren L. Spontaneous rupture of liver and spleen with severe intraabdominal bleeding during streptokinase treatment of deep venous thrombosis. Vasa 1977;6:369–371.

17. Arnesen H, Höiseth A, Ly B. Streptokinase or heparin in the treatment of deep vein thrombosis. Acta Med Scand 1982;211:65–68.
18. Elliot MS, Immelman EJ, Jeffery P, et al. A comparative randomised trial of heparin versus streptokinase in the treatment of acute proximal venous thrombosis: an interim report of a prospective trial. Br J Surg 1979;66:838–843.
19. Kakkar VV, Paes TRF, Murray WJG. Does thrombolytic therapy prevent the post-phlebitic syndrome. In: Negus D, Jantet G, eds. Phlebology 85. London: John Libbey, 1986:481.
20. Kadji H. Traitment chirurgical des thromboses veineuse hautes des membres inferieurs. A propos de 186 cas [These]. Marseille: Université de Marseille, 1980.
21. Plate G, Einarsson E, Ohlin P, Jensen R, Qvarfordt P, Eklöf B. Thrombectomy with temporary arteriovenous fistula in acute iliofemoral venous thrombosis. J Vasc Surg 1984;1:867–876.
22. Juhan C, Cornillon B, Tobiana F, Schlama S, Barthelemy P, Denjean-Massia JP. Patency after iliofemoral and iliocaval venous thrombectomy. Ann Vasc Surg 1987;1:529–533.
23. Einarsson E, Albrechtsson U, Eklöf B. Thrombectomy and temporary AV-fistula in iliofemoral vein thrombosis. Technical considerations and early results. Inter Angiol 1986;5:65–70.
24. Läwen A. Weitere Ehrfahrung über operative Thrombenentfernung bei Venenthrombose. Zentralbl Chir 1938;64:961–968.
25. Dos Santos JC. La phlebographie directe. Conception, technique, premier resultats. J Int Chir 1938;3:625.
26. Gregoire R. La phlebite bleu. (Phlegmasia coerulea dolens). Press Med 1938; 46:1313–1315.
27. Audier M, Haimovici H. Les gangrenes des membres d'origine veineuse. Press Med 1938;46:1403–1406.
28. Mahorner H, Castleberry JW, Coleman WO. Attempts to restore function in major veins which are the site of massive thrombosis. Ann Surg 1957;146:510–522.
29. DeWeese JA, Jones TI, Lyon J, Dale WR. Evaluation of thrombectomy in the management of iliofemoral venous thrombosis. Surgery 1960;47:140–159.
30. Haller JA, Abrams BL. Use of thrombectomy in the treatment of acute iliofemoral venous thrombosis in forty-five patients. Ann Surg 1963;158:561–569.
31. Fogarty TJ, Dennis D, Krippaehne WW. Surgical management of iliofemoral venous thrombosis. Am J Surg 1966;112:211–217.
32. Mavor GE, Galloway JMD. Iliofemoral venous thrombosis. Pathological considerations and surgical management. Br J Surg 1969;56:45–59.
33. Lansing AM, Davis WM. Five year follow-up study of iliofemoral venous thrombectomy. Ann Surg 1968;168:620–628.
34. Gillot C, Imbert P. Les thromboses ilio-caves. Rapport au 82e Congrès Francais de Chirurgie. Paris: Masson, 1980.
35. Kunlin J. Les greffes veineuses. 15 Congress of International Surgical Society. Lisbon: 1953;15:875–907.
36. Christenson J, Einarsson E, Eklöf B. Infection complications after thrombectomy in deep venous thrombosis. Acta Chir Scand 1977;143:431–434.
37. Basmajian JV. The distribution of the valves in the femoral, external iliac and common iliac vein and their relation to varicose veins. Surg Gynecol Obstet 1952;95:537–542.
38. Winter G, Weber H, Loeprecht H. Surgical treatment of iliofemoral vein thrombosis: technical aspects. Possible secondary interventions. Inter Angiol 1989;8:188–193.
39. Eklöf B. Temporary arteriovenous fistula in reconstruction of iliac vein obstruction using PTFE grafts. In: Eklöf B, Gjöres JE, Thulesius O, Bergqvist D, eds. Controversies in management of venous disorders. London: Butterworths, 1989:280–290.

40. Einarsson E, Eklöf B, Kuenzig M, von Mecklenburg C, Schwartz SI. Scanning electron microscopy and Evans blue staining for assessing endothelial trauma and reconstitution after venous thrombectomy. Scan Electron Microsc 1984;1:273–278.
41. Endrys J, Eklöf B, Neglén P, Zyka I, Peregrin J. Percutaneous closure of femoral arteriovenous fistula after venous thrombectomy. J Cardiovasc Intervent Radiol 1989;12:226–229.
42. Piquet P, Tournigand P, Josso B, Mercier C. Traitement chirurgical des thromboses iliocaves: exigences et resultats. In: Kieffer E, ed. Chirurgie de la vein cave inferieur et de ses branches. Paris: Expansion Scientifique Francaise, 1985:210–216.
43. Vollmar JF, Hutschenreiter S. Surgical treatment of acute thromboembolic disease: the role of vascular endoscopy. In: Veith F, ed. Current critical problems in vascular surgery. St. Louis: Quality Medical Publishing Company, 1989:154–160.
44. Plate G, Åkesson H, Einarsson E, Ohlin P, Eklöf B. Long-term results of venous thrombectomy combined with a temporary arteriovenous fistula. Europ J Vasc Surg 1990;4:483–489.
45. Browse NL, Burnand KG, Thomas ML. Deep vein thrombosis: treatment. In: Browse NL, Burnand KG, Thomas ML, eds. Diseases of the veins. London: Edward Arnold, 1988:501–541.
46. Kniemeyer HW. Personal communication, 1987.
47. Einarsson E, Albrechtsson U, Eklöf B, Norgren L. Follow-up evaluation of venous morphologic factors and function after thrombectomy and temporary arteriovenous fistula in thrombosis of iliofemoral vein. Surg Gynecol Obstet 1986;163:111–116.
48. Lindhagen J, Haglund M, Haglund U, Holm J, Scherstén T. Iliofemoral venous thrombectomy. J Cardiovasc Surg 1978;19:319–327.
49. Goto H, Wada T, Matsumoto A, Matsumura H, Soma T. Iliofemoral venous thrombectomy. Follow-up studies of 88 patients. J Cardiovasc Surg 1980;21:341–346.
50. Kistner RL, Sparkuhl MD. Surgery in acute and chronic venous disease. Surgery 1979;85:31–43.
51. Masuda EM, Kistner RL, Ferris EB. Long-term effects of superficial femoral vein ligation: thirteen-year follow-up. J Vasc Surg 1992;16:741–749.
52. Röder OC, Lorentzen JE, Buchardt-Hansen HJ. Venous thrombectomy for iliofemoral thrombosis. Early and long-term results in 46 consecutive cases. Acta Chir Scand 1984;150:31–34.
53. Akesson H, Brudin L, Dahlström JA, Eklöf B, Ohlin P, Plate G. Venous function assessed during a 5 year period after acute iliofemoral venous thrombosis treated with anticoagulation. Europ J Vasc Surg 1990;4:43–48.
54. Bradham RR, Buxton JT. Thrombectomy for acute iliofemoral venous thrombosis. Surg Gynecol Obstet 1964;119:1271–1275.
55. O'Donnell TF Jr, Browse NL, Burnand KG, Thomas ML. The socioeconomic effects of an iliofemoral thrombosis. J Surg Res 1977;22:483–488.

section VI

Venous Trauma

chapter 35

Diagnosis and Management of Venous Trauma

David L. Gillespie, Norman M. Rich, James M. Goff, Sean D. O'Donnell, and Mark R. Jackson

Although diagnosis can be a challenge, the issue of whether injured veins should be repaired or ligated has remained controversial in civilian and military hospitals around the world (1–6, 8–10, 12–22, 26, 27, 30–33, 35, 38, 41, 44–46). Managing injured extremity veins may not appear initially to be as dramatic as managing arterial injuries; however, bleeding from injured veins can be even more difficult to control. Acute venous hypertension, associated with interruption of a major vein, particularly in the lower extremities, can be a significant problem. Chronic venous insufficiency can be the potential long-term sequela associated with interruption of a major vein in the lower extremities.

An early civilian report on the management of injured veins came from Gaspar and Treiman in Los Angeles in 1960 (9). There has been a proliferation of civilian reports over the past 16 years since the report by Mullins, et al., from Detroit in 1980 (25). This interest was stimulated in part by the American military experience in Southeast Asia during the Vietnam War from 1965–1971 (33–47, 49). Hobson has combined his vast experience, first with the military and later in civilian practice, with the latest valuable report made to the 1996 annual meeting of the American Venous Forum (19). Despite the controversy, there is increasing agreement that a more aggressive approach should be taken for the repair of large-caliber lower extremity veins, particularly the popliteal vein. Appreciation of normal anatomic variation and physiologic changes produced by venous injuries should be considered in their management (37).

Experience gained during armed conflicts has shown that large numbers of casualties with similar injuries treated over a short period of time provide a unique opportunity for the evaluation of new approaches in the management of vascular injury. This was demonstrated by the emphasis placed upon arterial repair during the Korean conflict, and again in Vietnam with the repair of venous injuries (19, 44, 50). The repair of injured veins appeared to be reasonably successful both in the immediate postoperative period and throughout an extended follow-up. This was corroborated through experimental research aimed at understanding the pathophysiology associated with acute venous interruption. Early fears that there might be an increased incidence of thrombophlebitis and/or pulmonary embolism have been strongly refuted both in civilian and military reports over the past 35 years.

NOTES OF HISTORICAL INTEREST

It is recognized that there are a number of excellent reviews on the development of vascular surgery; however, specific emphasis and additional detailed information with extensive references can be found in Rich and Spencer's Vascular Trauma and Hobson, et al.'s, Venous Trauma: Pathophysiology, Diagnosis and Surgical Management (19, 42). In the early 19th Century, Travers and Guthrie closed a small venous laceration and were credited with one of the earliest clinical venous repairs. In 1982, Shede became the first to accomplish successful lateral suture repair of a venous laceration in a human when he repaired a femoral venous laceration. He recommended this approach for clinical management of similar venous injuries. In 1877, Eck, a Russian surgeon, made an important contribution in his experimental work with the first successful anastomosis of two vessels, creating a lateral communication between the inferior vena cava and the portal vein. In 1889, Kümmel is reported to have performed the first clinical end-to-end anastomosis of a vein when he repaired an injured femoral vein. In 1897, Murphy of Chicago documented the first successful clinical end-to-end anastomosis of an artery at the same time that he repaired a common femoral venous laceration. He believed that similar approaches could be utilized in successful repair of both arteries and veins. Carrel and Guthrie made a number of outstanding contributions to the understanding of the principles of vascular surgery at the turn of the century. They were interested in suturing venous lacerations at the time of arterial reconstructions.

Soubbotitch, during the Balkan Wars of 1911 and 1912, repaired veins as well as arteries; however, his patients had arteriovenous fistulas and false aneurysms that were later recognized and repaired. Surgical leaders came to Belgrade from many European capitals to witness the pioneering efforts of Soubbotitch and his colleagues. In World War I, only a few years later, however, there were few reports of the repair of injured veins, probably largely due to the changes in weaponry in 1915 from the old shrapnel shells to the high explosive artillery rounds. Without blood banking and antibiotics, it was emphasized that "life over limb" was critically important. In 1918, Goodman, serving with the American Expeditionary Force, wrote that it had been possible to perform successful lateral suture repair in five patients with lower extremity venous injuries. There were four repairs of popliteal and superficial femoral veins. In 1917, Makins documented the experience of the British Army, reporting that injured veins were considered to be of minor importance. He stressed that ligation was preferable to repair. When an arterial injury required ligation, he also proposed ligating the associated vein even if it was uninjured (42). Weglowski (46) also recommended the repair of injured veins, first from his experience serving with the Russian

Army and later when he became the Polish Surgeon General. This information was only recently brought to the attention of the English-speaking world by Shumacker. The experience remained essentially the same during World War II except for the emphasis that there was no benefit from ligating the concomitant injured vein when injured arteries required ligation.

Hughes and Spencer provided the leadership during the Korean Conflict (1950–53) in recognizing that there was merit in repairing injured veins in select patients. Hughes noted that the majority of venous injuries were managed by ligation and also that there were resulting degrees of venostasis. He observed that there were several patients with severe venostasis who required amputations after ligation of injured major veins. Hughes reported that there was an increased interest in repairing injured veins to avoid these complications. Thrombosis did occur in early repairs, with fewer complications than those following ligation. It was this early experience by these investigators and others in the Korean War that stimulated the increased interest in repairing injured veins during the Vietnam War.

From 1965 through 1972, there were an increasing number of clinical reports from the Vietnam experience that substantiated the observations during the Korean War. There was a specific emphasis on repairing the injured popliteal vein, as well as the injured popliteal artery. A retrospective study of 125 failures of repair of injured popliteal arteries demonstrated that acute venous hypertension was a significant factor, leading to amputation in at least 19 of the patients (38). Nearly 78% of the patients in this series had concomitant venous injury. Surgeons in Vietnam became increasingly impressed with the additional risk factors involved with combined arteriovenous injuries in the popliteal area (49). Sullivan and his colleagues at the 12th Evacuation Hospital emphasized the early influence of repair of injured popliteal veins on the overall treatment of popliteal vascular injuries. Their report remains extremely important. The Vietnam Vascular Registry, established at Walter Reed General Hospital in 1966, collected data regarding American casualties in Southeast Asia and established early evidence for the value of repairing injuries of major veins of the lower extremity. Also, it was substantiated that ligation of these injured veins could lead to chronic venous insufficiency (36, 37, 40–42). The Vietnam Vascular Registry had the additional responsibility of providing long-term followup of the American casualties (34, 44). There was a question initially regarding the incidence of venous injuries. The initial report from the Vietnam Vascular Registry included 500 patients with 718 vascular injuries, of which 194 were venous injuries (27%). It was recognized and emphasized that this was lower than the true incidence of venous injuries because many surgeons did not document venous injuries. In a subsequent interim review from the Vietnam Vascular Registry, the incidence of documented concomitant venous injuries in 1000 acute arterial injuries in 1970 was nearly 38%. This was also believed to be less than the actual number. Additional research and follow-up were stimulated by these retrospective studies and an additional report in 1974 emphasized that a more aggressive approach should be taken in the repair of larger caliber lower extremity injured veins. It was established that the incidence of acute venous hypertension could be lowered and that long-term sequelae of chronic venous hypertension could be prevented. In 1975, a subsequent report of 110 isolated popliteal venous injuries corroborated this conclusion. This report remains of significant value because of the unique nature of the injuries in relatively large numbers (40). Contrary views were developed from civilian experience in the early 1980s, particularly by the reports of Mullins and colleagues from Detroit and Timberlake and Kerstein from New Orleans. Nevertheless, there were equally encouraging reports from a variety of locations regarding the repair of injured veins, emphasized by the Chicago report by Meyers and highlighted by the 1996 report from Newark by Hobson's group.

ETIOLOGY AND INCIDENCE

In both civilian and military experience, venous injuries have been recognized and documented with increasing frequency since the initial series by Gaspar and Treiman from Los Angeles County Hospital. Their report spanned a 10-year period during which 51 venous injuries were seen in 228 patients with vascular injuries, a 22% incidence (9). The superficial femoral vein was the most frequently injured vein (n = 9). Both the inferior vena cava and the internal jugular vein were injured eight times. A representative example of civilian experience came from Hobson and coworkers in 1983 in their report of 262 major vascular injuries treated at the New Jersey University Hospital between January 1979 and February 1983 of which 81 were venous injuries (31%) (20). The femoral venous system was injured most frequently (30%). The superficial femoral vein was injured 15 times and the common femoral vein was injured nine times. The largest number of injuries were associated with gunshot wounds in 16 patients, shotgun wounds in four, blunt trauma with two, a stab wound in one, and a sharp object in one. From the Lincoln Hospital in New York City, Agarwal and colleagues documented their experience in managing 115 civilian venous injuries over a 6-year period beginning in 1979 (1); 75% of the total of the venous injuries involved the internal and external jugular veins, femoral and iliac veins, and the inferior vena cava. Again, gunshot wounds accounted for the majority, involving 52%. Stab wounds were associated with 36%, blunt trauma with 7%, and shotgun wounds with 5%. In a prospective study reported to the American Surgical Association in 1987, Meyer and colleagues from Cook County Hospital and the University of Illinois in Chicago identified iatrogenic injuries to the venous system associated with invasive diagnostic and therapeutic techniques (24). Of 36 patients with major extremity venous injuries treated with reconstruction over a 27-month period, 34 patients (94%) also had major arterial injuries that required repair. Table 35.1 identifies the mechanisms of injury; the majority resulted from gunshot wounds, underscoring the violence occurring in major cities in the United States.

With armed conflict continuing throughout the world the incidence of venous injuries has been significant enough to warrant attention to the variety of missiles accounting for these injuries, including fragments from various exploding devices as well as bullets. It is ironic that renewed fighting in the Balkans during the early 1990s has added to the broad experience, as documented by Lovric and colleagues from Osijek Hospital in Croatia (23). He described 44 venous injuries caused by a combination of exploded fragments and gunshot wounds over a 1-year period. Combined arterial injuries occurred at the same level in 34 patients. Fifty percent of the venous injuries were managed by ligation with lateral suture repair per-

TABLE 35-1

MECHANISM OF VENOUS INJURY IN 36 PATIENTS

	Number	Percent
Gunshot	24	67
Laceration/stab	6	17
Shotgun	4	11
Blunt injury	2	5

(Reproduced by permission from Meyer JP, Walsh J, Schuler J, et al. The early fate of venous repair following civilian vascular trauma; a clinical hemodynamic and venographic assessment. Ann Surg 1987;206:458–464.)

formed in 36.4%, and the remainder were managed by end-to-end anastomosis or synthetic prosthesis interposition. Lovric's report clearly illustrates the need for continued attention to the timely management of venous trauma.

DIAGNOSIS OF VENOUS INJURY

Venous injury is usually not as obvious as arterial injury, with the latter associated frequently with bright red blood spurting from a wound. Also, the absence of distal pulses, the warmth and color of an extremity, and the development of neurologic deficits that mark arterial injury are not associated with venous injuries nor are there many other signs and symptoms. Although there may be severe venous hemorrhage with large hematomas, there may be only a steady flow of dark blood from a wound or a hematoma that develops rather slowly. Hemorrhagic shock can be common with major venous injuries, and it should be remembered that arterial injury can be a part of the multiple injury complex contributing to exsanguinating hemorrhage.

Roentgenograms have been of value in identifying offending missiles and associated fractures that may have caused venous injuries and these are important in the routine evaluation of injured patients. Phlebography, the term preferred to venography, remains a valuable tool in determining the location and extent of venous injury with or without associated thrombus. Gerlock and associates emphasize the valuable information obtained from venography in patients with venous injuries in their civilian experience (10). Doppler ultrasonography has been useful and this approach has been extended in recent years to color-flow duplex ultrasonography. This is a practical, noninvasive diagnostic tool in evaluating patients with interrupted veins; it is also helpful in determining the presence of thrombus, adding to its value for long-term follow-up. This approach may nonetheless have limited practical application in the injured patient. A variety of other techniques ranging from impedance plethysmography to phleborheography and radionucleotide studies have had even more limited value in managing patients with multiple injuries. All these studies have demonstrated value in long-term follow-up of patients with injured veins with or without associated thrombosis.

PATHOPHYSIOLOGY

Although early observations were documented by Montgomery in 1932, and later by Barcia and his colleagues, investigators at Walter Reed Army Institute of Research contributed significantly to the body of knowledge augmenting previous information. Information had also come from studies by Haimovici and coauthors in 1970, with a review of experimental and clinical evaluations of grafts in the venous system (13). The immediate decrease in femoral arterial flow as part of the hemodynamics of acute venous occlusion in the experimental model was emphasized at Walter Reed Army Institute of Research in the canine hind limb where femoral venous ligation resulted in a 50–75% reduction in femoral arterial flow and marked increases in venous pressure and peripheral resistance (17). Hobson and coworkers noted that there was a return to baseline in approximately 72 hours, which was critically important for the clinical observation and management of venous injuries. Hiratzka and Wright discussed the results of grafts in the venous system in a review in 1978 (15). Additional clinical observations were corroborated by experimental data.

MANAGEMENT OF VENOUS INJURIES

Surgical intervention may frequently be required in the management of injured veins. Control of hemorrhage is initially very important and digital pressure or compressive bandages over injured veins can be a successful temporary treatment (19, 44). Prevention of air embolism through the disrupted venous system can also be established by this temporary control. The management of injured patients with multiple injuries should include appropriate supportive measures with infusion of electrolyte solutions and whole blood, as well as utilization of antibiotics if indicated. Rapid exposure can be established through longitudinal incisions along the course of injured veins. This will provide adequate exposure for proximal and distal access to the vein to control hemorrhage. Stabilization of fractures must be accomplished and other major injuries documented and treated appropriately. Because there is a high incidence of arterial injury associated with injured veins, there is a frequent question as to which vessel should be repaired initially. Obviously, it is most important to repair the injured artery as soon as possible to minimize anoxia in the distal extremity. In a number of clinical situations, however, it may be more expeditious to repair the venous injury first, usually by lateral suture to establish hemostasis and permit better exposure for the arterial repair. This approach can also ensure the prevention of air embolism through the venous system. Copious saline irrigation can assist in the removal of foreign material and better exposure of the injured vessels. Adequate debridement is important in removing nonviable tissue and foreign material that might be a nidus for infection in the early postoperative period. Digital pressure for control of hemorrhage can be complemented by pressure with stick sponges. A proximal temporary tourniquet can provide simple atraumatic control of hemorrhage. Utilizing vascular tape to encircle vessels both proximal and distal to the area of injury on the vein and partial occluding vascular clamps can be useful in controlling hemorrhage from lacerations. Partial occluding clamps can be particularly helpful in managing tangential injuries of large veins.

Removal of thrombus from the injured veins both proximally and distally prior to repair is important. Gentle pressure peripherally toward the area of injury can extrude thrombus. A balloon catheter can also be manipulated to gently assist in retrieving residual thrombus; however, there may be difficulty in inserting the balloon catheter retrograde because of competent venous valves. These valves should be protected if at all possible. Heparinization, either local or systemic, can be utilized to help prevent additional propagation of thrombus, particularly if thrombus is known to be present already or if the venous occlusion has developed over a period of hours.

Meticulous surgical technique is mandatory for successful venous reconstruction (19, 39, 44). This has been demonstrated experimentally and in clinical practice. Meticulous surgical technique is more critical in management of injured veins than of injured arteries. Fine synthetic suture (6–0 or 7–0) on a small needle (C-1, BV-1) minimizes bleeding from the repair site. If a continuous suture line is utilized, less tension is applied than in an arterial anastomosis to prevent circular constriction. Leaving loops of a continuous line somewhat loose in a venous repair may create a few leaks, but bleeding usually ceases with mild pressure applied for a few minutes. Interrupted sutures lessen the risk of constricting the anastomotic line. Autogenous venous patch grafts may be useful in preventing constriction at the repair site. If there is significant loss of venous tissue, a replacement conduit may be required; however, this is much more challenging than repair by lateral suture, patch angioplasty, or end-to-end anastomosis. Insertion of a vascular graft should be considered only if the patient's general condition is stable, remembering the adage of "life over limb." Autogenous veins are the only satisfactory grafts for the venous system to date. The use of compilation grafts to create a diameter compatible with the injured veins has been employed with increasing frequency and success, particularly the spiral vein graft (7, 19, 20, 44, 50).

Recently, the group from UMDNJ-Newark presented their experience in managing 100 patients sustaining lower extremity venous injuries. In this series, 45 of the patients underwent complex venous repairs: six spiral grafts, eight panel grafts, eight reversed saphenous vein interposition grafts, eight end-to-end repairs, and 15 vein patches. The remaining 55 injuries were treated with ligation ($n = 27$) or lateral venorrhaphy ($n = 28$) (29).

Completion phlebography in the operating room is an important adjunctive measure and repeated phlebograms have been helpful in the early postoperative period to determine the success of repair (19, 31, 44). Color-flow duplex ultrasonography may also be valuable in these situations for noninvasive evaluation.

RESULTS OF LIGATION AND REPAIR

The debate as to whether a venous injury should be repaired or ligated has raged for the last few decades. Initial reaction to the idea of traumatic venous repair fueled speculation of an increased incidence of thrombophlebitis and/or pulmonary embolism. These concerns, however, have been refuted by both the Vietnam experience as outlined through the Vietnam Vascular Registry and numerous recent civilian reports over the past 16 years (19, 44). The extensive experimental work at Walter Reed Army Institute of Research allowed a better understanding of the pathophysiology associated with acute venous hypertension (50). Further clinical research stimulated by these basic science activities provided additional data at Walter Reed (44). The long-term follow-up of the Vietnam casualties provided a unique opportunity through the Registry, with 110 combat casualties sustaining isolated popliteal venous injuries as outlined in Table 35.2 (40). There was no increase in the incidence of thrombophlebitis or pulmonary embolism with attempted venous repair in this important study. There was no statistically significant difference in the frequency of these potential complications whether the veins were ligated or repaired. Nevertheless, significant edema remained in 51% of the patients who had ligation of the injured veins in contrast to the 13% incidence in the patients who had been treated by repair of the injured vein whether or not the repair was initially successful. A complementary study of 51 Vietnam casualties included the repair of larger lower extremity veins by autogenous interposition venous grafts. Again, there was favorable experience in the long-term follow-up. In this series, only one patient developed thrombophlebitis and the condition was transitory. There was no clinical detection of pulmonary embolism. Again, there was a relatively low residual edema rate (approximately 12%) following venous repairs.

In 1980, Mullins, Lucas, and Ledgerwood in Detroit reviewed the natural history after ligation of venous injuries in their civilian experience in 46 patients (25). They challenged the more aggressive approach to the repair of injured veins, noting that the majority of their patients (40 of 46) were discharged free of lower extremity swelling and the other six patients had only mild edema. Their follow-up in 39 patients revealed no edema in 30 patients, mild edema requiring no treatment in one patient, and moderate edema necessitating support stockings in eight patients (Table 35.3). Subsequently, there have been others who have challenged or championed the more aggressive approach to the repair of injured veins. Feliciano and colleagues at the Ben Taub Hospital in Houston emphasized that polytetrafluoroethylene (PTFE) grafts had limited value in the repair of injured veins (8).

Several reports on the success of repairing injured veins were challenged by Timberlake and colleagues as outlined in Table 35.4. Their group from Tulane

TABLE 35-2

INCIDENCE OF EDEMA FOLLOWING LIGATION AND REPAIR OF INJURED POPLITEAL VEINS

Management	Number	With Edema	Percent
Ligation	57	29	50.9
Repair	53	7	13.2

(Modified from Rich NM, Hobson RW II, Collins GJ Jr, Andersen CA. The effect of acute popliteal venous interruption. Ann Surg 1976;183:365.)

TABLE 35-3

EDEMA AT DISCHARGE AND FOLLOW-UP IN 46 PATIENTS AFTER LIGATION OF MAJOR LOWER EXTREMITY VEINS

		Edema*	
Vessel (no.)	**No.**	**Discharge**	**Follow-up**
Popliteal (5)	4	0	0
	0	0	1+
Common iliac (3)	2	0	0
	1	0	2+
Profunda femoral (6)	5	0	0
	1	0	†
Superficial femoral (13)	5	0	0
	5	0	†
	2	1+	0
	1	0	2+
Common femoral (8)	5	0	0
	2	0	2+
	1	1+	2+
External iliac (5)	3	0	†
	1	0	2+
Vena cava (6)	3	0	0
	2	1+	2+
	1	1+	0

*Edema graded as follows: 0 = none; 1+ = minimal; 2+ = moderate, requiring support hose; 3+ = severe, causing scaling or ulceration; 4+ = massive, causing ischemia.

†No follow-up.

(Reproduced by permission from Mullins RJ, Lucas CE, Ledgerwood AM. The natural history following venous ligation for civilian injuries. J Trauma 1980;20:737–743.)

University managed 184 patients with major venous injury (49). There were 43 patients with isolated venous injury, of whom 31 were treated by ligation. In the remaining 141 patients, there was combined arterial and venous injury. Eighty-three percent (117) had ligation of the injured vein. Follow-up of the patients from 1 month to 9 years identified no permanent sequelae of the venous ligation although extremity edema developed in as many of 32% of the patients, regardless of whether the vein was ligated or repaired. In all their patients, the edema resolved within 12 weeks and there was no extremity lost after ligation of a venous injury. In a recent follow-up to this study, the Tulane group has now reviewed the records of 322 patients suffering venous trauma. In this most recent review, the authors reaffirm the concept that repair of venous injuries is not mandatory for limb salvage. Although they found a slightly higher incidence of transient edema (<12 weeks) in patients with isolated venous injuries, treatment by ligation did not result in any significant long-term morbidity or limb loss. This was also found to

TABLE 35-4

METHODS OF TREATMENT AND RESULTS IN 43 PATIENTS WITH ISOLATED VENOUS INJURY

Vein Injured (no.)	Average Follow-up (mos.)	Treatment	Adjunctive Fasciotomy	Sequelae		
				None	Transient Edema	Permanent Edema
Popliteal (9)	18.8	Ligation (4)	3	3	2	0
		Repair (5)	3	5	0	0
Femoral (23)	26.5	Ligation (17)	2	12	5	0
		Repair (6)	0	4	2	0
Iliac (8)	21.9	Ligation (6)	0	4	2	0
		Repair (2)	0	1	1	0
Vena cava (3)	24.3	Ligation (3)	0	2	1	0
		Repair (0)	0	0	0	0

(Reproduced by permission from Timberlake GA, O'Connell RC, Kerstein MD. Venous injuries: to repair or ligate, the dilemma. J Vasc Surg 1986;4:533–538.)

be the case in patients with combined arterial and venous injuries even at the popliteal level. The authors do concede that, despite their success with popliteal vein ligation, a more aggressive approach to venous repair in this area is warranted (48).

At the University of North Carolina in Chapel Hill, Blumoff and associates analyzed their management of 17 patients with major femoral venous injuries, of whom 10 had concomitant arterial injuries. Venous repair was performed in seven patients with satisfactory functional result. In five patients who also had concomitant arterial injuries, however, there was chronic venous insufficiency following venous ligation manifested by stasis dermatitis, secondary varicose veins, pedal edema, and venous ulceration (4). Long-term patency of venous repairs was analyzed by Phifer, et al. (28), in five patients with six venous reconstructions studied by phlebography at 6–20 years. They demonstrated venous patency with functioning valves in asymptomatic patients and no evidence of clinical venous insufficiency in all but one case, which had been repaired in 1962 with a Teflon graft, as identified in Table 35.5. The Chicago study of Meyer and colleagues, with 36 venous reconstructions with concomitant arterial repair in most cases, is outlined in Table 35.6. There were no perioperative deaths and the limb salvage rate was 100%, with all 34 major arterial repairs patent at the time of discharge from the hospital. Phlebography performed on the seventh postoperative day demonstrated that 61% (22 repairs) remained patent (Table 35.6) (24). Lateral venous repair had a significantly lower thrombosis rate (21%) than did interposition vein grafting (59%). These authors found that the clinical evaluation was 67% accurate in assessing patency of venous repair and that the noninvasive evaluation was 53% accurate.

Finally, the recent results from the UMDNJ-Newark group reveal an impressive experience with some of the more complex venous repairs. These grafts were

TABLE 35-5

FOLLOW-UP VENOGRAPHIC FINDING IN SIX VENOUS REPAIRS

Type of repair	Follow-up (years)	Findings at repair site
Teflon graft (superficial femoral vein)	20	Occluded
Lateral suture repair (common femoral vein)	5	Patent
Saphenous vein graft	11	Patent
End-to-end anastomosis	10	Patent
Lateral suture repair	8	Patent
Autogenous vein patch graft	6	Patent

(Reproduced by permission from Phifer TJ, Gerlock AJ, Rich NM, McDonald JC. Long-term patency of venous repairs demonstrated by venography. J Trauma 1985;25:342–346.)

used primarily to reconstruct iliac or common femoral vein injuries. These authors report a 75% patency for reversed autogenous saphenous vein interposition grafts and a 50% patency rate for panel and spiral grafts upon follow-up at 0.5–9 years. Although patency was lower than desired, alternatives for reconstruction of these large veins are limited (29).

SUMMARY

Considerable interest in the management of injured veins, particularly in the lower extremities, developed during the American experience in the Vietnam War (1965–71). Increasing numbers of civilian reports on the management of ve-

TABLE 35-6

METHODS OF VASCULAR REPAIR AND EARLY OUTCOME IN 36 PATIENTS

Type of repair (no.)	Venography findings: Patent	Venography findings: Occluded
Venous Repair		
Lateral repair (6)	5	1
End-to-end (4)	4	0
Vein patch (9)	6	3
Vein graft (15)	6	9
Paneled vein graft (2)	1	1
Total	22	14

(Reproduced by permission from Meyer JP, Walsh J, Schuler J, et al. The early fate of venous repair following civilian vascular trauma; a clinical hemodynamic and venographic assessment. Ann Surg 1987;206:458–464.)

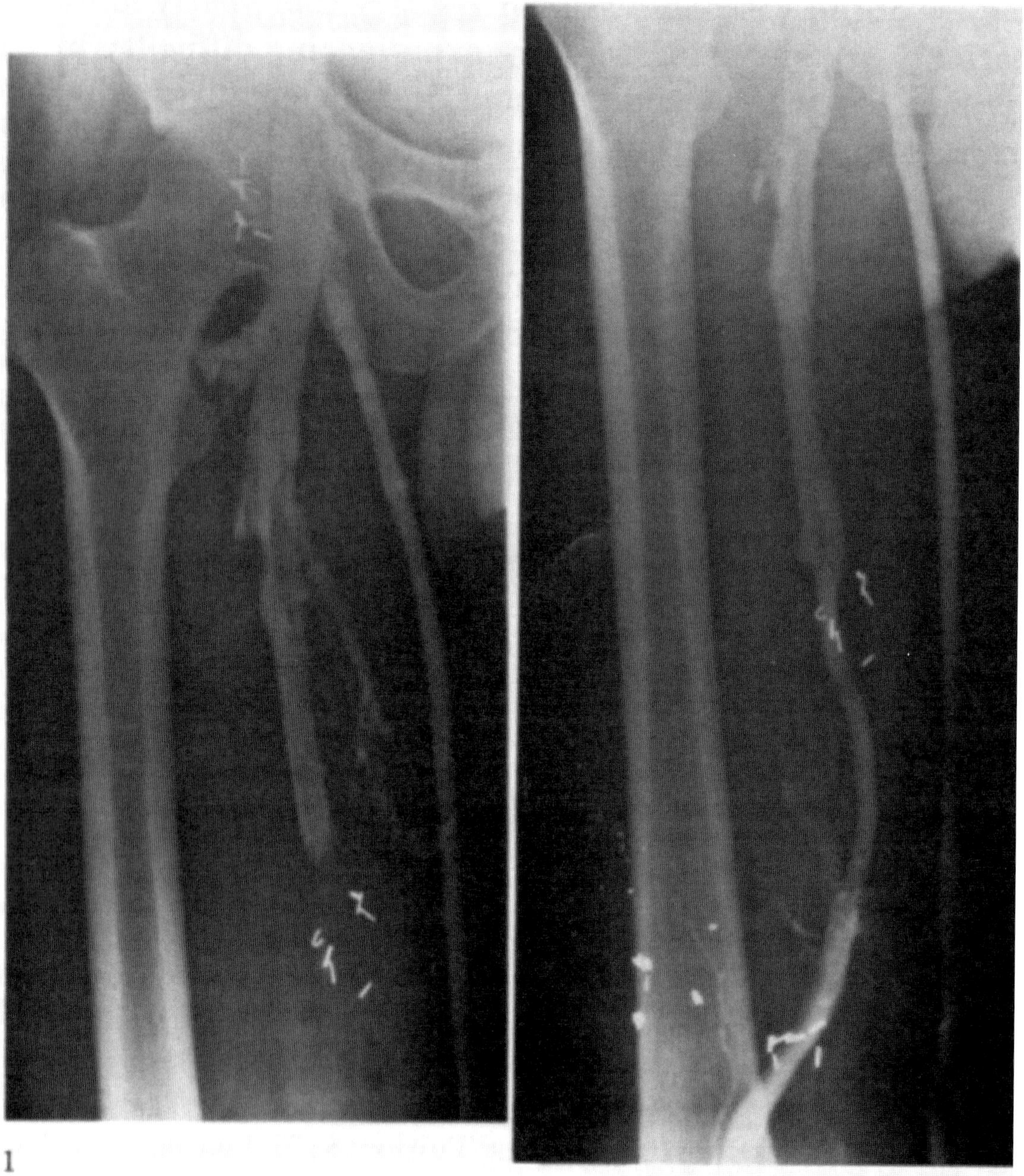

FIG. 35–1. (*left*) Venogram 1 week after surgery demonstrates occlusion of a saphenous vein interposition graft with thrombosis extending into the superficial femoral vein. The second venogram (*right*), performed 6 weeks postoperatively, demonstrates full recanalization of the venous interposition graft. (Reproduced by permission from Blumoff RL, Proctor HJ, Johnson G Jr. Recanalization of a saphenous vein interposition venous graft. J Trauma 1981;21:407–408.)

nous injuries in the United States have added additional valuable information over the past 16 years (26). Despite the continuing controversy and lack of long-term follow-up of a large number of patients, it appears that there is merit in repairing many of the larger caliber lower extremity veins that are injured, particularly the popliteal vein when it is a single return conduit, assuming that the patient's general condition will permit. It has been demonstrated both clinically and experimentally that this approach will help prevent acute venous hypertension with loss of an extremity initially and subsequent chronic venous hypertension with long-term disability. Figure 35.1 identifies the recovery potential that exists even if the initial venous repair fails. In contrast to the thrombosis that develops in the arterial system and will not recanalize, recanalization is the rule in the venous system. There can be patent valves above and below the rather localized area of thrombosis, which is an important consideration in the venous system. Recanalization can prevent problems of chronic venous insufficiency. Late sequelae of acute venous hypertension with the gradual development of chronic venous hypertension may not be demonstrable for 10–15 years, as shown in the long-term follow-up through the Vietnam Vascular Registry. Recent follow-up of a patient from the Registry at 28 years postligation of the superficial femoral vein, who has suffered with ulceration for the last 15 years, illustrates the need for competent and lifelong follow-up (11) (Fig. 35.2). There has not been a similar expe-

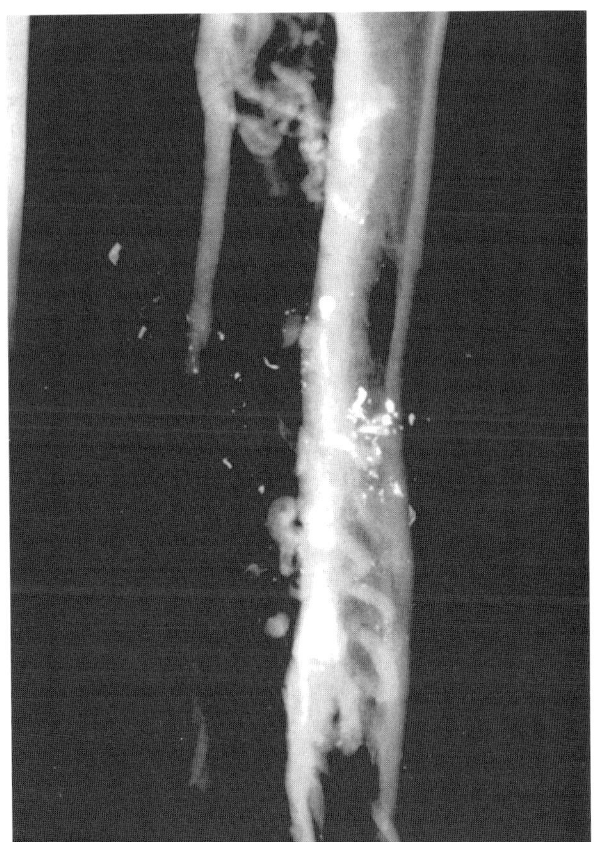

FIG. 35–2. Descending venogram 15 years after ligation of traumatic injury to superficial femoral vein. (Reproduced by permission from Goff JM, Gillespie DL, Rich NM. Long-term follow-up of military superficial femoral vein injury: a case report from the Vietnam Vascular Registry. Proceedings of the Eighth American Venous Forum; 1996 February 23–25; San Diego. San Diego, CA: American Venous Forum, 1996.)

rience to support a more aggressive approach in general in upper extremity veins; however, it should be appreciated that a return pathway must remain patent, as noted in the replantation of extremities and as originally identified in the 17th Century when the circulation was first described. There are obvious differences in military and civilian wounds, with the former having a more extensive soft tissue destruction and obliteration of collateral veins and lymphatics. These differences might account for the generally acceptable results with venous ligation in the civilian trauma experience. Civilian gunshot wounds, unfortunately, are being seen more frequently in the United States with an increasing similarity to the military-type wounds. Also, terrorist activities and limited warfare involving civilian populations have added additional insult to the civilian casualties. Finally, there is a significant difference in the venous anatomy when compared to the arterial anatomy, with the former being much more variable. It is important to know the details of the clinical situation. We must not forget the lessons of the past, and we must continue to analyze our experience in the management of injured veins under a variety of conditions.

REFERENCES

1. Agarwal N, Shah PM, Clauss RH, Reynolds DM, Stahl WM. Experience with 115 civilian venous injuries. J Trauma 1982;22:827–832.
2. Bergan JJ, Yao JST, eds. Symposium on venous problems in honor of Geza de Takats. Chicago: Yearbook Medical Publishers, 1978.
3. Blumoff RL, Proctor HJ, Johnson G Jr. Recanalization of a saphenous vein interposition venous graft. J Trauma 1981;21:407–408.
4. Blumoff RL, Powell T, Johnson G Jr. Femoral venous trauma in a university referral center. J Trauma 1982;22:703–705.
5. Borman KR, Jones GH, Snyder WH 3d. A decade of lower extremity venous trauma: patency and outcome. Am J Surg 1987;154:608–612.
6. Brigham RA, Eddleman WL, Clagett GP, Rich NM. Isolated venous injury produced by penetrating trauma to the lower extremity. J Trauma 1983;23:255–257.
7. Doty DB, Baker WH. Bypass of superior vena cava with spiral vein graft. Ann Thorac Surg 1976;22:490–493.
8. Feliciano DV, Mattox KL, Graham JM, Bitondo CG. Five-year experience with PTFE grafts in vascular wounds. J Trauma 1985;25:71–82.
9. Gaspar MR, Treiman RL. The management of injuries to major veins. Am J Surg 1960;100:171–175.
10. Gerlock AJ Jr, Thal ER, Snyder WH 3d. Venography in penetrating injuries of the extremities. AJR 1976;126:1023–1027.
11. Goff JM, Gillespie DL, Rich NM. Long-term follow-up of military superficial femoral vein injury: a case report from the Vietnam Vascular Registry. Proceedings of the Eighth American Venous Forum; 1996 February 23–25; San Diego. San Diego, CA: American Venous Forum, 1996.
12. Graham JM, Mattox KL, Beall AC Jr. Portal venous system injuries. J Trauma 1978;18:419–422.
13. Haimovici H, Hoffert PW, Zinicola N, Steinman C. An experimental and clinical evaluation of grafts in the venous system. Surg Gynecol Obstet 1970;131:1173–1186.
14. Hardin WD Jr, Adinolfi MF, O'Connell RC, Kerstein MD. Management of traumatic peripheral vein injuries: primary repair or vein ligation. Am J Surg 1982;144:235–238.

15. Hiratzka LF, Wright CB. Experimental and clinical results of grafts in the venous system: a current review. J Surg Res 1978;25:542–561.
16. Hobson RW 2d, Croom RD, Rich NM. Influence of heparin and low molecular weight dextran on the patency of autogenous vein grafts: vein grafts in the venous system. Ann Surg 1973;178:773–776.
17. Hobson RW 2d, Howard EW, Wright CB, Collins GJ, Rich NM. Hemodynamics of canine femoral venous ligation: significance in combined arterial and venous injuries. Surgery 1973;74:824–829.
18. Hobson RW 2d, Wright CB. Peripheral side to side arteriovenous fistula: hemodynamics and application in venous reconstruction. Am J Surg 1973;126:411–414.
19. Hobson RW 2d, Rich NM, Wright CB, eds. Venous trauma; pathophysiology, diagnosis and surgical management. Mount Kisco, NY: Futura Publishing, 1983.
20. Hobson RW, Yeager RA, Lynch TG, et al. Femoral venous trauma: techniques for surgical management and early results. Am J Surg 1983;146:220–4.
21. Jacobson JH, Haimov J. Venous revascularization of the arm: report of three cases. Surgery 1977;81:599–604.
22. Jamil Z, Padberg FT. Femoral venous trauma: techniques for surgical management and early results. Am J Surg 1983;146:220.
23. Lovrić Z, Wertheimer B, Candrlic K, et al. War injuries of major extremity vessels. J Trauma 1994;36:248–251.
24. Meyer JP, Walsh J, Schuler J, et al. The early fate of venous repair following civilian vascular trauma; a clinical hemodynamic and venographic assessment. Ann Surg 1987;206:458–464.
25. Mullins RJ, Lucas CE, Ledgerwood AM. The natural history following venous ligation for civilian injuries. J Trauma 1980;20:737–743.
26. Nypaver TJ, Schuler JJ, McDonnell P, et al. Long-term results of venous reconstruction after vascular trauma in civilian practice. J Vasc Surg 1992;16:762–768.
27. Pappas PJ, Haser PB, Teehan EP, et al. Outcome of complex venous reconstructions in trauma patients. Proceedings of the Eighth American Venous Forum; 1996 February 23–25; San Diego. San Diego, CA: American Venous Forum, 1996.
28. Phifer TJ, Gerlock AJ, Vekovius WA, Rich NM, McDonald JC. Amputation risk factors in concomitant superficial femoral artery and vein injuries. Ann Surg 1984;199:241–243.
29. Phifer TJ, Gerlock AJ, Rich NM, McDonald JC. Long-term patency of venous repairs demonstrated by venography. J Trauma 1985;25:342–346.
30. Quast DC, Shirkey AL, Fitzgerald JB, Beall AC Jr, DeBakey ME. Surgical correction of injuries to the vena cava; an analysis of sixty-one cases. J Trauma 1965;5:1–10.
31. Rich NM, Hughes CW. Vietnam Vascular Registry: a preliminary report. Surgery 1969;65:218–226.
32. Rich NM, Baugh JH, Hughes CW. Acute arterial injuries in Vietnam: 1,000 cases. J Trauma 1970;10:359–369.
33. Rich NM, Hughes CW, Baugh JH. Management of venous injuries. Ann Surg 1970;171:724–730.
34. Rich NM, Sullivan WG. Clinical recanalization of an autogenous vein graft in the popliteal vein. J Trauma 1972;12:919–920.
35. Rich NM, Hobson RW 2d, Wright CB, Fedde CW. Repair of lower extremity venous trauma: a more aggressive approach required. J Trauma 1974;14:639–652.
36. Rich NM, Jarstfer BS, Geer TM. Popliteal artery repair failure: causes and possible prevention. J Cardiovasc Surg 1974;15:340–351.
37. Rich NM, Hobson RW 2d, Wright CB, Swan KG. Techniques of venous repair. In: Swan KG, Hobson RW 2d, Reynolds DG, Rich NM, Wright CB, eds. Symposium on venous surgery in the lower extremities. St Louis: Warren H. Green Publishers, 1975;243–256.
38. Rich NM, Hobson RW 2d, Collins GJ Jr, Anderson CA. The effect of acute popliteal venous interruption. Ann Surg 1976;183:365–368.

39. Rich NM, Collins GJ, Andersen CA, McDonald PT. Autogenous venous interposition grafts in repair of major venous injuries. J Trauma 1977;17:512–520.
40. Rich NM, Collins GJ Jr, Andersen CA, McDonald PT, Ricotta JJ. Venous trauma: successful venous reconstruction remains an interesting challenge. Am J Surg 1977;134:226–230.
41. Rich NM, Hobson RW 2d, Wright CB. Historical aspects of direct venous reconstruction. In: Bergan JJ, Yao JTS, eds. Symposium on venous problems in honor of Geza de Takats. Chicago: Year Book Medical Publishers, 1978:441–449.
42. Rich NM, Spencer FC. Vascular trauma. Philadelphia: WB Saunders, 1978.
43. Rich NM. Principles and indications for primary venous repair. Surgery 1982;91:492–496.
44. Rich NM. Venous injuries. In: Sabiston DC Jr, ed. Textbook of surgery. 13th ed. Philadelphia: WB Saunders, 1986:2009–2018.
45. Richardson JB Jr, Jurkovich GJ, Walker GT, Nenstiel R, Bone EG. A temporary arteriovenous shunt (Scribner) in the management of traumatic venous injuries of the lower extremity. J Trauma 1986;26:503–509.
46. Shumacker HB Jr. Ramuald Weglowski: neglected pioneer in vascular surgery. J Vasc Surg 1987;6:95–97.
47. Sullivan WG, Thorton FG, Baker LH, LaPlante ES, Cohen A. Early influence of popliteal vein repair in the treatment of popliteal vessel injuries. Am J Surg 1971;122:528–531.
48. Swan KG, Hobson RW, Reynolds DG, Rich NM, Wright CB, eds. Venous surgery in the lower extremities. St Louis: Warren H. Green Publishers, 1975:243–255.
49. Timberlake GA, O'Connell RC, Kerstein MD. Venous injuries: to repair or ligate, the dilemma. J Vasc Surg 1986;4:533–538.
50. Timberlake GA, Kerstein MD. Venous injury: to repair or ligate, the dilemma revisited. Am Surgeon 1995;61:139–145.

Index

Page numbers followed by *f* indicate figures; t indicates tables.